Lecture Notes in Computer Science 11663

More information about this series at http://www.springer.com/series/7412

Fakhri Karray · Aurélio Campilho ·
Alfred Yu (Eds.)

Image Analysis and Recognition

16th International Conference, ICIAR 2019
Waterloo, ON, Canada, August 27–29, 2019
Proceedings, Part II

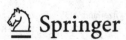

Springer

Editors
Fakhri Karray
University of Waterloo
Waterloo, ON, Canada

Aurélio Campilho
University of Porto
Porto, Portugal

Alfred Yu
University of Waterloo
Waterloo, ON, Canada

ISSN 0302-9743 ISSN 1611-3349 (electronic)
Lecture Notes in Computer Science
ISBN 978-3-030-27271-5 ISBN 978-3-030-27272-2 (eBook)
https://doi.org/10.1007/978-3-030-27272-2

LNCS Sublibrary: SL6 – Image Processing, Computer Vision, Pattern Recognition, and Graphics

This Springer imprint is published by the registered company Springer Nature Switzerland AG
The registered company address is: Gewerbestrasse 11, 6330 Cham, Switzerland

Preface

ICIAR 2019 was the 16th edition of the series of annual conferences on image analysis and recognition, offering a forum for participants to interact and present their latest research contributions in the theory, methodology, and applications of image analysis and recognition. ICIAR 2019, the International Conference on Image Analysis and Recognition, was held in Waterloo, Ontario, Canada, August 27–29, 2019. ICIAR is organized by AIMI, the Association for Image and Machine Intelligence, a not-for-profit organization registered in Ontario, Canada.

We received a total of 142 papers from 27 countries. Before the review process, all the papers were checked for similarity using a comparison database of scholarly work. The review process was carried out by members of the Program Committee and other reviewers. Each paper was reviewed by at least two reviewers (most articles received three professional reviews), and checked by the conference chairs. A total of 84 papers were finally accepted and appear in these proceedings. We would like to sincerely thank the authors for responding to our call, and to thank the reviewers for the careful evaluation and feedback provided to the authors. It is this collective effort that resulted in the strong conference program and high-quality proceedings.

We were very pleased to include four outstanding keynote talks: "Image Synthesis and Its Growing Role in Medical Imaging" by Professor Jerry Prince of Johns Hopkins University, USA; "Exploiting Data Sparsity and Machine Learning in Medical Imaging" by Professor Michael Insana, of the University of Illinois at Urbana Champaign, USA; "Knowledge Discovery: Can We Do Better than Deep Neural Networks" by Professor Ling Guan of Ryerson University, Toronto, Canada; and "Palmprint Authentication—Research and Development" by Professor David Zhang of Chinese University of Hong Kong (Shenzhen), Hong Kong. We would like to express our gratitude to our distinguished keynote speakers for accepting our invitation to share their vision and recent advances in their areas of expertise.

Besides the standard sessions, the program included five special sessions in the theory and applications of tools of image analysis and recognition:

- Image Analysis and Recognition for Automotive Industry
- Deep Learning on the Edge
- Medical Imaging and Analysis Using Deep Learning and Machine Intelligence
- Adaptive Methods for Ultrasound Beamforming and Motion Estimation
- Signal Processing Techniques for Ultrasound Tissue Characterization and Imaging in Complex Biological Media

We would like to thank the program co-chairs, Dr. Wail Gueaieb, of the University of Ottawa, and Dr. Shady Shehata of YourIKA Inc., who secured a high-quality program, Dr. Mark Crowley of the University of Waterloo and Dr. Chahid Ouali of YourIKA Inc., for helping with the local logistics with precious assistance from Nichola Harrilall, of the Waterloo AI Institute, and Dr. Khaled Hammouda, the publications chair and webmaster of the conference, for maintaining the website, managing the registrations, interacting with the authors, and preparing the proceedings. We are also grateful to Springer's editorial staff, for supporting this publication in the LNCS series. Additionally, we would like to thank the precious sponsorship and support of the Faculty of Engineering, at the University of Waterloo, notably, Dean Pearl Sullivan, the Faculty of Engineering at the University of Porto, the Institute for Systems and Computer Engineering, Technology and Science (INESC TEC), Portugal, the Waterloo AI Institute at the University of Waterloo, the Center for Pattern Analysis and Machine Intelligence at the University of Waterloo, and the Center for Biomedical Engineering Research at INESC TEC. We also appreciate the valuable co-sponsorship of the IEEE Computational Intelligence Society, Waterloo-Kitchener Chapter.

We were very pleased to welcome all the participants to ICIAR 2019. For those who were not able to attend, we hope this publication provides a good overview of the research presented at the conference, and we look forward to meeting you at the next ICIAR conference.

August 2019

Fakhri Karray
Aurélio Campilho
Alfred Yu

Organization

General Chairs

Fakhri Karray	University of Waterloo, Canada karray@uwaterloo.ca
Aurélio Campilho	University of Porto, Portugal campilho@fe.up.pt
Alfred Yu	University of Waterloo, Canada alfred.yu@uwaterloo.ca

Organizing Committee Chairs

Mark Crowley	University of Waterloo, Canada mcrowley@uwaterloo.ca
Chahid Ouali	YourIKA Inc., Canada chahid.ouali@gmail.com

Program Committee Chairs

Shady Shehata	YourIKA Inc., Canada shady.h.shehata@gmail.com
Wail Gueaieb	University of Ottawa, Canada wgueaieb@uottawa.ca

Industrial Liaison Chair

Alaa Khamis	GM-Canada alaakhamis@gmail.com

Publication and Web Chair

Khaled Hammouda	Waterloo, Canada khaledh@aimiconf.org

Supported and Co-sponsored by

AIMI – Association for Image and Machine Intelligence

Faculty of Engineering
University of Waterloo
Canada

CPAMI – Centre for Pattern Analysis and Machine Intelligence
University of Waterloo
Canada

Waterloo AI Institute
Canada

Center for Biomedical Engineering Research
INESC TEC – Institute for Systems and Computer Engineering, Technology and Science
Portugal

Department of Electrical and Computer Engineering
Faculty of Engineering
University of Porto
Portugal

IEEE Computational Intelligence Society
Kitchener-Waterloo Chapter

Program Committee

J. Alba-Castro	University of Vigo, Spain
L. Alexandre	University of Beira Interior, Portugal
H. Araujo	University of Coimbra, Portugal
G. Azzopardi	University of Groningen, The Netherlands
J. Batista	University of Coimbra, Portugal
R. Bernardes	University of Coimbra, Portugal
H. Bogunovic	Medical University Vienna, Austria
J. Boisvert	CNRC, Ottawa, Canada
F. Camastra	University of Naples Parthenope, Italy
A. Campilho	University of Porto, Portugal
C. Carvalho	INESC TEC, Portugal
P. Carvalho	INESC TEC, Portugal
F. Ciompi	Radboud University Medical Center, The Netherlands
A. Cunha	INESC TEC, Portugal
J. Debayle	Ecole Nationale Supérieure des Mines de Saint-Etienne (ENSM-SE), France
L. Demi	University of Trento, Italy
M. Dimiccoli	Institut de Robòtica i Informàtica Industrial (CSIC-UPC), Spain
L. Duong	École de Technologie Superieure, Canada
M. Ebrahimi	University of Ontario Institute of Technology, Canada
A. El Khatib	University of Waterloo, Canada
M. El-Sakka	University of Western Ontario, Canada
F. Falck	Imperial College London, UK
P. Fallavollita	University of Ottawa, Canada
J. Fernandez	CNB-CSIC, Spain
R. Fisher	University of Edinburgh, UK
D. Frejlichowski	West Pomeranian University of Technology, Szczecin, Poland
A. Galdran	INESC TEC, Portugal
M. García	University of Valladolid, Spain
V. Gonzalez-Castro	Universidad de Leon, Spain
G. Grossi	University of Milan, Italy
W. Gueaieb	University of Ottawa, Canada
M. Hassaballah	South Valley University, Egypt
F. Karray	University of Waterloo, Canada
F. Khalvati	University of Toronto, Canada
A. Khamis	General Motors of Canada, Canada
Y. Kita	National Institute AIST, Japan
R. Kolar	Brno University of Technology, Czech Republic
M. Koskela	CSC, IT Center for Science Ltd., Finland
A. Kuijper	TU Darmstadt & Fraunhofer IGD, Germany
H. Li	University of New Brunswick, Canada
J. Lorenzo-Ginori	Universidad Central Marta Abreu de Las Villas, Cuba

J. Marques	University of Lisbon, Portugal
M. Melkemi	Université de Haute Alsace, France
A. Mendonça	University of Porto, Portugal
Y. Miao	General Motors of Canada, Canada
P. Morrow	Ulster University, UK
M. Mueller	North Carolina State University, USA
M. Nasr	University of Waterloo, Canada
H. Ogul	Baskent University, Turkey
H. Oliveira	INESC TEC, Portugal
C. Ou	University of Waterloo, Canada
C. Ouali	University of Waterloo, Canada
E. Ovreiu	University Politehnica of Bucharest, Romania
X. Pardo	CiTIUS, Universidade de Santiago de Compostela, Spain
J. Pedrosa	INESC TEC, Portugal
M. Penedo	University of Coruña, Spain
P. Pina	University of Lisbon, Portugal
A. Pinho	University of Aveiro, Portugal
L. Prevost	ESIEA (Ecole d'ingénieurs du monde numérique), France
B. Remeseiro	Universidad de Oviedo, Spain
D. Riccio	University of Naples Federico II, Italy
H. Rivaz	Concordia University, Canada
J. Rodrigues	University of the Algarve, Portugal
N. Rodriguez	University of A Coruña, Spain
J. Rouco	University of A Coruña, Spain
K. Roy	North Carolina A&T State University, USA
R. Sablatnig	TU Wien, Austria
S. Saeedi	Imperial College, UK
A. Sappa	ESPOL Polytechnic University, Ecuador; Computer Vision Center, Spain
G. Schaefer	Loughborough University, UK
H. Sekkati	National Research Council of Canada, Canada
M. Shafiee	University of Waterloo, Canada
J. Silva	University of Porto, Portugal
P. Siva	Sportlogiq, Canada
N. Strisciuglio	University of Groningen, The Netherlands
S. Sural	Indian Institute of Technology, India
A. Taboada-Crispi	Universidad Central Marta Abreu de Las Villas, Cuba
F. Tortorella	Università degli Studi di Salerno, Italy
A. Uhl	University of Salzburg, Austria
M. Vento	Università di Salerno, Italy
K. Vermeer	Rotterdam Ophthalmic Institute, Rotterdam Eye Hospital, The Netherlands
E. Vrscay	University of Waterloo, Canada
Z. Wang	University of Waterloo, Canada

A. Wong	University of Waterloo, Canada
L. Xu	University of Waterloo, Canada
J. Xue	University College London, UK
A. Yu	University of Waterloo, Canada
P. Zemcik	Brno University of Technology, Czech Republic
B. Zhang	University of Macau, SAR China
H. Zhou	Queen's University Belfast, UK
R. Zwiggelaar	Aberystwyth University, UK

Additional Reviewers

T. Araújo	INESC TEC, Portugal
G. Aresta	INESC TEC, Portugal
D. Kumar	University of Waterloo, Canada
L. Yu	ASML, USA

Contents – Part II

Contents – Part I

Image Processing

Image Analysis

Deep Learning on the Edge

Foothill: A Quasiconvex Regularization for Edge Computing of Deep Neural Networks

Mouloud Belbahri, Eyyüb Sari, Sajad Darabi, and Vahid Partovi Nia(✉)

Huawei Noah's Ark Lab, Montreal, Canada
vahid.partovinia@huawei.com

Abstract. Deep neural networks (DNNs) have demonstrated success for many supervised learning tasks, ranging from voice recognition, object detection, to image classification. However, their increasing complexity might yield poor generalization error that make them hard to be deployed on edge devices. Quantization is an effective approach to compress DNNs in order to meet these constraints. Using a quasiconvex base function in order to construct a binary quantizer helps training binary neural networks (BNNs) and adding noise to the input data or using a concrete regularization function helps to improve generalization error. Here we introduce *foothill* function, an infinitely differentiable quasiconvex function. This regularizer is flexible enough to deform towards L_1 and L_2 penalties. Foothill can be used as a binary quantizer, as a regularizer, or as a loss. In particular, we show this regularizer reduces the accuracy gap between BNNs and their full-precision counterpart for image classification on ImageNet.

1 Introduction

Deep learning has seen a surge in progress, from training shallow networks to very deep networks consisting of tens to hundreds of layers. Deep neural networks (DNNs) have demonstrated success for many supervised learning tasks [14,16]. The focus has been on increasing accuracy, in particular for image, speech, and recently text tasks, where deep convolutional neural networks (CNNs) are applied. The resulting networks often include millions to billions parameters. Having too many parameters increases the risk of over-fitting and hence a poor model generalization after all. Furthermore, it is hard to deploy DNNs on low-end edge devices which have tight resource constraints such as memory size, battery life, computation power, etc. The need for models that can operate in resource-constrained environments becomes more and more important.

Quantization is an effective approach to satisfy these constraints. Instead of working with full-precision values to represent the parameters and activations, quantized representations use more compact formats such as integers or binary numbers. Often, binary neural networks (BNNs) are trained with heuristic methods [5,12]. However it is possible to embed the loss function with an appropriate

F. Karray et al. (Eds.): ICIAR 2019, LNCS 11663, pp. 3–14, 2019.
https://doi.org/10.1007/978-3-030-27272-2_1

regularization to encourage binary training [2]. Common regularizations encourage the weights to be estimated near zero. Such regularization are not aligned with the objective of training binary networks where the weights are encouraged to be estimated −1 or +1. Using a regularization function specifically devised for binary quantization [11], it is shown how to modify the objective function in back-propagation to quantize DNNs into one bit with a scaling factor using a quasiconvex base.

In deep learning regularization is sometimes hidden in heuristic methods during training. For instance, adding noise to the input data yields to generalization error improvement [1,13]. Data augmentation, and early stopping are some other heuristic regularizations widely applied in practice. A more theoretically sound regularization method is dropout [15], a widely-used method for addressing the problem of over-fitting. The idea is to drop units randomly from the neural network during training. It is known that dropout improves the test accuracy compared to conventional regularizers such as L_1 [18] and L_2 [15]. [19] proved that dropout is equivalent to an L_2-type regularizer applied after scaling the inputs.

Linear regression can be regarded as the simplest neural network, with no hidden layer and a linear activation function. Therefore, it is important to study regularization in linear regression context.

Inspired by the extensive research literature on regularization in the statistical community we introduce *foothill* as a quasiconvex function with attractive properties with strong potentials to be applied in practice in neural network quantization, training neural networks, linear regression, and robust estimation.

This function is a generalization of lasso and Ridge penalties and has a strong potential to be used in deep learning. First, we start studying attractive functional properties of foothill that motivates its use. Then, we demonstrate its application in neural networks binary quantization and neural networks training. Foothill is flexible enough to be used as a regularizer or even as a loss function.

2 Foothill Regularizer

Let us define the mathematical notation first. Denote univariate variables with lowercase letters, e.g. x, vectors with lowercase and bold letters, e.g. $\mathbf{x}$, and matrices with uppercase and bold letters, e.g. $\mathbf{X}$.

2.1 Definition

Define the foothill regularization function as

$$p_{\alpha,\beta}(x) = \alpha x \tanh\left(\frac{\beta x}{2}\right). \qquad (1)$$

where tanh(.) is the hyperbolic tangent function, $\alpha > 0$ is a shape parameter and $\beta > 0$ is a scale parameter. The function is symmetric about 0 (see Fig. 1, left panel). The first and the second derivatives (see Fig. 1, right panel) of foothill are

$$\frac{dp_{\alpha,\beta}(x)}{dx} = \alpha \tanh\left(\frac{\beta x}{2}\right) + \frac{1}{2}\alpha\beta x \,\mathrm{sech}^2\left(\frac{\beta x}{2}\right),$$
$$\frac{d^2 p_{\alpha,\beta}(x)}{d^2 x} = \frac{1}{2}\alpha\beta \,\mathrm{sech}^2\left(\frac{\beta x}{2}\right)\left\{2 - \beta x \tanh\left(\frac{\beta x}{2}\right)\right\},$$

where sech(.) is the hyperbolic secant function.

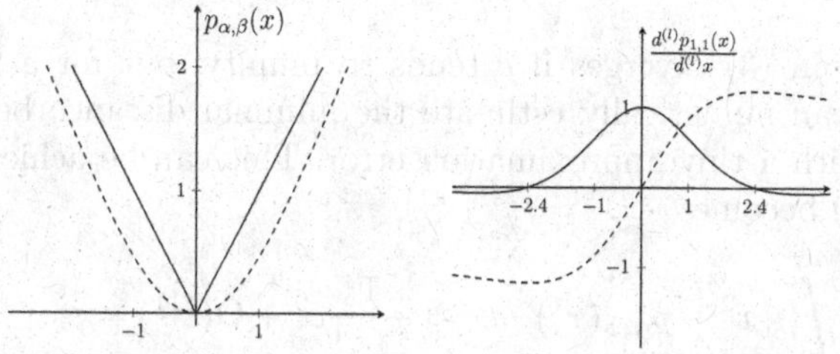

Fig. 1. Left panel: regularization function (1) for $\alpha = 1$, $\beta = 1$ (solid line) and $\alpha = 1$, $\beta = 50$ (dashed line). Right panel: the first (dashed line) and the second (solid line) derivatives of the regularization function (1) for $\alpha = 1$ and $\beta = 1$.

2.2 Properties

The regularization function (1) has several interesting properties. It is infinitely differentiable and symmetric about the origin,

$$p_{\alpha,\beta}(x) = p_{\alpha,\beta}(-x).$$

Also, it is flexible enough to approximate the lasso [18] and Ridge penalties [4] for particular values of α and β. The following properties suggest that this function could be considered as a quasiconvex alternative to the elastic net penalty [20].

Property 1. For $\alpha = 1$ and $\beta \to \infty$, the foothill penalty (1) converges to the lasso penalty.

Proof. For $x > 0$, it is easy to see that

$$\lim_{\beta\to+\infty} \tanh\left(\frac{\beta x}{2}\right) = 1,$$
$$\lim_{\beta\to+\infty} p_{\alpha,\beta}(x) = x.$$

Equivalently, for negative x, as $p_{\alpha,\beta}(x)$ is symmetric about the origin, then $\lim_{\beta\to+\infty} p_{\alpha,\beta}(x) = -x$, which is equivalent to $p_{\alpha,\beta}(x) \to |x|$ when $\beta \to +\infty$. ■

Property 2. For $\alpha > 0$, $\beta > 0$, and $\beta = 2/\alpha$ the foothill penalty (1) approximates the Ridge penalty in a given interval $[-c; c]$.

Proof. Let us study this property formally. Take the Taylor expansion of (1),

$$p_{\alpha,\beta}(x) \approx \frac{\alpha\beta}{2}x^2 - \frac{\alpha\beta^3}{24}x^4 + \frac{\alpha\beta^5}{240}x^6 + \mathrm{O}(x^8). \tag{2}$$

And, for a given $c > 0$,

$$\int_0^c \left(\frac{\alpha\beta}{2}x^2 - p_{\alpha,\beta}(x)\right)^2 dx \approx \frac{\alpha^2\beta^6}{5184}c^9 + \mathrm{O}(c^{11}). \tag{3}$$

The integral in (3) diverges if c tends to infinity, but for a finite positive number c, one can numerically estimate the minimal distance between the L_2 norm and (1) with a tiny approximation error. This can be achieved by taking $\beta = 2/\alpha$ and (3) becomes

$$\int_0^c \left(x^2 - p_{\alpha,\beta}(x)\right)^2 dx \approx \frac{1}{81\alpha^4}c^9 + \mathrm{O}(c^{11}) = \varepsilon_c. \tag{4}$$

For large values of α, the error ε_c is negligible, see for example Fig. 2 where the regularization function (1) approximates the Ridge penalty almost perfectly within $[-5; 5]$. Furthermore, for fixed parameters, note that

$$\lim_{x\to+\infty} p_{\alpha,\beta}(x) - \alpha x = 0, \quad \text{and} \quad \lim_{x\to-\infty} p_{\alpha,\beta}(x) + \alpha x = 0. \qquad \blacksquare$$

Hence it is also interesting to note that (1) behaves like a polynomial function for small values of x, and like a linear function for large values. Therefore, using it as a loss function (instead of a regularization), (1) behaves like the Huber loss used in practice for robust estimation [6]. Figure 2 shows that (1) is bounded between the Huber loss and the squared error loss.

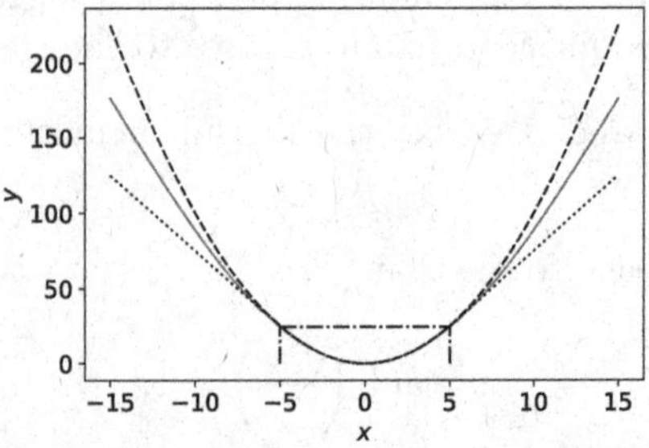

Fig. 2. Plots of the ridge, the foothill penalty with $\alpha = 16$ and $\beta = 0.125$ and twice the Huber loss. The solid blue line represents the foothill penalty, the dashed line represents the Ridge one (upper bound) and Huber (lower bound) is represented in dotted line. (Color figure online)

Property 3. Saddle points of $p_{\alpha,\beta}(x)$ are $x_0 \approx \pm 2.3994/\beta$ and $p_{\alpha,\beta}(x_0) = \frac{2\alpha}{\beta}$.

Proof. Indeed, the second order derivative vanishes at

$$2 - \beta x \tanh\left(\frac{\beta x}{2}\right) = 0,$$

which is solved by an iterative method for $\beta x \approx \pm 2.3994$. This implies

$$\beta x_0 \tanh\left(\frac{\beta x_0}{2}\right) = 2,$$

or equivalently

$$p_{\alpha,\beta}(x_0) = \frac{2\alpha}{\beta}.$$

■

Property 4. The function $p_{\alpha,\beta}(x)$ is quasiconvex.

Proof. It is straight forward to show that $p_{\alpha,\beta}(x)$ is decreasing from $-\infty$ to 0 and increasing from 0 to $+\infty$ and any monotonic function is quasiconvex (see Fig. 1, right panel). ■

Table 1 suggests that foothill has the flexibility to be used for feature selection regularizer such as the lasso or used only to shrink the estimator in order to prevent over-fitting like the Ridge. Finally, it also can be used as a loss function for robust regression as an alternative to the Huber loss.

Table 1. Relationship to other functions

	Shape α	Scale β	Function
Lasso	1	$+\infty$	$p_{\alpha,\beta}(x) = \lvert x \rvert$
Ridge	$+\infty$	$2/\alpha$	$p_{\alpha,\beta}(x) = x^2$
Huber	$< +\infty$	$2/\alpha$	$p_{\alpha,\beta}(x) = \alpha x \tanh\left(\frac{x}{\alpha}\right)$
Foothill	1	2	$p_{\alpha,\beta}(x) = x\tanh(x)$

3 Models

We start with motivating the use of foothill regularizer for binary quantization. Then, we study some properties in the linear regression context.

3.1 Binary Quantization

In BNNs, weights and activations are binarized using the non-differentiable sign function during the forward pass. It allows to compute dot product using xnor-popcount operations. However, we need to take the derivative of sign w.r.t. its input, which does not exist. Therefore, a gradient estimator is required [5]. The framework of BNN+ [2] introduces modified L_1 and L_2 regularizations functions which encourage the weights to concentrate around $\mu \times \{-1; +1\}$, where μ is a scaling factor. The modified L_1 and L_2 regularizations are defined as

$$R_1(x) = ||x| - \mu|, \tag{5}$$

$$R_2(x) = (|x| - \mu)^2. \tag{6}$$

We follow the generalization of [11] and modify (1) to construct a shifted regularization function $\tilde{p}_{\alpha,\beta}(x)$ as

$$\tilde{p}_{\alpha,\beta}(x) = p_{\alpha,\beta}\big(x - \mu\ \text{sign}(x)\big). \tag{7}$$

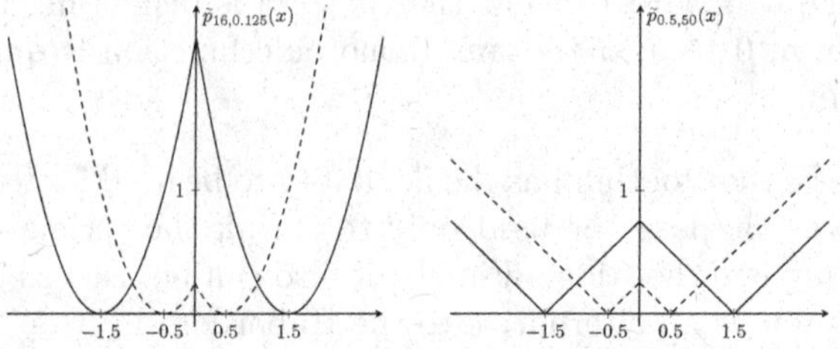

Fig. 3. Regularization functions for binary networks (7) with $\alpha = 16$ and $\beta = 0.125$ (left panel) and $\alpha = 0.5$ and $\beta = 50$ (right panel). Dashed line is $\mu = 0.5$ and solid line is $\mu = 1.5$. The scaling factor μ is trainable, as a result the regularization function adapts accordingly.

The regularization term is added to the loss function,

$$J(\mathbf{W}, \mathbf{b}) = L(\mathbf{W}, \mathbf{b}) + \lambda \sum_{h=1}^{H} \tilde{p}_{\alpha,\beta}(\mathbf{W_h}),$$

where $L(\mathbf{W}, \mathbf{b})$ is the cost function, $\mathbf{W}$ and $\mathbf{b}$ are the matrices of all weights and bias parameters in the network, $\mathbf{W_h}$ is the matrix of weights at layer h and H is the total number of layers. Here, $\tilde{p}_{\alpha,\beta}(.)$ is the binary quantizer (7). The regularization function is differentiable, so more convenient to implement in back-propagation. The parameters α and β could be defined for the whole network or per layer. In this case, each layer has its own regularization term.

Training the objective function $J(\mathbf{W}, \mathbf{b})$ quantizes the weights around $\pm\mu$ for large values of the regularization constant λ. Adding the regularization function to the objective function of a deep neural networks adds only one line to the back-propagation in order to estimate the scaling factors. Hence, while training, the regularization function adapts and the weights are encouraged towards $\mu \times \{-1; +1\}$ (see Fig. 3). We suggest starting training with $\lambda = 0$ and increasing λ with logarithmic rate as a function of the number of epochs [11,17]. The scaling factor and the number of scaling factors are important for BNNs to compete with full-precision networks. In practice, we use a scaling factor per neuron for fully-connected layers and a scaling factor per filter for convolutional layers. Without a scaling factor, the accuracy loss is large [5]. The scaling factors are applied after the fully-connected and convolutional layers which are performed using xnor-popcount operations during inference. In our experiments, we learn the scaling factors with back-propagation.

3.2 Regression

Suppose the response variable is measured with an additive statistical error ε and the relationship between the response and the predictors is fully determined by a linear function

$$\mathbf{y} = \mathbf{X}\boldsymbol{\theta} + \boldsymbol{\varepsilon}, \tag{8}$$

where $\mathbf{y}_{n\times 1}$ is the vector of observed response, $\mathbf{X}_{n\times p}$ is row-wise stacked matrix of predictors, $\boldsymbol{\theta}_{p\times 1}$ is the p-dimensional vector of coefficients, and $\boldsymbol{\varepsilon}_{n\times 1}$ is white noise with zero mean and a constant variance τ^2.

The penalized estimator with squared-loss function is defined as

$$\hat{\boldsymbol{\theta}} = \underset{\boldsymbol{\theta}}{\operatorname{argmin}} \ \frac{1}{2n} \|\mathbf{y} - \mathbf{X}\boldsymbol{\theta}\|_2^2 + \lambda \sum_{j=1}^{p} p_{\alpha,\beta}(\theta_j), \tag{9}$$

where $p_{\alpha,\beta}(.)$ is the regularization function (1). Here, λ is the regularization constant. Setting $\lambda = 0$ returns the ordinary least squares estimates, which performs no shrinking and no selection. For a given $\lambda > 0$ and finite α and β, the regression coefficients $\hat{\boldsymbol{\theta}}$ are shrunk towards zero, and for $\alpha = 1$, when $\beta \to +\infty$, (1) converges to the lasso penalty which sets some of the coefficients to zero (sparse selection), so does selection and shrinkage simultaneously.

To better understand the proposed penalty, we consider the orthogonal case where we assume that the columns of $\mathbf{X}$ in (8) are orthonormal, i.e. $\mathbf{X}^\top \mathbf{X} = n\mathbf{I}_p$. Therefore, the minimization problem of (9) is equivalent to estimating coefficients component-wise. Let $\hat{z}_j = \mathbf{x}_j^\top \mathbf{y}/n$ be the ordinary least squares estimate for $j = 1, ..., p$. Here, for fixed $\alpha > 0$ and a given scale parameter $\beta > 0$, this leads us to the univariate optimization problem

$$\underset{\theta_j}{\operatorname{argmin}} \ \left[\frac{1}{2}(\hat{z}_j - \theta_j)^2 + \lambda\alpha\theta_j \tanh\left(\frac{\beta\theta_j}{2}\right)\right]. \tag{10}$$

The numerical solutions of (10) with various values of α and β are shown in Fig. 4. When β is small, the solutions are smooth and by increasing β, the solutions become similar to ones of lasso.

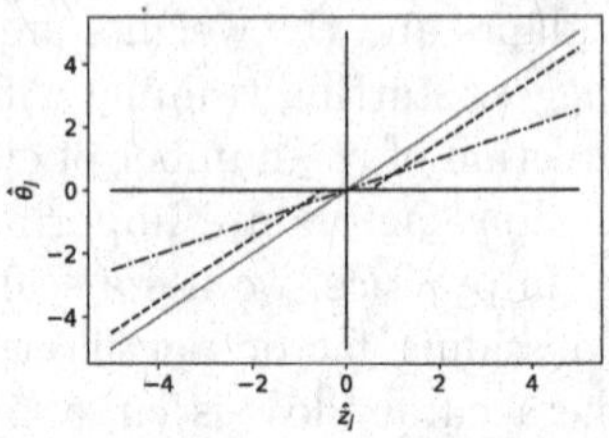

Fig. 4. Solution paths in the orthogonal design study according to the OLS estimator $\hat{z}_j$ for the foothill with $\alpha = 16$ and $\beta = 0.125$ (dashed and dotted line) and $\alpha = 1$ and $\beta = 50$ (dashed line), with $\lambda = 0.5$. The solid blue line represents the OLS estimator. (Color figure online)

Following [8] proof for Bridge regression [3], we show that under similar conditions and a fixed λ, the penalized estimator is $\sqrt{n}$-consistent.

Consider the linear model (8) and denote the penalized least squares function by

$$J_n(\boldsymbol{\theta}) = \frac{1}{2}(\mathbf{y} - \mathbf{X}\boldsymbol{\theta})^\top(\mathbf{y} - \mathbf{X}\boldsymbol{\theta}) + \lambda \sum_{j=1}^{p} p_{\alpha,\beta}(\theta_j).$$

Property 5. Assume that the matrix $\mathbb{E}[\mathbf{X}^\top\mathbf{X}] < \infty$ is positive definite. Let $\hat{\boldsymbol{\theta}}_n$ be the penalized estimator. $\hat{\boldsymbol{\theta}}_n$ is consistent if any given $\epsilon > 0$, there exist a large constant C such that

$$\Pr\left(\inf_{\|\mathbf{u}\|=C} J_n\left(\boldsymbol{\theta} + \frac{\mathbf{u}}{\sqrt{n}}\right) > J_n(\boldsymbol{\theta})\right) \geq 1 - \epsilon. \tag{11}$$

Proof. This implies there is a local minimizer such that $\|\hat{\boldsymbol{\theta}}_n - \boldsymbol{\theta}\| = O_P(\sqrt{n})$. Simple algebra shows that

$$\begin{aligned} D_n(\mathbf{u}) &:= J_n(\boldsymbol{\theta} + \frac{\mathbf{u}}{\sqrt{n}}) - J_n(\boldsymbol{\theta}) \\ &= \frac{1}{2}\mathbf{u}^\top \frac{\mathbf{X}^\top\mathbf{X}}{n}\mathbf{u} - \mathbf{u}^\top \frac{\mathbf{X}^\top(\mathbf{y} - \mathbf{X}\boldsymbol{\theta})}{\sqrt{n}} \\ &\quad + \lambda \sum_{j=1}^{p}\left(p_{\alpha,\beta}\left(\theta_j + \frac{u_j}{\sqrt{n}}\right) - p_{\alpha,\beta}(\theta_j)\right), \end{aligned}$$

which is minimized at $\sqrt{n}(\hat{\boldsymbol{\theta}}_n - \boldsymbol{\theta})$. By the strong law of large numbers and the central limit theorem, the first two terms converge to

$$\frac{1}{2}\mathbf{u}^\top\mathbb{E}[\mathbf{X}^\top\mathbf{X}]\mathbf{u} - \mathbf{u}^\top\mathbf{Z},$$

where $\mathbf{Z} \sim \mathcal{N}(\mathbf{0}, \boldsymbol{\Sigma})$ where $\boldsymbol{\Sigma} = \tau^2 \mathbb{E}[\mathbf{X}^\top \mathbf{X}]$. The third term can be rewritten as

$$\frac{\lambda}{\sqrt{n}} \sum_{j=1}^{p} \left(\frac{p_{\alpha,\beta}\left(\theta_j + \frac{u_j}{\sqrt{n}}\right) - p_{\alpha,\beta}(\theta_j)}{\frac{u_j}{\sqrt{n}}} \right) u_j,$$

and suppose that $\frac{\lambda}{\sqrt{n}} \to \lambda_0$. Therefore, when $n \to +\infty$, we have $\frac{u_j}{\sqrt{n}} \to 0$ so the third term of D_n converges to

$$\lambda_0 \sum_{j=1}^{p} \left(\frac{dp_{\alpha,\beta}(\theta_j)}{d\theta_j} \right) u_j.$$

For λ fixed, $\lambda_0 = 0$ and the first derivative of the regularization function is bounded, which means that $D_n(\mathbf{u})$ converges to

$$D(\mathbf{u}) = \frac{1}{2\tau^2} \mathbf{u}^\top \boldsymbol{\Sigma} \mathbf{u} - \mathbf{u}^\top \mathbf{Z},$$

which is convex and has a unique minimizer and hence,

$$\sqrt{n}(\hat{\boldsymbol{\theta}}_n - \boldsymbol{\theta}) \to_d argmin D(\mathbf{u}),$$

which shows that by choosing sufficiently large C, (11) holds and that $\hat{\boldsymbol{\theta}}_n$ is $\sqrt{n}$-consistent. ■

4 Application

In this section, we evaluate the performance of foothill on different applications. With two extra parameters, foothill is more flexible than L_1 and L_2. We believe that its flexibility helps fine-tuning.

4.1 Binary Quantization

In this section, we evaluate foothill's performance on a hard task. We use the shifted version from equation (7) in order to quantize a neural network. We quantize AlexNet architecture on ImageNet [9]. This dataset consists of ~1.2M training images, 50K validation images and 1000 classes. During training, images are resized to 256×256 and a random crop is applied to obtain 224×224 input size. Random horizontal flip is also used as a data augmentation technique. At test time, images are resized to 256×256 and a center crop is applied to get 224×224 size. For both steps, standardization is applied with mean $= [0.485, 0.456, 0.406]$ and std $= [0.229, 0.224, 0.225]$. Note that AlexNet architecture used for training BNNs is slightly modified from the original architecture as we need to change the order of some operation. For instance, pooling should not be performed after the binary activations. Therefore, we adopt the architecture described in [2] where batch normalization layers are added [7]. Weights and activations are quantized using the sign function for all convolutional and fully-connected layers except the first and the last ones which are kept to be in full-precision. We initialize the learning rate with 5×10^{-3} and divide it each 10 epochs alternatively, by 5 and by 2. We use $\lambda = 10^{-6} \times \log(t)$ where t is the current epoch and train the networks for 100 epochs. We compare our method to traditional binary networks.

Table 2. Comparison of top-1 and top-5 accuracies of quantized neural network using the lasso (5), Ridge (6) and foothill (7) modified regularizers to traditional BinaryNet [5] and XNOR-Net [12] on ImageNet dataset, using AlexNet architecture.

Method	Top-1 accuracy	Top-5 accuracy
$R_1(x)$	43.0%	67.5%
$\tilde{p}_{0.5,50}(x)$	44.4%	68.5%
$\tilde{p}_{0.75,50}(x)$	44.3%	68.4%
$R_2(x)$	42.9%	67.5%
$\tilde{p}_{100,0.02}(x)$	44.2%	68.5%
$\tilde{p}_{20,0.1}(x)$	**44.5%**	68.3%
BinaryNet	41.2%	65.6%
XNOR-Net	44.2%	69.2%
Full-precision	57.1%	80.3%

In Table 2, we report XNOR-Net performance from the original paper of [12] and the BinaryNet one from the implementation of [10], which is higher than the one reported in the original paper. We do not report the performance of [2] as they make use of a pre-trained model in their experiments, whereas we train the binary neural networks from scratch. We see that quantizing a neural network using foothill function as a regularization that pushes the weights towards binary values gives more accurate results for ImageNet dataset, better than L_1 and L_2 by more than 1.5%, which is a big gain for BNNs. Furthermore, for AlexNet architecture, our method beats the state of the art BinaryNet and XNOR-Net.

4.2 Regularization

We use AlexNet architecture augmented by batch normalization in order to compare foothill (1) to L_1 and L_2 regularizers on CIFAR-10. We train the network for 50 epochs using stochastic gradient descent optimizer with momentum 0.9 and a learning rate of 10^{-2} that is divided by 10 at epochs 20 and 30. The data preprocessing pipeline is the same as for ImageNet. For each experiment, the regularization constant λ is set to a value in $\{10^{-4}, 10^{-3}, 10^{-2}\}$.

The results reported in Table 3 and Fig. 5 empirically demonstrate the flexibility of foothill against L_1 and L_2. Our regularization function is less sensitive to the choice of λ. For instance, L_1-regularized AlexNet's accuracy can have 34.16% difference depending on which λ has been used for training while foothill with $\alpha = 0.5$ and $\beta = 50$ regularized AlexNet's accuracy difference ranges in 4.96%.

Table 3. Regularized AlexNet top-1 accuracies on CIFAR-10 test set, using different λ values. Our implementation of the non-regularized AlexNet achieves 88.63% accuracy.

λ	$L_1(x)$	$p_{0.5,50}(x)$	$p_{0.75,50}(x)$	$L_2(x)$	$p_{16,0.125}(x)$	$p_{20,0.1}(x)$
10^{-4}	89.75%	89.53%	**90.24%**	88.61%	88.73%	89.12%
10^{-3}	81.74%	**90.55%**	90.05%	89.51%	89.30%	89.44%
10^{-2}	55.59%	85.60%	84.78%	89.99%	89.86%	**90.21%**

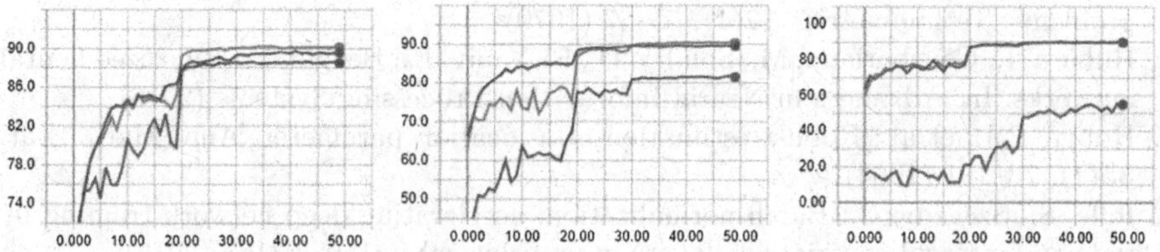

Fig. 5. From left to right, $\lambda = 10^{-4}, 10^{-3}, 10^{-2}$ validation curves for L_1 (blue), L_2 (red) and the best foothill regularizer (orange). The validation curves show the robustness of foothill in comparison with L_1 with respect to λ. (Color figure online)

5 Conclusion

Here we developed a new function, called foothill, that can be used as a binary quantizer, as a regularizer, or a loss function.

Most of the deep networks includes millions of parameters that requires extensive resources to be implemented in realtime. A modified version of foothill can be used to quantize deep networks and ultimately run neural networks to low power edge devices, such as wearable devices, cell phones, wireless base stations, etc. Network quantization yields to accuracy degradation. Recent studies [5,12] suggest proper training of weights controls the accuracy loss. The shift version of foothill has the potential of pushing heuristic training towards a more clear and formalized training using regularization. Our numerical results confirm this assumption since our implementation of a quantized neural network using foothill regularizer beats L_1 and L_2 regularizers and XNOR-Net, which is the state of the art binary quantization method.

As a regularizer foothill may encourage estimation shrinkage, sparse selection, or both depending on the values of its parameters. More concretely its parameters can be tuned to approximate both lasso (which implements sparse selection) and Ridge penalty (which implements shrinkage). Therefore foothill looks like a quasiconvex version of the elastic net which approximates the lasso and the Ridge. As a loss function, the behaviour of foothill is similar to the Huber loss.

Acknowledgements. We want to acknowledge technical discussions with Matthieu Courbariaux, Mohan Liu, and Alejandro Murua. This research was not possible without continuous support of Yanhui Geng and Li Zhou.

References

1. Bishop, C.M.: Training with noise is equivalent to tikhonov regularization. Neural Comput. **7**(1), 108–116 (1995)
2. Darabi, S., Belbahri, M., Courbariaux, M., Nia, V.P.: BNN+: improved binary network training. arXiv preprint arXiv:1812.11800 (2018)
3. Frank, L.E., Friedman, J.H.: A statistical view of some chemometrics regression tools. Technometrics **35**(2), 109–135 (1993)
4. Hoerl, A.E., Kennard, R.W.: Ridge regression: biased estimation for nonorthogonal problems. Technometrics **12**(1), 55–67 (1970)
5. Hubara, I., Courbariaux, M., Soudry, D., El-Yaniv, R., Bengio, Y.: Binarized neural networks. In: Advances in Neural Information Processing Systems (2016)
6. Huber, P.J., et al.: Robust estimation of a location parameter. Ann. Math. Stat. **35**(1), 73–101 (1964)
7. Ioffe, S., Szegedy, C.: Batch normalization: accelerating deep network training by reducing internal covariate shift. arXiv preprint arXiv:1502.03167 (2015)
8. Knight, K., Fu, W.: Asymptotics for lasso-type estimators. Ann. Stat. **28**, 1356–1378 (2000)
9. Krizhevsky, A., Sutskever, I., Hinton, G.E.: Imagenet classification with deep convolutional neural networks. In: Advances in Neural Information Processing Systems, pp. 1097–1105 (2012)
10. Lin, X., Zhao, C., Pan, W.: Towards accurate binary convolutional neural network. In: Advances in Neural Information Processing Systems, pp. 345–353 (2017)
11. Nia, V.P., Belbahri, M.: Binary quantizer. J. Comput. Vis. Imaging Syst. **4**(1), 3 (2018)
12. Rastegari, M., Ordonez, V., Redmon, J., Farhadi, A.: XNOR-Net: imagenet classification using binary convolutional neural networks. In: Leibe, B., Matas, J., Sebe, N., Welling, M. (eds.) ECCV 2016. LNCS, vol. 9908, pp. 525–542. Springer, Cham (2016). https://doi.org/10.1007/978-3-319-46493-0_32
13. Rifai, S., Glorot, X., Bengio, Y., Vincent, P.: Adding noise to the input of a model trained with a regularized objective. arXiv preprint arXiv:1104.3250 (2011)
14. Simonyan, K., Zisserman, A.: Very deep convolutional networks for large-scale image recognition. arXiv preprint arXiv:1409.1556 (2014)
15. Srivastava, N., Hinton, G., Krizhevsky, A., Sutskever, I., Salakhutdinov, R.: Dropout: a simple way to prevent neural networks from overfitting. J. Mach. Learn. Res. **15**(1), 1929–1958 (2014)
16. Szegedy, C., et al.: Going deeper with convolutions. In: Proceedings of the IEEE Conference on Computer Vision and Pattern Recognition, pp. 1–9 (2015)
17. Tang, W., Hua, G., Wang, L.: How to train a compact binary neural network with high accuracy? In: Thirty-First AAAI Conference on Artificial Intelligence (2017)
18. Tibshirani, R.: Regression shrinkage and selection via the lasso. J. Roy. Stat. Soc. Series B **58**, 267–288 (1996)
19. Wager, S., Wang, S., Liang, P.S.: Dropout training as adaptive regularization. In: Advances in Neural Information Processing Systems, pp. 351–359 (2013)
20. Zou, H., Hastie, T.: Regularization and variable selection via the elastic net. J. Roy. Stat. Soc. Series B **67**(2), 301–320 (2005)

NetScore: Towards Universal Metrics for Large-Scale Performance Analysis of Deep Neural Networks for Practical On-Device Edge Usage

Alexander Wong[1,2(✉)]

[1] Waterloo Artificial Intelligence Institute, University of Waterloo, Waterloo, ON, Canada
a28wong@uwaterloo.ca
[2] DarwinAI Corp., Waterloo, ON, Canada

Abstract. Much of the focus in the design of deep neural networks has been on improving accuracy, leading to more powerful yet highly complex network architectures that are difficult to deploy in practical scenarios, particularly on edge devices such as mobile and other consumer devices given their high computational and memory requirements. As a result, there has been a recent interest in the design of quantitative metrics for evaluating deep neural networks that accounts for more than just model accuracy as the sole indicator of network performance. In this study, we continue the conversation towards universal metrics for evaluating the performance of deep neural networks for practical on-device edge usage. In particular, we propose a new balanced metric called **NetScore**, which is designed specifically to provide a quantitative assessment of the balance between accuracy, computational complexity, and network architecture complexity of a deep neural network, which is important for on-device edge operation. In what is one of the largest comparative analysis between deep neural networks in literature, the NetScore metric, the top-1 accuracy metric, and the popular information density metric were compared across a diverse set of 60 different deep convolutional neural networks for image classification on the ImageNet Large Scale Visual Recognition Challenge (ILSVRC 2012) dataset. The evaluation results across these three metrics for this diverse set of networks are presented in this study to act as a reference guide for practitioners in the field. The proposed NetScore metric, along with the other tested metrics, are by no means perfect, but the hope is to push the conversation towards better universal metrics for evaluating deep neural networks for use in practical on-device edge scenarios to help guide practitioners in model design for such scenarios.

Keywords: Performance analysis · Deep neural networks · On-device · Edge usage

---

Supported by Natural Sciences and Engineering Research Council of Canada (NSERC), the Canada Research Chairs program, Nvidia, and DarwinAI.

F. Karray et al. (Eds.): ICIAR 2019, LNCS 11663, pp. 15–26, 2019.
https://doi.org/10.1007/978-3-030-27272-2_2

1 Introduction

There has been a recent urge in both research and industrial interests in deep learning [4], with deep neural networks demonstrating state-of-the-art performance in recent years across a wide variety of applications. In particular, deep convolutional neural networks [5,6] has been shown to outperform other machine learning approaches for visual perception tasks ranging from image classification [19] to object detection [22] and segmentation [11]. One of the key driving factors behind the tremendous recent successes in deep neural networks has been the availability of massive computing resources thanks to the advances and proliferation of cloud computing and highly parallel computing hardware such as graphics processing units (GPUs). The availability of this wealth of computing resources has enabled researchers to explore significantly more complex and increasingly deeper neural networks that has resulted in significant performance gains over past machine learning methods. For example, in the realm of visual perception, the depth of deep convolutional neural networks with state-of-the-art accuracies have reached hundreds of layers, hundreds of millions of parameters in size, and billions of calculations for inferencing.

While the ability to build such large and complex deep neural networks has led to a constant increase in accuracy, the primary metric for performance widely leveraged for evaluating networks, it has also created significant barriers to the deployment of such networks for practical edge device usage. The practical deployment bottlenecks associated with the powerful yet highly complex deep neural networks in research literature has become even more visible in recent years due to the incredible proliferation of mobile devices, consumer devices, and other edge devices and the increasing demand for machine learning applications in such devices. As a result, the design of deep neural networks that account for more than just accuracy as the sole indicator of network performance and instead strike a strong balance between accuracy and complexity has very recently become a very hot area of research focus, with a number of different deep neural network architectures designed specifically with efficiency in mind [14,18,26,28,33,34,36].

One of the key challenges in designing deep neural networks that strikes a strong balance between accuracy and complexity for practical usage lies in the difficulties with assessing how well a particular network architecture is striking that balance. As previous mentioned, using accuracy as the sole metric for network performance does not provide the proper indicators of how efficient a particular network is in practical scenarios such as deployment on mobile devices and other consumer devices. As a result, there has been a recent interest in the design of quantitative metrics for evaluating deep neural networks that accounts for more than just model accuracy. In particular, it is generally desirable to design such metrics in a manner that is as hardware vendor agnostic as possible so that different network architectures can be compared to each other in a consistent manner. One of the most widely cited metrics in research literature for assessing the performance of deep neural networks that accounts for both accuracy and architectural complexity is the information density metric proposed by [1], which attempts to measure the relative amount of accuracy captured within one of the most basic building blocks of a deep neural network: a parameter. More specifically, the information density ($D(\mathcal{N})$) of a deep neural network $\mathcal{N}$ is defined as the accuracy of the deep neural network (denoted by $a(\mathcal{N})$) divided by the number of parameters needed for representing it (denoted by $p(\mathcal{N})$),

$$D(\mathcal{N}) = \frac{a(\mathcal{N})}{p(\mathcal{N})} \quad (1)$$

While highly effective for giving a good general idea of the balance between accuracy and architectural complexity (which also acts as a good indicator for memory requirements), the information density metric does not account for the fact that, depending on the design of the network architecture, the architecture complexity does not necessarily reflect the computational requirements for performing network inference (e.g., MobileNet [14] has more parameters than SqueezeNet [18] but has lower computational requirements for network inference). Therefore, the exploration and investigation towards universal performance metrics that account for accuracy, architectural complexity, and computational complexity is highly desired as it has the potential to improve network model search and design.

In this study, we continue the conversation towards universal metrics for evaluating the performance of deep neural networks for practical usage. In particular, we propose a new balanced metric called **NetScore**, which is designed specifically to provide a quantitative assessment of the balance between accuracy, computational complexity, and network architecture complexity of a deep neural network. This paper is organized as follows. Section 2 describes the proposed NetScore metric and the design principles around it. Section 3 presents and discusses experimental results that compare the NetScore, information density, and top-1 accuracy across 60 different deep convolutional neural networks for image classification on the ImageNet Large Scale Visual Recognition Challenge (ILSVRC 2012) dataset [25], making this one of the largest comparative studies between deep neural networks.

2 NetScore: Design Principles

The proposed NetScore metric (denoted here as Ω) for assessing the performance of a deep neural network $\mathcal{N}$ for practical usage can be defined as:

$$\Omega(\mathcal{N}) = 20 \log \left(\frac{a(\mathcal{N})^{\alpha}}{p(\mathcal{N})^{\beta} m(\mathcal{N})^{\gamma}} \right) \quad (2)$$

where $a(\mathcal{N})$ is the accuracy of the network, $p(\mathcal{N})$ is the number of parameters in the network, $m(\mathcal{N})$ is the number of multiply–accumulate (MAC) operations performed during network inference, and α, β, γ are coefficients that control the influence of accuracy, architectural complexity, and computational complexity of the network on Ω. A number of design principles were taken into consideration in the design of the proposed NetScore metric, which is described below.

2.1 Model Accuracy Representation

In the NetScore metric, the obvious incorporation of the model accuracy $a(\mathcal{N})$ of the network $\mathcal{N}$ into the metric is in the numerator of the ratio, as an increase in accuracy should naturally lead to an increase in the metric, similar to the information density metric [1]. We further introduce a coefficient α in the proposed NetScore metric to provide better control over the influence of model accuracy on the overall metric. In particular, we set $\alpha = 2$ to better emphasize the importance of model accuracy in assessing the overall performance of a network in practical usage, as deep convolutional neural networks that have unreasonably low model accuracy remain unusable in practical scenarios, regardless how small or fast the network is. In this study, the unit used for $a(\mathcal{N})$ is in percent top-1 accuracy on the ILSVRC 2012 dataset [25].

2.2 Model Architectural and Computational Complexity Representations

Taking inspiration from the information density metric [1], we represent the architectural complexity of a deep neural network by the number of parameters $p(\mathcal{N})$ in the network $\mathcal{N}$ and incorporate it in the denominator of the ratio. As such, the architecture complexity of the network is inversely proportional to the metric Ω, where an increase in architectural complexity results in a decrease in Ω. In addition, we incorporate the computational complexity of the deep neural network as an additional factor in the denominator of the ratio to be taken into consideration for assessing the overall performance of a network for practical usage, which is particularly important in operational scenarios such as inference on mobile devices and other consumer devices where computational power is limited. To represent the computational complexity of the network $\mathcal{N}$ in a manner that is relatively hardware vendor agnostic, thus enabling a more consistent comparison between networks, we chose to leverage the number of multiply–accumulate (MAC) operations necessary for performing network inference. Given that the computational bottleneck associated with performing network inference on a deep neural network is predominantly in the computation of MAC operations, the number of MAC operations $m(\mathcal{N})$ is a good proxy for the computational complexity of the network. By incorporating both architectural and computational complexity, the proposed NetScore metric can better quantify the balance between accuracy, memory requirements, and computational requirements in practical usage. Furthermore, we introduce two coefficients (β and γ, respectively) to provide better control over the influence of architectural and computational complexity on the overall metric. In particular, we set $\beta = 0.5$ and $\gamma = 0.5$ since, while architectural and computational complexity are both very important factors to assessing the overall performance of a network in practical scenarios, the most important metric remains the model accuracy given that, as eluded to before, networks with unreasonably low model accuracy are not useful in practical scenarios regardless of size and speed.

Given these coefficients, NetScore is in the units of squared percentage accuracy per root parameter per root MAC operation, and represents the capacity of a network architecture to utilize its full learning and computing capacity.

2.3 Logarithmic Scaling

One of the difficulties with comparing the overall performance of different deep neural networks with each other is their great diversity in their model accuracy, architectural complexity, and computational complexity. This makes the dynamic range of the performance metric quite large and unwieldy for practitioners to compare for model search and design purposes. To account for this large dynamic range, we take inspiration from the field of signal processing; in particular, the logarithmic scale commonly used to express the ratio between one value of a property to another. In the proposed NetScore metric, we transform the ratio between the model accuracy property ($a(\mathcal{N})$) and the model architectural and computational complexity ($p(\mathcal{N})$ and $m(\mathcal{N})$) into the logarithmic scale to reduce the dynamic range to within a more readily interpretable range.

3 Experimental Results and Discussion

To get a better sense regarding the overall performance of the huge wealth of deep convolutional neural networks introduced in research literature in the context of practical usage, we perform a large-scale comparative analysis across a diverse set of 60 different deep convolutional neural networks designed for image classification using the following quantitative performance metrics: (i) top-1 accuracy, (ii) information density, and (iii) the proposed NetScore metric. The dataset of choice for the comparative analysis in this study is the ImageNet Large Scale Visual Recognition Challenge (ILSVRC 2012) dataset [25], which consists of 1000 different classes. To the best of the author's knowledge, this comparative analysis is one of the largest in research literature and the hope is that the results presented in this study can act as a reference guide for practitioners in the field.

The set of deep convolutional neural networks being evaluated in this study are: AlexNet [19], AmoebaNet-A (4, 50) [23], AmoebaNet-A (6, 190) [23], AmoebaNet-A (6, 204) [23], AmoebaNet-B (3, 62) [23], AmoebaNet-B (6, 190) [23], AmoebaNet-C (4, 50) [23], AmoebaNet-C (6, 228) [23], CondenseNet (G = C = 4) [16], CondenseNet (G = C = 8) [16], DenseNet-121 (k = 32) [17], DenseNet-169 (k = 32) [17], DenseNet-161 (k = 48) [17], DenseNet-201 (k = 32) [17], DPN-131 [2], GoogleNet [31], IGC-L100M2 [35], IGC-L16M16 [35], IGC-L100M2 [35], Inception-ResNetv2 [30], Inceptionv2 [32], Inceptionv3 [32], Inceptionv4 [30], MobileNetv1 (1.0-224) [14], MobileNetv1 (1.0-192) [14], MobileNetv1 (1.0-160) [14], MobileNetv1 (1.0-128) [14], MobileNetv1 (0.75-224) [14], MobileNetv2 [26], MobileNetv2 (1.4) [26], NASNet-A (4 @ 1056) [38], NASNet-A (6 @ 4132) [38], NASNet-B (4 @ 1536) [38], NiN [20], OverFeat [27], PNASNet-5 (4, 216) [21], PolyNet [37], PreResNet-152 [13], PreResNet-200 [13], PyramidNet-101 (alpha = 250) [9], PyramidNet-200 (alpha = 300) [9], PyramidNet-200 (alpha = 450) [9], ResNet-152 [12], ResNet-50 [12], ResNet-101 [12], ResNeXt-101, SENet [15], ShuffleNet (1.5) [36], ShuffleNet (x2) [36], SimpleNet [10], SqueezeNet [18], SqueezeNetv1.1 [18], SqueezeNext (1.0-23v5) [7], SqueezeNext (2.0-23) [7], SqueezeNext (2.0-23v5) [7], TinyDarkNet [24], VGG16 [29], Xception [3], ZynqNet [8].

In this study, the units used for $p(\mathcal{N})$ and $m(\mathcal{N})$ for two of the quantitative performance metrics (information density and the proposed NetScore metric) are in M-Params (millions of parameters) and G-MACs (billions of MAC operations), respectively, given that most modern deep convolutional neural networks are within those architectural and computational complexity ranges.

3.1 Top-1 Accuracy

The top-1 accuracies across 60 different deep convolutional neural networks for the ILSVRC 2012 dataset is shown in Fig. 1. It can be clearly observed that significant progress has been made in the design of deep convolutional neural networks for image classification over the past six years, with the difference between the deep convolutional neural network with the highest top-1 accuracy in this study (i.e., AmoebaNet-C (6, 228)) and that of AlexNet exceeding 25%. It is also interesting to see that more recent developments in efficient deep convolutional neural networks such as MobileNetv1, MobileNetv2, and ShuffleNet all have top-1 accuracies that exceed VGG-16, the third largest tested network evaluated in the study that was also the state-of-the-art just four years ago, thus further illustrating the improvements in network design over the past few years.

3.2 Information Density

The information densities across 60 different deep convolutional neural networks for the ILSVRC 2012 dataset is shown in Fig. 2. It can be clearly observed that the deep convolutional neural networks that were specifically designed for efficiency (e.g., MobileNetv1, MobileNetv2, ShuffleNet, SqueezeNet, Tiny DarkNet, and SqueezeNext) have significantly higher information densities compared to networks that were designed purely with accuracy as a metric. More specifically, the SqueezeNext (1.0-23v5), Tiny DarkNet, and the SqueezeNet family of networks had the highest information density by a wide margin compared to the other tested deep convolutional neural networks, which can be attributed to their significantly lower architectural complexity in terms of number of network parameters. Another notable observation from the results in Fig. 2 is that the dynamic range of the information density metric is quite large across the diverse set of 60 deep convolutional neural networks evaluated in this study.

3.3 NetScore

The NetScore across 60 different deep convolutional neural networks for the ILSVRC 2012 dataset is shown in Fig. 3. Similar to the trend observed in Fig. 2,

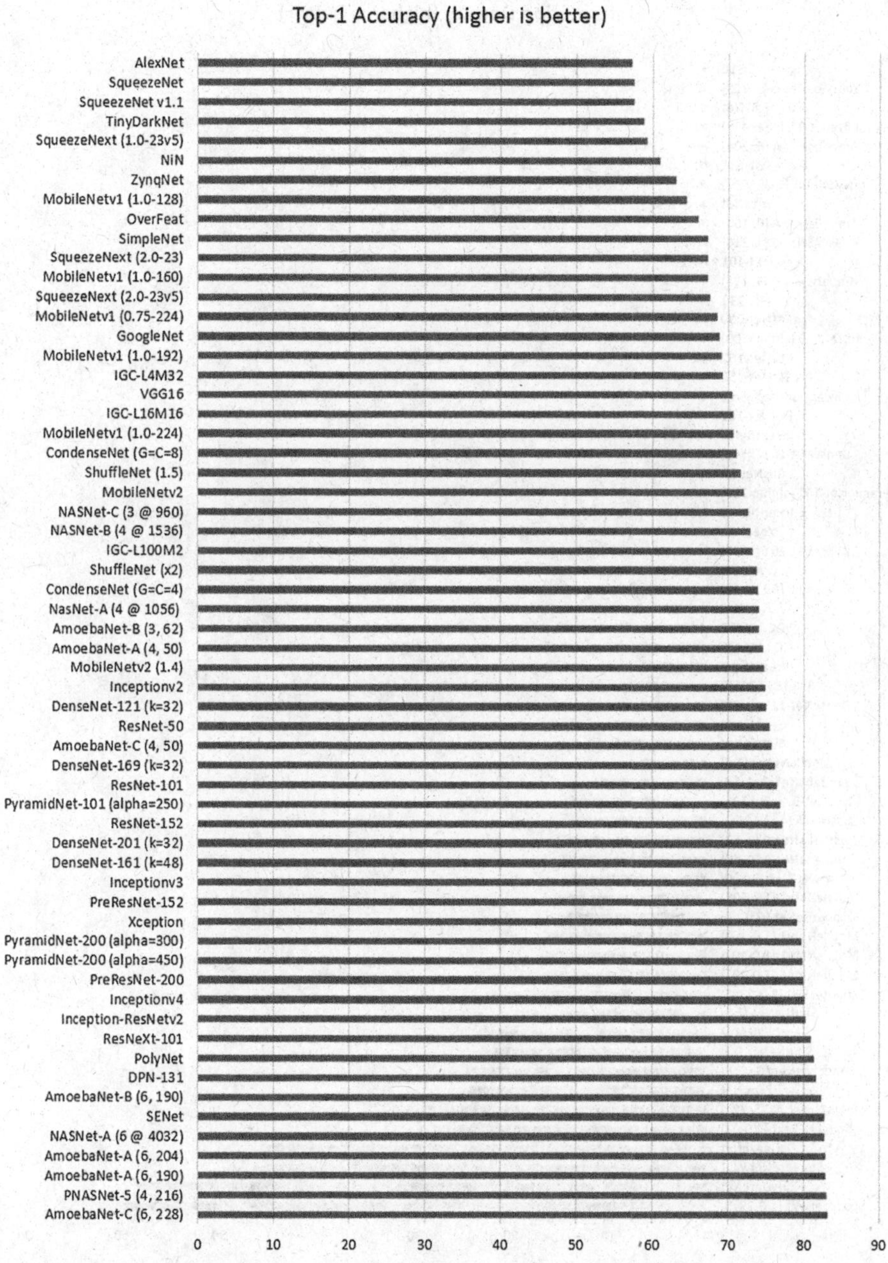

Fig. 1. Top-1 accuracy across 60 different deep convolutional neural networks for the ILSVRC 2012 dataset.

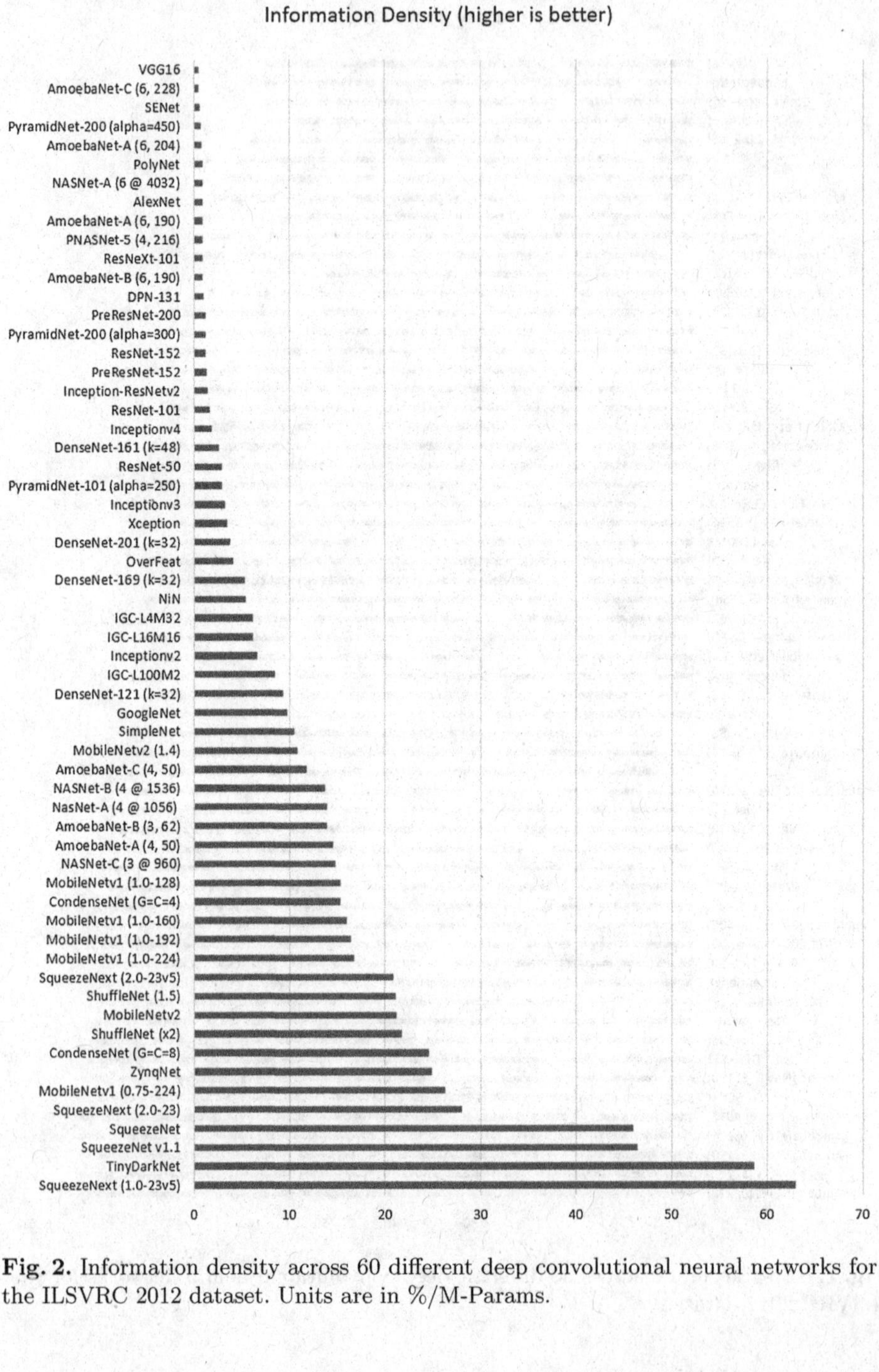

Fig. 2. Information density across 60 different deep convolutional neural networks for the ILSVRC 2012 dataset. Units are in %/M-Params.

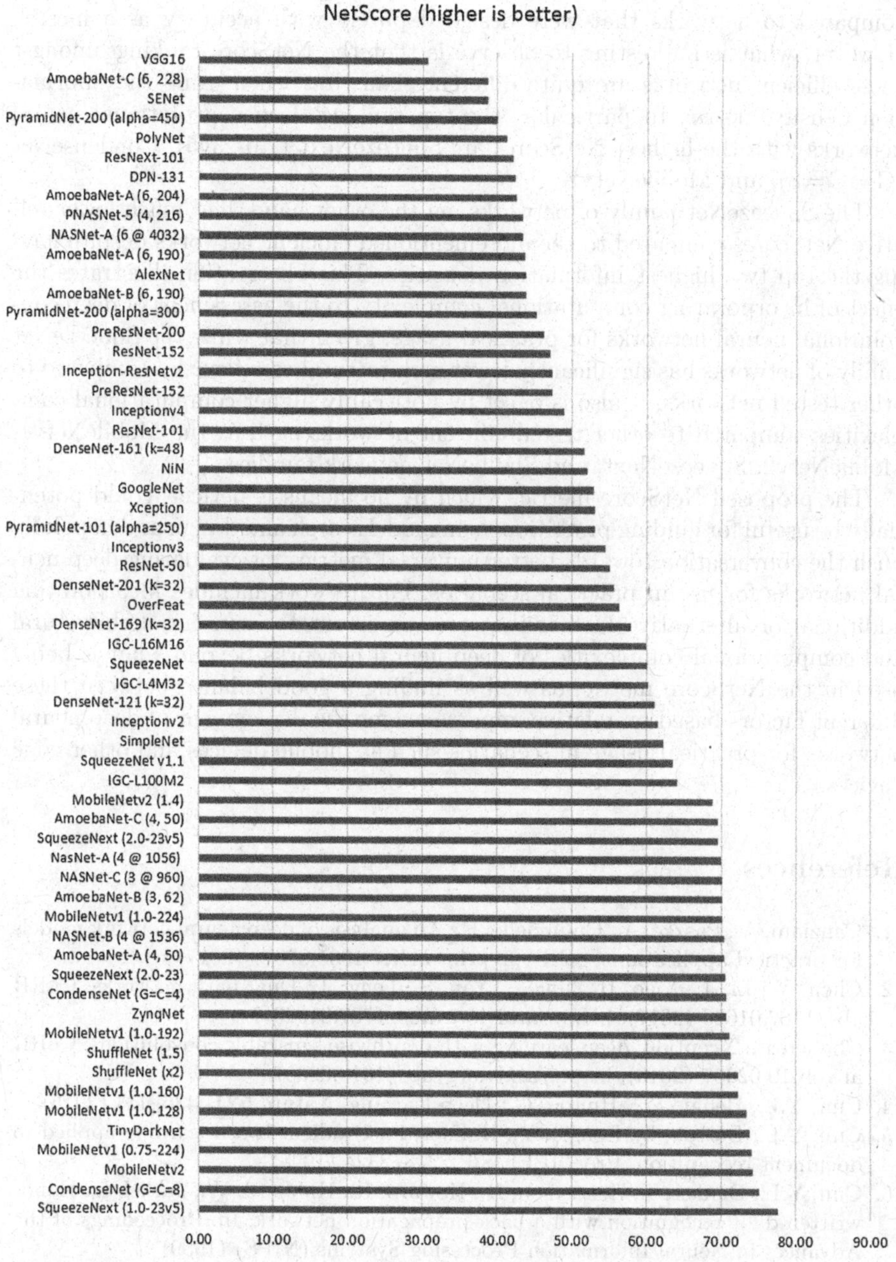

Fig. 3. NetScore across 60 different deep convolutional neural networks for the ILSVRC 2012 dataset.

it can be clearly observed that many of the deep convolutional neural networks that were specifically designed for efficiency have significantly higher NetScores compared to networks that were designed purely with accuracy as a metric. However, what is interesting to observe is that the NetScore ranking amongst these efficient networks are quite different than that when using the information density metric. In particular, the top ranking deep convolutional neural networks with the highest NetScores are SqueezeNext (1.0-23v5), CondenseNet (G = C = 8), and MobileNetv2.

The SqueezeNet family of networks, on the other hand, had much lower relative NetScores compared to the aforementioned efficient networks despite having the top two highest information densities. This observation illustrates the effect of incorporating computational complexity to the assessment of deep convolutional neural networks for practical usage, given that while the SqueezeNet family of networks has significantly lower architectural complexities compared to other tested networks, it also is offset by noticeably higher computational complexities compared to other tested efficient networks such as the MobileNetv1, MobileNetv2, SqueezeNext, and ShuffleNet network families.

The proposed NetScore metric, which by no means is perfect, could potentially be useful for guiding practitioners in model search and design and hopefully push the conversation towards better universal metrics for evaluating deep neural networks for use in practical scenarios. Future work includes incorporating additional or alternative factors that are important to assessing architectural and computational complexities of deep neural networks beyond what is being used in the NetScore metric, as well as finding a good balance between these different factors based on relative importance for the deployment of deep neural networks for practical usage in scenarios such as mobile devices and other edge devices.

References

1. Canziani, A., Paszke, A., Culurciello, E.: An analysis of deep neural network models for practical applications. arXiv preprint arXiv:1605.07678 (2017)
2. Chen, Y., Li, J., Xiao, H., Jin, X., Yan, S., Feng, J.: Dual path networks. CoRR abs/1707.01629 (2017). http://arxiv.org/abs/1707.01629
3. Chollet, F.: Xception: deep learning with depthwise separable convolutions. CoRR abs/1610.02357 (2016). http://arxiv.org/abs/1610.02357
4. Cun, Y.L., Bengio, Y., Hinton, G.: Deep learning. Nature **521**, 436–444 (2015)
5. Cun, Y.L., Bottou, L., Bengio, Y., Haffner, P.: Gradient-based learning applied to document recognition. Proc. IEEE **86**, 2278–2324 (1998)
6. Cun, Y.L., Denker, J., Henderson, D., Howard, R., Hubbard, W., Jackel, L.: Handwritten digit recognition with a back-propagation network. In: Proceedings of the Advances in Neural Information Processing Systems (NIPS) (1989)
7. Gholami, A., et al.: Squeezenext: hardware-aware neural network design. CoRR abs/1803.10615 (2018). http://arxiv.org/abs/1803.10615
8. Gschwend, D.: ZynqNet: an FPGA-accelerated embedded convolutional neural network (2016). https://github.com/dgschwend/zynqnet

9. Han, D., Kim, J., Kim, J.: Deep pyramidal residual networks. CoRR abs/1610.02915 (2016). http://arxiv.org/abs/1610.02915
10. HasanPour, S.H., Rouhani, M., Fayyaz, M., Sabokrou, M.: Lets keep it simple, using simple architectures to outperform deeper and more complex architectures. CoRR abs/1608.06037 (2016). http://arxiv.org/abs/1608.06037
11. He, K., Gkioxari, G., Dollar, P., Girshick, R.: Mask R-CNN. In: ICCV (2017)
12. He, K., Zhang, X., Ren, S., Sun, J.: Deep residual learning for image recognition. CoRR abs/1512.03385 (2015). http://arxiv.org/abs/1512.03385
13. He, K., Zhang, X., Ren, S., Sun, J.: Identity mappings in deep residual networks. CoRR abs/1603.05027 (2016). http://arxiv.org/abs/1603.05027
14. Howard, A., et al.: Mobilenets: efficient convolutional neural networks for mobile vision applications. arXiv preprint arXiv:1704.04861 (2017)
15. Hu, J., Shen, L., Sun, G.: Squeeze-and-excitation networks. CoRR abs/1709.01507 (2017). http://arxiv.org/abs/1709.01507
16. Huang, G., Liu, S., van der Maaten, L., Weinberger, K.Q.: Condensenet: an efficient densenet using learned group convolutions. CoRR abs/1711.09224 (2017). http://arxiv.org/abs/1711.09224
17. Huang, G., Liu, Z., Weinberger, K.Q.: Densely connected convolutional networks. CoRR abs/1608.06993 (2016). http://arxiv.org/abs/1608.06993
18. Iandola, F., Han, S., Moskewicz, M., Ashraf, K., Dally, W., Keutzer, K.: Squeezenet: Alexnet-level accuracy with 50x fewer parameters and <0.5 MB model size. arXiv preprint arXiv:1602.07360 (2016)
19. Krizhevsky, A., Sutskever, I., Hinton, G.: Imagenet classification with deep convolutional neural networks. In: NIPS (2012)
20. Lin, M., Chen, Q., Yan, S.: Network in network. CoRR abs/1312.4400 (2013). http://arxiv.org/abs/1312.4400
21. Liu, C., et al.: Progressive neural architecture search. CoRR abs/1712.00559 (2017). http://arxiv.org/abs/1712.00559
22. Liu, W., et al.: SSD: single shot multibox detector. In: Leibe, B., Matas, J., Sebe, N., Welling, M. (eds.) ECCV 2016. LNCS, vol. 9905, pp. 21–37. Springer, Cham (2016). https://doi.org/10.1007/978-3-319-46448-0_2
23. Real, E., Aggarwal, A., Huang, Y., Le, Q.V.: Regularized evolution for image classifier architecture search. CoRR abs/1802.01548 (2018). http://arxiv.org/abs/1802.01548
24. Redmon, J.: Tiny darknet (2016). https://pjreddie.com/darknet/tiny-darknet/
25. Russakovsky, O., et al.: Imagenet large scale visual recognition challenge. Int. J. Comput. Vis. **115**(3), 211–252 (2015)
26. Sandler, M., Howard, A., Zhu, M., Zhmoginov, A., Chen, L.: Mobilenetv 2: inverted residuals and linear bottlenecks. arXiv preprint arXiv:1704.04861 (2017)
27. Sermanet, P., Eigen, D., Zhang, X., Mathieu, M., Fergus, R., LeCun, Y.: Overfeat: integrated recognition, localization and detection using convolutional networks. CoRR abs/1312.6229 (2013). http://arxiv.org/abs/1312.6229
28. Shafiee, M., Li, F., Chwyl, B., Wong, A.: Squishednets: squishing squeezenet further for edge device scenarios via deep evolutionary synthesis. In: NIPS (2017)
29. Simonyan, K., Zisserman, A.: Very deep convolutional networks for large-scale image recognition. CoRR abs/1409.1556 (2014). http://arxiv.org/abs/1409.1556
30. Szegedy, C., Ioffe, S., Vanhoucke, V.: Inception-v4, inception-resnet and the impact of residual connections on learning. CoRR abs/1602.07261 (2016). http://arxiv.org/abs/1602.07261
31. Szegedy, C., et al.: Going deeper with convolutions. CoRR abs/1409.4842 (2014). http://arxiv.org/abs/1409.4842

32. Szegedy, C., Vanhoucke, V., Ioffe, S., Shlens, J., Wojna, Z.: Rethinking the inception architecture for computer vision. CoRR abs/1512.00567 (2015). http://arxiv.org/abs/1512.00567
33. Wong, A., Shafiee, M.J., Jules, M.S.: muNet: a highly compact deep convolutional neural network architecture for real-time embedded traffic sign classification. CoRR abs/1804.00497 (2018). http://arxiv.org/abs/1804.00497
34. Wong, A., Shafiee, M.J., Li, F., Chwyl, B.: Tiny SSD: a tiny single-shot detection deep convolutional neural network for real-time embedded object detection. CoRR abs/1802.06488 (2018). http://arxiv.org/abs/1802.06488
35. Zhang, T., Qi, G., Xiao, B., Wang, J.: Interleaved group convolutions for deep neural networks. CoRR abs/1707.02725 (2017). http://arxiv.org/abs/1707.02725
36. Zhang, X., Zhou, X., Lin, M., Sun, J.: Shufflenet: an extremely efficient convolutional neural network for mobile devices. CoRR abs/1707.01083 (2017). http://arxiv.org/abs/1707.01083
37. Zhang, X., Li, Z., Loy, C.C., Lin, D.: Polynet: a pursuit of structural diversity in very deep networks. CoRR abs/1611.05725 (2016). http://arxiv.org/abs/1611.05725
38. Zoph, B., Vasudevan, V., Shlens, J., Le, Q.V.: Learning transferable architectures for scalable image recognition. CoRR abs/1707.07012 (2017). http://arxiv.org/abs/1707.07012

Real-Time Person Re-identification at the Edge: A Mixed Precision Approach

Mohammadreza Baharani(✉), Shrey Mohan, and Hamed Tabkhi

Electrical and Computer Engineering Department, Energy Production and Infrastructure Center (EPIC), The University of North Carolina-Charlotte, Charlotte, NC 28223, USA
{mbharan,smohan7,htabkhiv}@uncc.edu

Abstract. A critical part of multi-person multi-camera tracking is person re-identification (re-ID) algorithm, which recognizes and retains identities of all detected unknown people throughout the video stream. Many re-ID algorithms today exemplify state of the art results, but not much work has been done to explore the deployment of such algorithms for computation and power constrained real-time scenarios. In this paper, we study the effect of using a light-weight model, MobileNet-v2 for re-ID and investigate the impact of single (FP32) precision versus half (FP16) precision for training on the server and inference on the edge nodes. We further compare the results with the baseline model which uses ResNet-50 on state of the art benchmarks including CUHK03, Market-1501, and Duke-MTMC. The MobileNet-V2 mixed precision training method can improve both inference throughput on the edge node, and training time on server 3.25× reaching to 27.77 fps and 1.75×, respectively and decreases power consumption on the edge node by 1.45×, while it deteriorates accuracy only 5.6% in respect to ResNet-50 single precision on the average for three different datasets. The code and pre-trained networks are publicly available. (https://github.com/TeCSAR-UNCC/person-reid)

Keywords: Person re-identification · MobileNet-V2 · ResNet-50 · Real-time multi-target multi-camera tracking · Edge node · Triplet-loss

1 Introduction

Real-time Multi-target Multi-Camera Tracking (MTMCT) is a task of positioning different unknown people on different camera views at a constrained amount of time. The results of this task can be beneficial to video surveillance, smart stores, and behavior analysis and anomaly detection. The core of MTMCT is person re-identification (re–ID) algorithm which retrieves person identities regardless of their poses and camera views.

Ideally, system re-identification should happen in real-time fashion at edge nodes. However, the most of recently proposed methods in literature [6,17,20,23]

This research was supported by the National Science Foundation (NSF) under Award No. 1831795.

F. Karray et al. (Eds.): ICIAR 2019, LNCS 11663, pp. 27–39, 2019.
https://doi.org/10.1007/978-3-030-27272-2_3

used ResNet-50 [7] as a backbone of their method, which is computationally expensive and targeted at the server side. One approach to reducing the computation complexity is to leverage light-weight network models such as MobileNet-V2 [11], even though these networks might not meet the real-time demands due to limited hardware resources and memory bandwidth at the edge node. Lowering accuracy and quantization can relive the pressure on both memory bandwidth and computation throughput [1,14]. However, to the best of our knowledge, the effect of quantization on final accuracy has not been studied for object re-identification approaches based on deep learning paradigms.

In this paper, we proposed a scalable and light-weight architecture based on the MobileNet-V2 to meet a predefined timing and power budget. We have also studied the effect of quantization and mixed training on two ResNet-50 and MobileNet-V2 network architecture in details. Specifically, our contribution is summarized as follows:

- We proposed a re-identification architecture based on light-weight MobileNet-V2, and we compare the results against the ResNet-50 in respect of accuracy.
- We also studied the effect of mixed precision training approach on both ResNet-50 and MobileNet-V2. We investigated which layers of networks should be quantized to be able to train the network. Our finding is orthogonal to other object re-identification based on deep learning methods and can be applied to improve their performance.
- We evaluated final system performance concerning throughput and power consumption on Nvidia Xavier board and discussed in details.

The rest of this article is organized as the following: Sect. 2 briefly reviews the previous person re–ID approaches. Section 3 presents our re–ID methods based on MobileNet-V2 and mixed precision for real-time inference. Section 4 presents the experimental results including comparison with existing approaches, and finally Sect. 5 concludes this article.

2 Related Works

There has been an increasing amount of research in the domain of object detection and tracking in recent years. With the problem of multi-object detection and tracking comes another one, which is re-identifying the same objects throughout the frames in the video precisely as the accuracy of tracking highly depends on it. Hence, in this section, we will be reviewing some of the recent work done for person re-id.

Classical computer vision approaches like those in [21] which are based on covariance descriptors which augment various feature representations of an image like RGB, Hue-Saturation-Value (HSV), local binary patterns, etc. over a mean Riemannian matrix (introduced by Bak et al. [2]) from multi-shot images to find similarities between different images have been done. Similar approaches were adopted in [15] for real-time embedded computation but the authors do not provide with any accuracy evaluation.

In [3], Oliveira et al. generate a unique signature for each object which comprises interest points and color features for the object and calculates the similarity between different signatures using Sum of Quadratic Differences(SQD). Similar classical approaches are demonstrated by [9] and [5], which uses Biologically Inspired Features (BIF) and k-shortest path algorithm. Classical techniques are promising; however, with the boom in deep learning algorithms and plethora of computational power all thanks to the top of the line GPUs, they are even surpassing human level recognition for re-id.

Modern deep learning techniques like Alignedreid [23], extract features from ROI using CNNs as base networks and then divide the feature map into local and global features intuitively dividing the ROI into horizontal sections and matching each section with the other images. Xiaoke et al. in [27], use videos instead of separate frames to learn the inter-video and intra-video distances between people in them effectively creating triplet pairs. Tong et al. [22] proposed an Online Instance Matching(OIM) loss paradigm which uses a Look Up Table(LUT) for labeled objects and a cicular queue for unlabelled objects and learns to re-id people on the go.

Yantao et al. in [18] formulate the problem of person re-id into a graph neural network problem, with each node denoting a pair of images whose similarity and dissimilarities are learned through a message passing technique between the nodes. Siamese network is used to compute similarity metric between pairs. Authors in [12] introduce spatiotemporal attention models to learn key spatial features of objects throughout the video.

Almost all the works as mentioned above are novel and state of the art, however, they all use very complicated and deep networks which would hinder their performance in real-time scenarios. In next section, we propose a lightweight system with reasonably high accuracy on the state of the art benchmarks.

3 Mixed Precision Real-Time Person Re-identification

In this section, we discuss two ResNet-50 and MobileNet-V2 architectures. Then we continue to explain the loss function, and in the last, we give an introduction about mixed precision training, and we elaborate more on network layers and loss precision partitioning.

3.1 Background

In this section, we will give an introduction for two ResNet-50, MobileNet-V2 networks. Since the ResNet-50 is massively used for state-of-art person re-id, we consider it as baseline for our evaluation in experimental results (Sect. 4).

Residual Network (ResNet). Observing the difficulty of optimizing deeper convolutional networks for the task of image recognition and image localization, authors in [7] came up with the idea of using shortcut connections which they called residual connections claiming that such connections will help deeper

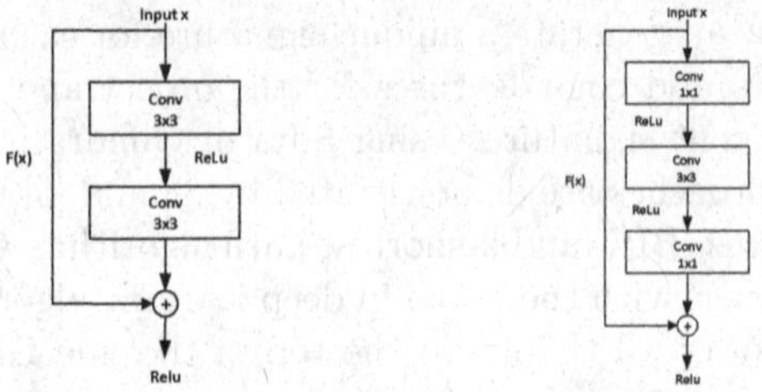

(a) Basic building block

(b) Bottleneck block

Fig. 1. Structural components of ResNet

stacked networks to learn efficiently. They use the baseline VGG nets [19] architecture, which uses 3x3 convolution blocks, and translate it to a 34 layer plain network and a 34 layer residual network (ResNet) for initial experimentation. They further evaluate the results on deeper ResNets with 50, 101 and 152 layers with the latter achieving a minimum error rate on the ImageNet [4] dataset for recognition.

Figure 1(a) shows the basic building block of a ResNet. After every two convolution blocks, there is an input residual mapping added to the output of the blocks which then goes to the ReLu activation layer. The function $F(x)$ is an identity function prevents the residual mapping in adding any additional parameters to the network. Figure 1(b) shows a bottleneck block for ResNet 50/101/152 where a three stack layer replaces a two stack layer. The idea for introducing a bottleneck block is to reduce training time constraints for deeper networks, without adding any additional parameters.

For object re-identification, we used a pre-trained ResNet-50 model on ImagNet dataset. We also removed the last Fully Connected (FC) layer at the end of the network used for classification and added a 2D average pooling with the kernel size of (16, 8) in order to make the output of the network in the shape of a 1D vector with size of 2048 as an embedded appearance features. In contrast to [17], we did not add any additional FC to prevent increasing the computational complexity at the edge node.

Mobile Network (Mobilenet). Most deep convolution networks have a huge number of parameters and operations making them unsuitable for use in mobile and embedded platforms. Authors in [10], developed light-weight deep convolution network which they called MobileNets. They effectively break down a standard convolution into a depthwise and pointwise convolution operation reducing the computational complexity of the net. They also introduce two hyper-parameters, width multiplier and resolution multiplier, which alter the thickness of intermediate layers and resolution of the inputs respectively. They evaluate their model on ImageNet dataset with other state of the art light-weight networks. Following the same trend in [11], MobileNet-V2 were introduced, which incorporated linear bottleneck layers and inverted residual connections into the previous network reducing the multiply-add operations and number of parameters further but increasing the accuracy.

In Fig. 2(a), the normal convolution filters can be seen with the shape of $K \times K \times M \times N$, where K is the size of the filter, M is the input channels, and N is output channels. Andrew et al. [4], transform this convolution into depthwise filtering, Fig. 2(b), where each filter is applied to each channel individually and pointwise combination, Fig. 2(c), where a 1×1 filter transforms the filtered features into a new feature map. They show the reduced computation cost and parameters with this approach. MobileNet has 28 layers including depthwise and pointwise layers separately with batch normalization and ReLu activation function. Width multiplier alpha scales the input and output channels by $\alpha \times M$ and $\alpha \times N$. Resolution multiplier does the same thing with the input image resolution hence scaling the computation expense and accuracy trade-off.

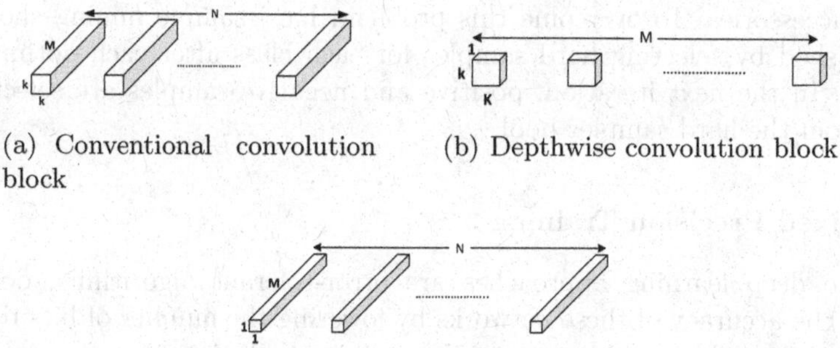

(a) Conventional convolution block (b) Depthwise convolution block

(c) Pointwise convolution block

Fig. 2. Different MobileNet-V2 convolution blocks

We also used a pre-trained MobileNet-V2 model on ImagNet dataset. We removed the classification layer (FC) at the end of the network used for classification and added again a 2D average pooling with the kernel size of (8, 4) in order to make the output of the network in the shape of a 1D vector with size of 1280 as an embedded appearance features.

3.2 Triplet-Loss Function

Alexander et al. in [8], rekindles the triplet loss network for person re-identification (re-id) with their work. The underlying architecture of a triplet loss network consists of three identical networks which transform the cropped Region of Interest(ROI) into embeddings on a lower dimensional space. One ROI has to be the anchor image, second has to be a positive sample of the anchor and third a negative sample. The basic concept here is to minimize the distance between the anchor and the positive samples and maximize the distance between the anchor and the negative samples in the lower dimensional embedding space. To facilitate such learning, a suitable loss function is used after the embeddings are extracted from the ROIs:

$$Loss = \sum_{i=1}^{n} \left[\alpha + \| f_i^a - f_i^p \|^2 - \| f_i^a - f_i^n \|^2 \right]_+, \tag{1}$$

where α is margin, f^a, f^p, and f^n are embedded appearance feature of anchor, positive, and negative samples for the class i, respectively. Minimizing $Loss$ function will force all samples of class i to be inside of hypersphere of radius α. The dimension of the hypersphere is equal to the size of the output of our networks (2048 for ResNet-50, and 1280 for MobileNet-V2). Now a drawback here is that the network might only learn easy samples and not hard samples, i.e., hard positives and hard negatives, and be biased towards the easy ones. An example of hard positives is when a person may change his/her clothes and an example of a hard negative is two different persons wearing the same colored clothes/accessories. To overcome this problem, hard sample mining should be accomplished by selecting hard samples for each class after each optimization iteration. In the next iteration, positive and negative samples are selected for class i from the hard samples pool.

3.3 Mixed Precision Training

Since the deep learning approaches are error-tolerant algorithms, designers decrease the accuracy of these networks by lowering the number of bits required to represents weights and biases, and they minimize the introduced error caused by quantization by training the network with reduced precision. However, half precision training needs to overcome two critical challenges of mapping numbers which are too small to be represented in half precision, and vanishing gradient due to limited precision representation. In [14], they address these problems FP32 master copy of weights, and gradient scaling method during the back-propagation respectively.

For networks used for person identification, we partitioned networks in two single, and half precision categories. We used Apex[1] to assign error-friendly operations, such as convolution and General Matrix Multiply (GeMM) operation, to half precision. During our experiment, we realized if we map the inputs of batch normalization layers in both networks to half precision, training does not converge. We also realized that the loss calculation should also be accomplished in single precision since hard samples are extracted based on loss function and the average distance between anchors and their positives and negatives instances. Lowering the accuracy at loss function will lead to weak hard positives and negatives pool.

[1] https://github.com/NVIDIA/apex.

4 Experimental Results

We evaluate the performance and accuracy of the two ResNet-50 and MobileNet-V2 networks in this section. We also describe the testing data-sets, the hardware setups, training time, accuracy, throughput, and power consumption for both single and half precision for each network on three datasets.

4.1 Learning Parameters and Datasets

We used DukeMTMC-reID [16,25], CUHK03 [13], and Market1501 [24] for evaluating the performance of two networks with different training methods. Table 1 summarizes the hyper parameters of our network. We updated the baseline framework for person re-ID[2] in order to support mixed precision training and different network models. We used the combined version of training sets of all three datasets to have better generalization at test phase. We decreased learning rate exponentially after 150 epochs and used Adam optimizer to train both networks.

Table 1. The training parameters

Item	Description	Value
1	Batch size	128
2	IDs per batch	32
3	Instances per ID	4
4	Initial learning rate	2×10^{-4}
5	Input shape (H × W)	(256 × 128)
6	Epoch	300
7	Margin	0.3

4.2 Accuracy

Figure 3 compares the accuracy results for baseline and ResNet-50 half precision. The Re-Ranking (RR) [26] method can improve the mAP on the average of 12% for both half and single precision. The CUHK03 benefits the highest improvement by applying the RR method among other datasets. Based on the results, we can realize that half precision only degrades 0.9% on the average concerning single precision for all three CMC-(1, 5) and mAP.

Figure 4 depicts the MobileNet-V2 model performance for both single and half precision in a similar approach. As we can see single precision negligibility deteriorate the CMC-1 performance for 0.5%. Based on side by side CMC-1 comparison on Fig. 5 for both ResNet-50 and MobileNet-V2 network, we can

[2] https://github.com/huanghoujing/person-reid-triplet-loss-baseline.

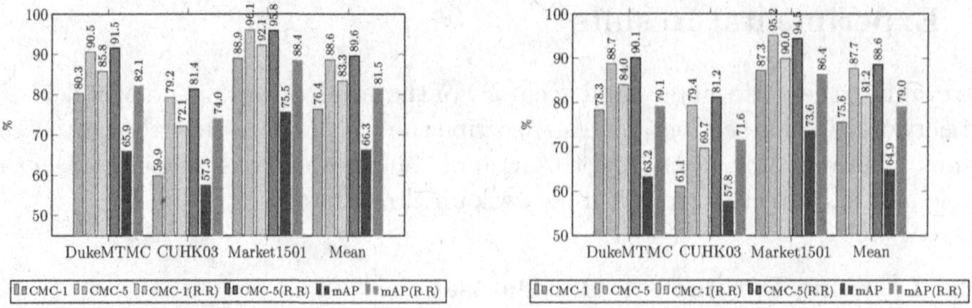

(a) Single Precision (b) Mixed Precision

Fig. 3. ResNet-50 accuracy evaluation on three different benchmarks. We trained the model for two different precision configuration, one single precision (a) and mixed precision (b).

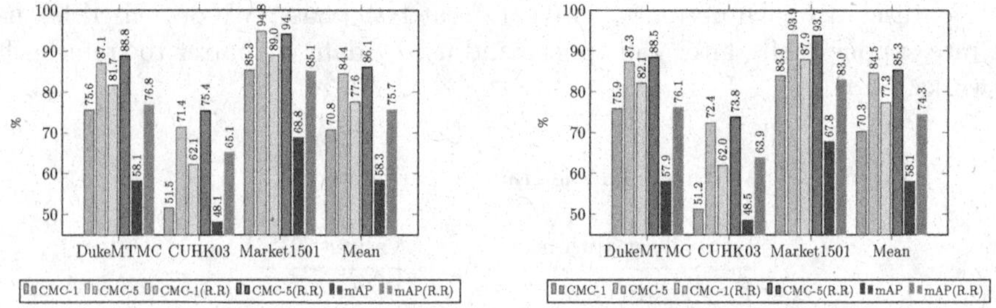

(a) Single Precision (b) Mixed Precision

Fig. 4. MobileNetV2 accuracy evaluation on three different benchmarks. We trained the model for two different precision configuration, one single precision (a) and mixed precision (b).

realize that the MobileNet-V2 half precision is negligibly 5.6% less than baseline. We also compare the results qualitatively in Fig. 6. We selected randomly three queries from each dataset and sorted the nearest objects based on Euclidean distance from the gallery considering the embedded appearance feature extracted without applying the RR method.

4.3 Training Time

We used the system described in Table 2 to train two ResNet-50 and MobileNet-V2 networks. Table 3 shows the results of training time on the server for different system configuration. As we can observe, half precision can improve training time to 1.20× on the average for both networks, and MobileNet-V2 half precision can upgrade it to 1.75× with respect to the baseline model.

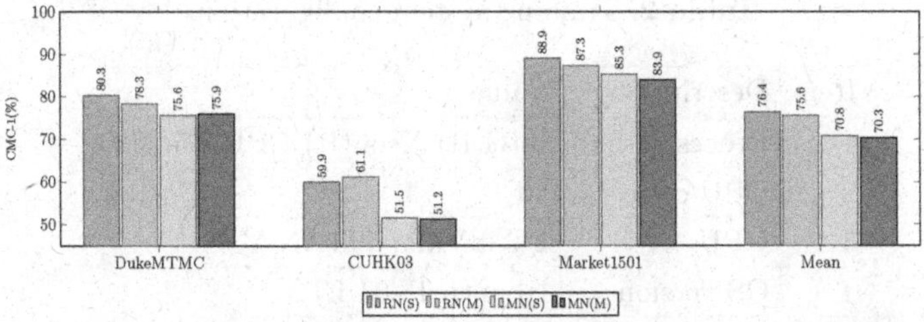

Fig. 5. A CMC-1 Comparison of two networks ResNet50 (RN) and MobileNetV2 (MN) for three different training and inference approaches.

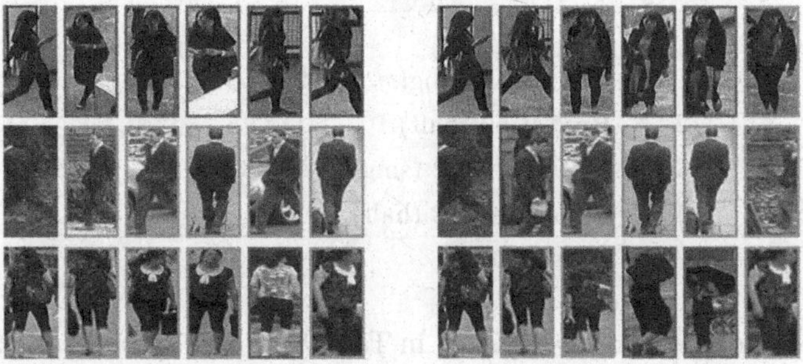

(a) ResNet-50: Single precision (left), half precision (right)

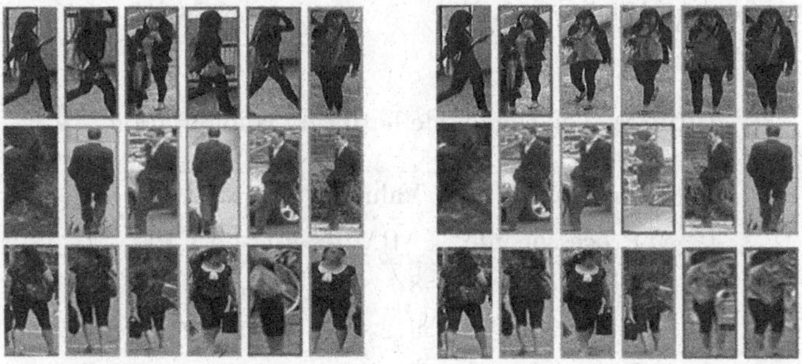

(b) MobileNet-V2: Single precision (left), half precision (right)

Fig. 6. A qualitative comparison of two networks with different precision. The images without the bounding box in each sample are queries, and five images in front of it are the first five ranked samples in the gallery. We marked true and false detected with green and red boxes respectively.

4.4 Edge Node Evaluation

We evaluated system performance in respect to power consumption and inference time on Nvidia Xavier embedded node. Table 4 summarizes the hardware resources on this board. We extracted the Open Neural Network eXchange (ONNX) format representation of all four network configurations and uploaded

Table 2. Training system configuration

Item	Description	Value
1	Processor info	Intel(R) Xeon(R) CPU E5-2640
2	CPU cores	40
3	GPUs	2 × nVidia TITAN V
4	OS version	Ubuntu 18.04 LTS
5	Memory	96GB/94.2GB Available

Table 3. Training elapsed time of two networks with different precision

Item	Description	Value (mins)
1	ResNet-50 (single)	242.65
2	ResNet-50 (half)	174.45
3	MobileNet-V2 (single)	140.3
4	MobileNet-V2 (half)	138.1

them on the edge side. As it is depicted in Table 5, we can reach to 18.92× model size compression ratio over the baseline model for MobileNet-V2 half precision. We mapped the half-precision types of both networks on Deep Learning Accelerators (DLA) and single precision to GPU Volta cores. We also set the Xavier power mode to MAX-N[3].

Table 4. The edge node hardware configuration

Item	Description	Value
1	Processor info	ARM v8.2 64-bit CPU
2	CPU cores	8
3	GPUs	512-Core Volta GPU
4	DL accelerators	2
5	OS version	Ubuntu 18.04 LTS
6	Memory	16GB/15.4GB Available

The inference time (Table 6) and power consumption (Table 7) is acquired for the batch size of 16. We obtained both timing performance and power consumption only for extracting features, and we did not consider model loading and other pre-processing tasks. MobileNet-V2 half precision improves the inference throughput 3.25× and reaches to 27.77 fps, while it only consumes 6.48 W.

[3] https://developer.nvidia.com/embedded/jetson-agx-xavier-dl-inference-benchmarks.

Table 5. Model sizes of two networks.

Network	Model Size (MB)		Improvement(×)	
	Single precision	Mixed precision	Per same model	Over the baseline
ResNet-50	94.6	47.7	1.98	18.92
MobileNetV2	9.4	5.0	1.88	

Table 6. Throughput performance on Nvidia Xavier.

Network	Throughput (fps)		Improvement (×)	
	Single precision	Mixed precision	Per same model	Over the baseline
ResNet-50	8.54	21.71	2.54	3.25
MobileNetV2	20	27.77	1.38	

Table 7. Power consumption on Nvidia Xavier.

Network	Power (W)		Improvement (×)	
	Single precision	Mixed precision	Per same model	Over the baseline
ResNet-50	9.45	7.86	1.2	1.45
MobileNetV2	6.48	6.48	1	

As the hardware warm-up was same for both MobileNet-V2 half-precision and single precision, we did not observe any power consumption improvement for this network.

5 Conclusion

In this paper, we present a light-weight person re-identification method based on MobileNet-V2. We even improved the performance of the edge node to the next level by mapping models to half precision. The experimental results elucidate that mixed precision training can achieve real-time re-identifying persons at the frame rate of 27.77 per second by only consuming 6.48 W. Our finding of network partitioning for mixed precision training is orthogonal to other person re-identification based on deep learning paradigm and can be applied to improve the overall system performance.

References

1. Baharani, M., Noori, H., Aliasgari, M., Navabi, Z.: High-level design space exploration of locally linear neuro-fuzzy models for embedded systems. Fuzzy Sets Syst. **253**, 44–63 (2014)

2. Bąk, S., Corvee, E., Brémond, F., Thonnat, M.: Multiple-shot human re-identification by mean riemannian covariance grid. In: 2011 8th IEEE International Conference on Advanced Video and Signal Based Surveillance (AVSS), pp. 179–184 (2011)
3. de Oliveira, I.O., de Sousa Pio, J.L.: Object reidentification in multiple cameras system. In: 2009 Fourth International Conference on Embedded and Multimedia Computing, pp. 1–8 (2009)
4. Deng, J., Dong, W., Socher, R., Li, L.: Imagenet: a large-scale hierarchical image database. In: 2009 IEEE Conference on Computer Vision and Pattern Recognition, pp. 248–255 (2009)
5. Fleuret, F., Ben Shitrit, H., Fua, P.: Re-identification for improved people tracking. In: Gong, S., Cristani, M., Yan, S., Loy, C. (eds.) Person Re-Identification, pp. 309–330. Springer, London (2014). https://doi.org/10.1007/978-1-4471-6296-4_15
6. Fu, Y., et al.: Horizontal pyramid matching for person re-identification. In: Proceedings of the Association for the Advancement of Artificial Intelligence (AAAI) (2019)
7. He, K., Zhang, X., Ren, S., Sun, J.: Deep residual learning for image recognition. In: 2016 IEEE Conference on Computer Vision and Pattern Recognition (CVPR), pp. 770–778 (2016)
8. Hermans, A., Beyer, L., Leibe, B.: In defense of the triplet loss for person re-identification. CoRR abs/1703.07737 (2017)
9. Hirzer, M., Beleznai, C., Roth, P.M., Bischof, H.: Person re-identification by descriptive and discriminative classification. In: Heyden, A., Kahl, F. (eds.) SCIA 2011. LNCS, vol. 6688, pp. 91–102. Springer, Heidelberg (2011). https://doi.org/10.1007/978-3-642-21227-7_9
10. Howard, A.G., et al.: Mobilenets: Efficient convolutional neural networks for mobile vision applications. CoRR abs/1704.04861 (2017)
11. Jacob, B., et al.: Quantization and training of neural networks for efficient integer-arithmetic-only inference. In: 2018 IEEE Conference on Computer Vision and Pattern Recognition, CVPR 2018, Salt Lake City, UT, USA, 18–22 June 2018, pp. 2704–2713 (2018)
12. Li, S., Bak, S., Carr, P., Wang, X.: Diversity regularized spatiotemporal attention for video-based person re-identification. In: 2018 IEEE/CVF Conference on Computer Vision and Pattern Recognition, pp. 369–378 (2018)
13. Li, W., Zhao, R., Xiao, T., Wang, X.: Deepreid: deep filter pairing neural network for person re-identification. In: CVPR (2014)
14. Micikevicius, P., et al.: Mixed precision training. In: International Conference on Learning Representations (2018)
15. Mier y Terán, A.R., Lacassagne, L., Zahraee, A.H., Gouiffès, M.: Real-time covariance tracking algorithm for embedded systems. In: 2013 Conference on Design and Architectures for Signal and Image Processing, pp. 104–111 (2013)
16. Ristani, E., Solera, F., Zou, R., Cucchiara, R., Tomasi, C.: Performance measures and a data set for multi-target, multi-camera tracking. In: European Conference on Computer Vision workshop on Benchmarking Multi-Target Tracking (2016)
17. Ristani, E., Tomasi, C.: Features for multi-target multi-camera tracking and re-identification. In: Conference on Computer Vision and Pattern Recognition (2018)
18. Shen, Y., Li, H., Yi, S., Chen, D., Wang, X.: Person re-identification with deep similarity-guided graph neural network. In: The European Conference on Computer Vision (ECCV), September 2018

19. Simonyan, K., Zisserman, A.: Very deep convolutional networks for large-scale image recognition. In: International Conference on Learning Representations (2015)
20. Sun, Y., Zheng, L., Yang, Y., Tian, Q., Wang, S.: Beyond part models: person retrieval with refined part pooling (and a strong convolutional baseline). In: Proceedings of the European Conference on Computer Vision (ECCV), pp. 480–496 (2018)
21. y Terán, A.R.M., Gouiffès, M., Lacassagne, L.: Covariance descriptor multiple object tracking and re-identification with colorspace evaluation. In: ACCV Workshops (2012)
22. Xiao, T., Li, S., Wang, B., Lin, L., Wang, X.: Joint detection and identification feature learning for person search. In: 2017 IEEE Conference on Computer Vision and Pattern Recognition (CVPR), pp. 3376–3385 (2017)
23. Zhang, X., et al.: Alignedreid: surpassing human-level performance in person re-identification. arXiv preprint arXiv:1711.08184 (2017)
24. Zheng, L., Shen, L., Tian, L., Wang, S., Wang, J., Tian, Q.: Scalable person re-identification: a benchmark. In: IEEE International Conference on Computer Vision (2015)
25. Zheng, Z., Zheng, L., Yang, Y.: Unlabeled samples generated by GAN improve the person re-identification baseline in vitro. In: Proceedings of the IEEE International Conference on Computer Vision (2017)
26. Zhong, Z., Zheng, L., Cao, D., Li, S.: Re-ranking person re-identification with k-reciprocal encoding (2017)
27. Zhu, X., Jing, X., You, X., Zhang, X., Zhang, T.: Video-based person re-identification by simultaneously learning intra-video and inter-video distance metrics. IEEE Trans. Image Process. **27**(11), 5683–5695 (2018)

Product Recommendation Through Real-Time Object Recognition on Image Classifiers

Nelson Forte de Souza Junior[1(✉)], Leandro Augusto da Silva[2(✉)], and Mauricio Marengoni[2(✉)]

[1] Luizalabs, Magazine Luiza, Sao Paulo, Brazil
nelson@luizalabs.com
[2] Faculdade de Computacao e Informatica, Universidade Presbiteriana Mackenzie, Sao Paulo, Brazil
{mauricio.marengoni,leandroaugusto.silva}@mackenzie.br

Abstract. With the development of e-commerce in the past years and its growing overlap over the classic way of doing business, many computational and statistical methods were researched and developed to make recommendations for products belonging to the store catalog. Often the data used in recommendation methods involves user interactions, being images and video types of information somewhat unexplored. This work, which we call Xanathar, proposes to extend such paradigm with real-time in-video recommendations for 25 classes of products, using image classifiers and feeding video streams to a modified *ResNet-50* network processed on GPU, achieving a top-5 error of 5.17% and running at approximately 60 frames per second. Therefore, describing objects in the scene and proposing related products in-screen, directing user buying experience and creating an immersive and intensive purchase environment.

Keywords: Deep learning · Convolutional neural networks · Computer vision · Video product recommendation · E-commerce

1 Introduction

The commercial relationship between companies and customers has changed significantly in the past twenty years, mainly due to the development of online commerce platforms or internet-only firms. Before this paradigm shift, word of mouth product recommendations was the fundamental manner to advertise goods and services. Since most of the time online commerce hits a global coverage of customers, the amount of data that can be collected from customer interactions is vast and can describe user buying preferences [13]. Recommendation algorithms uses this data in many ways to show product recommendations

Supported by Magazine Luiza.

F. Karray et al. (Eds.): ICIAR 2019, LNCS 11663, pp. 40–51, 2019.
https://doi.org/10.1007/978-3-030-27272-2_4

to customers [20], but images are a type of data seldom used and video are even more rare. Considering the human-like image classification capabilities of current network architectures [6], hardware advances and the ubiquity of mobile devices with video capture, we can expand the type of data used for product recommendations to a new multimedia domain, therefore the usage of prerecorded or real-time video streams depicts a brand-new and unexplored form of product advertising. The current work, which we call **Xanathar**, accomplishes the aforementioned video based product recommendations with orders of magnitude faster than [1] and more accurate than [15].

1.1 Proposal

Devices that take pictures are ubiquitously with almost every buyer and mobile cameras present on devices like smartphones can be used to digitize a natural scene containing consumer goods. Also the TV or videos posted to online video services are a source of data for this type of recommendation. Analyzing the real-time scene captured and finding objects related to the product catalog of an arbitrary retailer is a new way of recommending products. Therefore, the purpose of Xanathar is to perform image classification on video streams, based on a convolutional neural network (CNN) called *ResNet-50* [7] with small changes on its architecture like *Leaky ReLU* [9] as the activation function and *Adam* [10] as the optimizer. Network weights was achieved by training with annotated images from selected classes available on ImageNet image database [4]. Architecture choice on this type of real-time application is guided by two metrics: resulting frames per second and accuracy. Using the mentioned architecture is possible to make real-time overlaid on video recommendations to customers only using user self generated prerecorded or real-time videos. Since the current work is focused on image classifiers for subsequent product recommendation, the localization of recognized objects is not important, thus recognizing its presence on a frame should be sufficient. Regarding this, real-time object recognition and localization architectures as proposed by [15] are not required.

1.2 Related Work

Image classification and object recognition on images or video were addressed in several works. On image classification, [11] presented a CNN achieving top-5 error rate of 18.9%. The top-n error rate is the default for measuring accuracy of these network predictions, describing the prediction likelihood of the top-n results. Improvements on accuracy with deepening of the network were introduced in [19]. With other specialized layers, [19] could achieve a top-5 error rate of 7.5% on ImageNet database. The CNN went deeper in [21], decreasing even further the error rate and accomplishing a top-5 error of 3.1%, although with increased classification time. The state-of-the-art image classifiers are [1,2], obtaining respectively a top-5 error rate of 3% and 3.7%. These network architectures has impressive low error rates, but can be really slow on classification time, which is not suitable for real-time applications like classifying online video streams or image classification in milliseconds. Real-time classifiers like [16] has higher error rates, but faster classification time. As a region proposal network, which describes object's position on scene, [16] was trained with PASCAL VOC database [5] using mAP metric. The mAP, or *mean average precision*, describes how precise the predicted bounding boxes of detected objects are overlapped with actual own predetermined one. [16] attained a mAP of 70.4% with recognition time of 0.2 s. Another real-time recognizer is known as YOLO [15], with a mAP of 66.4% and recognition time of 0.04 s. For the mentioned static image classification networks, the main differences between [11,19,21] resides on the number and type of layers used. [11] has 5 convolutional layers followed by max-pooling ending with dense layers, [19] is deep as 26 convolutional blocks and [21] has more than 95 convolutional layers. Visual search and recommendation presented on [18] depicts searching by image on retail product catalog with accuracy of 84.04%, but it's not suitable for video recognition as it was build to be an image search engine. Although none of the mentioned related works are focused on product recommendation based on video, they are some of the state-of-the-art approaches for general object recognition and recommendation based on images.

2 Methodology

2.1 Image Database

To train the convolutional network and obtain the weights that will be used in the classification, a subset of the image database ImageNet [4] was used, containing *synsets* related to product categories commonly sold on e-commerce, for instance consumer goods like *toaster* or *iron*. A *synset* is synonym that groups words into sets of related meaning [14]. A complete list of the *synsets* used on network's training phase can be analyzed on Table 1.

Table 1. The twenty five selected synsets used to train the network related to consumer goods.

ImageNet selected subset of synsets				
fridge	stove	blender	fryer	mixer
microwave	toaster	purifier	coffeepot	cooktop
refrigerator	vase	espresso maker	rack	couch
chair	dinning table	cabinet	armchair	wardrobe
iron	washer	dishwasher	tv	crock pot

All input images from ImageNet were converted to have the same dimensions (224 × 224). The training and test base images was first stored in an HDF5 [22] file as rank-3 tensors and shape 224 × 224 × 3, i.e., the RGB channels have been preserved. At least one dimension of the original image have 224 pixels, hence the majority of images in the database has suffered with minimal distortions, due to enlarging or reduction of these dimensions. Total samples on this database is 25048. The hierarchy built for image retrieval in the HDF5 file can be seen in Fig. 1.

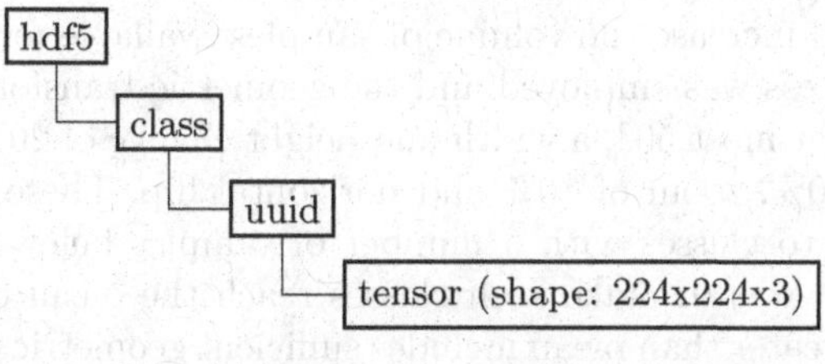

Fig. 1. The tree's organization with the tensors representing images. Each synset receives an integer numeric identifier describing the class which the object is part of, followed by an *universal unique identifier* [12], which determines the uniqueness of image. Finally, we have the image tensor itself, with dimensions $224 \times 224 \times 3$.

To retrieve these images, the image's URLs contained in each synsets received a request and its tensors saved on the mentioned HDF5 file. Each class gained a constant unique integer identifier for posterior training and class identification, for instance *microwave* → 1, *refrigerator* → 2 and so on. Samples of images in the database can be seen on Fig. 2. From the samples, 80% were separated for CNN training (10% of this for validation), leaving 20% for testing.

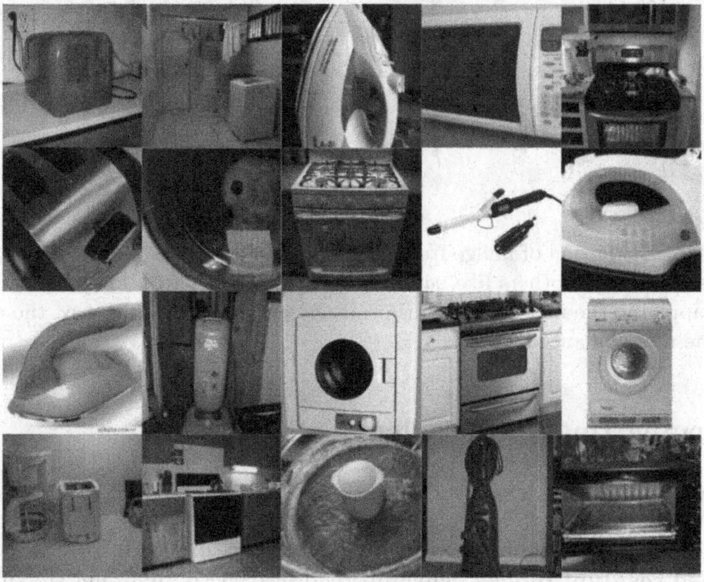

Fig. 2. Twenty random image samples that are stored in the image base, from the total of 25048. In this visualization, it is possible to perceive the different geometric transformations that the images in classes may have.

2.2 Data Augmentation

Image retrieval and their grouping into classes caused an uneven distribution of sample quantities in each group (see Fig. 3). The unbalanced distribution may lead to under-fitting of the model for classes near the minima of this distribution. To standardize and increase the volume of samples available for training, a *data augmentation* process was employed and the geometric transformations applied were a rotation of at most 50°, a width and height change of 20%, shear left and right of at most 30%, zoom of 10% and horizontal flip. These transformations were only applied to classes with a number of samples below the distribution mean and the goal was to make such classes reach the mean quantity. Classes with sample size greater than mean includes sufficient geometric transformations.

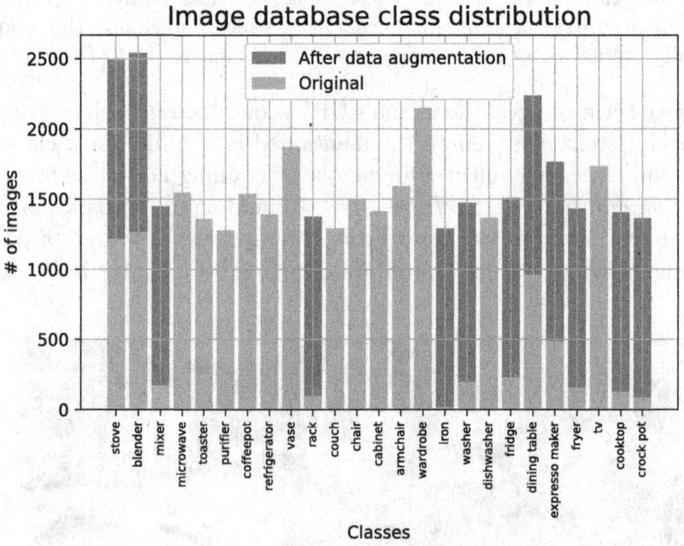

Fig. 3. Class distribution of image frequencies. Since some classes like *mixer* and *fryer* has fewer samples than others like *vase* and *purifier*, classes with low frequencies were expanded applying the mentioned transformations in Sect. 2.2. This way, the distribution became more balanced.

3 Learning Image Classifiers

3.1 Training

To avoid accuracy degradation in training, it is possible to introduce blocks of layers called **residual blocks**, which instead of directly mapping the output of one layer to the next, maps it to a *residual*. If the calculated residuals do not address an error E less than the current one, the identity-function is applied to the block, transferring it to the next one, and this process is repeated in the following layers. Consider $\mathcal{H}(\mathbf{x})$ as the mapping between layers, also the existence of a new mapping $\mathcal{F}(\mathbf{x})$ such that $\mathcal{F}(\mathbf{x}) \mapsto \mathcal{H}(\mathbf{x}) - \mathbf{x}$, which $\mathcal{F}(\mathbf{x})$ is a residual mapping to fit instead of a direct one. Thus, $\mathcal{F}(\mathbf{x})$ becomes $\mathcal{F}(\mathbf{x}) + \mathbf{x}$ in the case of an optimal mapping [7]. This explains that each calculated residual works as an *error minimizing* gate between layers, hence only layers that directs the overall error to a minimum are employed in a batch and is easier to drive a residual to zero than stack nonlinear layers [7]. An instance of a sample residual block can be visualized in Fig. 4.

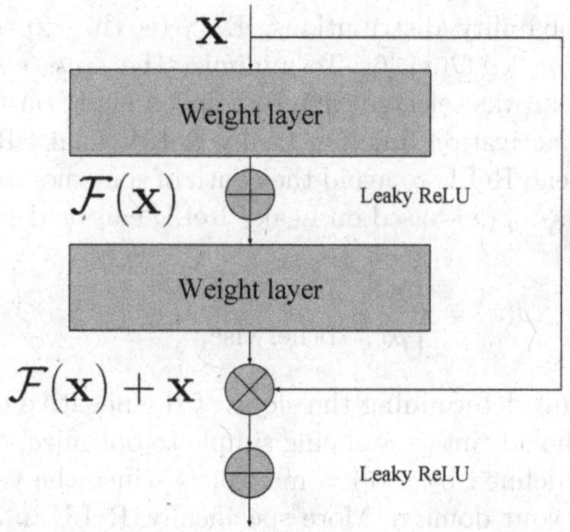

Fig. 4. Example of a residual block. The input tensor $\mathbf{x}$ being mapped to $\mathcal{F}(\mathbf{x})$ and depending on the residual, its identity function $\mathbf{I}$ is calculated and a decision point is computed. If the residual decreases, the direct next one layer are calculated. Otherwise, it works like a gate and some layers forward starts its weight update, instead of the next one.

The convolutional network architecture used for training is similar to that proposed by [7] and known as *ResNet-50*. It is constituted of 50 residual blocks, using as activation function the *Leaky ReLU* instead of *ReLU* from the original architecture. At the end, a dense network (*multi-layer perceptron*) was used, followed by a *softmax* activation function. The stochastic algorithm *Adam* [10] was employed for cost function optimization, with hyper-parameters defined by $\epsilon = 10^{-3}$, $\rho_1 = 0,9$, $\rho_2 = 0,999$ e $\delta = 10^{-8}$. For weight initialization, the *variance scaling* technique was employed, with samples drawn from an uniform distribution calculated by Eq. 1

$$\phi = \sqrt{3\frac{1}{n}} \tag{1}$$

and based on the number of inputs n in the weight tensor. To normalize data between residual blocks, a *batch normalization* [8] process was applied. The convolution operation used in this architecture was the *cross correlation* [6] which measures the similarity between two arbitrary functions $f(x)$ e $g(x)$ during a time window t [23]. Since time domain is not present in images, cross correlation between tensors **K** and **I** are defined by Eq. 2

$$(\mathbf{I} * \mathbf{K})(i, j) = \sum_m \sum_n \mathbf{I}(i + m, j + n)\mathbf{K}(m, n) \tag{2}$$

The cost function chosen was the *cross entropy*, which is described by Eq. 3

$$H(P, Q) = -\mathbb{E}_{x \sim P} \log Q(x), \tag{3}$$

where P and Q are probability distributions, $\mathbb{E}_{x \sim P}$ is the expectation with respect to $P(x)$ of function $\log Q(x)$ [6]. To minimize the *cross entropy*, *Adam* [10] optimization algorithm was selected, due to a speed boost on training time over other methods. The activation function Leaky ReLU (Leaky Rectified Linear Unit) was chosen instead ReLU to avoid the death of some neurons and given the nature of the task [9]. A $\varphi(x)$ based on Leaky ReLU can be defined by Eq. 4

$$\varphi(x) = \begin{cases} x, & \text{if } x > 0 \\ \rho x, & \text{otherwise,} \end{cases} \tag{4}$$

where ρ is a small constant determining the slope of the negative domain. This activation function has the advantage of being simple to optimize, as well as the original *ReLU* function, defined by $\varphi(x) = \max\{0, x\}$, since the two are differential in at least part of your domain. More specifically, ReLU in at least half, Leaky ReLU in all non-zero domain. Pooling layers were used in the beginning and ending of the architecture, respectively a *max-pooling* and *global average*

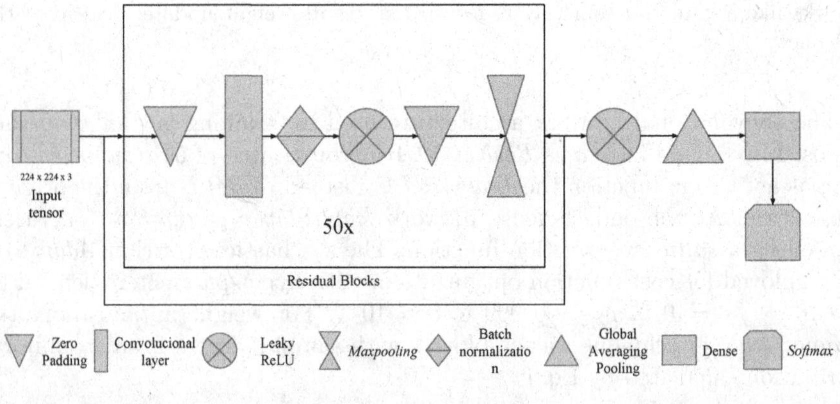

Fig. 5. The architecture of convolutional network used in training, which is known by *ResNet-50* [7]. It is composed by 50 residual blocks containing convolutional layers, applying convolution operations with changing shapes throughout the network followed by batch normalization. After that, a dense network performs the task of learning the classifications associated with the resulting tensors, ending on a *softmax* layer, giving a special case of multinomial distribution over the classes.

pooling. A dense layer at the end learns features associated to each class and a *softmax* layer depicts the distribution of input images to classes. The network has a total of 177 layers. The network's architecture is presented schematically on Fig. 5.

In the architecture used, the training ended after 122 h and 121 epochs, using a batch size of 16 and a NVIDIA® GTX 1060 GPU for acceleration. The portion of image database separated for validation was used at this training phase at the end of each epoch, to validate the network's cost function decay on the current epoch.

3.2 Classification

As a real-time video recommendation system, the actual network demands a sub-second classification time, preferable below 0.04 s per frame, since video streams below 24 *frames per second* (fps) or above 120 fps are respectively not recognized as a fluid video or even perceived by human eyes [17]. Thus, in Xanathar, prerecorded video streams lower than 60 fps are speed up and higher are slowed down, therefore no speed correction are applied. For video streams originating from video cameras, the classification time is bounded by the device fps capturing or hardware capabilities. For the mentioned video sources (prerecorded or video cameras), audio are discarded from the stream. Overall classification speed varies depending on the hardware accelerator used. The video resolution has no influence on the classification time due to down-scaling: every frame are resized to the same dimensions of input images on training phase, which is 224 × 224 pixels (RGB channels preserved). Tests with the full frame resolution was performed and the overall error rate remained unchanged, only increasing drastically

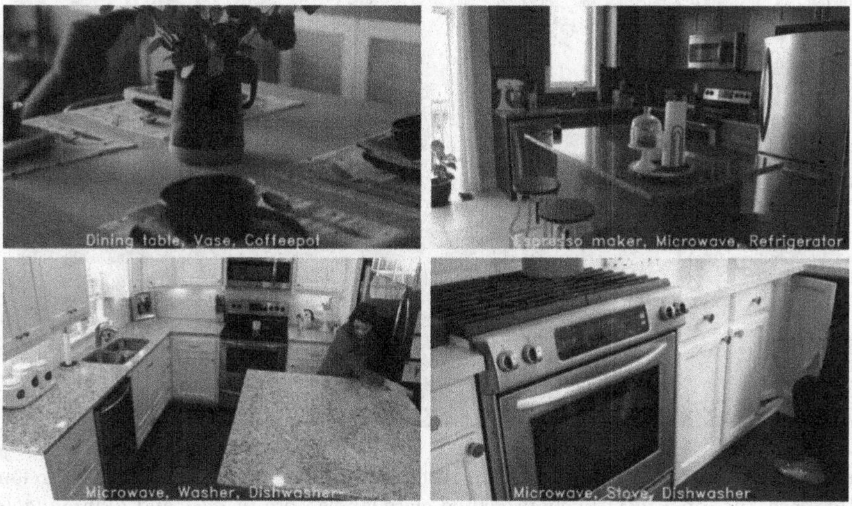

Fig. 6. Four samples of different video sources with top-3 recognized classes indicated. The most likely class labels of each frame is depicted below the frame. All video sources represented here were loaded from prerecorded video files.

the classification time. Five resolutions were tried to verify the network performance: 360p, 480p, 720p, 1080p and 4 K with respectively classification times (in seconds) of 0.030 s, 0.095 s, 0.324 s, 0.545 s and 1.174 s. Video-frame samples of recognized objects are presented on Fig. 6.

4 Results

Confronting the trained model against the test data set, it was possible to calculate a top-1 error of 21.41 and a top-5 error of 5.17. Xanathar achieves a frame classification in 0.016 s, classifying approximately at 60 fps. The comparison with other systems can be seen on Table 2. A final result of the system can be analyzed in Fig. 7.

4.1 Recommendation

Once the object has been recognized, we have its most likely class, which was based on the metadata entries described in Table 1. These entries enable the search for text similarity, using recognized class text labels to perform a search on the product catalog, looking for products with similar titles to the recognized

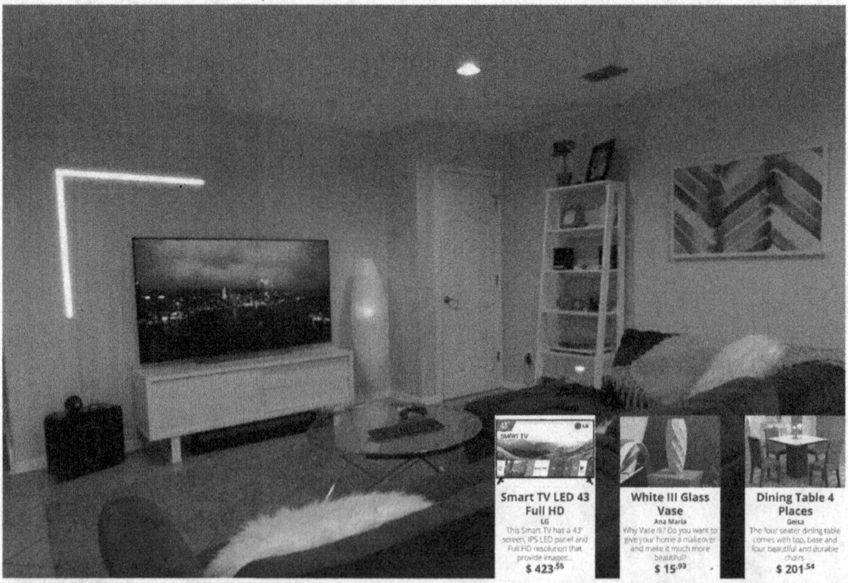
Smart TV LED 43 Full HD
LG
This Smart TV has a 43" screen, IPS LED panel and Full HD resolution that provide images...
$ 423.55
White III Glass Vase
Ana Maria
Why Vase III? Do you want to give your home a makeover and make it much more beautiful?
$ 15.93
Dining Table 4 Places
Geisa
The four seater dining table comes with top, base and four beautiful and durable chairs
$ 201.54

Fig. 7. Frame example of three product recommendations overlaid in a video stream. In this case, the top-3 most likely predicted class labels were *tv*, *vase* and *dinning table*. In possession of these class labels, the system can start the search for product titles which contains similar text to labels. Prices and descriptions of products are stored on an external catalog. Recommendations are preserved in the video stream for about five seconds if there is a change of objects in the scene. If class labels remains the same, no change in recommendations presented happens.

Table 2. Comparison of top-1 and top-5 error rate (classification networks) alongside with mAP (localization and/or real-time networks) against the *ResNet-50* based architecture used in Xanathar. Using *ResNet-50* to the classification task, was possible to achieve higher accuracy with lower classification time. The main reason to describe the two different metrics like top-n and mAP is due to the resulting nature of each network. [15,16] returns bounding boxes locating the object and [1,2,7,19] results likely classes which the image or frame may belongs.

Network	precision-1 (%)	precision-2 (%)	time (sec.)
YOLO [15]		mAP: 66.4	0.04
Faster R-CNN [16]		mAP: 70.4	0.2
VGG-19 [19]	top-1: 24.4	top-5: 7.5	4
MultiGrain [1]	top-1: 15.7	top-5: 3	4.1
Oct-ResNet-152+SE [2]	top-1: 17.1	top-5: 3.7	3.9
Xanathar	**top-1: 21.41**	**top-5: 5.17**	**0.016**

classes. More specifically, the title based recommendation uses text similarity algorithms like Jaro–Winkler and Damerau—Levenshtein distance [3] to compare recognized class labels over indexed product titles. The class labels are generated by the network on every frame, but the search for products with similar title from the class identified only happens every five seconds, selecting the most stable classes, or the ones that changes less. The option to change recommendation overlay at most every five seconds was made to maintain user's visibility of recommended products information. In this case, a customer that wants to keep some recommendation on the screen naturally will sustain the desired product at the center of video stream.

5 Conclusions

Classifying objects on video streams in real-time is a task that is bounded by processing time, since a common video stream has 30 or more frames per second, with varying resolutions, reaching not rarely 4096 × 2160 pixels per frame. Therefore, objects in a frame must be recognized in no more than 0.04 s to maintain the flow and be perceived by human eyes with fluidity. To achieve low classification error rate and accomplish the high frame rate needs, the ResNet-50 [7] network was chosen (with minor modifications) due its low top-5 error rate and classification speed. Several other network architectures were compared and the total time to perform classification on some of these architectures demonstrated as been a problem, since it took much more than the 0.04 s to classify a frame, damaging the video fluidity. Not all network architectures are suitable to run in real-time applications and hardware choices for processing each frame and classify objects are also important, as the speed of 0.016 s per frame of Xanathar was achieved with GPUs. Accuracy is also important, as the classification precision defines the quality of the recommendation and how the customer will react to it.

Hence, customers will only interact positively with these recommendations if the recommended products are correct, which is granted by the achieved low top-5 error rate of 5.17% of Xanathar. With the in-screen recommendations overlaid to the video, customers can quickly search for similar wanted products or receive product advertisements for what is been watched on TV or online video channels.

References

1. Berman, M., Jégou, H., Vedaldi, A., Kokkinos, I., Douze, M.: Multigrain: a unified image embedding for classes and instances. arXiv preprint. arXiv:1902.05509 (2019)
2. Chen, Y., et al.: Drop an octave: reducing spatial redundancy in convolutional neural networks with octave convolution. arXiv preprint. arXiv:1904.05049 (2019)
3. Cohen, W., Ravikumar, P., Fienberg, S.: A comparison of string metrics for matching names and records. In: KDD Workshop on Data Cleaning and Object Consolidation, vol. 3, pp. 73–78 (2003)
4. Deng, J., Dong, W., Socher, R., Li, L.J., Li, K., Fei-Fei, L.: ImageNet: a large-scale hierarchical image database. In: 2009 IEEE Conference on Computer Vision and Pattern Recognition, CVPR 2009, pp. 248–255. IEEE (2009)
5. Everingham, M., Van Gool, L., Williams, C.K., Winn, J., Zisserman, A.: The PASCAL visual object classes (VOC) challenge. Int. J. Comput. Vision **88**(2), 303–338 (2010)
6. Goodfellow, I., Bengio, Y., Courville, A., Bengio, Y.: Deep Learning, vol. 1. MIT Press, Cambridge (2016)
7. He, K., Zhang, X., Ren, S., Sun, J.: Deep residual learning for image recognition. In: Proceedings of the IEEE Conference on Computer Vision and Pattern Recognition, pp. 770–778 (2016)
8. Ioffe, S., Szegedy, C.: Batch normalization: accelerating deep network training by reducing internal covariate shift. arXiv preprint. arXiv:1502.03167 (2015)
9. Jarrett, K., Kavukcuoglu, K., LeCun, Y., et al.: What is the best multi-stage architecture for object recognition? In: 2009 IEEE 12th International Conference on Computer Vision, pp. 2146–2153. IEEE (2009)
10. Kingma, D.P., Ba, J.: Adam: a method for stochastic optimization. arXiv preprint. arXiv:1412.6980 (2014)
11. Krizhevsky, A., Sutskever, I., Hinton, G.E.: Imagenet classification with deep convolutional neural networks. In: Advances in Neural Information Processing Systems, pp. 1097–1105 (2012)
12. Leach, P., Mealling, M., Salz, R.: A universally unique identifier (UUID) URN namespace. Technical rep. (2005)
13. Linden, G., Smith, B., York, J.: Amazon. com recommendations: item-to-item collaborative filtering. IEEE Internet Comput. **7**(1), 76–80 (2003)
14. Miller, G.A.: WordNet: a lexical database for English. Commun. ACM **38**(11), 39–41 (1995)
15. Redmon, J., Divvala, S., Girshick, R., Farhadi, A.: You only look once: unified, real-time object detection. In: Proceedings of the IEEE Conference on Computer Vision and Pattern Recognition, pp. 779–788 (2016)
16. Ren, S., He, K., Girshick, R., Sun, J.: Faster R-CNN: towards real-time object detection with region proposal networks. In: Advances in Neural Information Processing Systems, pp. 91–99 (2015)

17. Scharnowski, F., Hermens, F., Herzog, M.H.: Bloch's law and the dynamics of feature fusion. Vision Res. **47**(18), 2444–2452 (2007)
18. Shankar, D., Narumanchi, S., Ananya, H., Kompalli, P., Chaudhury, K.: Deep learning based large scale visual recommendation and search for e-commerce. arXiv preprint. arXiv:1703.02344 (2017)
19. Simonyan, K., Zisserman, A.: Very deep convolutional networks for large-scale image recognition. arXiv preprint. arXiv:1409.1556 (2014)
20. Sivapalan, S., Sadeghian, A., Rahnama, H., Madni, A.M.: Recommender systems in e-commerce. In: World Automation Congress (WAC), pp. 179–184. IEEE (2014)
21. Szegedy, C., Ioffe, S., Vanhoucke, V., Alemi, A.A.: Inception-v4, inception-ResNet and the impact of residual connections on learning. In: AAAI, vol. 4, p. 12 (2017)
22. The HDF Group: Hierarchical Format, version 5 (1997–2018). http://www.hdfgroup.org/HDF5/
23. Welch, L.: Lower bounds on the maximum cross correlation of signals (corresp.). IEEE Trans. Inf. Theory **20**(3), 397–399 (1974)

Visual Inspection with Federated Learning

Xu Han, Haoran Yu, and Haisong Gu(✉)

VisionX Foundation, San Jose, USA
harrygu@visionx.org

Abstract. In industrial applications of AI, challenges for visual inspection include data shortage and security. In this paper, we propose a Federated Learning (FL) framework to address these issues. This method is incorporated with our novel Dataonomy^{SM} approach which can overcome the limited size of industrial dataset in each inspection task. The models pre-trained in the server can continuously and regularly update, and help each client upgrade its inspection model over time. The FL approach only requires clients to send to the server certain information derived from raw images, and thus does not sacrifice data security. Some preliminary tests are done to examine the workability of the proposed framework. This study is expected to bring the field of automated inspection to a new level of security, reliability, and efficiency, and to unlock significant potentials of deep learning applications.

Keywords: Visual Inspection · Federated Learning · Dataonomy^{SM}

1 Introduction

Visual inspection of products is a common task across the industry. In China alone, there are more than 60 million workers for it. In order to improve the quality of product and reduce the cost, machine vision has been used for a long time. Traditional automated vision technologies [1] such as pattern matching have made great progresses on measurement and presence detection. However, they typically require extensive development and expertise to build a specialized algorithm for each type of surface or structure. Recently, Deep Learning (DL) based approach has become an attractive alternative [2–4], which has proven to be successful in inspection applications. It is convenient to implement and generic enough to have similar models applied to different industries, and thus shows promising potentials in the automated inspection field.

One of the biggest challenges for applying DL-based approach to the industry is the lack of data samples for classification tasks of defect detection. In practice, a common approach [2] is to use the weights of lower layers of a convolutional neural network (CNN) that is pre-trained on large datasets with an existing architecture, for example, VGG [5], Inception [6], or others, and retrain the on top layers of the classifier on the datasets of a specific task. However, a public model trained on a variety of image classes may not be sensitive enough for transfer learning for defect inspection on material surfaces. Recent advances in transfer learning [7, 8] show that it is possible to

F. Karray et al. (Eds.): ICIAR 2019, LNCS 11663, pp. 52–64, 2019.
https://doi.org/10.1007/978-3-030-27272-2_5

quantify how a DL model can help another task. Previously, we proposed a novel approach named Dataonomy^{SM} [6], which can be used to train the classifier for a specific task with relatively small data samples. In this study, we extend the Dataonomy^{SM} approach into building cross-industry base models for transfer learning, instead of focusing on defection of single type of product or industry. The advantage of this is that it can allow clients from a new industry to quickly deploy a base model and perform acceptable automated inspection while the service provider (server) can work on improving the model as new datasets are continuously generated from the clients.

Another significant issue regarding all traditional approaches in automated surface inspection is that they all involve the modeler directly analyzing the raw image dataset or a similar version of that dataset that exposes the private information that manufacturers wish to protect. In those cases, if the modeler is from an external party, then the data security will be at risk, which hinders the development of this industry. Fortunately, Federated Analysis/Federated Learning [9, 10] (FL) has been researched recently, encompassing applications like autonomous driving, analytics of mobile phone data, etc. It is basically a computational framework that is based on a network with data distributed on edge devices. In FL, the model training (or data analytics if it is FA) is done on the original devices (edges) that store the data, e.g. IoT devices, mobile phones, instead of in the server, thus allowing the data to stay in the user devices with only the model information to be sent to the server. In this study, we propose a novel FL framework for the model training for automated inspections to ensure data security of clients.

In order to practically apply the Federated Learning with deep learning models, which typically require significant amount of data to train, one problem, which is the data (with labels) scarcity of each individual client, may pose a challenge to model training. This can be addressed by the Dataonomy^{SM} approach earlier introduced. In fact, Dataonomy^{SM} and its following transfer learning procedure are perfectly compatible with the FL framework, and are incorporated in our framework.

The following consists of Sect. 2: Dataonomy^{SM} for cross-industry applications Sect. 3: our Federated Learning framework, Sect. 4: Experiments, and finally Sect. 5: Conclusion.

2 Dataonomy^{SM} for Cross-Industry Applications

2.1 Dataonomy^{SM} Approach Workflow

Dataonomy^{SM} as an important method used in our FL framework, which can help address the difficulty posed by the scarcity of data on the local client side performing deep learning training. In our previously proposed workflow of defect inspection in [7], as shown in Fig. 1a and b, the Dataonomy^{SM} approach is used to prepare big datasets for the base model of specific industry, which is later used for transfer learning to obtain final model for defect inspection.

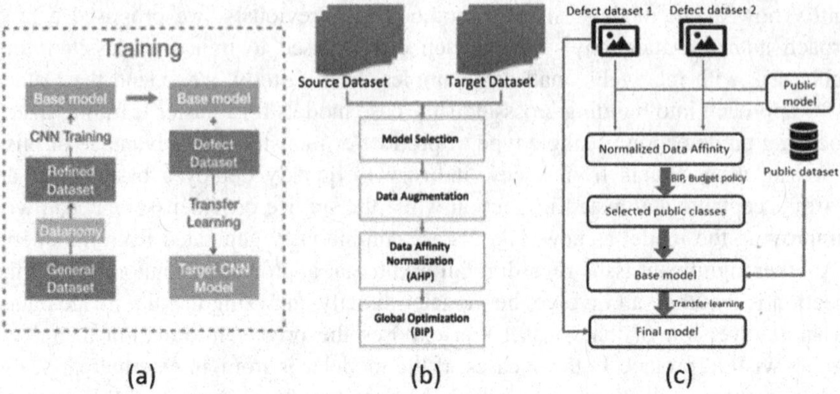

Fig. 1. Framework of the Dataonomy^{SM} approach. (a) Basic training workflow using Dataonomy^{SM}; (b) Detailed steps in Dataonomy^{SM} (c) Cross-industry training using Dataonomy^{SM}

Briefly, the Dataonomy^{SM} approach itself involves using a pretrained public available CNN model, e.g. Inception V3, to test the defect dataset, and obtain the mean probability of the defect dataset to be classified as each class in the public dataset, e.g. ImageNet. Then the probabilities will be used in the data augmentation process to quantify how well the differences between defect classes in the defect dataset can be related to each class in the public dataset. With a normalized affinity matrix [11], the final step is to obtain a global mapping scheme to maximize the performance across all defect classes, while minimizing the supervision. We achieve the selection problem using Binary Integer Programming (BIP) [12].

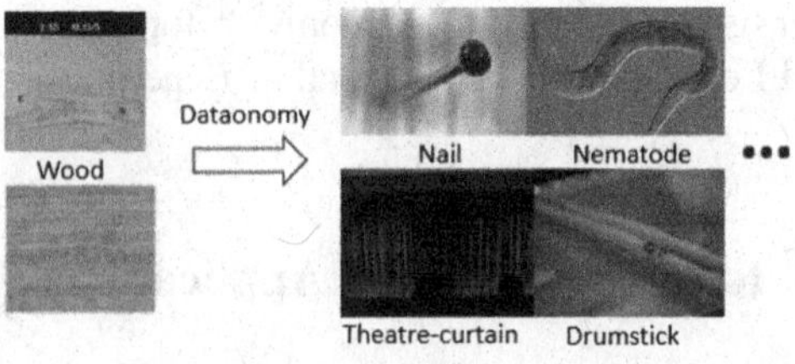

Fig. 2. Dataonomy^{SM} ranking of public classes for wood dataset [13].

To give some examples, Fig. 2 shows how public dataset classes in ImageNet are ranked for a wood [13] surface defect dataset using Dataonomy^{SM}.

This works perfectly for obtaining a base model for a single type of surface material of a specific industry. For cross-industry applications, we need to create a base model that is shared by defect datasets from different industries. The workflow of Dataonomy^{SM} is thus extended into what is shown in Fig. 1c.

Basically, a cross-industry base model which will later be used for transfer learning in clients' local computers, will be trained by a blend of public dataset classes that are highly related to each industry's surface defect data. In other words, for each industry, there will be a group of dataset classes, which are highly relevant (with high affinity) to it, included in the total of selected classes for the base model training. Certain selected classes may have high relevance to multiple industries. As shown in Fig. 1c, the defect dataset of each industry first undergoes data augmentation and AHP separately. Then the normalized data affinity from all industries are appended together as the affinity matrix P. Given this information, the BIP method under a budget policy for cross-industry application is applied to obtain the selected classes for base model training.

2.2 Budget Policy for Cross-Industry Base Model

Normally the numbers of sample from different industries are unbalanced. The budget policy is aimed at balancing the number of selected classes for each industry, while having the selected classes for different industries balanced in a way that the differences in the training difficulty, available defect data size, and importance among different industries are considered. The BIP method is applied to select the best set of classes among the 1000 classes in ImageNet to train the base model. A vector x is defined, in which each binary element x_i represents class i to be either included in the base model training ($x_i = 1$) or excluded ($x_i = 0$). The BIP problem becomes

$$\text{maximize} \quad \boldsymbol{c}^T\boldsymbol{x}$$

$$\text{subject to} \quad \boldsymbol{Ax} \leq \boldsymbol{b}$$

$$\boldsymbol{x} = \{0,1\}^N$$

where N is the total number of classes in the public dataset and equals 1000 for ImageNet. $\boldsymbol{c}$ is a vector, in which each element c_i is defined as a coefficient that quantifies the overall benefit of selecting class i, which is dependent on the affinities of class i to the target tasks ($p_{i,t}$), the importance of each target task in the final application (r_t), and a balance factor of accessible data size among different defect datasets (q_t). as given below:

$$c_i = \sum_{t=1}^{T} -r_t q_t p_{i,t} \tag{1}$$

where t represents a specific target defect detection task, T is the total number of target tasks, and

$$q_t = \frac{n_t^{-1}}{\sum_1^T n_k^{-1}} \tag{2}$$

is used to counter the imbalance of different defect datasets, so that the one with smaller data, which is assumingly more difficult to train in the transfer learning, will be more favored (or compensated) in determining the selection of related classes from the public dataset by having a higher weight for its closely related class.

The problem is constrained by the budget policy, in which the total amount of training budget of the base model cannot exceed a number M, e.g. 50, 100. Hence, the matrix A and b will satisfy:

$$a_{1,j} = l_j = 1 \tag{3}$$

$$b_1 = M \tag{4}$$

Where l_j is the cost of adding class j, which is assumed to be uniformly 1 in this study. Only one row for A and b is needed at this point. However, depending on the actual situation, more constraints can be added.

Note that this BIP design will only work under the premise that the base model trained with more classes will yield better predictions monotonically. A small number of 50 classes should be a safe one for that premise in most cases, as the model is a deep network that requires large training data. However, as the number of classes reaches a certain value, the quality may increase or reduce. The range of the number of classes in which class number still has a benefit can only be determined empirically by experiments. In our specific case, 50 classes is not too high a number that would otherwise negatively affect the prediction power of the final defect inspection model.

Finally, the cross-industry base model can be created by retraining the model with the new set of classes selected in the BIP process. This will be used for transfer learning to obtain the final defect model. The details for how this is implemented in business operations will be described in the next section on Federated Learning.

An example of the public data classes selected for the training of the cross-industry model of wood [13] and texture datasets [14] are given in Fig. 3.

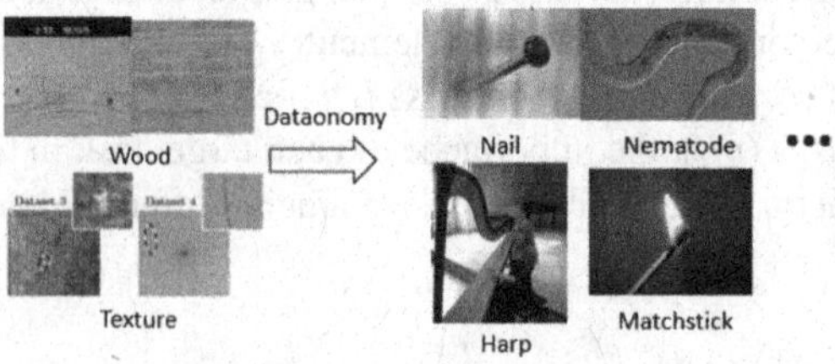

Fig. 3. Illustration of cross-industry Dataonomy^{SM} results for wood [13] and texture datasets [14].

3 Federated Learning Framework

3.1 Basic Framework

In the Federated Learning framework of our study, the server is the organization or individual that designs the model structures and provide service to manufacturers on automated inspection. Each client is one of inspection sites in production lines in a manufacturer that need high quality algorithms for its own specific inspection task. Some manufacturers may have hundreds of similar inspection sites, each of which is a client that undergoes separate communication with the server to obtain and update its inspection model. Note that each production line may have some different inspection task with another, so each line will need a different model.

The typical procedure for handling multiple clients in a manufacturing company is described here, as shown in Fig. 4. It includes three stages for a full cycle of service: Deploy, Server Model Update, and Client Model Update. After each cycle, there will be updates to the server and client models, with help of new image data collected from clients. The three stages are described in detail below.

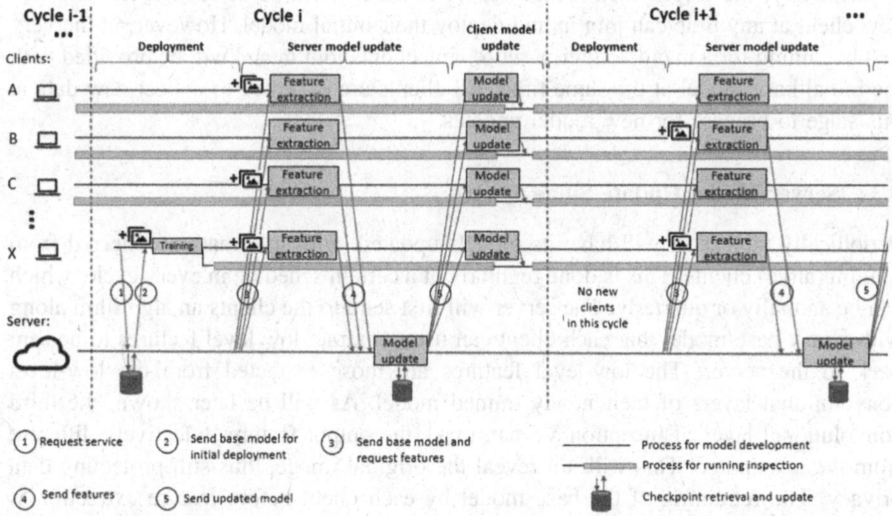

Fig. 4. Illustration of the workflow of Visual Inspection using Federated Learning.

3.2 Deployment Stage

As a client firstly requests service, the client sends a request to the server for a new model for their inspection task, along with some basic information regarding their data. The server will then analyze whether it is possible to finally obtain a model for the inspection or what approach to make. Typically, if the new client is of a new industry to the server, or there is no surface type similar enough in precedented cases done in the server before for the new client, then a generalized cross-industry base model will be given to be deployed directly for the production line as an initial solution. Otherwise, if the new client is a similar production line of an old client that has a customized model readily available (updated from the last cycle), then the new client will be given that model as the base model to train on its available data and directly run its surface inspection tasks with high accuracy.

As illustrated in Fig. 4, the existing inspection sites (A, B, C,…) of the manufacturer at Cycle i have already been running their models. They do not need any further operations in this stage. Client X is a new installation in the production line that firstly joined at some time point during the Deployment stage of Cycle i. Client X needs to send a request to the server. The server approves it based on the client's data type and local computer settings and responds by providing X with the initial base model for it. At any time during this stage of this cycle, which is typically in the order of months, if there is any other new client, it will be given a base model right after the request as well. Once the base model is received, the client will conduct the transfer learning with limited sample data locally and start the process of automated surface inspection.

Basically, the Deployment Stage covers most of the time of each cycle, and any new client at any time can join in and deploy their initial model. However, in the very first beginning for a manufacturer, a set of new clients join in and will be provided with the initial base model at the same time. All clients are expected to collect new data at this stage to prepare for new model updates.

3.3 Server Model Update Stage

Periodically the server will have its models updated, with information collected from running(alive) clients. This is done regularly at a certain schedule in every cycle, which can be annually or quarterly. The server will first send to the clients an algorithm along with a new base model that each client can use to extract low level features to be sent back to the server. The low-level features are those extracted from the low-level convolutional layers of their newly trained model. As will be later shown, the third convolutional layer of Inception V3 can make the output features effectively different from the raw image. This will not reveal the original image, thus still protecting data privacy. The retraining of the base model by each client before feature extraction is optional for the clients. The client can also directly use the base model sent by the server and extract image features from a designated convolutional layer. The retraining may add minor uncertainties to the later model training by the server but will add protection to clients' data. If the client does not have new image data generated at this moment, then it does not need to send back the feature data, as the case for Client B in Cycle i in Fig. 4.

After the server received all the feature data from the clients, the feature data will be fed into a truncated CNN that has the layers used by the clients removed and starts from the next higher-level layer. The server will conduct a set of procedures which can include the Dataonomy^{SM} process or other advanced methods to update the new base model in the server, with more weight on the new image features, rather than the initial cross-industry model. The lower level convolutional layers in the previous version will be added back to the truncated CNN after the latter is updated, in order to reconstruct the full CNN model. Note that even if one client possesses only a small dataset (hundreds of images), it can still be provided with a model update with reasonable quality, since the updated base model can be applied to each client.

3.4 Client Model Update Stage

In this stage, the server will send the updated base models to all the clients and each client will train its new model locally with a small size of raw data at minimal time cost. The clients will then deploy their final models in their inspection systems. After this short stage, the clients and the server will proceed to the Deployment stage of the next cycle.

4 Experiments

4.1 Experimental Setup

Preliminary experiments were done to examine the feasibility of the proposed Dataonomy^{SM} approach and the implementation of the FL framework. We will demonstrate our trained models including two models for single industry, and a cross-industry base model developed with Dataonomy^{SM} approach, used in deriving two specialized models.

For the development of the cross-industry base model, one dataset is the DAGM-2007 dataset [14] which consists of 8050 images for training, in which 1046 images contain defects; and 8050 images for testing, in which 1054 images contain defects. In our experiment, we split the training dataset into two parts, 80% for training and 20% for validation during the training stage. The example image for each class contained in this dataset is shown in Fig. 5a.

Another dataset we used in the experimental study is the Wood Defect Dataset provided by Silvén et al. in [13]. Since the dataset fails to provide the wood images without defect, we collect the positive examples from the Internet. Samples images are shown in Fig. 5b. The wood data as well used the 80%/20% training and test data split.

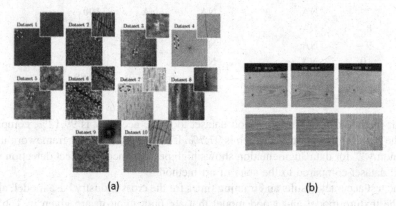

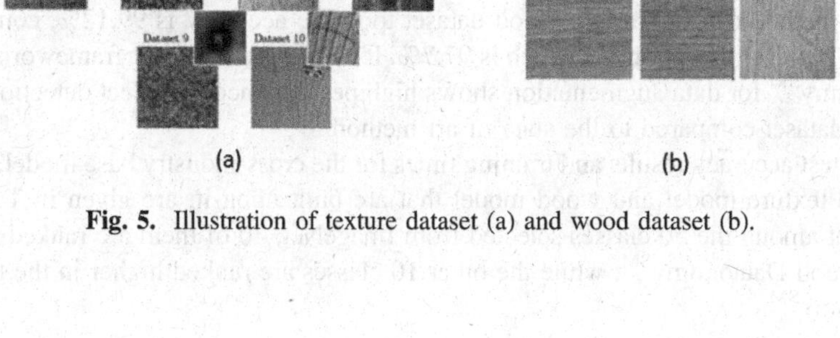

Fig. 5. Illustration of texture dataset (a) and wood dataset (b).

Our experiment for retraining the Inception V3 using ImageNet data subset ran on computer with eight GeForce GTX 1080 Ti graphics card as a server machine. For the transfer learning of the classifier for defect detection was ran on computer with one GeForce GTX 1080 Ti graphics card as a client machine.

A texture model was built on single industry base model, for which Inception V3 is trained through 500 classes in ImageNet selected by Dataonomy^{SM} analysis of texture data. Weights in all layers are freed to retrain in the transfer learning process. A wood model is also built on a similar manner.

For the cross-industry model, the texture and wood data were used together with Dataonomy^{SM} approach described in Sect. 2, and we selected 50 classes for the retraining of the Inception V3 model. Then we applied transfer learning to train a model for each of the wood and texture datasets.

4.2 Results

As shown in Table 1, the texture model that was built on single-industry base models show superior accuracy when compared with previous studies [15, 16].

Table 1. Accuracy results for the texture data defect detection model.

No.	TiBa2011 [15]	Muto et al. [16]		This study
		SVM	DNN	
1	91.5	99.33	100	**100**
2	99.9	100	100	**100**
3	98.7	98.66	49.38	**99.83**
4	96.8	99.63	98.75	**100**
5	NA	NA	NA	**99.83**
6	NA	NA	NA	**99.65**
7	NA	NA	NA	**100**
8	NA	NA	NA	**99.57**
9	NA	NA	NA	**100**
10	NA	NA	NA	**99.91**
Ave.	NA	NA	NA	**99.88**

Our method can be used in wood dataset too. The accuracy is 99.12%, compared with the build-in Inception V3 which is 97.7%. It can be seen that our framework using Dataonomy^{SM} for data augmentation shows high performance on defect detection with limited dataset compared to the state of art method.

The test accuracy results and training times for the cross-industry base model, along with the texture model and wood model that are built upon it, are given in Table 2. Note that among the 50 classes selected from ImageNet, 40 of them are ranked higher in the wood Dataonomy^{SM}, while the other 10 classes are ranked higher in the texture Dataonomy^{SM}.

Table 2. Models involved in the cross-industry approach (all trained on 8 GPU).

Model	Accuracy	Training time
Base model	85.5%	6.6 h
Wood model	100.0%	6 min
Texture model	99.7%	54 min

From Table 2, we see that the base model trained to have correlations with two different industries can be used to obtain high quality models for the defect inspection tasks of each industry. The time cost of each model is also satisfyingly low, which allows our server in the Federated Learning Framework to efficiently update the models and have them ready for the clients. The simulated FL process in one cycle for 4 clients on wood dataset gives the estimate of the time cost and data size involved as shown in Table 3.

Table 3. Federated Learning process time cost and data size involved in one cycle.

Stage	Client computing cost	Client data size	Server training cost	Server data size
Deployment	1 min (few layers)	1.0 MB (42 images) and 92 MB (base model)	NA	NA
Server update	48 min (all layers)	23.3 MB (1573 images) and 92 MB (model)	19 h	5.2 GB (features) and 368 MB (models)
Client update	2 min (few layers)	1.0 MB (42 images) and 92 MB (base model)	NA	NA

Some sample results of the features extracted from the first layer of the Inception V3 neural network are shown in Fig. 6. It can be seen that the first convolutional layer features do not show the same image as the raw one, though certain channels show close resemblance. This should be enough for most cases to protect data privacy in defect inspection applications. However, to make the image more unrecognizable from the raw ones, the client may extract features from a higher level layer to send to the server, as shown in Fig. 7.

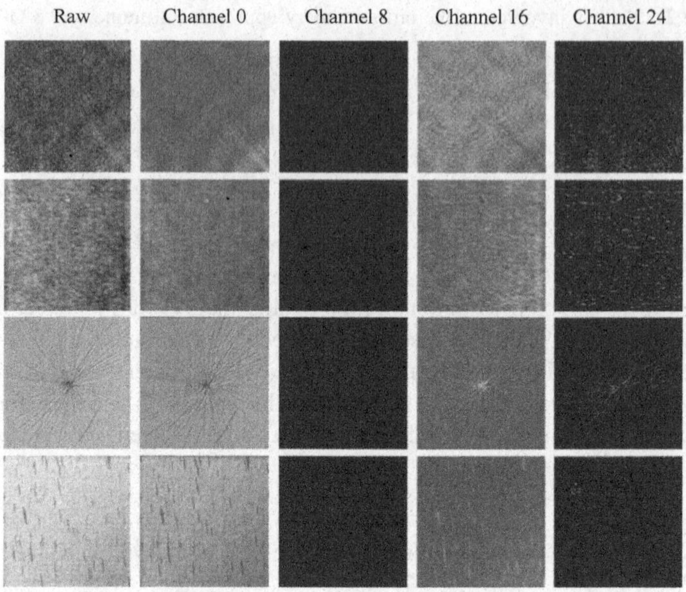

Fig. 6. 4 Raw images of the texture data (shown in the 1st column of the plot) and their extracted features from 4 different feature channels of the first convolutional layer of the pre-trained Inception V3 model. Each row shows the raw data and features of one image.

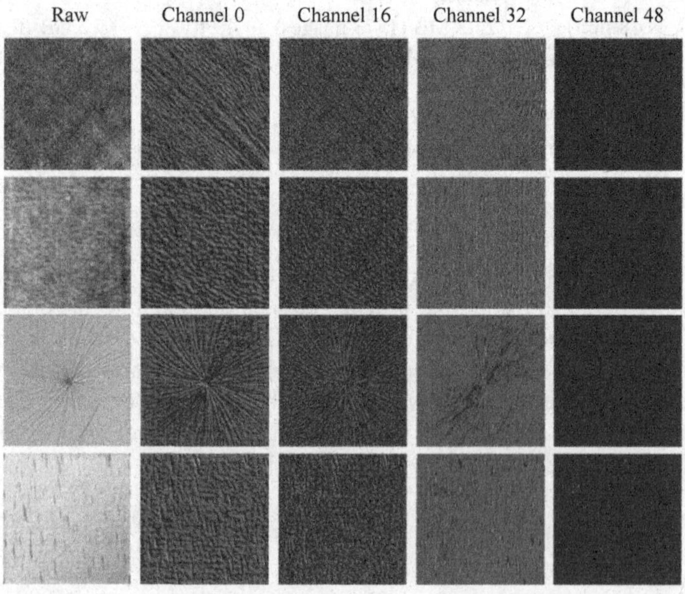

Fig. 7. 4 Raw images of the texture data (shown in the 1st column of the plot) and their extracted features from 4 different feature channels of the third convolutional layer of the pretrained Inception V3 model. Each row shows the raw data and features of one image.

5 Conclusion

We have presented a novel framework of using Federated Learning method and Dataonomy^{SM} to provide manufactures with the service in automated defect inspection without sacrificing data privacy and demanding large datasets. The feasibility of the cross-industry modelling and its efficiency in the FL framework is also demonstrated by experiments. Our framework can protect clients' data privacy by training models without directly accessing their raw data, but instead using extracted features from intermediate layers of the CNN model. The framework allows both fast model deployment for new clients and continuous model updates that does not require large dataset generated by an individual client. We will extend the framework as the distributed AI computing to serve various industries, with sustained/efficient improvement of model quality and quick model deployment in the near future.

References

1. Xie, X.: A review of recent advances in surface defect detection using texture analysis techniques. Electron. Lett. Comput. Vis. Image Anal. **7**(3), 1–25 (2008)
2. Ren, R., Hung, T., Tan, K.C.: A generic deep-learning-based approach for automated surface inspection. IEEE Trans. Cybern. **48**(3), 929–940 (2018)
3. Yu, Z., Wu, X., Gu, X.: Fully convolutional networks for surface defect inspection in industrial environment. In: Liu, M., Chen, H., Vincze, M. (eds.) ICVS 2017. LNCS, vol. 10528, pp. 417–426. Springer, Cham (2017). https://doi.org/10.1007/978-3-319-68345-4_37
4. Weimer, D., Scholz-Reiter, B., Shpitalni, M.: Design of deep convolutional neural network architectures for automated feature extraction in industrial inspection. CIRP Ann. **65**(1), 417–420 (2016)
5. Simonyan, K., Zisserman, A.: Very deep convolutional networks for large-scale image recognition. In: Computer Vision and Pattern Recognition. arXiv:1409.1556 (2014)
6. Szegedy, C., Vanhoucke, V., Loffe, S., Shlens, J., Wojna., Z.: Rethinking the Inception architecture for computer vision. In: Computer Vision and Pattern Recognition. arXiv:1512.00567 (2015)
7. Xu, W., Zhu, Y., Sun, K., Wang, D., Gu, H.: Visual Defect Inspection Across Industry, Proceeding of Vision Engineering workshop (ViEW2018), Tokyo, Japan (2018). ISBN 978-4-9907468-8-92018
8. Zamir, A.R., Sax. A., Shen. W., Guibas L., Malik J., Savarese S.: Tasknonomy: disentangling task transfer learning. In: Computer Vision and Pattern Recognition. arXiv: 1804.08328 (2018)
9. McMahan, H.B., Moore, E., Ramage, D., Hampson, S., Arcas, B.A.: Communication-efficient learning of deep networks from decentralized data. In: Proceedings of the 20th International Conference on Artificial Intelligence and Statistics, pp. 1273–1282 (2017)
10. McMahan, H.B., Ramage, D.: Federated learning: collaborative machine learning without centralized training data, April 2017. https://ai.googleblog.com/2017/04/federated-learning-collaborative.html. Google AI Blog
11. Saaty, R.W.: The analytic hierarchy process–what it is and how it is used. Math. Model. **9**(3–5), 161–176 (1987)
12. https://www.mathworks.com/help/optim/examples/office-assignments-by-binary-integer-programming.html

13. Silvén, O., Niskanen, M., Kauppinen, H.: Wood inspection with non-supervised clustering. Mach. Vis. Appl. **13**(5–6), 275–285 (2003)
14. https://hci.iwr.uni-heidelberg.de/node/3616. Accessed 10 Apr 2017
15. Timm, F., Barth, E.: Non-parametric texture defect detection using Weibull features. In: Proceedings of SPIE 7877, Image Processing: Machine Vision Applications, San Francisco Airport (2011)
16. Muto, K., Matsubara, T., Koshimizu, H.: Proposal of local feature vector focusing on the differences among neighboring ROI's. In: International Workshop on Advanced Image Technology (IWAIT), pp. 1–3. IEEE, Chiang Mai (2018)

Recognition

Looking Under the Hood: Visualizing What LSTMs Learn

Dhruva Patil, Bruce A. Draper(✉), and J. Ross Beveridge(✉)

Colorado State University, Fort Collins, USA
{dkpatil,draper,ross}@cs.colostate.edu

Abstract. Recurrent Neural Networks are a state of the art method for modeling sequential data. Unfortunately, the practice of RNNs is ahead of the theory. We lack any method for summarizing or analyzing what a network has learned, once it's trained. This paper presents two methods for visualizing concepts learned by RNNs in the domain of action recognition. The first method shows the sensitivity of joints over time. The second generates synthetic videos that maximize the responses of a class label or hidden unit given a set of anatomical constraints. These techniques are combined in a visualization tool called *SkeletonVis* to help developers and users gain insights into models embedded in RNNs for action recognition.

Keywords: LSTM · Action recognition · Visualizations · Saliency maps

1 Introduction

Recurrent Neural Networks (RNNs) such as Long Short Term Memory (LSTM) networks [20], have been successful in many applications involving sequential data. Examples can be found in text classification [5], image and video captioning [2,13], speech recognition [7,12], and action and gesture recognition [22,26,27]. The success of these deep learning models lies in the complex feature representations they learn from training data and encode as combinations of weights in memory.

Unfortunately, the practice of deep learning is ahead of the theory. There is currently no way of summarizing what a trained RNN has learned. All that a developer knows is the accuracy with which the network labels the validation data. This can lead to surprises when networks learn properties of the input data other than what the designer intended and/or the user assumes. As a result, we lack confidence in even high-performing networks when they are deployed in applications where the input might differ from the training data, or where the cost of failure is high. We need methods to visualize what recurrent nets learn. This paper presents two methods for visualizing concepts learned by RNNs in the domain of activity recognition. Activity recognition has the advantage that the inputs are sequences of 3D human poses (also called skeletons). This provides

F. Karray et al. (Eds.): ICIAR 2019, LNCS 11663, pp. 67–80, 2019.
https://doi.org/10.1007/978-3-030-27272-2_6

a framework for visualizing results and anatomical constraints for generating synthetic inputs. The first visualization method shows the *sensitivity* of joints over time, extending the work by Li et al. [15]. Sensitivity is the normalized partial derivative of an output signal with respect to a given joint, where the output may either be a class label or the output of a specific hidden unit. For example, when analyzing an LSTM trained to recognize throwing motions we see that it is sensitive to the positions and motions of the arms, which is not a surprise, but also the upward motion of the spine. In essence, the LSTM has learned that throwing requires an upward movement of the entire body, which otherwise the user may not know.

The second visualization method generates synthetic videos that maximize the responses of a class label or hidden unit within a set of known anatomical constraints. This yields different insights from the first method. For example, the response of one hidden unit to throws is maximized when the subject begins as low to the ground as possible. The goal of such visualizations is to show users what the system has learned, and therefore how it might respond to novel inputs.

The visualization techniques presented in this paper are presented as case studies in the context of LSTMs, but can be applied to most recurrent networks, including Gated Recurrent Unit networks (GRUs [8]). For LSTMs, we present a visualization tool called *SkeletonVis*. This tool can be used over the web to view LSTM networks we have trained on the NTU activity data set, or downloaded and applied to LSTMs trained by users on data sets of their choice.

In summary, the contributions of this paper are:

1. A technique for visualizing the sensitivity of an LSTM class label or hidden unit responses to specific joints in pose data.
2. A technique for generating synthetic videos that elicit maximal responses by class labels or hidden units.
3. A software tool called *SkeletonVis* for visualizing LSTMs.
4. Case studies of using SkeletonVis to probe the properties of trained networks.

2 Prior Literature

The computer vision literature includes many methods for visualizing features learned by convolutional neural networks. See [28] for an up-to-date survey and [1] for an interactive summary of visualization techniques in CNNs. This paper builds on two concepts in CNN visualizations, namely saliency maps by Simoyan and Zisserman [21] and activation maximization by Mahendran and Vedaldi [17]. This paper extends their techniques to recurrent networks.

Recently, RNN researchers have introduced techniques like attention mechanism that change the underlying network architecture to study specific properties of the input data. However, the model-driven properties still remain under explored. Diagnostic visualizations of RNN models are better established in the field of natural language processing than computer vision. See [3,15,23,25] for a brief survey. However, the input to all the above methods is a single character or word, embedded into a vector. This is significantly different from the input to LSTMs in an action recognition system.

The input to an action recognition LSTM is a 3D skeleton pose over time. Interpreting how relations over time within a video are modeled is particularly difficult. The two main techniques used to understand models in skeleton based action recognition are spatio-temporal attention mechanism [22] and co-occurrence of joints [27]. The spatio-temporal approach [22] helps us understand the importance given by the model to joints and time frames in a sequence. Unfortunately, as with the attention approach, the original model is altered. The co-occurrence of joints approach reveals correlations of joints in an action sequence without changing the model, but the hidden states of the LSTM are not explored. Our approach aims to interpret hidden states directly. The approach in [15] uses saliency heatmaps to highlight the network's ability to understand negative sentiment in text. Our approach shows that the network is able to focus on the most informative joints in an action by assigning them a higher saliency.

As part of visualization, we generate synthetic skeletons that conform to anatomical constraints. 3D pose estimation techniques have a similar need. Tripathy et al. [24] propose a constrained Kalman filter to denoise joint coordinates obtained from Kinect sensors. Our approach integrates the bone length constraints proposed in this paper. Dabral et al. [9] model joint angle limits and bone length limits as a loss function that strongly penalizes joints that deviate from valid angular limits. While our approach does not consider a loss function minimization, their formulation of joint angle limits is used below. There are pose estimation papers that go farther: [10] discriminates joint types (ball joints vs. hinge joints). Akhter and Black [4] formulate priors to eliminate invalid poses by pose-conditioned joint angle limits. Such constraints may be added to our techniques in the future.

3 Approach

We propose two approaches to visualizing what a trained RNN has learned. The first is a gradient-based saliency approach that illustrates the relevance of a joint to a class label or hidden unit. The approach is inspired by the saliency maps in [15], which use heat maps to visually demonstrate the importance of words. The second approach shows synthetic skeletons that maximize the hidden state activations of class labels or selected neurons. To make these techniques easy to use, we consolidate them into a visualization tool called *SkeletonVis*. SkeletonVis allows users to gain insights into the workings of their trained models in order to increase (or decrease) their confidence in a network's abilities.

Figure 1 show the architecture of a recurrent network used for skeleton-based action recognition. The input is a sequence of skeleton poses over time; the output is a vector of class label probabilities. Opening up the architecture, the recurrent network is a one-layer LSTM cell, similar to [22,26]. This is followed by a fully-connected (FC) layer and a softmax layer. The FC layer takes as input the outputs of the LSTM's hidden units h, and has one output unit for every class in the data set. The softmax layer converts the FC outputs into label probabilities.

The rest of this section describes our techniques in more detail. Section 3.1 explains how joint saliency is calculated. Section 3.2 describes how skeletons are generated to maximize a class label or hidden state output. A brief overview of the SkeletonVis tool is explained in Sect. 3.3.

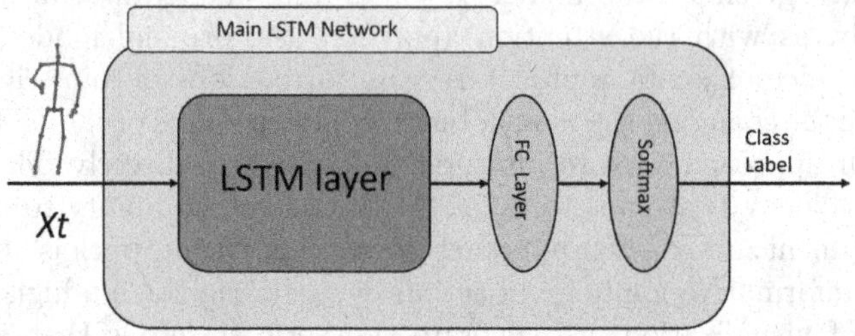

Fig. 1. The LSTM architecture used for the experiments in this paper. It is followed by a single hidden layer converting hidden unit responses into label responses, and then a softmax layer converting label responses into probabilities.

3.1 Gradient-Based Saliency

Gradients help us understand the contribution of each individual input unit to the final output of a network. This technique has been used extensively to find localized class-discriminative visual explanations in images for CNN models [21] and to find important words in text mining [15]. In skeleton-based action recognition, saliency measures the contribution of every body joint to the decision about a particular class of action.

For the model shown in Fig. 1, we first explore the gradient of the response h_u of hidden unit u with respect to dimension d of joint j. Note that we are considering the partial derivative of h_u with respect to the pose input $\mathrm{x_t}$ and not the previous hidden state input $\mathrm{h_{t\text{-}1}}$. We are therefore measuring the sensitivity of a particular pose value in time, not the combined impact of a joint over time.

We denote the gradient $\mathrm{g^u_{t,j,d}}$ as:

$$g^{\mathrm{u}}_{\mathrm{t,j,d}} = \frac{\delta h^{\mathrm{u}}_{\mathrm{t}}}{\delta x_{\mathrm{t,j,d}}} \tag{1}$$

where $\mathrm{x_t}$ and $\mathrm{h^u_t}$ are the pose input and hidden state output of neuron u at time instance t, respectively. The absolute value of $\mathrm{g^u_{t,j,d}}$ denotes the sensitivity of the input joint to the final output hidden state. Thus, we denote sensitivity $\mathrm{S^u_{t,j,d}}$ as:

$$S^u_{t,j,d} = |g^u_{t,j,d}| \tag{2}$$

For any particular time t, joint j and dimension d, the sensitivity $\mathrm{S}^{\mathrm{u}}_{\mathrm{t,j,d}}$ is a scalar. When there are joints with very little motion across the data set, i.e. body parts that don't move, their sensitivity can become very large due to random sensor noise. Hence, we normalize sensitivity across a sequence as:

$$S'^{u}_{t,j,d} = \frac{\sigma_{x_{t,j,d}}}{\sigma_{h^u_t}} * S^{u}_{t,j,d} \tag{3}$$

where $\mathrm{S}'^{\mathrm{u}}_{\mathrm{t,j,d}}$ denotes the normalized sensitivity for dimension d of joint j for neuron u at time t. $\sigma_{x_{t,j,d}}$ denotes the standard deviation of the pose input $\mathrm{x_{j,d}}$ over t, and $\sigma_{h^u_t}$ denotes the standard deviation of $\mathrm{h^u}$ over t. We will refer to the normalized sensitivity $\mathrm{S}'^{\mathrm{u}}_{\mathrm{j,d}}$ for the rest of this paper.

Sensitivity is a scalar value for each dimension of a joint in the skeleton pose. For a given time t, we denote the summation of sensitivities across the X, Y and Z dimensions of a joint as the final contribution of the joint to the hidden state of the neuron. Thus:

$$S'^{\mathrm{u}}_{\mathrm{t,j}} = \sum_{d=1}^{3} S'^{\mathrm{u}}_{\mathrm{t,j,d}} \tag{4}$$

Equation 4 measures the sensitivity of a hidden unit u to input joint j at time t. To understand the impact of a joint not just on a single hidden unit but on the overall class response we take the product of the normalized joint sensitivities with their magnitudes in the weight matrix column of the FC layer for the respective class. The weights in the FC layer indicate the final effect of a hidden unit in the classification of an input sequence. The weight matrix has dimensions (H, C) where H is the number of hidden neurons in the LSTM and C is the number of classes in the data set. The final sensitivity map is represented as an aggregation of the weighted sensitivities of all neurons for the class under consideration and can be written as:

$$S'_{\mathrm{t,j}} = \sum_{u=1}^{H} S'^{\mathrm{u}}_{\mathrm{t,j}} * |W^{\mathrm{u}}_{\mathrm{c}}| \tag{5}$$

where $|W^{\mathrm{u}}_{\mathrm{c}}|$ is the magnitude of the weight of neuron u for class c. This result is visually represented in SkeletonVis as a sequential colormap with darker values for large sensitivities and lighter values for small ones.

3.2 Activation Maximization

Sensitivity visualization shows a user what body parts are having the most influence over a class label or the response of a hidden unit. Activation maximization, on the other hand, generates synthetic inputs that maximize the response of a class label or hidden unit. The idea is to warn users about inputs that the network might never have encountered but which would cause the network to generate a strong response for a particular class label.

Activation maximization is implemented by hill-climbing. We begin with any input sequence that receives class label c. Starting with this input, we calculate the gradient of the fully connected layer for class c with respect to the input:

$$d^{\mathrm{c}}_{\mathrm{t,i}} = \frac{\delta o_{\mathrm{c}}}{\delta x_{\mathrm{t,i}}} \tag{6}$$

where $\mathrm{d}^{\mathrm{c}}_{\mathrm{t,i}}$ denotes the gradient of the output for class c with respect to the input pose x_i at time t. Note that this gradient is obtained for all neurons in the LSTM cell for input x_i and time t and is therefore a vector of length H, where H is the number of hidden units in the LSTM.

The gradient $d^c_{t,i}$ is a weighted sum of the gradients of every hidden unit u with respect to the input pose x_i at time t. This can also be written as:

$$d^{\mathrm{c}}_{\mathrm{t,i}} = \sum_{u=1}^{H} W^{\mathrm{u}}_{\mathrm{c}} * \frac{\delta h^{\mathrm{u}}_{\mathrm{t}}}{\delta x_{\mathrm{t,i}}} \tag{7}$$

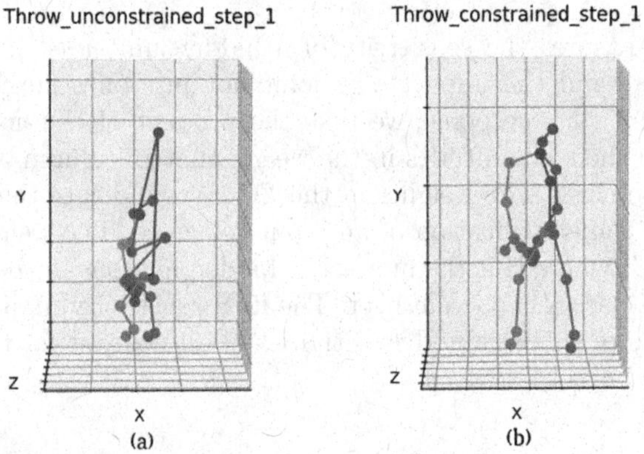

Fig. 2. Why anatomical constraints matter. Frame (a) shows a skeleton after one iteration of activation maximization without anatomical constraints. Frame (b) shows it after one iteration with constraints.

The value of $d^c_{t,i}$ is used to update input pose x_t for the next iteration. Unfortunately, the LSTM treats every input feature $x_{t,j,d}$ as independent. The gradient update calculated by Eq. 7 alters the data to increase the networks response, but the result may look nothing like a human skeleton. Figure 2(a) shows the input pose updated according to the gradient in Eq. 7. The human form is unrecognizable. The middle of the spine has been moved to the top, elongating the spine and giving it an unrealistic degree of curvature. Other joints have been moved in odd ways as well, resulting in a non-human shape.

In many ways, this situation is analogous to what happens when activation maximization is applied to convolutional neural networks performing image classification. Activation maximization produces "images" that fool the CNN, but look like white noise to human observers [6,11,18]. In our case, activation maximization produces "skeletons" that don't look like skeletons. Fortunately, in action recognition, unlike general image recognition, human anatomy provides constraints that can be used to alter how poses are updated.

To produce valid skeletons, we apply two types of constraints, *bone length constraints* and *pairwise angle constraints*. We are aware that the constraints below are not exhaustive. At this stage, we rely on a few, important constraints for conceptualization.

For a frame f, we construct a state vector s_f as:

$$\mathbf{s_f} = [x_0, x_1..x_N, y_0, y_1..y_N, z_0, z_1..z_N] \tag{8}$$

Thus, $\mathrm{s_f}$ is a $N \times 3$ dimension vector, where N is the number of joints. The bone length $\mathrm{b_{i,j}}$ between any two connected pair of joints is given by the Euclidean distance between the joints:

$$b_{\mathrm{i,j}} = \sqrt{(x_{\mathrm{i}} - x_{\mathrm{j}})^2 + (y_{\mathrm{i}} - y_{\mathrm{j}})^2 + (z_{\mathrm{i}} - z_{\mathrm{j}})^2} \tag{9}$$

For Kinect version 2, there are 25 joints and 24 pairs of connected joints (bones). We consider the reference bone length $\mathrm{b_{i,j}}$ to be the mean of $b_{i,j,t}$ over the input video sequence. The bone length constraint is defined as:

$$\|(s_{\mathrm{f}} + d') \cdot A_{\mathrm{i,j}}\| / \sqrt{2} - b_{\mathrm{i,j}} = 0 \tag{10}$$

where $\mathrm{A_{i,j}}$ is a 75×75 dimension matrix. For example, for joints (0,1) the A matrix will be represented as:

$$\begin{matrix} & 0 & 1 & ...25 & 26 & ...50 & 51 & ...74 \end{matrix}$$

$$\mathbf{A_{0,1}} = \begin{bmatrix} 1 & -1 & ..0 & 0 & ...0 & 0 & 0 \\ -1 & 1 & ..0 & 0 & ...0 & 0 & 0 \\ 0 & 0 & ..1 & -1 & ...0 & 0 & 0 \\ 0 & 0 & ..-1 & 1 & ...0 & 0 & 0 \\ 0 & 0 & ..0 & 0 & ...1 & -1 & 0 \\ 0 & 0 & ..0 & 0 & ...-1 & 1 & 0 \\ 0 & 0 & ..0 & 0 & ...0 & 0 & 0 \end{bmatrix}$$

In addition to preserving bone lengths between connected pairs, certain joint angle constraints are also imposed on skeletons. Inspired by the joint angle limits in [9], we propose three joint constraints and four joints constraints.

The conditions for three joint angle constraints are as follows: Let $\mathbf{v_{sb,sm}}$ and $\mathbf{v_{ss,sm}}$ be two unit vectors, in this case the vectors from spine mid to spine base and spine mid to spine shoulder. We constrain the angle between $\mathbf{v_{sb,sm}}$ and $\mathbf{v_{ss,sm}}$ to be between 160° and 180°. Mathematically, this is expressed as:

$$-0.93969 \geqslant (v_{\mathrm{sb,sm}} \cdot v_{\mathrm{ss,\,sm}}) \geqslant -1 \tag{11}$$

Similarly we constrain the angle made by the spine top and the two shoulders to be between 110° and 180°, the angle made by the spine base with the hips to be between 100° and 180°, and the angle made by the wrist with the elbow and hand joint to be between 90° and 180°. We formulate similar angle constraints with four joints. Let $\mathbf{v_{rh,sb}}$, $\mathbf{v_{lh,sb}}$ and $\mathbf{v_{sm,sb}}$ be three unit vectors from spine base to right hip, spine base to left hip and spine base to spine mid, respectively. We define the vector $\mathbf{n_{rh,sb,lh}}$ as the normal vector to the plane defined by $\mathbf{v_{rh,sb}}$ and $\mathbf{v_{lh,sb}}$.

$$n_{\mathrm{rh,sb,lh}} = (v_{\mathrm{rh,sb}} \times v_{\mathrm{lh,sb}}) \tag{12}$$

For the four joints to be in a valid position, we restrict the vectors $\mathbf{n_{rh,sb,lh}}$ and $\mathbf{v_{sm,sb}}$ to be between 0° and 90°. Mathematically this is written as:

$$1 \geqslant (n_{\mathrm{rh,sb,lh}} \cdot v_{\mathrm{sm,sb}}) \geqslant 0 \tag{13}$$

All the constraint equations (bone lengths, three joint angles and four joint angles) are grouped and denoted as C. We then find the update d' that optimizes:

$$\text{minimize} \quad (d - d')^2 \quad \text{subject to} \quad C. \tag{14}$$

We then add this constrained update d' to the current skeleton pose and iterate to hill climb in the space of valid skeletons. Figure 2(b) shows the skeleton updated with one iteration of the constrained gradient.

Equation 14 modifies the input (i.e. the sequence of skeleton poses) to increase the label response while generating skeletons that satisfy the anatomical constraints. As shown in Fig. 2(b), the first update yields a more extreme motion that optimizes, in this case, the *throw* action. If we continue the gradient updates until convergence, we get a skeleton that maximizes the class response for the sequence. Unfortunately, the skeleton that optimizes the class response still fails to look like a skeleton, despite adhering to the constraints imposed on it. Figure 5 shows a skeleton that optimizes the response but does not look like a valid skeleton. We could add more constraints, for example by requiring that the skeleton be supported rather than floating in mid-air, but at the moment these unrealistic optima provide a warning about inputs that generate strong false responses, while earlier stages in the optimization show us more realistic motions that strengthen the response.

3.3 SkeletonVis

We aggregate sensitivity analysis and activation maximization into an interactive visualization tool called *SkeletonVis*. This tool is intended to help users better understand models learned by LSTMs. SkeletonVis can be used over the web to see visualizations of previously trained networks, or it can be downloaded and run locally to examine the user's own LSTM networks. Users can log on to http://www.cs.colostate.edu/~vision/skvis_toolset/index.php to view the existing case studies or download the source code from the same site to run it locally.

Figure 3 shows SkeletonVis as it appears over the web. On top, the system summarizes the model and data information, showing the number of data samples, classes, and hidden neurons in the model, as well as the Kinect version used

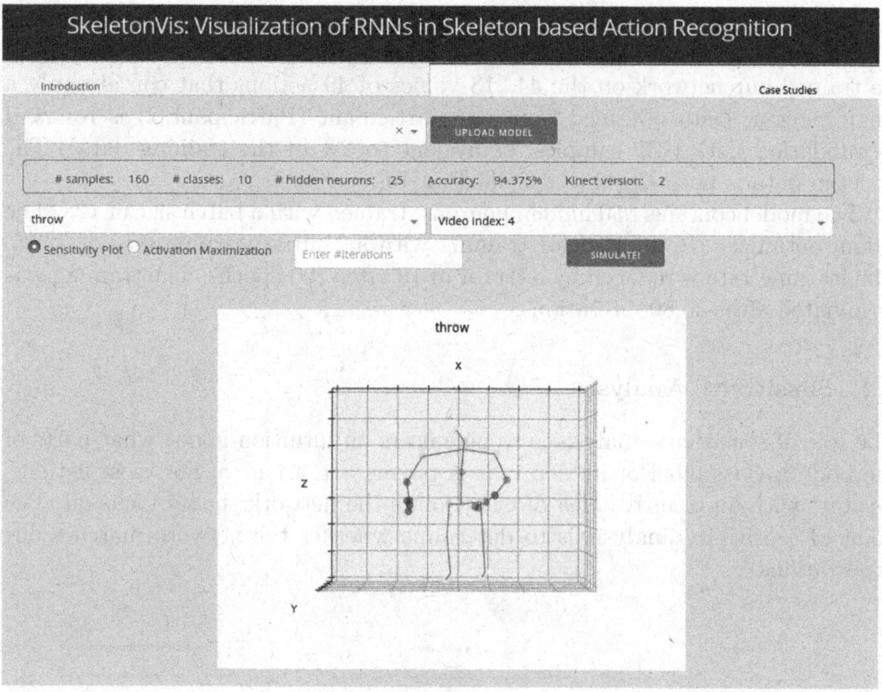

Fig. 3. The SkeletonVis tool, as it appears to LSTM developers and users.

and the classification accuracy of the system. Users select the class or hidden unit they want to inspect, and an input video to visualize. Users also choose whether to visualize sensitivity or activation maximization, and in the case of activity maximization how many optimization iterations to apply. In the next section, we present case studies using this tool.

4 Case Studies

This section provides examples of using the visualization techniques described above to analyze LSTM networks. In particular, we trained LSTM networks on two data sets, NTU-RGBD action recognition data set [19] and SYSU data set [14], and analyzed what was learned using SkeletonVis. Although the network is modern and relatively good at action recognition, we remind the reader that focus of this paper is on the analysis of the network, not the network's accuracy.

4.1 An LSTM Trained on NTU-RGBD Data Set

For our first case studies, we trained a single-layer LSTM network on the NTU-RGBD data set [19]. This dataset contains 56,880 video samples of RGB-D videos and skeleton data captured using a Kinect v2. There are 60 action classes performed by 40 participants and seen from multiple viewpoints. Cross Subject (CS) and Cross View (CV) are the standard modes of evaluation. For simplicity, we trained our network on the 44,213 videos of 49 actions that contain only a single person. Data obtained from one participant (Participant 2) is reserved as validation data (739 samples, equivalent to 2% of the training data). The skeleton data is normalized as specified in [19].

The model contains 150 hidden neurons, trained with a batch size of 128. The Adam optimizer [16] is used for training with an initial learning rate of 0.005. The learning rate is reduced by a factor of 10 after 100 epochs. The training was terminated after 25,800 iterations.

4.2 Sensitivity Analysis

The role of sensitivity analysis is to give users an intuition about what parts of the body a class label or hidden unit is paying attention to. For most actions, we start with an intuitive idea of what joints the network should focus on. The point of sensitivity analysis is to determine whether the network matches our expectations.

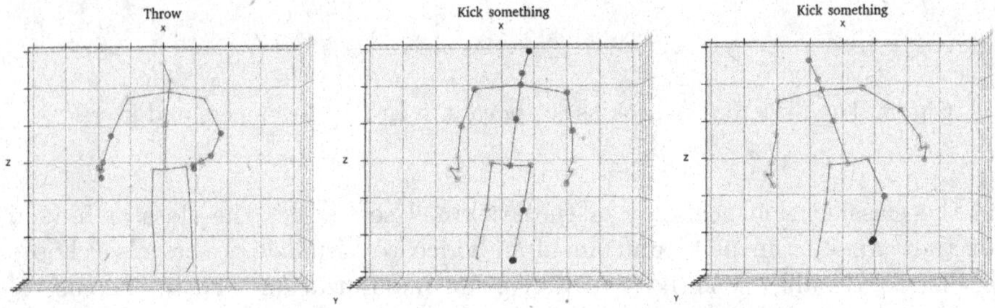

Fig. 4. Sensitivity visualizations of frames extracted from throw and kick actions. (a) shows the sensitivity of joints from an early frame of a throwing motion. (b) shows the sensitivities from an early frame of a kicking motion, while (c) shows a later frame from the same kicking video.

Figure 4(a) shows the sensitivity plot of one frame in a *throw* action. As we expected, the arms are highly sensitive. However, the mid-spine joint is unexpectedly sensitive, too. It has roughly the same sensitivity as the hands and elbows in the initial frames of the action. The *throw* label seems to be sensitive to it because throwing includes a vertical movement of the torso in all the training samples.

Parts (b) and (c) of Fig. 4 show frames from a *kick* action. With kicking, we expect attention to be focused on the knees and feet. The actual story is more dynamic. In the early frames of the video, the LSTM is sensitive to the spine, shoulders and elbows as well as the knees and left foot. As the kicking motion progresses, the LSTM becomes less sensitive to the upper body and focuses on the foot instead. This seems to emphasize the starting pose, since most NTU kicks begin from a standing position. It may also be that people tend to spread their arms slightly at the beginning of a kick for balance.

4.3 Activation Maximization

In addition to sensitivity analysis, SkeletonVis shows synthetic videos produced by activation maximization. Figure 5 concentrates on a single frame from each of two throwing videos. The actual skeleton for each frame shown on the left. The middle shows this skeleton after one iteration of activation maximization. The right shows the final local optima reached after 12 iterations.

We learn different things from the second and third columns of Fig. 5. The second columns teaches us how to make the *throw* response stronger through exaggeration, in this case by putting the participant in a more crouched position, with their left arm more curled and their left shoulder dipped. The feet are also shown as more splayed, but we know that *throw* is not very sensitive to the positions of the feet, so presumably this difference is unimportant.

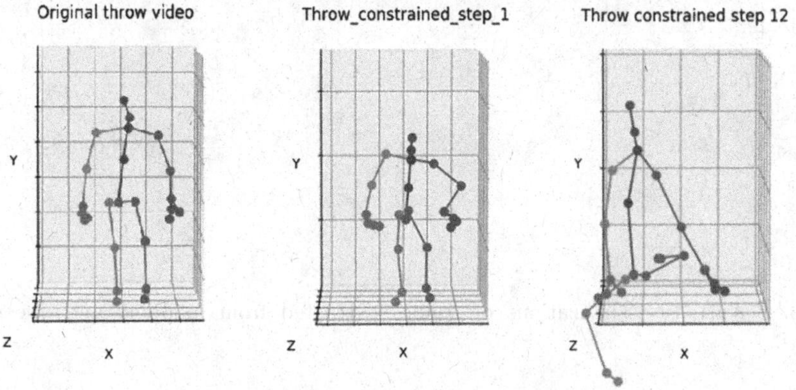

Fig. 5. Figure shows the progression of skeleton

The third column of Fig. 5, on the other hand, warns us about non-sensical videos that could fool us. For the *throw* motion, activation maximization converges to a local optimum that might be described as a floating contortionist. Although the bone and angle constraints are satisfied, the skeleton is extremely contorted and floating in mid-air. This is clearly not feasible, yet it maximizes the *throw* response and suggests a possible source of false responses.

4.4 An LSTM Trained on SYSU Data Set

The SYSU dataset [14] contains 480 video samples of RGB-D videos and skeleton data captured using a Kinect v1, rendering skeletons with 20 joints. There are

12 action classes performed by 40 participants. We evaluate the system using one cross validation, with 20 training subjects and 20 testing subjects. Skeleton data is normalized as in the NTU-RGBD data set.

The model consists of 200 hidden neurons, trained with a batch size of 64. The Adam optimizer [16] is used for training with an initial learning rate of 0.005. The learning rate is reduced by a factor of 10 after 60 epochs. The training was terminated after 3,000 iterations.

Figure 6 shows frames from two similar actions: *mopping* and *sweeping.* To differentiate these actions, the model focuses on the movement of the legs in the sweeping action, and the lowered position of the head in the mopping action. Thus these joints have unexpectedly high sensitivities, in addition to the expected high sensitivities of the arms. The position and orientation of the spine seems to be a differentiating factor in most of the samples of the two actions.

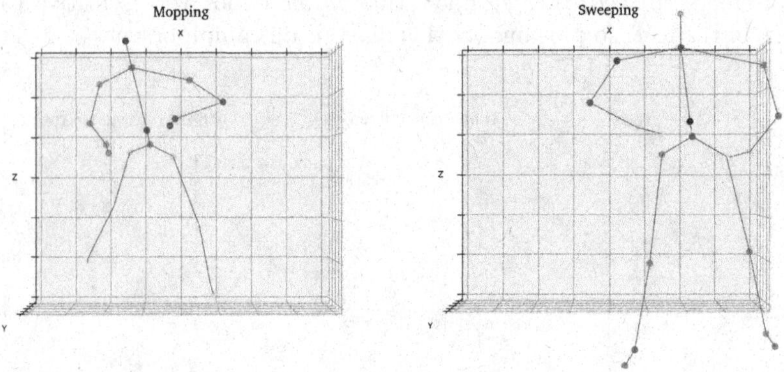

Fig. 6. Sensitivity visualizations of frames extracted from mopping and sweeping actions.

5 Conclusions and Future Work

Recurrent Neural Networks are a state of the art method for modeling sequential data. However, the internal workings of these models are often treated as black boxes by the researchers using them. This paper provide insights into models learned by RNNs through visualization. Sensitivity, reveals the most relevant joints in an action. We observe that while the joints we expect to be important generally are important, there is often more to the story. For example, throwing may include an upward trajectory of the torso, while kicking may be recognized in part by the starting pose. Using one (or a few) iterations of activation maximization, we show how the response of a video can be strengthened by exaggerating a motion, thus providing intuitions about the idealized form of an action. At the same time, by running activation maximization to convergence we produce impossible inputs that can fool an RNN. We aggregate these techniques into an interactive visualization tool called SkeletonVis, which we are making available so that RNN developers and users can gain insights into these enigmatic networks.

In the future, we plan to improve the anatomical constraints underlying activation maximization. We will add temporal constraints to eliminate implausible accelerations, and volume constraints to prevent body parts from passing inside each other. Lastly, multi-layer LSTMS are becoming common, and we intend to explore feature abstractions from higher layers.

Acknowledgements. This work was supported by the U.S. Defense Advanced Research Projects Agency and the U.S. Army Research Office under contract #W911NF-15-1-0459.

References

1. https://distill.pub
2. Aafaq, N., Gilani, S., Liu, W., Mian, A.: Video description: a survey of methods, datasets and evaluation metrics (2018) arXiv:1806.00186v1
3. Karpathy, A., Johnson, J., Li, F.: Visualizing and understanding recurrent networks (2015). coRR, abs/1506.02078
4. Akhter, I., Black, M.J.: Pose-conditioned joint angle limits for 3D human pose reconstruction. In: CVPR 2015 (2015)
5. Allahyari, M., Pouriyeh, S., Assefi, M., Safaei, S., Trippe, E.D., Gutierrez, J.B.: A brief survey of text mining: classification, clustering and extraction techniques (2017). arXiv:1707.02919v2
6. Bendale, A., Boult, T.E.: Towards open set deep networks (2015). arXiv:1511.06233v1
7. Chiu, C.C., et al.: State-of-the-art speech recognition with sequence-to-sequence models (2017). arXiv:1712.01769v6
8. Cho, K., van Merrienboer, B., Bahdanau, D., Bengio, Y.: On the properties of neural machine translation: encoder-decoder approaches (2014). arXiv:1409.1259
9. Dabral, R., Mundhada, A., Kusupati, U., Afaque, S., Sharma, A., Jain, A.: Learning 3D human pose from structure and motion (2018). arXiv:1711.09250v2
10. Engell-Nørregård, M., Erleben, K.: Estimation of joint types and joint limits from motion capture data. In: WSCG 2009 (2009)
11. Goodfellow, I.J., Shlens, J., Szegedy, C.: Explaining and harnessing adversarial examples (2015). arXiv:1412.6572v3
12. Graves, A., Mohamed, A.R., Hinton, G.: Speech recognition with deep recurrent-neural networks. In: IEEE International Conference on Acoustics, Speech and Signal Processing, pp. 6645–6649. IEEE (2013)
13. Hossain, M., Sohel, F., Shiratuddin, M.F., Laga, H.: A comprehensive survey of deep learning for image captioning (2018). arXiv:1810.04020v2
14. Hu, J.-F., Zheng, W.-S., Zhang, J., Lai, J.-H.: Jointly learning heterogeneous features for RGB-D activity recognition. In: IEEE Conference on Computer Vision and Pattern Recognition, pp. 5344–5352 (2015)
15. Li, J., Chen, X., Hovy, E., Jurafsky, D.: Visualizing and understanding neural models in NLP. coRR, abs/1506.01066v2 (2016)

16. Kingma, D.P., Ba, J.L.: Adam: a method for stochastic optimization (2015). arXiv:1412.6980v9
17. Mahendran, A., Vedaldi, A.: Visualizing deep convolutional neural networks using natural pre-images (2016). arXiv:1512.02017v3
18. Nguyen, A., Yosinski, J., Clune, J.: Deep neural networks are easily fooled: High confidence predictions for unrecognizable images (2015). arXiv:1412.1897v4
19. Shahroudy, A., Liu, J., Ng, T., Wang, G.: NTU RGB+D: a large scale dataset for 3D human activity analysis. In: IEEE Conference on Computer Vision and Pattern Recognition, pp. 1010–1019 (2016)
20. Hochreiter, S., Schmidhuber, J.: Long short-term memory. Neural Comput. **9**(8), 1735–1780 (1997)
21. Simonyan, K., Vedaldi, A., Zisserman, A.: Deep inside convolutional networks: visualising image classification models and saliency maps. Technical report, GMD - German National Research Institute for Computer Science, Technical report (2001)
22. Song, S., Lan, C., Xing, J., Zeng, W., Liu, J.: An end-to-end spatio-temporal attention model for human action recognition from skeleton data. In: AAAI Conference on Artificial Intelligence, pp. 4263–4270 (2017)
23. Strobelt, H., Gehrmann, S., Huber, B., Pfister, H., Rush, A.M.: Visual analysis of hidden state dynamics in recurrent neural networks, coRR, abs/1606.07461 (2016)
24. Tripathy, S.R., Chakravarty, K., Sinha, A., Chatterjee, D., Saha, S.K.: Constrained Kalman filter for improving kinect based measurements (2017)
25. Ming, Y., Cao, S., Zhang, R., Li, Z., Chen, Y.: Understanding hidden memories of recurrent neural networks. coRR, abs/1710.10777v1 (2017)
26. Zhang, P., Lan, C., Xing, J., Zeng, W., Xue, J., Zheng, N.: View adaptive recurrent neural networks for high performance human action recognition from skeleton data (2017). arXiv:1703.08274v2
27. Zhu, W., et al.: Co-occurrence feature learning for skeleton based action recognition using regularized deep LSTM networks. In: Proceedings of the Thirtieth AAAI Conference on Artificial Intelligence (AAAI-16) (2016)
28. Qin, Z., Yu, F., Liu, C., Chen, X.: How convolutional neural networks see the world - a survey of convolutional neural network visualization methods. Math. Found. Comput. **1**(2), 149–180 (2018)

Information Fusion via Multimodal Hashing with Discriminant Canonical Correlation Maximization

Lei Gao(✉) and Ling Guan

Department of Electrical and Computer Engineering, Ryerson University, Toronto, Canada
iegaolei@gmail.com, lguan@ee.ryerson.ca

Abstract. In this paper, we introduce an effective information fusion method using multimodal hashing with discriminant canonical correlation maximization. As an effective computation method of similarity between different inputs, multimodal hashing technique has attracted increasing attentions in fast similarity search. In this paper, the proposed approach not only finds the minimum of the semantic similarity across different modalities by multimodal hashing, but also is capable of extracting the discriminant representations, which minimize the between-class correlation and maximize the within-class correlation simultaneously for information fusion. Benefiting from the combination of semantic similarity across different modalities and the discriminant representation strategy, the proposed algorithm can achieve improved performance. A prototype of the proposed method is implemented to demonstrate its performance in audio emotion recognition and cross-modal (text-image) fusion. Experimental results show that the proposed approach outperforms the related methods, in terms of accuracy.

Keywords: Information fusion · Multimodal hashing · Discriminant canonical correlation maximization · Audio emotion recognition · Cross-modal fusion

1 Introduction

The advancement in multimedia content analysis and sensing technology have enabled and encouraged the design and development of computationally effective and economically feasible multimodal systems for a broad spectrum of applications [1–3]. Since multimodal data contain rich information about the semantics presented in the sensory and media data, valid interpretation and integration of multimodal information is recognized as a central issue for the successful utilization of multimedia in a wide range of applications. Therefore, information fusion is becoming an increasingly important research topic. However, for information fusion, one of the major concerns lies in the identification of the discriminatory representations between different modalities. To solve this problem, a wide variety of methods have been proposed [4–6].

F. Karray et al. (Eds.): ICIAR 2019, LNCS 11663, pp. 81–93, 2019.
https://doi.org/10.1007/978-3-030-27272-2_7

Since hashing has fast query speed and low storage cost, it has been widely applied to similarity search works. Recently, more and more attentions have been focused on multimodal hashing in multimedia data with modalities [7–9]. For instance, we can obtain a medical image from the same organ with different physical processes such as Computed Tomography (CT) and Magnetic Resonance Imaging (MRI).

It is widely acknowledged that there are two main categories of multimodal hashing methods: *cross-modal hashing* (CMH) and *multi-source hashing* (MSH). The method of MSH is also named multiple feature hashing with the purpose of studying better codes by leveraging auxiliary views than unimodal hashing [7]. Recently, there has been extensive focus on the method of CMH, since only one view is needed for a query point in CMH. For instance, all the tasks of image-to-image, text-to-image, and image-to-text retrieval can be performed by CMH [10].

CMH methods are further grouped into two classes: *unsupervised* CMH and *supervised* CMH based on the usage of supervised information or not. For unsupervised CMH methods, mostly relying on canonical correlation analysis (CCA) [11], it maps two different views into a common latent space to explore the maximum between two variables. For *supervised* CMH method, it utilizes supervised information for hashing, leading to improved performance on different tasks. Although the existing supervised methods have achieved promising results in many real applications, they only account for the similarity across different modalities, completely ignoring the data structure and discriminant representation within each modality.

In this paper, a multimodal hashing with discriminant canonical correlation maximization is proposed for information fusion. The main contributions of the presented method are summarized as follows.

1. Since multi-source fusion is a special case of multimodal fusion, the proposed method in this paper can be used for CMH and MSH, simultaneously.

2. In this paper, the similarity across different modalities from multimodal hashing is applied to information fusion.

3. The proposed method is able to synchronously minimize the between-class correlation and maximize the within-class correlation of multimodal variables, revealing the intrinsic structure and discriminant representations from different multimodal hashing information.

4. Not only the intrinsic structures and discriminant representation are considered, but also the semantic similarity across different modalities is utilized, improving the final performance.

The remainder of this paper is organized as follows: Sect. 2 introduces the proposed multimodal hashing with discriminant canonical correlation maximization. In Sect. 3, implementation of the proposed method for audio emotion recognition and cross-modal fusion is presented. The experimental results and analysis are given in Sect. 4. Conclusions are drawn in Sect. 5.

2 The Proposed Method

In this section, we introduce the proposed method for information fusion. In the following, we first briefly describe the fundamentals of existing supervised multimodal hashing (SMH) method, and then formulate the proposed method.

2.1 The Existing SMH Method

Let $x^* = [x_1{}^*, ..., x_N{}^*]^T \in R^{N\times m}$ and $y^* = [y_1{}^*, ..., y_N{}^*]^T \in R^{N\times p}$ be two sets of variables as the entries, and N denotes the number of training samples. Then, m and p are the dimensions of feature space in each variable set, respectively.

As a supervised method, semantic labels for each training entity in SMH are available. The labels are represented by the label vectors $\{l_1, l_2 ..., l_N \,|l_i \in \{0,1\}^c\}$, where c is the total number of classes. Then, $l_{i,k}$ denotes the ith entity belongs to the kth class. Otherwise, $l_{i,k} = 0$. For the method of SMH, its goal is to learn two hashing functions for two different entries: $f(x_i{}^*) : R^m \to \{-1,1\}^L$ and $g(y_i{}^*) : R^p \to \{-1,1\}^L$, where L is the length of the binary hash code. These two hashing functions map the original data in the corresponding entry into a common hamming space. Although there are a great number of functions which can be used to define $f(x^*)$ and $g(y^*)$, we utilize the following functions

$$\begin{aligned} f(x^*) &= \mathrm{sgn}(x^* W_{x^*}), \\ g(y^*) &= \mathrm{sgn}(y^* W_{y^*}), \end{aligned} \tag{1}$$

where $sgn()$ denotes the element-wise sign function, $W_{x^*} \in R^{m\times L}$ and $W_{y^*} \in R^{p\times L}$ are the projected matrices. Therefore, the solution to the SMH is to find the projected matrices W_{x^*} and W_{y^*} with the minimum of the semantic similarity across different modalities.

2.2 The Proposed Multimodal Hashing with Discriminant Canonical Correlation Maximization (MH-DCCM)

Let $U \in R^{N\times c}$ be the matrix to store the class label information with $U_{i,k} = l_{i,k}$, where $U_{i,k}$ stands for the element at the ith row and kth column in the matrix U. Then, the similarity matrix is written as follows

$$S = UU^T \tag{2}$$

Since the value of sgn function satisfies the following relation

$$\mathrm{sgn} \in \{-1, 1\}, \tag{3}$$

therefore

$$\mathrm{sgn} \cdot \mathrm{sgn} \in [-1, 1]. \tag{4}$$

Hence, the element-wise linear transformation is applied to S to get S',

$$S' = 2S - \mathbf{1} \cdot \mathbf{1}^T \tag{5}$$

where $S' \in R^{N \times N}$ and the value of $S' \in [-1, 1]$.
The mean vector of x^* and y^* is written as follows:

$$x_M = \frac{1}{N}\sum_{i=1}^{N} x_i{}^*, y_M = \frac{1}{N}\sum_{i=1}^{N} y_i{}^* \tag{6}$$

Then $x = [x_1{}^* - x_M, ..., x_N{}^* - x_M]^T$ and $y = [y_1{}^* - y_M, ..., y_N{}^* - y_M]^T$ are two zero-mean sets, which are written as follows

$$\begin{aligned} x^T \cdot \mathbf{1} = \mathbf{0} \in R^m, \\ y^T \cdot \mathbf{1} = \mathbf{0} \in R^p \end{aligned} \tag{7}$$

where

$$\mathbf{1} = [1, 1, \cdots 1]^{\mathbf{T}} \in R^{N \times 1} \tag{8}$$

Let

$$x = [x_1{}^{(1)}, x_2{}^{(1)} \cdots x_{n_1}{}^{(1)}, \cdots x_1{}^{(c)}, x_2{}^{(c)} \cdots x_{n_c}{}^{(c)}]^T \in R^{N \times m} \tag{9}$$

$$y = [y_1{}^{(1)}, y_2{}^{(1)} \cdots y_{n_1}{}^{(1)}, \cdots y_1{}^{(c)}, y_2{}^{(c)} \cdots y_{n_c}{}^{(c)}]^T \in R^{N \times p}, \tag{10}$$

and

$$e_{n_d} = [\underbrace{0, 0, \cdots 0}_{\sum_{u=1}^{d-1} n_u}, \underbrace{1, 1, \cdots 1}_{n_d} \underbrace{0, 0, \cdots 0}_{N - \sum_{u=1}^{d} n_u}]^T \in R^{N \times 1} \tag{11}$$

where $x_j{}^{(d)}$ and $y_j{}^{(d)}$ denote the jth sample in the dth class, respectively. n_d is the total number of samples in the dth class, which satisfies the following relation

$$\sum_{d=1}^{c} n_d = N \tag{12}$$

Then, the within-class correlation matrix $C_{w_{xy}}$ can be written as [5]:

$$\begin{aligned} C_{w_{xy}} &= \sum_{d=1}^{c} \sum_{h=1}^{n_d} \sum_{g=1}^{n_d} x_h{}^{(d)T} y_g{}^{(d)} \\ &= \sum_{d=1}^{c} (e_{n_d}{}^T x)^T (e_{n_d}{}^T y) \\ &= x^T A y \end{aligned} \tag{13}$$

where

$$A = \begin{bmatrix} \begin{pmatrix} H_{n_1 \times n_1} & \cdots & 0 \\ \vdots & H_{n_d \times n_d} & \vdots \\ 0 & \cdots & H_{n_c \times n_c} \end{pmatrix} \end{bmatrix} \in R^{N \times N} \tag{14}$$

where $H_{n_d \times n_d}$ is in the form of $n_d \times n_d$ and all the elements in $H_{n_d \times n_d}$ are unit values. Similarly, the between-class correlation matrix $C_{b_{xy}}$ is in the form of [5]:

$$\begin{aligned} C_{b_{xy}} &= \sum_{\substack{d=1 \\ d \neq q}}^{c} \sum_{q=1}^{c} \sum_{h=1}^{n_d} \sum_{g=1}^{n_q} {x_h}^{(d)T} {y_g}^{(q)} \\ &= \sum_{d=1}^{c} \sum_{q=1}^{c} \sum_{h=1}^{n_d} \sum_{g=1}^{n_q} {x_h}^{(d)T} {y_g}^{(q)} - \sum_{d=1}^{c} \sum_{h=1}^{n_d} \sum_{g=1}^{n_d} {x_h}^{(d)T} {y_g}^{(d)} \\ &= (x^T \bullet \mathbf{1})(\mathbf{1}^T \bullet y) - x^T A y \\ &= \mathbf{0} - x^T A y \\ &= -x^T A y \end{aligned} \tag{15}$$

where $\mathbf{1} = [1, 1, \cdots 1]^{\mathbf{T}} \in R^{N \times 1}$. The discriminant function is formulated as the following expression:

$$\widetilde{C_{xy}} = C_{w_{xy}} - C_{b_{xy}} \tag{16}$$

Substituting Eqs. (13) and (15) into (16) yields:

$$\widetilde{C_{xy}} = C_{w_{xy}} - C_{b_{xy}} = x^T A y - (-x^T A y) = 2x^T A y \tag{17}$$

Therefore, the optimal discriminant function is written as the following optimization problem:

$$\arg\max_{W_x, W_y} {W_x}^T \widetilde{C_{xy}} W_y \tag{18}$$

Since A is a symmetric matrix, Eq. (18) is further expressed as follows

$$\begin{aligned} &\arg\max_{W_x, W_y} {W_x}^T \widetilde{C_{xy}} W_y \\ &= \arg\max_{W_x, W_y} 2{W_x}^T x^T A y W_y \\ &= \arg\max_{W_x, W_y} 2(x W_x)^T A (y W_y) \\ &= \arg\max_{W_x, W_y} 2(A^{1/2} x W_x)^T (A^{1/2} y W_y) \end{aligned} \tag{19}$$

Furthermore, for canonical correlation analysis, two sets of variables x and y should satisfy the following constrained condition to guarantee the first projection is uncorrelated with the second projection (canonical property):

$$\begin{aligned} {W_x}^T x^T A x W_x &= N I_L \\ {W_y}^T y^T A y W_y &= N I_L \end{aligned} \tag{20}$$

where I_L denotes an identity matrix of size $L \times L$.
In this paper, the mapping functions $f(x)$ and $g(y)$ are defined as follows:

$$\begin{aligned} f(x) &= \mathrm{sgn}(A^{1/2} x W_x), \\ g(y) &= \mathrm{sgn}(A^{1/2} y W_y), \end{aligned} \tag{21}$$

Based on multimodal hashing and discriminant correlation maximization methods, the objective function of the proposed multimodal hashing with discriminant correlation maximization is to find the minimum of the semantic similarity across different modalities shown as follows

$$\min_{W_x,W_y} \left\| \mathrm{sgn}(A^{1/2}xW_x)\mathrm{sgn}(A^{1/2}yW_y)^T - LS' \right\|^2 \tag{22}$$

Based on the spectral relaxation algorithm in [12], Eq. (22) is formulated as follows

$$\min_{W_x,W_y} \left\| (A^{1/2}xW_x)(A^{1/2}yW_y)^T - LS' \right\|^2 \tag{23}$$

subject to

$$\begin{array}{l} (A^{1/2}xW_x)^T A^{1/2}xW_x = NI_L \\ (A^{1/2}yW_y)^T A^{1/2}yW_y = NI_L \end{array} \tag{24}$$

Equation (23) is further written as follows

$$\begin{array}{l} \min_{W_x,W_y} \left\| (A^{1/2}xW_x)(A^{1/2}yW_y)^T - LS' \right\|^2 \\ = min(tr\{[(A^{1/2}xW_x)(A^{1/2}yW_y)^T - LS'] \\ [(A^{1/2}xW_x)(A^{1/2}yW_y)^T - LS']^T\}) \\ = min(tr\{[(A^{1/2}xW_x)(A^{1/2}yW_y)^T(A^{1/2}yW_y)(A^{1/2}xW_x)^T] \\ -2L[(A^{1/2}xW_x)^T S'(A^{1/2}yW_y)] + [L^2(S')^T S']\}) \\ = min(tr\{[(A^{1/2}xW_x)(NI_L)(A^{1/2}xW_x)^T]\} \\ -tr\{2L[(W_x{}^T x^T A^{1/2})S'(A^{1/2}yW_y)]\} + tr\{[L^2(S')^T S']\}) \\ = min(Ntr\{[(A^{1/2}xW_x)(I_L)(A^{1/2}xW_x)^T]\} - \\ Ltr\{2[(W_x{}^T x^T A^{1/2})S'(A^{1/2}yW_y)]\} + L^2 tr\{[(S')^T S']\}) \\ = min(-Ltr\{2[(W_x{}^T x^T A^{1/2})S'(A^{1/2}yW_y)]\} + LN^2 + \\ L^2 tr\{[(S')^T S']\}) \end{array} \tag{25}$$

where $tr()$ denotes the trace of a matrix. Since LN^2 and $L^2tr\{[(S')^TS']\}$ are const, Eq. (25) can be expressed as follows

$$\begin{array}{l} \max_{W_x,W_y} tr\{2[(W_x{}^T x^T A^{1/2})S'(A^{1/2}yW_y)]\} \\ s.t. \\ (A^{1/2}xW_x)^T A^{1/2}xW_x = NI_L \\ (A^{1/2}yW_y)^T A^{1/2}yW_y = NI_L \end{array} \tag{26}$$

After that, we apply the method of Lagrange multiplier to transform Eq. (26) into:

$$\begin{array}{l} J(W_x, W_y) = tr\{2[(W_x{}^T x^T A^{1/2})S'(A^{1/2}yW_y)]\} - \\ \frac{\lambda}{2}\{[(A^{1/2}xW_x)^T A^{1/2}xW_x) + (A^{1/2}yW_y)^T A^{1/2}yW_y] - 2NI_L\} \end{array} \tag{27}$$

Let

$$\frac{\partial J(W_x, W_y)}{\partial W_x} = 0 \tag{28}$$

and

$$\frac{\partial J(W_x, W_y)}{\partial W_y} = 0, \tag{29}$$

Equation (26) is further written as follows

$$\begin{bmatrix} 0 & R_{xy} \\ R_{yx} & 0 \end{bmatrix} W = \lambda \begin{bmatrix} R_{xx} & 0 \\ 0 & R_{yy} \end{bmatrix} W \tag{30}$$

where

$$R_{xx} = x^T A x, \tag{31}$$

$$R_{yy} = y^T A y, \tag{32}$$

$$R_{xy} = x^T A^{1/2} S' A^{1/2} y, \tag{33}$$

$$R_{yx} = R_{xy}{}^T, \tag{34}$$

$$W = \begin{bmatrix} W_x \\ W_y \end{bmatrix}. \tag{35}$$

Then, Eq. (30) can be solved as the generalized eigenvalue (GEV) problem. In summary of the discussion so far, the proposed multimodal hashing with discriminant canonical correlation maximization (MH-DCCM) algorithm is given below:

Algorithm 1 The Proposed MH-DCCM Algorithm

Require:

* Extracted data/information from multimodal sources to form the zero-mean sets x and y;

* Use the label information of samples from sets x and y to form A and S';

Ensure:

* Compute the matrixes R_{xx}, R_{yy}, R_{xy} and R_{yx}.

* Compute the eigenvalues and eigenvectors of Eq. (30).

return W_x and W_y.

---

3 Feature Extraction and Classification

In this section, the feature extraction and classification are presented in two applications ranging from multi-source information fusion in audio emotion recognition to multimodal information fusion in cross-modal (text-image) fusion.

3.1 Multi-source Information Fusion

Due to a special case of multimodal fusion, multi-source fusion utilizes different features extracted from the same modality data but with different extraction methods, highly likely carrying complementary information. Therefore, it would lead to better performance for different tasks.

Audio Emotion Recognition. Audio is one of the most essential and natural verbal channels to transmit human affective states and it is easily accessible for emotion recognition. Hence, the performance of audio emotion recognition has also been investigated by numerous works in the literature [13,14]. Currently, Prosodic and Mel-frequency cepstral coefficient (MFCC) are widely used in audio emotion recognition [15,16].

In this paper, the fusion of Prosodic and MFCC features is investigated. The two features are extracted as follows:

(a) 25-dimensional: Prosodic features used in [15].
(b) 65-dimensional: MFCC features (the mean, median, standard deviation, max, and range of the first 13 MFCC coefficients).

3.2 Multimodal Information Fusion

Multimodal information fusion refers to a process which achieves more reliable and robust analysis performance by integrating multimodal data sources [17]. It has drawn increasingly extensive interest in both research and industrial sectors, in a plethora of applications such as security and surveillance, video streaming, education and training, healthcare, and human computer interaction (HCI).

Cross-Modal (Text-Image) Fusion. In the paper, we extract the bag-of-visual SIFT feature vector from images [7] and Latent Dirichlet Allocation (LDA) feature vector from texts [18], which are shown as follows:

(c) 128-dimensional: bag-of-visual SIFT feature vector.
(d) 10-dimensional: Latent Dirichlet Allocation feature vector.

3.3 Classification

In this paper, we use the recognition algorithm proposed in [19], which can be written as follows:

Given two sets of features, represented by feature matrices

$$X^1 = [{x^1}_1, {x^1}_2, {x^1}_3, ...{x^1}_d] \tag{36}$$

and

$$X^2 = [{x^2}_1, {x^2}_2, {x^2}_3, ...{x^2}_d] \tag{37}$$

$dist[X^1 X^2]$ is defined as

$$dist[X^1 X^2] = \sum_{j=1}^{d} \|{x^1}_j - {x^2}_j\|_2 \tag{38}$$

where $\|a - b\|_2$ denotes the Euclidean distance between the two vectors a and b.

Let the feature matrices of the N training samples as $F_1, F_2, ...F_N$ and each sample belongs to some class C_i $(i = 1, 2...c)$, then for a given test sample I, if

$$dist[I, F_l] = \min_j dist[I, F_j](j = 1, 2...N) \tag{39}$$

and

$$F_l = C_i \tag{40}$$

the resulting decision is $I = C_i$.

4 Experimental Results and Analysis

To evaluate the effectiveness of the proposed discriminant multimodal hashing method, we implement experiments on Ryerson Multimedia Lab (RML) [15] and eNTERFACE (eNT) [16] audio emotion database for multi-source information fusion, and the Wiki dataset for cross-modal fusion, respectively.

4.1 Multi-source Fusion

The RML database consists of samples speaking six different languages (English, Mandarin, Urdu, Punjabi, Persian, and Italian) from eight subjects to express the six principal emotions-*angry, disgust, fear, surprise, sadness* and *happiness.* The audio samples are recorded at a sampling rate of 22050 Hz. The eNT database contains samples from 43 subjects, also expressing the six basic emotions, with a sampling rate of 48000 Hz for audio channel.

During the experiments, 456 audio samples of eight subjects from RML database and 456 audio samples of ten subjects from eNT database are utilized, respectively. Both of the audio samples are divided into training and testing subsets including 360 and 96 samples each. With the purpose of benchmark, the accuracy of utilizing Prosodic and MFCC features is first evaluated and tabulated in Table 1. The recognition accuracy is calculated as the ratio of the number of correctly classified samples over the total number of testing samples.

Table 1. Results of audio emotion recognition with the single feature

Database	Feature	Accuracy
RML	Prosodic	51.04%
RML	MFCC	37.50%
eNT	Prosodic	50.21%
eNT	MFCC	39.58%

To demonstrate the effectiveness of the proposed MH-DCCM method, the methods of Fisher Discriminant Analysis (FDA) [20], CCA [11], discriminant

CCA (DCCA) (a special case of DMCCA [5]), labeled CCA (LCCA) (a special case of LMCCA [21]), Semantic Correlation Maximization Multimodal Hashing (SCMMH) [7] with the same Prosodic and MFCC features, and deep learning based method Alexnet [22] are implemented on the same two datasets for comparison and the optimal accuracies are given in Tables 2 and 3, respectively.

Table 2. The optimal accuracy with different methods on RML database

Method	The optimal accuracy
FDA [20]	56.25%
CCA [11]	53.13%
DCCA [5]	63.54%
LCCA [21]	59.38%
SCMMH *(L = 32)* [7]	62.50%
Alexnet (Pre-trained) [22]	59.46%
Alexnet (Fine-tuned) [22]	66.17%
The proposed MH-DCCM method *(L = 32)*	**67.56%**

Table 3. The optimal accuracy with different methods on eNT database

Method	The optimal accuracy
FDA [20]	53.13%
CCA [11]	63.54%
DCCA [5]	67.71%
LCCA [21]	64.58%
SCMMH *(L = 32)* [7]	71.88%
Alexnet (Pre-trained) [22]	51.33%
Alexnet (Fine-tuned) [22]	78.08%
The proposed MH-DCCM method *(L = 32)*	**78.13%**

From Tables 2 and 3, it is observed that the performance of fusion methods is better than the single feature. Moreover, since the between-class correlation and within-class correlation are introduced to the proposed multimodal hashing method simultaneously, it outperforms the statistical machine learning based methods–CCA, DCCA, LCCA, SCMMH, and the deep learning based method.

4.2 Cross-Modal Fusion

For cross-modal (image-text) information fusion, we conduct experiments on the Wiki dataset. There are a total of 2866 documents which are image-text pairs and annotated with semantic labels of 10 categories. A random split was used to produce a training set of 2173 documents, and a test set of 693 documents.

As a benchmark, the performance of using the bag-of-visual SIFT feature vector and Latent Dirichlet Allocation feature vector is first evaluated shown in Table 4.

Table 4. Results of cross-modal fusion with the single feature

Database	Feature	Accuracy
Wiki	bag-of-visual SIFT	27.56%
Wiki	Latent Dirichlet Allocation	56.28%

To further demonstrate the effectiveness of the proposed discriminant multimodal hashing, comparison with CCA [11], discriminant CCA (DCCA) [5], labeled CCA (LCCA) [21], and Semantic Correlation Maximization Multimodal Hashing (SCMMH) [7], is conducted on the Wiki database for comparison and the optimal accuracies are tabulated in Table 5.

Table 5. The optimal accuracy with different methods on Wiki database

Method	The optimal accuracy
CCA [11]	58.73%
DCCA [5]	62.34%
LCCA [21]	61.62%
SCMMH *($L = 32$)* [7]	63.35%
The proposed MH-DCCM method *($L = 32$)*	**67.10%**

From the above experimental results, again, the accuracy of fusion methods is generally better than the single feature. On the other hand, clearly, the discriminant power of the proposed method provides a more effective modelling of the relationship between different features and cross-modal data, achieving better performance than the related methods.

5 Conclusions

In this paper, we have proposed an effective multimodal hashing with discriminant canonical correlation maximization method. The proposed method is applied to multi-source and multimodal information fusion problems in audio emotion recognition and cross-modal fusion. Benefiting from the discriminant power and semantic similarity across different modalities, it improves the final performance and achieves higher accuracy than the related methods.

References

1. Guan, L., Wang, Y., Zhang, R., Tie, Y., Bulzacki, A., Ibrahim, M.: Multimodal information fusion for selected multimedia applications. Int. J, Multimedia Intell. Secur. **1**(1), 5–32 (2010)
2. Balazs, J.A., Velsquez, J.D.: Opinion mining and information fusion: a survey. Inf. Fusion **27**, 95–110 (2016)
3. Ma, J., Ma, Y., Li, C.: Infrared and visible image fusion methods and applications: a survey. Inf. Fusion **45**, 153–178 (2019)
4. Suk, H.-I., Lee, S.-W.: A novel bayesian framework for discriminative feature extraction in brain-computer interfaces. IEEE Trans. Pattern Anal. Mach. Intell. **35**(2), 286–299 (2013)
5. Gao, L., Qi, L., Chen, E., Guan, L.: Discriminative multiple canonical correlation analysis forvinformation fusion. IEEE Trans. Image Process. **27**(4), 1951–1965 (2018)
6. Zhang, J.G., Huang, K.Q., et al.: Df2Net: a discriminative feature learning and fusion network for RGB-D indoor scene classification. In: 2018 AAAI, pp. 7041–7048 (2018)
7. Zhang, D., Li, W.-J.: Large-scale supervised multimodal hashing with semantic correlation maximization. In: 2014 AAAI, vol. 1, pp. 1–7 (2014)
8. Jin, L., Li, K., Hao, H., Qi, G.-J., Tang, J.: Semantic neighbor graph hashing for multimodal retrieval. IEEE Trans. Image Process. **27**(3), 1405–1417 (2018)
9. Tang, J., Li, Z.: Weakly supervised multimodalhashing forscalablesocial imageretrieval. IEEE Trans. Circuits Syst. Video Technol. **28**(10), 2730–2741 (2018)
10. Zhen, Y., Yeung, D.-Y.: A probabilistic model for multimodal hash function learning. In: Proceedings of the 18th ACM SIGKDD International Conference on Knowledge Discovery and Data Mining, pp. 940–948 (2012)
11. Wei, Y., et al.: Cross-modal retrieval with cnn visual features: a new baseline. IEEE Trans. Cybern. **47**(2), 449–460 (2017)
12. Torralba, A., Fergus, R., Weiss, Y.: Small codes and large image databases for recognition. In: 2008 CVPR, pp. 1–8 (2008)
13. Zeng, Z., Pantic, M., Roisman, G.I., Huang, T.S.: A survey of affect recognition methods: audio, visual, and spontaneous expressions. IEEE Trans. Pattern Anal. Mach. Intell. **31**(1), 39–58 (2009)
14. Wollmer, M., Kaiser, M., Eyben, F., Schuller, B.R., Rigoll, G.: LSTM-modeling of continuous emotions in an audio-visual affect recognition framework. Image Vis. Comput. **31**(2), 153–163 (2013)
15. Wang, Y., Guan, L.: Recognizing human emotional state from audiovisual signals. IEEE Trans. Multimedia **10**(5), 936–946 (2008)
16. Wang, Y., Guan, L., Venetsanopoulos, A.N.: Kernel cross-modal factor analysis for information fusion with application to bimodal emotion recognition. IEEE Trans. Multimedia **14**(3), 597–607 (2012)
17. Zeshui, X., Zhao, N.: Information fusion for intuitionistic fuzzy decision making: an overview. Inf. Fusion **28**, 10–23 (2016)
18. Blei, D.M., Ng, A.Y., Jordan, M.I.: Latent dirichlet allocation. J. Mach. Learn. Res. **3**, 993–1022 (2003)
19. Shekar, B.H., Sharmila Kumari, M., Mestetskiy, L.M., Dyshkant, N.F.: Face recognition using kernel entropy component analysis. Neurocomputing **74**(6), 1053–1057 (2011)

20. Cho, S., Jiang, J.: Optimal fault classification using fisher discriminant analysis in the parity space for applications to NPPs. IEEE Trans. Nucl. Sci. **65**(3), 856–865 (2018)
21. Gao, L., Zhang, R., Qi, L., Chen, E., Guan, L.: The labeled multiple canonical correlation analysis for information fusion. IEEE Trans. Multimedia **21**(2), 375–387 (2019)
22. Zhang, S., Zhang, S., Huang, T., Gao, W., Tian, Q.: Learning affective features with a hybrid deep model for audio-visual emotion recognition. IEEE Trans. Circuits Syst. Video Technol. **28**(10), 3030–3043 (2018)

Unsupervised Variational Learning of Finite Generalized Inverted Dirichlet Mixture Models with Feature Selection and Component Splitting

Kamal Maanicshah[1(✉)], Samr Ali[2], Wentao Fan[3], and Nizar Bouguila[1]

[1] Concordia Institute for Information Systems Engineering, Concordia University, Montreal, Quebec H3G 1M8, Canada
k_mathin@encs.concordia.ca, nizar.bouguila@concordia.ca

[2] Department of Electrical and Computer Engineering, Concordia University, Montreal, Quebec H3G 1M8, Canada
al_samr@encs.concordia.ca

[3] College of Computer Science and Technology, Huaqiao University, Xiamen 361021, Fujian, China
fwt@hqu.edu.cn

Abstract. Variational learning of mixture models has proved to be effective in recent research. In this paper, we propose a generalized inverted Dirichlet based mixture model with an incremental variational algorithm. We incorporate feature selection and a component splitting approach for model selection within the variational framework. This helps us estimate the complexity of the data efficiently concomitantly eliminating the irrelevant features. We validate our model with two challenging applications; image categorization and dynamic texture categorization.

Keywords: Unsupervised learning · Generalized inverted Dirichlet · Variational learning · Component splitting · Feature selection

1 Introduction

Image analysis plays a pivotal role in making crucial decisions, such as in industrial automation involving computer vision. Clustering images from different categories is an essential task in image analysis as it helps to learn the underlying patterns in the data. One of the best known methods for clustering is mixture models [11]. The basic idea of a mixture model is to estimate the parameters of a mixture of distributions that closely represent the data. Gaussian Mixture Models (GMM) have been used in the industry for many practical applications for some time now. However, not all data can be represented by Gaussian distributions. For example, proportional data can be better modeled by generalized

F. Karray et al. (Eds.): ICIAR 2019, LNCS 11663, pp. 94–105, 2019.
https://doi.org/10.1007/978-3-030-27272-2_8

inverted Dirichlet (GID) mixture models [2,3]. The efficiency of the models presented in these papers motivates us to explore more possibilities with generalized inverted Dirichlet mixture models.

When it comes to building a mixture model, the method we use to estimate the parameters of the model plays an phenomenal role. The most common method used is the maximum likelihood estimation (MLE) as in [4]. However, the MLE based Expectation Maximization (EM) algorithms can get stuck in global minima which leads to a wrong estimate of the parameters. An alternative is using the Bayesian approach [13], but this method is computationally expensive and convergence is not guaranteed. Variational estimation on the other hand may be used with a guarantee to converge. In our work we use the variational estimation method proposed in [10]. This paper also explores the idea of using a method called component splitting which involves splitting a component based on a split criteria. This solves the problem of model selection. The added advantage of this method is that it happens within the variational framework.

It is a well known fact that, given a dataset, not all the features contribute to the clustering process. This makes feature selection a very important process in model design. We also incorporate the feature selection process within the variational learning framework for increased efficiency. One such algorithm is presented in [5]. The model built this way offers very good flexibility and provides a better fit to the data. Since both model selection and feature selection are done within the same algorithm it saves much of the computational time. This is the approach we use in this paper. We validate the efficiency of our proposed model with two challenging applications; image and dynamic texture clustering.

The rest of the paper is organized as follows: the statistical model is introduced in Sect. 2, the variational approach is described in Sect. 3, the experimental results are outlined in Sect. 4 and Sect. 5 concludes the paper.

2 The Mathematical Model

Assume we have a set $\mathcal{Y}$ of N random positive vectors, $\mathcal{Y} = (\boldsymbol{Y}_1; \boldsymbol{Y}_2, ..., \boldsymbol{Y}_N)$ having D dimensions such that $\boldsymbol{Y}_i = (Y_{i1}, Y_{i2}, ..., Y_{iD})$. If we consider each vector to be drawn from a mixture of M GID distributions, then the probability density function apropos to the jth component is given by:

$$p(\boldsymbol{Y}_i \mid \boldsymbol{\alpha}_j, \boldsymbol{\beta}_j) = \prod_{d=1}^{D} \frac{\Gamma(\alpha_{jd} + \beta_{jd})}{\Gamma(\alpha_{jd})\Gamma(\beta_{jd})} \frac{Y_{id}^{\alpha_{jd}-1}}{\left(1 + \sum_{l=1}^{d} Y_{il}\right)^{\gamma_{id}}} \tag{1}$$

where, $\boldsymbol{\alpha} = (\boldsymbol{\alpha}_1, \boldsymbol{\alpha}_2, ..., \boldsymbol{\alpha}_M)$ with $\boldsymbol{\alpha}_j = (\alpha_{j1}, \alpha_{j2}, ..., \alpha_{jD})$, $\boldsymbol{\beta} = (\boldsymbol{\beta}_1, \boldsymbol{\beta}_2, ..., \boldsymbol{\beta}_M)$ with $\boldsymbol{\beta}_j = (\beta_{j1}, \beta_{j2}, ..., \beta_{jD})$ and $\gamma_{jd} = \beta_{jd} + \alpha_{jd} - \beta_{j(d+1)}$ represent the mixture parameters of the GID distribution such that, $\alpha_{jd} > 0$ and $\beta_{jd} > 0$. If $\boldsymbol{\pi} = (\pi_1, \pi_2, ..., \pi_j)$ indicates the mixing coefficients of the M components then, the mixture model is given by:

$$p(\boldsymbol{Y}_i \mid \boldsymbol{\pi}, \boldsymbol{\alpha}, \boldsymbol{\beta}) = \sum_{j=1}^{M} \pi_j p(\boldsymbol{Y}_i \mid \boldsymbol{\alpha}_j, \boldsymbol{\beta}_j) \tag{2}$$

It is to be noted that all elements of $\boldsymbol{\pi}$ must be positive and sum to one. Now, as proved in [2], we can factorize GID distribution as a product of inverted beta distribution since it does not change the underlying model. So, Eq. 2 can be represented as:

$$p(\mathcal{X} \mid \pi, \alpha, \beta) = \prod_{i=1}^{N} \left(\sum_{j=1}^{M} \pi_j \prod_{l=1}^{D} p_{iBeta}(X_{il} \mid \alpha_{jl}, \beta_{jl}) \right) \tag{3}$$

Where, $p_{iBeta}(X_{il} \mid \alpha_{jl}, \beta_{jl})$ depends on parameters, α_{jl} and β_{jl} and is given by:

$$p_{iBeta}(X_{il} \mid \alpha_{jl}, \beta_{jl}) = \frac{\Gamma(\alpha_{jl} + \beta_{jl})}{\Gamma(\alpha_{jl})\Gamma(\beta_{jl})} \frac{X_{il}^{\alpha_{jl}-1}}{(1 + X_{il})^{\alpha_{jl}+\beta_{jl}}} \tag{4}$$

with $\mathcal{X} = (X_1, X_2, ..., X_N)$ where $\boldsymbol{X}_i = (X_{i1}, X_{i2}, ..., X_{iD})$, $X_{i1} = Y_{i1}$ and $X_{il} = \frac{Y_{il}}{1+\sum_{k=1}^{l-1} Y_{ik}}$ for $l > 1$. Next, we construct a latent variable, $\mathcal{Z}$ given by $\mathcal{Z} = (\boldsymbol{Z}_1, \boldsymbol{Z}_2, ..., \boldsymbol{Z}_N)$ with $\boldsymbol{Z}_i = (Z_{i1}, Z_{i2}, ..., Z_{iM})$ that follows the constraints, $Z_{ij} \epsilon \{0, 1\}$, and $\sum_{j=1}^{M} Z_{ij} = 1$. This is the indicator matrix defined by $Z_{ij} = 1$ if $\boldsymbol{X}_i$ belongs to component j and 0 if not. Based on this, we can write $p(\mathcal{Z} \mid \boldsymbol{\pi}) = \prod_{i=1}^{N} \prod_{j=1}^{M} \pi_j^{Z_{ij}}$.

Moreover, feature selection is an essential process in a mixture model as some features in the data do not necessarily have importance in clustering. The performance of the model is better when these features are removed. In our work we use the approach proposed in [5] where we approximate the irrelevant features by considering a distribution over it. Hence, the features follow the following distribution:

$$p(X_{il} \mid \phi_{il}, \alpha_{il}, \beta_{il}, \lambda_l, \tau_l) \simeq \big(iBeta(X_{il} \mid \alpha_{jl}, \beta_{jl})\big)^{\phi_{il}} \big(iBeta(X_{il} \mid \lambda_l, \tau_l)\big)^{1-\phi_{il}} \tag{5}$$

Here, $\phi_{il} = 0$ if feature l is irrelevant for j^{th} and 1 if relevant. In our case we consider the irrelevant features to follow an inverted beta distribution $iBeta(X_{il} \mid \lambda_l, \tau_l)$. Since ϕ_{il} is a binary latent variable we can write the prior distribution of $\boldsymbol{\phi}$ as:

$$p(\boldsymbol{\phi} \mid \epsilon) = \prod_{i=1}^{N} \prod_{l=1}^{D} \epsilon_{l_1}^{\phi_{il}} \epsilon_{l_2}^{1-\phi_{il}} \tag{6}$$

where, $\epsilon_{l_1} = p(\phi_{il} = 1)$ and $\epsilon_{l_2} = p(\phi_{il} = 0)$ since ϕ_{il} is a Bernoulli variable. $\boldsymbol{\epsilon} = (\epsilon_1, \epsilon_2, ...\epsilon_D)$ represent the probabilities that the features are relevant or not (i.e. feature saliencies), where $\boldsymbol{\epsilon}_l = (\epsilon_{l_1}, \epsilon_{l_2})$ and $\epsilon_{l_1} + \epsilon_{l_2} = 1$. In our model, the irrelevant features are modeled globally and model selection is done locally. For the local model selection we use the algorithm proposed in [6]. According to this algorithm, we initially start with two components and then we breakup the current set of components into two partitions. One is called *free components* and the other is called *fixed components*. The crux of the algorithm is that we consider the fixed components are already a better fit to the data and we only estimate the parameters for the remaining free components. For example, if we take $M - s$ to be the number of fixed components that represents the data very well, then we only estimate the parameters for s components to check if they give a better fit to the data. Let's say, $\boldsymbol{\pi}^* = \{\pi_j^*\}$ represents the mixing coefficients of the fixed components and $\boldsymbol{\pi} = \{\pi_j\}$ represents the mixing coefficients of the free components. These mixing coefficients claims the usual constraint that they are positive and $\sum_{j=1}^{s} \pi_j + \sum_{j=s+1}^{M} \pi_j^* = 1$. Based on this information we can write $p(\mathcal{Z} \mid \boldsymbol{\pi}, \boldsymbol{\pi}^*)$ as:

$$p(\mathcal{Z} \mid \boldsymbol{\pi}, \boldsymbol{\pi}^*) = \prod_{i=1}^{N} \left[\prod_{j=1}^{s} \pi_j^{Z_{ij}} \prod_{j=s+1}^{M} \pi_j^{*Z_{ij}} \right] \tag{7}$$

Following [6] we choose a non standard Dirichlet distribution as a prior for $\boldsymbol{\pi}_j^*$ which is given by:

$$p(\boldsymbol{\pi}^*) = (1 - \sum_{k=1}^{s} \pi_k)^{-M+s} \frac{\Gamma(\sum_{j=s+1}^{M} c_j)}{\prod_{j=s+1}^{M} \Gamma(c_j)} \prod_{j=s+1}^{M} (\frac{\pi_j^*}{1 - \sum_{k=1}^{s} \pi_k})^{c_j - 1} \tag{8}$$

As a final step, we choose a prior distribution to model the parameters $\boldsymbol{\alpha}, \boldsymbol{\beta}, \boldsymbol{\lambda}$ and $\boldsymbol{\tau}$. Gamma distribution is a perfect choice as GID is also from an exponential family. Hence, assuming the parameters are independent we define the priors for the parameters as, $p(\boldsymbol{\alpha}) = \mathcal{G}(\boldsymbol{\alpha} \mid \boldsymbol{u}, \boldsymbol{\nu}), p(\boldsymbol{\beta}) = \mathcal{G}(\boldsymbol{\beta} \mid \boldsymbol{p}, \boldsymbol{q}), p(\boldsymbol{\lambda}) = \mathcal{G}(\boldsymbol{\lambda} \mid \boldsymbol{g}, \boldsymbol{h})$ and $p(\boldsymbol{\tau}) = \mathcal{G}(\boldsymbol{\tau} \mid \boldsymbol{s}, \boldsymbol{t})$, where $\mathcal{G}(\boldsymbol{x} \mid \boldsymbol{a}, \boldsymbol{b}) = \frac{b^a}{\Gamma(a)} x^{a-1} e^{-bx}$. All the hyperparameter vectors $\boldsymbol{u}, \boldsymbol{v}, \boldsymbol{p}, \boldsymbol{q}, \boldsymbol{g}, \boldsymbol{h}, \boldsymbol{s}$ and $\boldsymbol{t}$ are positive in the above equations. Summarizing all the unknown variables, we introduce $\Theta = \{\mathcal{Z}, \boldsymbol{\alpha}, \boldsymbol{\beta}, \boldsymbol{\lambda}, \boldsymbol{\tau}, \boldsymbol{\phi}, \boldsymbol{\pi}^*\}$. Now, the joint distribution is given by:

$$\begin{aligned}
p(\mathcal{X}, \Theta \mid \boldsymbol{\pi}, \boldsymbol{\epsilon}) =& p(\mathcal{X} \mid \mathcal{Z}, \boldsymbol{\alpha}, \boldsymbol{\beta}, \boldsymbol{\lambda}, \boldsymbol{\tau}, \boldsymbol{\phi}) p(\boldsymbol{\phi} \mid \boldsymbol{\epsilon}) p(Z \mid \boldsymbol{\pi}, \boldsymbol{\pi}^*) \\
& \times p(\boldsymbol{\pi}^* \mid \boldsymbol{\pi}) p(\boldsymbol{\alpha}) p(\boldsymbol{\beta}) p(\boldsymbol{\lambda}) p(\boldsymbol{\tau}) \\
=& \prod_{i=1}^{N} \prod_{j=1}^{M} \left\{ \prod_{l=1}^{D} \left[\frac{\Gamma(\alpha_{jl} + \beta_{jl})}{\Gamma(\alpha_{jl}) \Gamma(\beta_{jl})} \frac{X_{il}^{\alpha_{jl}-1}}{(1 + X_{il})^{\alpha_{jl}+\beta_{jl}}} \right]^{\phi_{il}} \right. \\
& \left. \times \left[\frac{\Gamma(\lambda_l + \tau_l)}{\Gamma(\lambda_l) \Gamma(\tau_l)} \frac{X_{il}^{\lambda_l - 1}}{(1 + X_{il})^{\lambda_l + \tau_l}} \right]^{1-\phi_{il}} \right\}^{Z_{ij}} \times \prod_{i=1}^{N} \prod_{l=1}^{D} \epsilon_{l_1}^{\phi_{il}} \epsilon_{l_2}^{1-\phi_{il}} \\
& \times \prod_{i=1}^{N} \left[\prod_{j=1}^{s} \pi_j^{Z_{ij}} \prod_{j=s+1}^{M} \pi_j^{*Z_{ij}} \right] \times \left(1 - \sum_{k=1}^{s} \pi_k \right)^{-M+s} \\
& \times \frac{\Gamma(\sum_{j=s+1}^{M} C_j)}{\prod_{j=s+1}^{M} \Gamma(C_j)} \prod_{j=s+1}^{M} \left(\frac{\pi_j^*}{1 - \sum_{k=1}^{s} \pi_k} \right)^{C_j - 1} \\
& \times \frac{\nu_{jl}^{u_{jl}}}{\Gamma(u_{jl})} \alpha_{jl}^{u_{jl}-1} e^{-\nu_{jl}\alpha_{jl}} \times \frac{q_{jl}^{p_{jl}}}{\Gamma(p_{jl})} \beta_{jl}^{p_{jl}-1} e^{-q_{jl}\beta_{jl}} \\
& \times \frac{h_l^{g_l}}{\Gamma(g_l)} \lambda_{jl}^{g_l - 1} e^{-h_l \lambda_l} \times \frac{t_l^{s_l}}{\Gamma(s_l)} \tau_l^{s_l - 1} e^{-t_l \tau_l}
\end{aligned} \tag{9}$$

Figure 1 shows the graphical model of the dependencies between the different parameters.

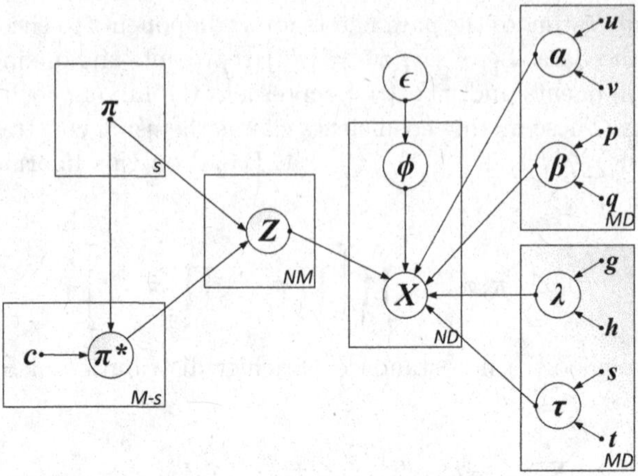

Fig. 1. Graphical representation of finite GID mixture model with feature selection and component splitting. The circles denote the random variables and the conditional dependencies between the variables are indicated by the arcs. The number in the bottom right corner of the platesindicates the dimension of the variables inside

3 Variational Learning

In this section we describe the variational learning approach that we use to estimate the parameters of the GID mixture model with feature selection and component splitting. The main drawback of the Bayesian approach is that the computation of $p(\Theta \mid \mathcal{X})$ is complex and is sometimes intractable. To overcome this problem, we use the variational approach as proposed in [7] where we determine the posterior probability by approximating another distribution $\mathcal{Q}(\Theta)$. We can say that two distributions are exactly equal if the Kulllback-Leibler (KL) divergence between the two distributions is equal to 0. The KL divergence between $\mathcal{Q}(\Theta)$ and the true posterior $p(\Theta \mid \mathcal{X})$ can be written as:

$$KL(\mathcal{Q} \mid\mid P) = -\int \mathcal{Q}(\Theta) \ln\left(\frac{p(\Theta \mid \mathcal{X}, \pi)}{\mathcal{Q}(\Theta)}\right) d\Theta = \ln\, p(\mathcal{X} \mid \pi) - \mathcal{L}(\mathcal{Q}) \quad (10)$$

This equation clearly shows that, $KL(\mathcal{Q} \mid\mid P)$ is equal to 0 when the lower bound $\mathcal{L}(\mathcal{Q}) = \int \mathcal{Q}(\Theta) \ln\left(\frac{p(\mathcal{X}, \Theta \mid \pi)}{\mathcal{Q}(\Theta)}\right) d\Theta$ is maximum. Since in our case the parameters are independent, by using mean field approximation [14] we can factorize $\mathcal{Q}(\Theta)$ as $\mathcal{Q}(\Theta) = \prod_k \mathcal{Q}_k(\Theta_k)$. This means, we maximize $\mathcal{L}(\mathcal{Q})$ with respect to each parameter $\mathcal{Q}_k(\Theta_k)$ whose general expression is given by:

$$\mathcal{Q}_k(\Theta_k) = \frac{exp\langle \ln\, p(\mathcal{X}, \Theta)\rangle_{\neq k}}{\int exp\langle \ln\, p(\mathcal{X}, \Theta)\rangle_{\neq k} d\Theta} \quad (11)$$

where $\langle . \rangle_{\neq k}$ is the expectation irrespective of Θ_k. Based on Eq. 11, we can write the variational solutions for our model as:

$$\mathcal{Q}(\mathcal{Z}) = \prod_{i=1}^{N} \left[\prod_{j=1}^{s} r_{ij}^{Z_{ij}} \prod_{j=s+1}^{M} r_{ij}^{*Z_{ij}} \right], \ \mathcal{Q}(\boldsymbol{\phi}) = \prod_{j=1}^{M} \prod_{l=1}^{D} f_{il}^{\phi_{il}} (1 - f_{il})^{1-\phi_{il}} \tag{12}$$

$$\mathcal{Q}(\boldsymbol{\pi}^*) = (1 - \sum_{k=1}^{s} \pi_k)^{-M+s} \frac{\Gamma(\sum_{j=s+1}^{M} c_j^*)}{\prod_{j=s+1}^{M} \Gamma(c_j^*)} \prod_{j=s+1}^{M} (\frac{\pi_j^*}{1 - \sum_{k=1}^{s} \pi_k})^{c_j^* - 1} \tag{13}$$

$$\mathcal{Q}(\boldsymbol{\alpha}) = \prod_{j=1}^{M} \prod_{l=1}^{D} \mathcal{G}(\alpha_{jl} \mid u_{jl}^*, \nu_{jl}^*), \ \mathcal{Q}(\boldsymbol{\beta}) = \prod_{j=1}^{M} \prod_{l=1}^{D} \mathcal{G}(\beta_{jl} \mid p_{jl}^*, q_{jl}^*) \tag{14}$$

$$\mathcal{Q}(\boldsymbol{\lambda}) = \prod_{l=1}^{D} \mathcal{G}(\lambda_l \mid g_l^*, h_l^*), \ \mathcal{Q}(\boldsymbol{\tau}) = \prod_{l=1}^{D} \mathcal{G}(\tau_l \mid s_l^*, t_l^*) \tag{15}$$

provided,

$$r_{ij} = \frac{\tilde{r}_{ij}}{\sum_{j=1}^{s} \tilde{r}_{ij} + \sum_{j=s+1}^{M} \tilde{r}_{ij}^*}, \ r_{ij}^* = \frac{\tilde{r}_{ij}^*}{\sum_{j=1}^{s} \tilde{r}_{ij} + \sum_{j=s+1}^{M} \tilde{r}_{ij}^*} \tag{16}$$

$$\ln \tilde{r}_{ij} = \ln \pi_j + \sum_{l=1}^{D} \Bigg\{ \langle \phi_{il} \rangle \Big[\tilde{\mathcal{R}}_{jl} + (\overline{\alpha}_{jl} - 1) \ln X_{il} - (\overline{\alpha}_{jl} + \overline{\beta}_{jl}) \ln (1 + X_{il}) \Big]$$
$$+ \langle 1 - \phi_{il} \rangle \Big[\tilde{\mathcal{F}}_l + (\overline{\lambda}_l - 1) \ln X_{il} - (\overline{\lambda}_l + \overline{\tau}_{jl}) \ln (1 + X_{il}) \Big] \Bigg\} \tag{17}$$

$$\ln \tilde{r}_{ij}^* = \langle \ln \pi_j^* \rangle + \sum_{l=1}^{D} \Bigg\{ \langle \phi_{il} \rangle \Big[\tilde{\mathcal{R}}_{jl} + (\overline{\alpha}_{jl} - 1) \ln X_{il} - (\overline{\alpha}_{jl} + \overline{\beta}_{jl}) \ln (1 + X_{il}) \Big]$$
$$+ \langle 1 - \phi_{il} \rangle \Big[\tilde{\mathcal{F}}_l + (\overline{\lambda}_l - 1) \ln X_{il} - (\overline{\lambda}_l + \overline{\tau}_{jl}) \ln (1 + X_{il}) \Big] \Bigg\} \tag{18}$$

$$c_j^* = \sum_{i=1}^{N} r_{ij}^* + c_j, \quad f_{il} = \frac{f_{il}^{(\phi_{il})}}{f_{il}^{(\phi_{il})} + f_{il}^{(1-\phi_{il})}} \tag{19}$$

$$f_{il}^{(\phi_{il})} = exp \Bigg\{ \langle \ln \epsilon_{l_1} \rangle + \sum_{j=1}^{M} \langle Z_{ij} \rangle \Big[\tilde{\mathcal{R}}_{jl} + (\overline{\alpha}_{jl} - 1) \ln X_{il} - (\overline{\alpha}_{jl} + \overline{\beta}_{jl}) \ln (1 + X_{il}) \Big] \Bigg\} \tag{20}$$

$$f_{il}^{(1-\phi_{il})} = exp \Bigg\{ \langle \ln \epsilon_{l_2} \rangle + \Big[\tilde{\mathcal{F}}_l + (\overline{\lambda}_l - 1) \ln X_{il} - (\overline{\lambda}_l + \overline{\tau}_l) \ln (1 + X_{il}) \Big] \Bigg\} \tag{21}$$

$$\begin{aligned}\tilde{\mathcal{R}} =& \ln\frac{\Gamma(\overline{\alpha}+\overline{\beta})}{\Gamma(\overline{\alpha})\Gamma(\overline{\beta})} + \overline{\alpha}\big[\psi(\overline{\alpha}+\overline{\beta}) - \psi(\overline{\alpha})\big](\langle \ln\alpha\rangle - \ln\overline{\alpha}) \\ &+ \overline{\beta}\big[\psi(\overline{\alpha}+\overline{\beta}) - \psi(\overline{\beta})\big](\langle \ln\beta\rangle - \ln\overline{\beta}) \\ &+ 0.5\overline{\alpha}^2\big[\psi'(\overline{\alpha}+\overline{\beta}) - \psi'(\overline{\alpha})\big]\langle(\ln\alpha - \ln\overline{\alpha})^2\rangle \\ &+ 0.5\overline{\beta}^2\big[\psi'(\overline{\alpha}+\overline{\beta}) - \psi'(\overline{\beta})\big]\langle(\ln\beta - \ln\overline{\beta})^2\rangle \\ &+ \overline{\alpha}\overline{\beta}\psi'(\overline{\alpha}+\overline{\beta})(\langle \ln\alpha\rangle - \ln\overline{\alpha})(\langle \ln\beta\rangle - \ln\overline{\beta}) \end{aligned} \tag{22}$$

$$\begin{aligned}\tilde{\mathcal{F}} =& \ln\frac{\Gamma(\overline{\lambda}+\overline{\tau})}{\Gamma(\overline{\lambda})\Gamma(\overline{\tau})} + \overline{\lambda}\big[\psi(\overline{\lambda}+\overline{\tau}) - \psi(\overline{\lambda})\big](\langle \ln\lambda\rangle - \ln\overline{\lambda}) \\ &+ \overline{\tau}\big[\psi(\overline{\lambda}+\overline{\tau}) - \psi(\overline{\tau})\big](\langle \ln\tau\rangle - \ln\overline{\tau}) \\ &+ 0.5\overline{\lambda}^2\big[\psi'(\overline{\lambda}+\overline{\tau}) - \psi'(\overline{\tau})\big]\langle(\ln\lambda - \ln\overline{\lambda})^2\rangle \\ &+ 0.5\overline{\tau}^2\big[\psi'(\overline{\lambda}+\overline{\tau}) - \psi'(\overline{\tau})\big]\langle(\ln\tau - \ln\overline{\tau})^2\rangle \\ &+ \overline{\lambda}\overline{\tau}\,\psi'(\overline{\lambda}+\overline{\tau})(\langle \ln\lambda\rangle - \ln\overline{\lambda})(\langle \ln\tau\rangle - \ln\overline{\tau}) \end{aligned} \tag{23}$$

$$\begin{aligned}u_{jl}^* =& u_{jl} + \sum_{i=1}^{N}\langle Z_{ij}\rangle\langle\phi_{il}\rangle\overline{\alpha}_{jl}\Bigg[\psi(\overline{\alpha}_{jl}+\overline{\beta}_{jl}) - \psi(\overline{\alpha}_{jl}) \\ &+ \overline{\beta}_{jl}\psi'(\overline{\alpha}_{jl}+\overline{\beta}_{jl})(\langle \ln\beta_{jl}\rangle - \ln\overline{\beta}_{jl})\Bigg] \end{aligned} \tag{24}$$

$$\nu_{jl}^* = \nu_{jl} - \sum_{i=1}^{N}\langle Z_{ij}\rangle\langle\phi_{il}\rangle \ln\frac{X_{il}}{1+X_{il}} \tag{25}$$

Similar to the calculation of u_{jl}^* and ν_{jl}^* we can calculate the hyperparameters $p_{jl}^*, q_{jl}^*, g_l^*, h_l^*, s_l^*$ and t_l^* as well. $\psi(.)$ and $\psi'(.)$ denote the digamma and trigamma functions, in the equations above. $\tilde{\mathcal{R}}$ and $\tilde{\mathcal{F}}$ in Eqs. 22 and 23 are the taylor series approximation of $\mathcal{R} = \langle \ln\frac{\Gamma(\alpha+\beta)}{\Gamma(\alpha)\Gamma(\beta)}\rangle$ and $\mathcal{F} = \langle \ln\frac{\Gamma(\lambda+\tau)}{\Gamma(\lambda)\Gamma(\tau)}\rangle$ since these equations are intractable [2]. The expected values mentioned in the equations above are given by:

$$\langle Z_{ij}\rangle = \begin{cases} r_{ij}, & \text{for } j = 1, ..., s \\ r_{ij}^*, & \text{for } j = s+1, ..., M \end{cases} \tag{26}$$

$$\overline{\alpha}_{jl} = \frac{u_{jl}^*}{\nu_{jl}^*},\ \langle \ln\alpha_{jl}\rangle = \psi(u_{jl}^*) - \ln\nu_{jl}^* \tag{27}$$

$$\langle(\ln\alpha_{jl} - \ln\overline{\alpha}_{jl})^2\rangle = \big[\psi(u_{jl}^*) - \ln u_{jl}^*\big]^2 + \psi'(u_{jl}^*) \tag{28}$$

$$\langle\phi_{il}\rangle = f_{il},\ \langle 1-\phi_{il}\rangle = 1 - f_{il} \tag{29}$$

$$\langle \pi_j^* \rangle = \left(1 - \sum_{k=1}^{s} \pi_k\right) \frac{\sum_{i=1}^{N} r_{ij}^* + c_j}{\sum_{i=1}^{N} \sum_{k=s+1}^{M} r_{ik}^* + c_k} \tag{30}$$

$$\langle \ln \pi_j^* \rangle = \ln\left(1 - \sum_{k=1}^{s} \pi_k\right) + \psi\left(\sum_{i=1}^{N} r_{ij}^* + c_j\right) - \psi\left(\sum_{i=1}^{N} \sum_{k=s+1}^{M} r_{ik}^* + c_k\right) \tag{31}$$

We can derive similar equations like in 27 and 28, for $\boldsymbol{\beta}, \boldsymbol{\lambda}$ and $\boldsymbol{\tau}$. π_j^* and π_j depend on each other and similarly for ϵ_{l_1} and ϵ_{l_2}. Hence, we equate the lower bound with respect to π_j and ϵ_{l_1} to zero to get:

$$\pi_j = \left(1 - \sum_{k=s+1}^{M} \langle \pi_k^* \rangle\right) \frac{\sum_{i=1}^{N} r_{ij}}{\sum_{i=1}^{N} \sum_{k=1}^{s} r_{ik}}, \quad \epsilon_{l_1} = \frac{1}{N} \sum_{i=1}^{N} f_{il} \tag{32}$$

According to our algorithm, the irrelevant features will have lower probabilities and hence will not be used in the clustering process. These features are eliminated in the learning process which increases the efficiency of the clustering algorithm. The model selection method using component splitting approach on the other hand follows a unique algorithm where we split a component pertaining to the relevant features into two called the free components. The remaining components are called the fixed components. We then run the variational algorithm on the free components locally without modifying the fixed components. At convergence, one of the three things might happen: (1) Both the components might have significant mixing coefficient and hence the new approximation is a better fit to the data. So the split is a success and both the components are retained. The algorithm starts splitting the new set of components from the beginning again. (2) Only one of the components is retained and the other is insignificant, i.e. the corresponding mixing coefficient fades out closer to 0. In this case the split test is a failure and the algorithm moves to split the next component. (3) The mixing weights of both the new components fades out to 0 which means they are redundant. We do not allow this split as it will lead to an infinite loop. It is obvious that the data should have more than one component for this idea to work. So we check this condition first. The algorithm stops when all the components in the current set fails the splitting test. The efficiency of the model lies in the fact that the model selection approach is applied only to the components of the relevant features which saves time.

4 Experimental Results

To evaluate our model we use two challenging datasets; the dynamic texture dataset (Dyntex) [15] and the Corel 10K dataset[1] for image categorization. We compare the results of our proposed variational GID mixture model (*varGIDMM*) with the standard benchmark of Gaussian mixture models based on maximum likelihood estimation (*GMM*) and variational approximation

[1] http://www.ci.gxnu.edu.cn/cbir/Dataset.aspx.

(*varGMM*). The initial values of the hyperparameters u, p, g, s and c is set to 1, that of ν and q is set to be 0.09 and that of h and t is set to be 0.06. These initiations were found to give the best results in our experiments.

4.1 Image Clustering

There has been a huge increase in the amount of images generated in recent years. With the increase in the volume of images, the need to categorize them based on analyzed patterns has been on the rise as well. Clustering the images hence plays a predominant role in categorizing the images. The efficiency of the use of bag of visual words features [8] is also imminent in recent years. To get the bag of visual words we first have to extract feature descriptors (scale invariant feature transform (SIFT) [12], histogram of Gaussians (HOG) [9], Speeded-up robust features (SURF) [1], etc.) from the images. We then use k-means clustering on the extracted descriptors with the k value indicating the number of features. The Corel 10K dataset which we choose for our application has about a 100 classes with 100 images per class. We choose 7 image classes from them corresponding to "Playing Cards", "Dolls", "Steam Tractors", "Paintings", "Easter Eggs", "Beads" and "Dinosaurs". Sample images from the dataset are shown in Fig. 2. It is to be noted that the use of seven categories is ease of representation. In our case we first extract SIFT feature descriptors from the images as it is found to give better results and then generate bag of visual words features from the descriptors. We feed this data as input to our model. The Confusion matrix pertaining to our model is shown in Fig. 3. Table 1 shows the accuracy of different models compared with ours. It clearly shows that our model outperforms *GMM* models by a large margin.

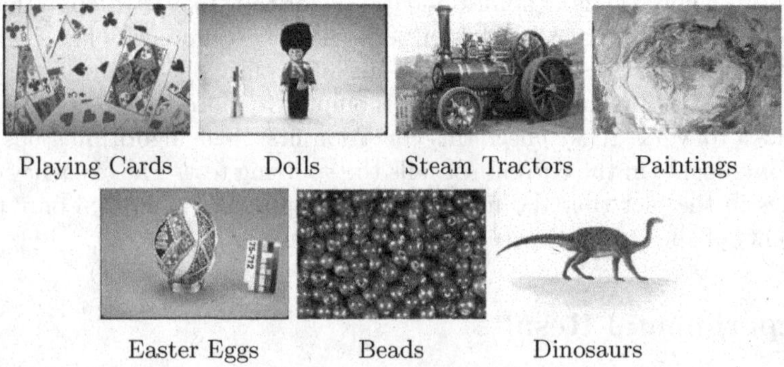

Fig. 2. Sample images from different categories of Corel 10K dataset

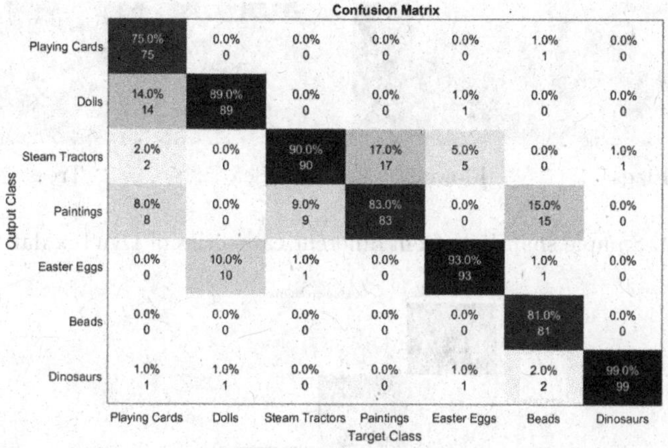

Fig. 3. Confusion matrix of Corel 10K dataset with varGIDMM

Table 1. Accuracy of different models on Corel 10K dataset

Method	Accuracy (%)
varGIDMM	87.41
varGMM	60.42
GMM	57.42

4.2 Dynamic Texture Clustering

Dynamic textures refers to textures in the temporal dimension. For example, videos of burning fire, turbulence, sea waves, etc. Dynamic textures play an important role in various applications such as dynamic background subtraction, video completion, etc. Hence clustering them is of prime importance as well. In the case of dynamic textures extracting local binary pattern (LBP) features makes more sense because LBP mainly divides an image into cells and constructs a histogram of features by comparing each cell with its neighboring cells. In our experiment we use 4 classes from the DynTex dataset, which are: Flags, Flowers, Sea and Trees. Examples of the four classes are shown in Fig. 4. We extract LBP features from each frame of every video in a class. This is used as input to our model. The confusion matrix indicating the results obtained with our model is shown in Fig. 5. The accuracy of the different models is shown in Table 2. The results show that the *varGIDMM* is better than the *GMM* models. Based on the number of frames assigned to a particular cluster we can predict to which cluster the video belongs to.

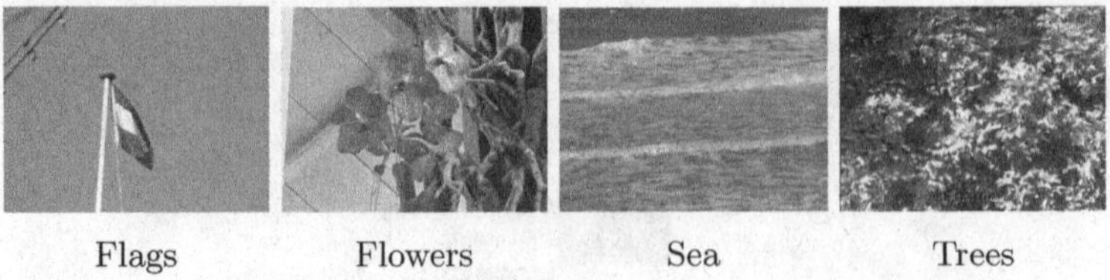

Fig. 4. Sample snapshots from different categories of DynTex dataset

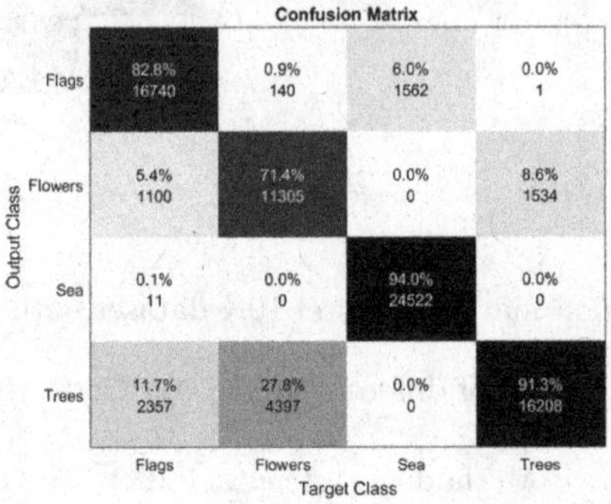

Fig. 5. Confusion matrix of DynTex dataset with varGIDMM

Table 2. Accuracy of different models on DynTex dataset

Method	Accuracy (%)
varGIDMM	86.10
varGMM	84.42
GMM	84.87

5 Conclusion

This article proposed an unsupervised learning approach using $GIDMM$ with feature selection and model selection. Using component splitting as a model selection method hand in hand with the feature selection process has proved to improve the efficiency of our algorithm as indicated by the results. Our model performed better than the GMM models by a large margin of over 25% in image categorization. The results with dynamic texture categorization also shows that our model is significantly better than the standard GMM models. The performance of the model is encouraging and can be applied to many other applications such as image segmentation and video categorization.

Acknowledgement. The completion of this research was made possible thanks to the Natural Sciences and Engineering Research Council of Canada (NSERC) and Concordia University Research Chair Tier 2.

References

1. Bay, H., Ess, A., Tuytelaars, T., Gool, L.V.: Speeded-up robust features (surf). Comput. Vis. Image Underst. **110**(3), 346–359 (2008). Similarity Matching in Computer Vision and Multimedia
2. Bdiri, T., Bouguila, N., Ziou, D.: Variational bayesian inference for infinite generalized inverted dirichlet mixtures with feature selection and its application to clustering. Appl. Intell. **44**(3), 507–525 (2016)
3. Bouguila, N., Mashrgy, M.A.: An infinite mixture model of generalized inverted dirichlet distributions for high-dimensional positive data modeling. In: Linawati, M.M.S., Neuhold, E.J., Tjoa, A.M., You, I. (eds.) Information and Communication Technology, ICT-EurAsia. Lecture Notes in Computer Science, vol. 8407, pp. 296–305. Springer, Heidelberg (2014). https://doi.org/10.1007/978-3-642-55032-4_29
4. Bouguila, N., Ziou, D., Vaillancourt, J.: Unsupervised learning of a finite mixture model based on the dirichlet distribution and its application. IEEE Tran. Image Process. **13**, 1533–1543 (2004)
5. Boutemedjet, S., Bouguila, N., Ziou, D.: A hybrid feature extraction selection approach for high-dimensional non-gaussian data clustering. IEEE Trans. Pattern Anal. Mach. Intell. **31**(8), 1429–1443 (2009)
6. Constantinopoulos, C., Likas, A.: Unsupervised learning of gaussian mixtures based on variational component splitting. IEEE Trans. Neural Networks **18**(3), 745–755 (2007)
7. Corduneanu., A., Bishop, C.M.: Variational Bayesian model selection for mixture distributions. In: Proceedings Eighth International Conference on Artificial Intelligence and Statistics (2001)
8. Csurka, G., Dance, C.R., Fan, L., Willamowski, J., Bray, C.: Visual categorization with bags of keypoints (2004)
9. Dalal, N., Triggs, B.: Histograms of oriented gradients for human detection. In: Proceedings IEEE Computer Society Conference Computer Vision and Pattern Recognition (CVPR 2005), vol. 1, pp. 886–893, June 2005
10. Fan, W., Bouguila, N.: A variational component splitting approach for finite generalized dirichlet mixture models. In: 2012 International Conference on Communications and Information Technology (ICCIT), pp. 53–57, June 2012
11. Fan, W., Bouguila, N.: Variational learning of a dirichlet process of generalized dirichlet distributions for simultaneous clustering and feature selection. Pattern Recogn. **46**(10), 2754–2769 (2013)
12. Lowe, D.G.: Distinctive image features from scale-invariant keypoints. Int. J. Comput. Vis. **60**(2), 91 (2004)
13. Ma, Z., Leijon, A.: Bayesian estimation of beta mixture models with variational inference. IEEE Trans. Pattern Anal. Mach. Intell. **33**(11), 2160–2173 (2011)
14. Opper, M., Saad, D.: Tutorial on Variational Approximation Methods. Neural Information Processing. Institute of Technology Press, Cambridge (2001)
15. Péteri, R., Fazekas, S., Huiskes, M.J.: DynTex: a comprehensive database of dynamic textures. Pattern Recogn. Lett. **31**(12), 1627–1632 (2010)

TPUAR-Net: Two Parallel U-Net with Asymmetric Residual-Based Deep Convolutional Neural Network for Brain Tumor Segmentation

Mahmoud Khaled Abd-Ellah[1], Ashraf A. M. Khalaf[2], Ali Ismail Awad[3,4](✉), and Hesham F. A. Hamed[2]

[1] Electronics and Communications Department, Al-Madina Higher Institute for Engineering and Technology, Giza, Egypt
eng_mahmoudkhaled@yahoo.com

[2] Faculty of Engineering, Minia University, Minia, Egypt
ashkhalaf@yahoo.com, hfah66@yahoo.com

[3] Department of Computer Science, Electrical and Space Engineering, Luleå University of Technology, Luleå, Sweden
ali.awad@ltu.se

[4] Faculty of Engineering, Al-Azhar University, P.O. Box 83513, Qena, Egypt

Abstract. The utilization of different types of brain images has been expanding, which makes manually examining each image a labor-intensive task. This study introduces a brain tumor segmentation method that uses two parallel U-Net with an asymmetric residual-based deep convolutional neural network (TPUAR-Net). The proposed method is customized to segment high and low grade glioblastomas identified from magnetic resonance imaging (MRI) data. Varieties of these tumors can appear anywhere in the brain and may have practically any shape, contrast, or size. Thus, this study used deep learning techniques based on adaptive, high-efficiency neural networks in the proposed model structure. In this paper, several high-performance models based on convolutional neural networks (CNNs) have been examined. The proposed TPUAR-Net capitalizes on different levels of global and local features in the upper and lower paths of the proposed model structure. In addition, the proposed method is configured to use the skip connection between layers and residual units to accelerate the training and testing processes. The TPUAR-Net model provides promising segmentation accuracy using MRI images from the BRATS 2017 database, while its parallelized architecture considerably improves the execution speed. The results obtained in terms of Dice, sensitivity, and specificity metrics demonstrate that TPUAR-Net outperforms other methods and achieves the state-of-the-art performance for brain tumor segmentation.

Keywords: Brain tumor segmentation · Computer-aided diagnosis · MRI images · Deep learning · Convolutional neural networks · TPUAR-Net · Parallel U-Net

F. Karray et al. (Eds.): ICIAR 2019, LNCS 11663, pp. 106–116, 2019.
https://doi.org/10.1007/978-3-030-27272-2_9

1 Introduction

The American Cancer Society has announced that the number of people with brain malignancies in the United States alone expanded by 23,880 new instances and caused an estimated 16,830 deaths in 2018 [1]. While the most recognized tumors of the cerebrum are gliomas, they can be low-grade, resulting in long life expectancy, or high-grade, causing short life expectancy [2]. Furthermore, as announced by the National Brain Tumor Foundation (NBTF), the number of individuals who die from brain tumors in advanced nations has increase by 300% in recent decades [3,4].

While a few tumors, such as meningiomas, can be segmented relatively effortlessly, others, such as glioblastomas and gliomas, are significantly more difficult to segment. These tumors with edema form expanded tentacle-like structures that are frequently diffuse and have inadequate contrast, which makes segmentation challenging. Their borders are frequently ill-defined and difficult to differentiate from healthy tissues. Moreover, tumors can appear anyplace in the skull and can have unique shapes and sizes [5]. The objective of brain tumor segmentation is to identify the area and extent of the tumor regions. The segmentation is achievable by recognizing areas that differ from ordinary tissues.

In spite of the fact that medical surgery is the most widely recognized form of brain tumor treatment, manual investigation requires considerable time and effort by radiologists and different specialists who must identify, localize and classify tumors from magnetic resonance imaging (MRI) images. MRI images are rich sources of data for brain tumor treatment and analysis, and they possess a larger number of characteristics than do other imaging methods [6]. Brain tumor segmentation from MRI images can greatly enhance diagnosis, treatment, and growth rate predictions.

The literature includes some deep learning-based segmentation methods that have been introduced to enhance brain tumor diagnosis. Pereira et al. [7] introduced an automatic brain tumor segmentation system based on a convolutional neural network (CNN) that used intensity normalization as a preprocessing step. Later, Pereira et al. in [8] presented a hierarchical study of brain tumor segmentation using a fully convolutional network (FCN) and MRI histograms. In [9], automatic brain image segmentation was proposed for 2D and 3D MRI patches using a deep neural network. Xiao et al. [10] proposed a segmentation method that used a deep learning network-based classification approach. First, a stacked auto-encoder network was used to extract features from the input; then, image patches were classified to create a binary image map. Subsequently, a morphological filter was used to produce the segmented tumor.

Havaei et al. [2] presented a brain tumor segmentation method that used a CNN. They applied a two-pathway architecture to efficiently train the CNN using global and local details. Casamitjana et al. [11] proposed a 3D CNN that combined global and local details from three different architectures. Zhao et al. [12] combined a fully convolutional neural network with conditional random fields (CRF) to efficiently segment brain tumors; this model was trained in three stages. In [13], a fully automatic 2D method based on U-Net with a comprehensive data augmentation technique was proposed for brain tumor segmentation. Wang et al. [14] explored a 3D U-Net network for brain tumor segmentation that included upsampling and downsampling paths with shortcut connections between them.

In this study, a new network structure called two parallel U-Net with asymmetric residual-based deep convolutional neural network (TPUAR-Net) is proposed for brain tumor segmentation. It involves two asymmetric parallel paths. Each path consists of a U-Net and different residuals of a deep convolutional neural network (DCNN). The proposed structure uses a DCNN with modified U-Net submodels, residual units, batch normalization, parametric rectified linear unit (PReLU), and skip connections. The model considers both the local shape and the context of tumors. The proposed method overcomes the problem of performing pixel arrangements without considering local label dependencies.

TPUAR-Net uses redesigned U-Net units with residual units to overcome the vanishing gradient problem. The residual units use different levels of skip connections to generate different features levels, allowing the network to learn both low- and high-level features. Parallel paths are used to decrease the processing time, and they provide good generalization by adding local and global features that improve the overall model performance. Furthermore, a weighted-loss function is applied in which the weights are computed in a per image manner.

The remainder of this paper is structured as follows. The structure of the proposed TPUAR-Net model is shown in Sect. 2. The implementation and performance evaluation phases are demonstrated in Sect. 3. Finally, conclusions and future work are provided in Sect. 4.

2 TPUAR-Net Architecture

The proposed TPUAR-Net model consists of two parallel paths; each path has down-sampling and up-sampling units, skip connections, and several residual units. The outputs of the lower and upper paths are concatenated and input to the next cascaded path in the network. Figure 1 shows a block diagram of the proposed TPUAR-Net model. The sequence of processes that occur in the proposed structure are explained in detail in the Simulation Sect. 3. The input to the proposed model consists of labeled batches from five categories fused together: enhancing tumor, non-enhancing tumor, edema, necrosis, and everything else, as shown in Fig. 2.

2.1 Preprocessing

The database used in this study (BRATS 2017) contains 3D MRI volumes with different spacings in the three dimensions and low isotropic resolution. Segmentation is performed on each 2D image (slice) using different image modalities (FLAIR, T2, T1, and T1C). Therefore, patches with a size of 128×128 were generated. The patches were centered on the classified pixel. Slices bordered with 0 pixels were ignored by taking only the interior pixels. Each input was arranged to contain patches with the four modalities.

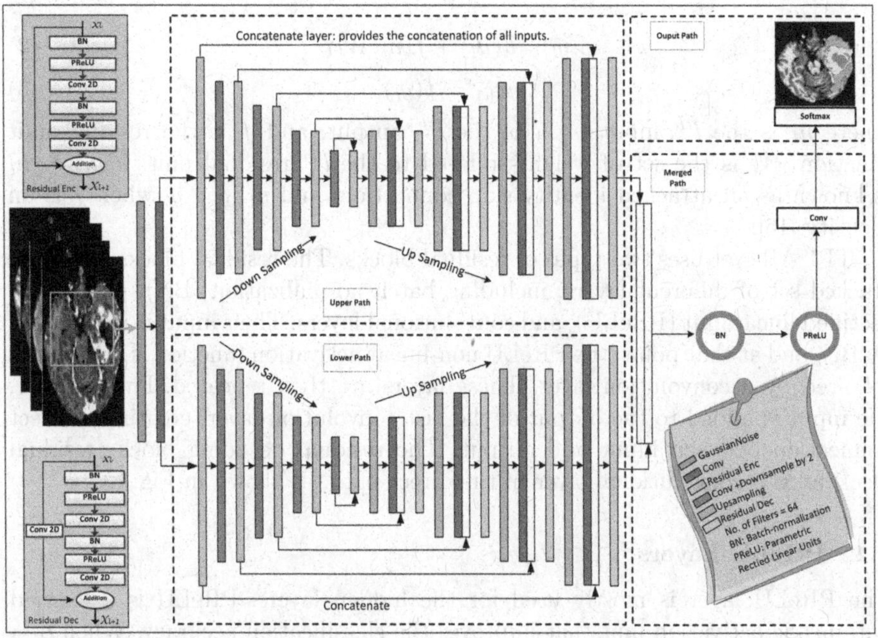

Fig. 1. A block diagram of the proposed TPARU-Net architecture for brain tumor segmentation.

2.2 Convolutional Layers

The main building block in the proposed TPUAR-Net architecture consists of convolutional layers. The input to each convolutional layer consists of the output of the previous layer, and the output feature maps (except for the input to first convolutional layer) are related to the number of modalities used. The feature plan calculation O_s is given in Eq. 1:

$$O_s = b_s + \sum_r W_{sr} * X_r, \tag{1}$$

where W_{sr} is the subkernel for the input channel, X_r is the rth input channel in the convolution sequence, and b_s is a bias term. A convolutional layer has the ability to learn the biases and weights of individual features that improve the data-driven, customized, and task-specific dense feature extractors.

2.3 Residual Blocks

The architecture contains many stacked residual blocks. Each residual block has a direct connection (skip connection) for propagating information, allowing it to propagate directly between blocks in both the forward and backward directions, as shown in Eqs. 2 and 3:

$$y_l = h(n_l) + f(n_l, W_l) \tag{2}$$

$$n_{l+1} = f(y_l), \tag{3}$$

where n_l is the lth input, n_{l+1} is the lth output, and f is the residual unit function. W_l is the set of weights related to the lth residual unit. $h(n_l) = n_l$ is known as an attached identity skip connection, and $n_{l+1} = y_l$ when f is an identity [15].

TPUAR-Net uses two types of residual blocks. The residual blocks contain a stacked set of different layers, including batch normalization (BN), parametric rectified linear unit (PReLU), and convolutional layers. Their input is normalized by BN, and at that point, the PReLU non-linear activation function is connected, followed by a convolution layer. These layers are then repeated. Furthermore, the input is added to the output of the last convolution layer, creating a direct connection between input and output. The residual decoding block (residual Dec.) adds a convolutional layer in the direct path, as shown in Fig. 1.

2.4 PReLU Layers

The PReLU layer is mostly used for the hidden layers. PReLU is a learned parametric activation unit that improves the classification accuracy. When $\alpha = 0$, this layer becomes a ReLU in which the input x and the output y are the same when input is greater than 0; otherwise, the output is equal to 0. When α is a learnable parameter, we refer to Eq. 4 as a PReLU operation, which requires only a small number of parameters [16]:

$$fy = \max(y, 0) + \alpha \min(y, 0). \tag{4}$$

2.5 Loss Function and Regularization

The loss function is characterized as the sum of the cross entropy for all the pixels in the image. Cross-entropy loss is used to measure the classification model performance, and it increases as the probability of the predicted label diverges from the true label as calculated in Eq. 5:

$$L_{ce}(y, \hat{y}) = y \log(\frac{y}{\hat{y}}) + (1 - y) \log(\frac{1 - y}{1 - \hat{y}}), \tag{5}$$

where $L_{ce}(y, \hat{y})$ is the cross entropy error between y (the desired output) and $\hat{y}$ (the predicted output) [17].

BN is used to regularize the values provided to the activation function and omit non-linearities as shown in Eq. 6. BN helps in training TPUAR-Net by smoothing the optimization plane, creating more stable gradients, faster optima, and making weight initialization easier due to the increased activation function viability. The regularization and weighted-loss functions prevent the network from becoming stuck in local minima and increase the model's performance:

$$\hat{x} = \frac{x - \mathrm{E}[x]}{\sqrt{\mathrm{Var}[x]}}, \tag{6}$$

where $\hat{x}$ represents the normalized activations, x is the layer input, $E[x]$ is the expected value, and $\mathrm{Var}[x]$ is the unbiased variance estimate [18]. Dropout is another regularization technique that randomly ignores selected neurons during training and prevents weight updating [8].

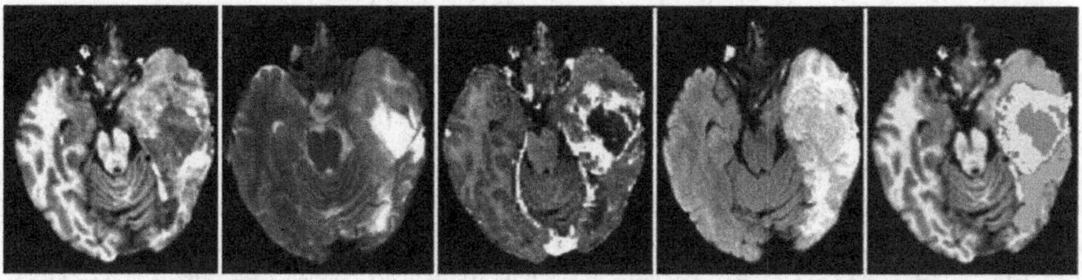

Fig. 2. The four MRI modalities are shown: from left to right, these are T1, T2, T1C, and FLAIR. These four modalities are used as inputs to the network. The last image shows the ground truth with Necrosis in ( ) color, Enhanced tumor in ( ) color, Nonenhanced tumor in ( ) color, and Edema in ( ) color. (Color figure online)

3 Simulation Experiments and Evaluation Metrics

The conducted simulation experiments are described in this section, and the evaluation process was applied using different metrics. The experimental method was created in Jupiter notebook and utilized the ipython, Tensorflow, and Keras toolkits. The proposed architecture was coded in Jupiter notebook utilizing the keras and Tensorflow toolkits. The computer was equipped with an Intel Core i7 processor running at 3.2 GHz, 24 GB of RAM, and an Ubuntu desktop 64-bit operating system.

3.1 Simulation Process and Scenario

The calculations and the sequence of the operations can be described as follows: Fused MRI image from the five different categories of images shown in Fig. 2 were prepared and provided as input to the model. Next, preprocessing was applied to reduce noise and enhance the image resolution. The two parallel calculation paths through the TPUAR-Net model were used to extract both local and global features from the input image. These features are accumulated and provided as the input to the remainder of the architecture.

Each of the upper and lower parallel paths contains both upsampling and downsampling processes with shortcut connections (skip connection) between them. Two different residual blocks were used in each of the upper and lower paths. One of the residual blocks is called the residual encoding block (Residual Enc.), and the other is called the residual decoding block (Residual Dec.). These blocks are shown on the far left side of Fig. 1.

Table 1. Distribution of images in the evaluation database.

		No. in training set		No. in testing set	
		HG	LG	HG	LG
BRATS 2017	No. of patients	60	40	50	20
	3D volume	240	160	200	80
	2D image	37200	24800	31000	12400
	Total 2D image	62000		43400	

A convolutional layer is applied after each residual block. The convolutional layer has a stride of 2 in the downsampling path. However, a standard convolutional layer is used in the upsampling path followed by an upsampling layer that duplicates the columns and rows of the data with a factor of 2. Then, the two parallel paths are merged by a concatenation layer, which takes a list of inputs with the same shape and returns a concatenation of all the inputs, providing one path, and a new cascaded path is launched until it reaches the segmented output. The merging path contains a BN layer connected to a PReLU layer and followed by a convolutional layer.

In the final stage of the output path, a fully connected layer with the softmax function is used to perform image classification. In the simulation, the architecture of the proposed model achieved accurate brain tumor segmentation from MRI images. The model addresses the pixelwise segmentation problem as a simple type of classification problem.

3.2 Input Dataset

The MRI image database used to evaluate the proposed tumor segmentation was extracted from the BRATS 2017 MRI database. The database consists of 75 low-grade (LG) and 210 high-grade (HG) patients with FLAIR, T2, T1, and T1C type MRI modalities. It was not possible to use the entire dataset because of the patch-per-pixel training strategy, which makes the dataset very large. Thus, a randomly selected number of patients were used for the training and testing datasets. The testing dataset was randomly selected from both LG and HG data. Table 1 lists the specifications for the training and testing databases, and a sample of the MRI images used in the experiments is shown in Fig. 2.

3.3 Evaluation Metrics

The system executed on the test set, and the predicted output was compared with the ground truth provided by expert radiologists. The tumor structures are grouped into 3 diverse tumor areas, largely due to convenient clinical applications. The tumor districts were characterized as complete tumors (including all types), core tumors (including all types except "edema"), and enhanced tumor

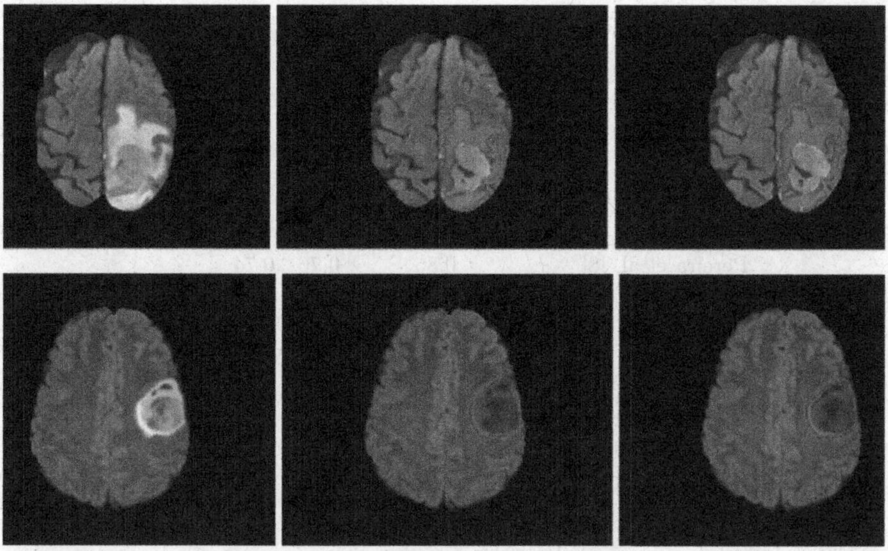

Fig. 3. Visual sample results from TPUAR-Net from the axial view. From left to right, the top row shows the FLAIR modality of an HG tumor, the ground truth, and the predicted image. The second row from left to right shows the FLAIR modality of an LG tumor, the ground truth, and the predicted image.

(including "the enhanced" images). We calculated the Dice, sensitivity and specificity metrics for all the tumor regions as shown in Eqs. 7, 8, and 9, respectively:

$$\textbf{Dice} = \frac{|P \cap T|}{(|P| + |T|)/2} \tag{7}$$

$$\textbf{Sensitivity} = \frac{|P \cap T|}{|T|} \tag{8}$$

$$\textbf{Specificity} = \frac{|P_0 \cap T_0|}{|T_0|} \tag{9}$$

where P is a positive segmented region and P_0 is a negative segmented region. Similarly, T represents the true ground truth, and T_0 represents the negative ground truth. $|P \cap T|$ is the intersecting area between P and T [2].

3.4 Accuracy Analysis

Reproductions of these tests were conducted to demonstrate the performance of the proposed network in fulfilling the tumor segmentation task. A comparison with different methods found in the literature is shown in Tables 2, 3, and 4. Clearly, the proposed system is superior to the others in terms of network size, specificity, sensitivity and Dice metrics. Figure 3 shows an example of the segmentation results. Although the network training time was not considered, the average testing time per MRI image was measured at 0.08 s.

Table 2. Dice score comparison of the proposed brain tumor segmentation approach with various state-of-the-art methods.

Methods	Dice score		
	Complete	Core	Enhancing
Havaei et al. [2]	0.88	0.79	0.73
Pereira et al. [7]	0.84	0.72	0.62
Pereira et al. [8]	0.85	0.76	0.74
Casamitjana et al. [11]	0.89	0.76	0.63
Zhao et al. [12]	0.87	0.83	0.76
Dong et al. [13]	0.86	0.86	0.65
Wang et al. [14]	0.86	0.76	0.73
Hai et al. [19]	0.85	0.81	0.72
Proposed TPUAR-Net	0.89	0.82	0.79

Table 3. Sensitivity comparison of the proposed brain tumor segmentation approach against various state-of-the-art methods.

Methods	Sensitivity		
	Complete	Core	Enhancing
Havaei et al. [2]	0.87	0.79	0.80
Pereira et al. [7]	0.89	0.83	0.81
Pereira et al. [8]	0.92	0.79	0.78
Casamitjana et al. [11]	0.86	0.73	0.66
Zhao et al. [12]	0.83	0.81	0.77
Hai et al. [19]	0.87	0.85	0.82
Proposed TPUAR-Net	0.89	0.84	0.81

Table 4. Specificity comparison of the proposed brain tumor segmentation approach against various state-of-the-art methods.

Methods	Specificity		
	Complete	Core	Enhancing
Havaei et al. [2]	0.89	0.79	0.68
Pereira et al. [7]	0.88	0.87	0.74
Pereira et al. [8]	0.80	0.78	0.74
Casamitjana et al. [11]	0.93	0.85	0.74
Zhao et al. [12]	0.92	0.87	0.77
Proposed TPUAR-Net	0.99	0.99	0.99

4 Conclusions and Future Work

In this paper we presented two parallel U-Net with asymmetric residual-based deep convolutional neural networks (TPUAR-Nets) for brain tumor segmentation from MRI images. The TPUAR-Net model offeres several advantages, including the possibility of considering both local and global features to learn both high-level and low-level features simultaneously. The deployment of the fully connected layer, the residual blocks, and the skip connection can overcome the vanishing gradient problem while achieving speed improvements in training and testing. The proposed tumor segmentation method was evaluated using 2D slices extracted from the BRATS 2017 dataset using 62000 and 43400 images for training and testing purposes, respectively. The TPUAR-Net architecture achieved promising results on the complete, core, and enhancing tumor areas, achieving a maximum Dice score of 0.89. The superiority of the proposed method stems from combining the global and local features in the two parallel networks. In future work, we will focus on improving the current architecture and possibly expanding to a 3D network architecture to perform 3D brain tumor segmentation.

References

1. Siegel, R.L., Miller, K.D., Jemal, A.: Cancer statistics. CA Cancer J. Clin. **68**(1), 7–30 (2018). https://doi.org/10.3322/caac.21442
2. Havaei, M., et al.: Brain tumor segmentation with deep neural networks. Med. Image Anal. **35**, 18–31 (2017). https://doi.org/10.1016/j.media.2016.05.004
3. Abd-Ellah, M.K., Awad, A.I., Khalaf, A.A.M., Hamed, H.F.A.: Classification of brain tumor MRIs using a kernel support vector machine. In: Li, H., Nykänen, P., Suomi, R., Wickramasinghe, N., Widén, G., Zhan, M. (eds.) WIS 2016. CCIS, vol. 636, pp. 151–160. Springer, Cham (2016). https://doi.org/10.1007/978-3-319-44672-1_13
4. Abd-Ellah, M.K., Awad, A.I., Khalaf, A.A.M., Hamed, H.F.A.: Two-phase multi-model automatic brain tumour diagnosis system from magnetic resonance images using convolutional neural networks. EURASIP J. Image Video Process. **2018**(1), 97 (2018). https://doi.org/10.1186/s13640-018-0332-4
5. Soltaninejad, M., et al.: Automated brain tumour detection and segmentation using superpixel-based extremely randomized trees in FLAIR MRI. Int. J. Comput. Assist. Radiol. Surg. **12**(2), 183–203 (2017). https://doi.org/10.1007/s11548-016-1483-3
6. Abd-Ellah, M.K., Awad, A.I., Khalaf, A.A.M., Hamed, H.F.A.: Design and implementation of a computer-aided diagnosis system for brain tumor classification. In: 2016 28th International Conference on Microelectronics (ICM), pp. 73–76, 17–20 December 2016. https://doi.org/10.1109/ICM.2016.7847911
7. Pereira, S., Pinto, A., Alves, V., Silva, C.A.: Brain tumor segmentation using convolutional neural networks in MRI images. IEEE Trans. Med. Imaging **35**(5), 1240–1251 (2016). https://doi.org/10.1109/TMI.2016.2538465
8. Pereira, S., Oliveira, A., Alves, V., Silva, C.A.: On hierarchical brain tumor segmentation in MRI using fully convolutional neural networks: a preliminary study. In: 2017 IEEE 5th Portuguese Meeting on Bioengineering (ENBENG), pp. 1–4, 16–18 February 2017. https://doi.org/10.1109/ENBENG.2017.7889452

9. de Brebisson, A., Montana, G.: Deep neural networks for anatomical brain segmentation. In: 2015 IEEE Conference on Computer Vision and Pattern Recognition Workshops (CVPRW), pp. 20–28, June 2015. https://doi.org/10.1109/CVPRW.2015.7301312
10. Xiao, Z., et al.: A deep learning-based segmentation method for brain tumor in MR images. In: 2016 IEEE 6th International Conference on Computational Advances in Bio and Medical Sciences (ICCABS), pp. 1–6 (2016). https://doi.org/10.1109/ICCABS.2016.7802771
11. Casamitjana, A., Puch, S., Aduriz, A., Vilaplana, V.: 3D convolutional neural networks for brain tumor segmentation: a comparison of multi-resolution architectures. In: Crimi, A., Menze, B., Maier, O., Reyes, M., Winzeck, S., Handels, H. (eds.) BrainLes 2016. Lecture Notes in Computer Science, vol. 10154, pp. 150–161. Springer, Cham (2016). https://doi.org/10.1007/978-3-319-55524-9_15
12. Zhao, X., Wu, Y., Song, G., Li, Z., Fan, Y., Zhang, Y.: Brain tumor segmentation using a fully convolutional neural network with conditional random fields. In: Crimi, A., Menze, B., Maier, O., Reyes, M., Winzeck, S., Handels, H. (eds.) BrainLes 2016. Lecture Notes in Computer Science, vol. 10154, pp. 75–87. Springer, Cham (2016). https://doi.org/10.1007/978-3-319-55524-9_8
13. Dong, H., Yang, G., Liu, F., Mo, Y., Guo, Y.: Automatic brain tumor detection and segmentation using u-net based fully convolutional networks. In: Valdés Hernández, M., González-Castro, V. (eds.) MIUA 2017. CCIS, vol. 723, pp. 506–517. Springer, Cham (2017). https://doi.org/10.1007/978-3-319-60964-5_44
14. Wang, G., Li, W., Ourselin, S., Vercauteren, T.: Automatic brain tumor segmentation using convolutional neural networks with test-time augmentation. In: Crimi, A., Bakas, S., Kuijf, H., Keyvan, F., Reyes, M., van Walsum, T. (eds.) BrainLes 2018. LNCS, vol. 11384, pp. 61–72. Springer, Cham (2019). https://doi.org/10.1007/978-3-030-11726-9_6
15. He, K., Zhang, X., Ren, S., Sun, J.: Identity mappings in deep residual networks. In: Leibe, B., Matas, J., Sebe, N., Welling, M. (eds.) ECCV 2016. LNCS, vol. 9908, pp. 630–645. Springer, Cham (2016). https://doi.org/10.1007/978-3-319-46493-0_38
16. He, K., Zhang, X., Ren, S., Sun, J.: Delving deep into rectifiers: surpassing human-level performance on ImageNet classification. In: 2015 IEEE International Conference on Computer Vision (ICCV), pp. 1026–1034 (2015). https://doi.org/10.1109/ICCV.2015.123
17. Miller, J.W., Goodman, R., Smyth, P.: On loss functions which minimize to conditional expected values and posterior probabilities. IEEE Trans. Inf. Theor. **39**(4), 1404–1408 (1993). https://doi.org/10.1109/18.243457
18. Ioffe, S., Szegedy, C.: Batch normalization: accelerating deep network training by reducing internal covariate shift. In: Proceedings of the 32nd International Conference on International Conference on Machine Learning, ICML 2015, vol. 37, pp. 448–456, 06–11 July 2015. http://dl.acm.org/citation.cfm?id=3045118.3045167, JMLR.org
19. Le, H.T., Pham, H.T.T.: Brain tumour segmentation using U-Net based fully convolutional networks and extremely randomized trees. Vietnam J. Sci. Technol. Eng. **60**(3), 19–25 (2018). https://doi.org/10.31276/VJSTE.60(3).191

Data Clustering Using Variational Learning of Finite Scaled Dirichlet Mixture Models with Component Splitting

Hieu Nguyen[1(✉)], Kamal Maanicshah[1], Muhammad Azam[2], and Nizar Bouguila[1]

[1] Concordia Institute for Information Systems Engineering, Concordia University, Montreal, Quebec H3G 1M8, Canada
{hi_guy,k_mathin}@encs.concordia.ca, nizar.bouguila@concordia.ca

[2] Department of Electrical and Computer Engineering, Concordia University, Montreal, Quebec H3G 1M8, Canada
mu_azam@encs.concordia.ca

Abstract. We have developed a variational learning approach for finite Scaled Dirichlet mixture model with local model selection framework. By gradually splitting the components, our model is able to reach convergence as well as obtain the optimal number of clusters. By tackling real life challenging problems including spam detection and object clustering, the proposed model's flexibility and performance are validated.

Keywords: Unsupervised learning · Finite mixture model · Scaled Dirichlet · Variational inference · Component splitting · Object clustering · Spam detection

1 Introduction

Data analysis is an essential process with influential impact in various decision-making fields. Emphasis is now increasingly added on the use of images and videos in advertising campaigns. One of the most widely used techniques is clustering, which originates from statistics and its main goal is assigning similar data points to the same group [11]. Furthermore, along with the rapid development of automation, clustering is immensely important for spam detection. In other words, being able to filter spam automatically could not only reduce frustration, but also avoid being exposed to harmful content [23].

Among the proposed solutions, finite mixture model approach has shown its effectiveness with different scopes and applications [5,13,20]. In order to represent data mathematically, it assumes that data are generated from a set of components with sub-populations and each instance belongs to one of them, then the posterior probabilities handle the clustering process [19]. Therefore, choosing a flexible distribution which could efficiently fit different types of data

F. Karray et al. (Eds.): ICIAR 2019, LNCS 11663, pp. 117–128, 2019.
https://doi.org/10.1007/978-3-030-27272-2_10

is decisive to the outcome of the model, and Dirichlet distribution family has proven to be superior than the well-known Gaussian distribution in terms of clustering analysis [2,3].

The proposed learning framework is based on variational Bayesian inference, which focuses on minimizing the difference between the true posterior distribution and the approximated one by maximizing the lower bound of the likelihood function with Kullback-Leibler (KL) divergence [12]. This method is able to both efficiently estimate the parameters and find the optimal number of components. Furthermore, it also overcomes two critical drawbacks of conventional Bayesian approach: computational intensity of Markov chain Monte Carlo and Laplace's approximation [4,14] and challenging convergence estimation [6]. Moreover, Bayesian techniques are already proven more efficient than maximum likelihood estimation (MLE) since MLE's convergence could correspond to local maxima.

Recent works on mixture models based on Scaled Dirichlet distribution have shown its modeling capabilities [7,21]. Therefore, the variational Bayesian inference for finite Scaled Dirichlet mixture model is proposed along with component splitting, a local model selection framework. The main idea is starting from two components and then gradually adding new components by splitting existing ones based on a predefined threshold. Several applications have been tested to validate the performance of proposed algorithm including spam detection and object clustering.

The rest of the paper is organized as follows. The finite Scaled Dirichlet mixture model is introduced in Sect. 2. Next, Sect. 3 describes the variational Bayesian learning process. Then, the experimental results are discussed in Sect. 4. Finally, the conclusion and some remarks are in Sect. 5.

2 Finite Scaled Dirichlet Mixture Model

Assuming a set of N D-dimensional vectors generated from Scaled Dirichlet distribution $\mathcal{X} = (\boldsymbol{X}_1, ..., \boldsymbol{X}_N)$. Then, the vectors follow the probability density function $p(\boldsymbol{X}_i \mid \boldsymbol{\alpha}, \boldsymbol{\beta})$:

$$p(\boldsymbol{X}_i \mid \boldsymbol{\alpha}, \boldsymbol{\beta}) = \frac{\Gamma(\alpha_+)}{\prod_{d=1}^{D} \Gamma(\alpha_d)} \frac{\prod\limits_{d=1}^{D} \beta_d^{\alpha_d} X_{id}^{\alpha_d - 1}}{\left(\sum\limits_{d=1}^{D} \beta_d X_{id}\right)^{\alpha_+}} \tag{1}$$

where $\Gamma(\cdot)$ is the Gamma function, $\boldsymbol{\alpha} = (\alpha_1, ..., \alpha_D)$, $\alpha_d > 0$ for $d = 1, ..., D$, $\boldsymbol{\beta} = (\beta_1, ..., \beta_D)$, $0 \leq \beta_d \leq 1$ for $d = 1, ..., D$, $\sum\limits_{d=1}^{D} \beta_d = 1$, and $\alpha_+ = \sum\limits_{d=1}^{D} \alpha_d$.

Then, the M-component finite Scaled Dirichlet mixture model (SDMM) is defined as follows:

$$p(\boldsymbol{X}_i \mid \boldsymbol{\pi}, \boldsymbol{\alpha}_j, \boldsymbol{\beta}_j) = \sum_{j=1}^{M} \pi_j p(\boldsymbol{X}_i \mid \boldsymbol{\alpha}_j, \boldsymbol{\beta}_j) \tag{2}$$

where $\boldsymbol{\pi} = (\pi_1, ..., \pi_M)$ is the vector of mixing coefficients with respect to each component, which are positive and sum to 1. Then, $\boldsymbol{\alpha}_j$ and $\boldsymbol{\beta}_j$ denote the distribution's parameters with respect to component j. So, the likelihood function is:

$$p\left(\mathcal{X} \mid \boldsymbol{\pi}, \boldsymbol{\alpha}_j, \boldsymbol{\beta}_j\right) = \prod_{i=1}^{N}\left[\sum_{j=1}^{M} \pi_j p\left(\boldsymbol{X}_i \mid \boldsymbol{\alpha}_j, \boldsymbol{\beta}_j\right)\right] \tag{3}$$

For each vector $\boldsymbol{X}_i$, a M-dimensional assigning vector $\boldsymbol{Z}_i = (Z_{i1}, ..., Z_{iM})$, where $Z_{ij} \in \{0, 1\}$, $\sum_{j=1}^{M} Z_{ij} = 1$ and $Z_{ij} = 1$ if $\boldsymbol{X}_i$ belongs to component j and 0, otherwise. The conditional probability $\mathcal{Z} = (\boldsymbol{Z}_1, ..., \boldsymbol{Z}_N)$ given $\boldsymbol{\pi}$ is:

$$p(\mathcal{Z} \mid \boldsymbol{\pi}) = \prod_{i=1}^{N}\prod_{j=1}^{M} \pi_j^{Z_{ij}} \tag{4}$$

So, the conditional probability of data set $\mathcal{X}$ with the class labels $\mathcal{Z}$ is as follows:

$$p(\mathcal{X} \mid \mathcal{Z}, \boldsymbol{\alpha}, \boldsymbol{\beta}) = \prod_{i=1}^{N}\prod_{j=1}^{M} p\left(\boldsymbol{X}_i \mid \boldsymbol{\alpha}_j, \boldsymbol{\beta}_j\right)^{Z_{ij}} \tag{5}$$

Where $\boldsymbol{\alpha} = (\boldsymbol{\alpha}_1, ..., \boldsymbol{\alpha}_M)$ and $\boldsymbol{\beta} = (\boldsymbol{\beta}_1, ..., \boldsymbol{\beta}_M)$. The estimation of the mixture parameters and finding the optimal number of components M is a crucial part of a mixture model. The next section provides details about the variational Bayesian inference along with component splitting.

3 Variational Learning with Component Splitting

3.1 Parameters Estimation

The use of component splitting is inherited from [8]. First, the mixture components are divided into two parts, *fixed* components and *free* components. While the $M - s$ fixed components already provided a reasonable fit for the data, the model selection process operates on the s free ones. Therfore, the prior distribution of Z can be rewritten as follows:

$$p(\mathcal{Z} \mid \boldsymbol{\pi}, \boldsymbol{\pi}^*) = \prod_{i=1}^{N}\left[\prod_{j=1}^{s} \pi_j^{Z_{ij}} \prod_{j=s+1}^{M} \pi_j^{*Z_{ij}}\right] \tag{6}$$

where $\boldsymbol{\pi} = \{\pi_j\}$ are the mixing coefficients of the free components, $\boldsymbol{\pi}^* = \{\pi_j^*\}$ are the mixing coefficients of the fixed ones, and their sum must be 1: $\sum_{j=1}^{s} \pi_j + \sum_{j=s+1}^{M} \pi_j^* = 1$. Considering π_j^* as a random variable, the prediction for optimal number of components is then computed solely on the free components by maximizing the marginal likelihood given $\{\pi_j\}$ Then, according to [8], we have prior distribution for $\boldsymbol{\pi}^*$:

$$p(\boldsymbol{\pi}^* \mid \boldsymbol{\pi}) = \left(1 - \sum_{k=1}^{s} \pi_k\right)^{-M+s} \frac{\Gamma(\sum_{j=s+1}^{M} c_j)}{\prod_{j=s+1}^{M} \Gamma(c_j)} \prod_{j=s+1}^{M} \left(\frac{\pi_j^*}{1 - \sum_{k=1}^{s} \pi_k}\right)^{c_j - 1} \tag{7}$$

We choose Gamma and Dirichlet distribution as priors for $\boldsymbol{\alpha}_{jd}$ and $\boldsymbol{\beta}_j$, respectively:

$$p(\alpha_{jd}) = \mathcal{G}(\alpha_{jd} \mid u_{jd}, v_{jd}) = \frac{v_{jd}^{u_{jd}}}{\Gamma(u_{jd})} \alpha_{jd}^{u_{jd}-1} e^{-v_{jd}\alpha_{jd}} \tag{8}$$

$$p(\boldsymbol{\beta}_j) = \mathcal{D}(\boldsymbol{\beta} j \mid h_j) = \frac{\Gamma\left(\sum_{d=1}^{D} h_{jd}\right)}{\prod_{d=1}^{D} \Gamma(h_{jd})} \prod_{d=1}^{D} \beta_{jd}^{h_{jd}-1} \tag{9}$$

where $h_j = (h_{j1}, ..., h_{jD})$, $\mathcal{G}(\cdot)$ and $\mathcal{D}(\cdot)$ represent Gamma and Dirichlet distributions, respectively; $\{u_{jd}\}$, $\{v_{jd}\}$, and $\{h_{jd}\}$ are hyperparameters, where $u_{jd} > 0$, $v_{jd} > 0$, and $h_{jd} > 0$. Therefore

$$p(\boldsymbol{\alpha}) = \prod_{j=1}^{M} \prod_{d=1}^{D} p(\alpha_{jd}),\ p(\boldsymbol{\beta}) = \prod_{j=1}^{M} \prod_{d=1}^{D} p(\beta_{jd}) \tag{10}$$

We have the joint distribution of all the random variables:

$$\begin{aligned}
p(\mathcal{X}, \Theta \mid \boldsymbol{\pi}) &= p(\mathcal{X} \mid \mathcal{Z}, \boldsymbol{\alpha}, \boldsymbol{\beta})\, p(\mathcal{Z} \mid \boldsymbol{\pi}, \boldsymbol{\pi}^*)\, p(\boldsymbol{\pi}^* \mid \boldsymbol{\pi})\, p(\boldsymbol{\alpha})\, p(\boldsymbol{\beta}) \\
&= \prod_{i=1}^{N} \prod_{j=1}^{M} \left[\pi_j \frac{\Gamma(\alpha_+)}{\prod_{d=1}^{D} \Gamma(\alpha_{jd})} \frac{\prod_{d=1}^{D} \beta_{jd}^{\alpha_{jd}} X_{id}^{\alpha_{jd}-1}}{\left(\sum_{d=1}^{D} \beta_{jd} X_{id}\right)^{\alpha_+}} \right]^{Z_{ij}} \times \prod_{i=1}^{N} \left[\prod_{j=1}^{s} \pi_j^{Z_{ij}} \prod_{j=s+1}^{M} \pi_j^{*Z_{ij}} \right] \\
&\times \left(1 - \sum_{k=1}^{s} \pi_k\right)^{-M+s} \times \frac{\Gamma\left(\sum_{j=s+1}^{M} c_j\right)}{\prod_{j=s+1}^{M} \Gamma(c_j)} \prod_{j=s+1}^{M} \left(\frac{\pi_j^*}{1 - \sum_{k=1}^{s} \pi_k}\right)^{c_j - 1} \\
&\times \prod_{j=1}^{M} \prod_{d=1}^{D} \frac{v_{jd}^{u_{jd}}}{\Gamma(u_{jd})} \alpha_{jd}^{u_{jd}-1} e^{-v_{jd}\alpha_{jd}} \times \frac{\Gamma\left(\sum_{d=1}^{D} h_{jd}\right)}{\prod_{d=1}^{D} \Gamma(h_{jd})} \prod_{d=1}^{D} \beta_{jd}^{h_{jd}-1}
\end{aligned} \tag{11}$$

where $\Theta = \{\mathcal{Z}, \boldsymbol{\alpha}, \boldsymbol{\beta}, \boldsymbol{\pi}^*\}$ is the set of unknown parameters. The model's graphical representation is shown in Fig. 1.

The goal is to find the true posterior distribution $p(\Theta \mid \mathcal{X}, \boldsymbol{\pi})$ by creating $Q(\Theta)$ as an approximated distribution to it. By applying the KL divergence, the difference between two distributions is computed as follows

$$\mathcal{L}(Q) = \ln\, p(\mathcal{X} \mid \boldsymbol{\pi}) - KL(Q \,\|\, P) \tag{12}$$

The maximum value of lower bound $\mathcal{L}(Q) = \int Q(\Theta) \ln\left(\frac{p(\mathcal{X}, \Theta \mid \boldsymbol{\pi})}{Q(\Theta)}\right) d\Theta$ is achieved when the KL divergence is zero. Since the true posterior is intractable,

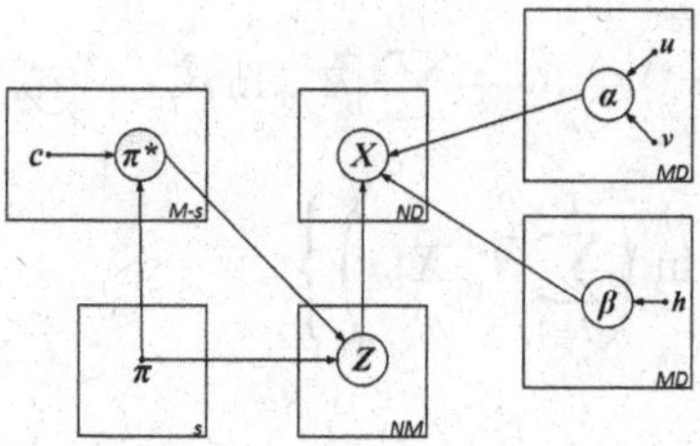

Fig. 1. Graphical demonstration of the finite Scaled Dirichlet mixture model with component splitting. Symbols in circles denote parameters and random variables, arcs describe the conditional dependencies of the variables, plates shows repetitions, and the numbers in the lower right corners of the plates explain the quantity of repetitions.

the mean field theory [22] is applied factorize $Q(\Theta)$ so that $Q(\Theta) = Q(\mathcal{Z})\, Q(\boldsymbol{\alpha})\, Q(\boldsymbol{\beta})\, Q(\boldsymbol{\pi}^*)$. The maximization of lower bound $\mathcal{L}(Q)$ with respect to each sub-distribution $Q_s(\Theta_s)$ is:

$$Q_s(\Theta_s) = \frac{exp\, \langle \ln\, p(\mathcal{X}, \Theta)\rangle_{j\neq s}}{\int exp\, \langle \ln\, p(\mathcal{X}, \Theta)\rangle_{j\neq s}\, d\Theta} \tag{13}$$

where $\langle\cdot\rangle_{j\neq s}$ denotes the expectation of the parameters with the exception of $j = s$. Then, (13) is used for updating the algorithm to reach convergence:

$$\mathcal{Q}(\mathcal{Z}) = \prod_{i=1}^{N}\left[\prod_{j=1}^{s} r_{ij}^{Z_{ij}} \prod_{j=s+1}^{M} r_{ij}^{*Z_{ij}}\right] \tag{14}$$

$$\mathcal{Q}(\boldsymbol{\pi}^*) = \left(1 - \sum_{k=1}^{s}\pi_k\right)^{-M+s} \frac{\Gamma\left(\sum_{j=s+1}^{M} c_j^*\right)}{\prod_{j=s+1}^{M}\Gamma\left(c_j^*\right)} \prod_{j=s+1}^{M}\left(\frac{\pi_j^*}{1-\sum_{k=1}^{s}\pi_k}\right)^{c_j^*-1} \tag{15}$$

$$Q(\boldsymbol{\alpha}) = \prod_{j=1}^{M}\prod_{d=1}^{D}\mathcal{G}\left(\alpha_{jd} \mid u_{jd}^*, v_{jd}^*\right),\ \ Q(\boldsymbol{\beta}) = \prod_{j=1}^{M}\prod_{d=1}^{D}\mathcal{D}\left(\beta_{jd} \mid h_{jd}^*\right) \tag{16}$$

where

$$r_{ij} = \frac{\tilde{r}_{ij}}{\sum_{j=1}^{s}\tilde{r}_{ij} + \sum_{j=s+1}^{M}\tilde{r}_{ij}^*},\ r_{ij}^* = \frac{\tilde{r}_{ij}^*}{\sum_{j=1}^{s}\tilde{r}_{ij} + \sum_{j=s+1}^{M}\tilde{r}_{ij}^*} \tag{17}$$

$$\begin{aligned}\tilde{r}_{ij} = exp\Bigg\{ &\ln\pi_j + \tilde{R}_j + \sum_{d=1}^{D}\left[\overline{\alpha}_{jd}\ln\overline{\beta}_{jd} + (\overline{\alpha}_{jd}-1)\ln X_{id}\right] \\ &- \sum_{d=1}^{D}\overline{\alpha}_{jd}\ln\left(\sum_{d=1}^{D}\overline{\beta}_{jd}X_{id}\right)\Bigg\}\end{aligned} \tag{18}$$

$$\tilde{r}_{ij}^* = exp\Bigg\{ \langle \ln \pi_j^* \rangle + \tilde{R}_j + \sum_{d=1}^{D} \left[\overline{\alpha}_{jd} \ln \overline{\beta}_{jd} + (\overline{\alpha}_{jd} - 1) \ln X_{id} \right] - \sum_{d=1}^{D} \overline{\alpha}_{jd} \ln \left(\sum_{d=1}^{D} \overline{\beta}_{jd} X_{id} \right) \Bigg\} \tag{19}$$

$$\begin{aligned} \tilde{R}_j = \ln \frac{\Gamma\left(\sum_{d=1}^{D} \overline{\alpha}_{jd}\right)}{\prod_{d=1}^{D} \Gamma\left(\overline{\alpha}_{jd}\right)} &+ \sum_{d=1}^{D} \overline{\alpha}_{jd} \left[\psi \left(\sum_{d=1}^{D} \overline{\alpha}_{jd} \right) - \psi\left(\overline{\alpha}_{jd}\right) \right] \left[\langle \ln \alpha_{jd} \rangle - \ln \overline{\alpha}_{jd} \right] \\ &+ \frac{1}{2} \sum_{d=1}^{D} \overline{\alpha}_{jd}^2 \left[\psi' \left(\sum_{d=1}^{D} \overline{\alpha}_{jd} \right) - \psi'\left(\overline{\alpha}_{jd}\right) \right] - \langle (\ln \alpha_{jd} - \ln \overline{\alpha}_{jd})^2 \rangle \\ &+ \frac{1}{2} \sum_{a=1}^{D} \sum_{b=1, a \neq b}^{D} \overline{\alpha}_{ja} \overline{\alpha}_{jb} \left\{ \psi' \left(\sum_{d=1}^{D} \overline{\alpha}_{jd} \right) (\langle \ln \overline{\alpha}_{ja} \rangle - \ln \overline{\alpha}_{ja}) \times (\langle \ln \overline{\alpha}_{jb} \rangle - \ln \overline{\alpha}_{jb}) \right\} \end{aligned} \tag{20}$$

$$c_j^* = \sum_{i=1}^{N} r_{ij}^* + c_j, \quad u_{jd}^* = u_{jd} + \varphi_{jd}, \quad v_{jd}^* = v_{jd} - \vartheta_{jd}, \quad h_{jd}^* = h_{jd} + \tau_{jd} \tag{21}$$

$$\varphi_{jd} = \sum_{i=1}^{N} \langle Z_{ij} \rangle \overline{\alpha}_{jd} \left[\psi \left(\sum_{d=1}^{D} \overline{\alpha}_{jd} \right) - \psi\left(\overline{\alpha}_{jd}\right) + \sum_{d \neq s}^{D} \psi' \left(\sum_{d=1}^{D} \overline{\alpha}_{jd} \right) \times \overline{\alpha}_{js} \left(\langle \ln \alpha_{js} \rangle - \ln \overline{\alpha}_{js} \right) \right] \tag{22}$$

$$\vartheta_{jd} = \sum_{i=1}^{N} \langle Z_{ij} \rangle \left[\ln \overline{\beta}_{jd} + \ln X_{id} - \ln \left(\sum_{d=1}^{D} \overline{\beta}_{jd} X_{id} \right) \right] \tag{23}$$

$$\tau_{jd} = \sum_{i=1}^{N} \langle Z_{ij} \rangle \left[\overline{\alpha}_{jd} - \overline{\alpha}_{jd} \overline{\beta}_{jd} \frac{X_{id}}{\sum_{d=1}^{D} \overline{\beta}_{jd} X_{id}} \right] \tag{24}$$

where $\psi(\cdot)$ and $\psi'(\cdot)$ denote the digamma and trigamma functions, respectively. The expectation of the aforementioned equations are

$$\langle Z_{ij} \rangle = r_{ij}, \quad \text{for } j = 1, ..., s, \langle Z_{ij} \rangle = r_{ij}^*, \quad \text{for } j = s+1, ..., M \tag{25}$$

$$\overline{\alpha}_{jd} = \langle \alpha_{jd} \rangle = \frac{u_{jd}}{v_{jd}}, \quad \langle \ln \alpha_{jd} \rangle = \psi(u_{jd}) - \ln v_{jd}, \quad \overline{\beta}_{jd} = \langle \beta_{jd} \rangle = \frac{h_{jd}}{\sum_{d=1}^{D} h_{jd}} \tag{26}$$

$$\left\langle \left(\ln \alpha_{jd} - \ln \overline{\alpha}_{jd} \right)^2 \right\rangle = \left[\psi(u_{jd}) - \ln u_{jd} \right]^2 + \psi'(u_{jd}) \tag{27}$$

$$\langle \pi_j^* \rangle = \left(1 - \sum_{k=1}^{s} \pi_k\right) \frac{\sum_{i=1}^{N} r_{ij}^* + c_j}{\sum_{k=s+1}^{M} \left(\sum_{i=1}^{N} r_{ik}^* + c_k\right)} \tag{28}$$

$$\langle \ln \pi_j^* \rangle = \ln \left(1 - \sum_{k=1}^{s} \pi_k\right) + \psi\left(\sum_{i=1}^{N} r_{ij}^* + c_j\right) - \psi\left(\sum_{i=1}^{N} \sum_{k=s+1}^{M} r_{ik}^* + c_k\right) \tag{29}$$

The estimation for the free mixing coefficients $\boldsymbol{\pi}$ is computed from the maximization of lower bound $\mathcal{L}(Q)$ and the variational updates for $\mathcal{Q}(\mathcal{Z})$, $\mathcal{Q}(\boldsymbol{\pi}^*)$, $\mathcal{Q}(\boldsymbol{\alpha})$, and $\mathcal{Q}(\boldsymbol{\beta})$. We have the derivative of $\mathcal{L}(Q)$ with respect to $\boldsymbol{\pi}$ after setting it to zero:

$$\pi_j = \left(1 - \sum_{k=s+1}^{M} \langle \pi_k^* \rangle\right) \frac{\sum_{i=1}^{N} r_{ij}}{\sum_{i=1}^{N} \sum_{k=1}^{s} r_{ik}} \tag{30}$$

3.2 Model Selection via Component Splitting

First, the algorithm starts with the variational learning without local model selection where $M = 2$. If the result has two components, the splitting process proceeds; otherwise, the algorithm ends if there is only one component. When the splitting test is passed, one of the components is split into two free components. Next, the model with local model selection operates on the free components while leaving the fixed ones intact. Two common possibilities could occur after the inference: first, both free components are kept due to their meaningful contribution to fit the data; second, only one component is kept while the insignificant one is removed. However, when there are some outliers in the data set, both the free components could end up being redundant, then this particular split is restored in order to avoid an infinite loop. Then, after each successful split, the number of components gradually increases until all the split tests fail.

4 Experimental Results

In this section, we discuss the performance of our proposed method (varSDMM) as compared to MLE-based Gaussian mixture model (GMM), variational Gaussian mixture model (varGMM), variational Dirichlet mixture model (varDMM). Two challenging real life applications are considered including spam email detection of both texts as well as images and image categorization consisting of textures and objects.

4.1 Spam Detection

For the past two decades, e-mail has become an essential means of communication, especially in the workplace environment. However, e-mails are also one of the most common target for network-based attacks namely phishing [16]. Spam emails containing not only texts, but also deceiving images combined with the evolve of various scam techniques are drawing increasing interest as a challenging task that needs immediate actions.

Table 1. Results on Spambase (%) using different models

Method	Accuracy	Precision	Recall	False positive rate
varSDMM	85.60	99.61	70.44	0.28
varDMM	83.84	97.23	69.06	1.99
GMM	73.08	73.24	72.75	26.59
varGMM	71.37	69.56	76.01	33.26

SIFT (Scale Invariant Feature transform) [18] is used for preprocessing the images. Then, all the $128D$ descriptors of SIFT are grouped into a corpus of local features. Next, we use K-means to cluster the collection to construct the visual words vocabulary, in which the centroids are the number of visual words.

The performance of each result is validated using four important measures: Accuracy ($\frac{TP+TN}{TP+TN+FP+FN}$), Precision ($\frac{TP}{TP+FP}$), Recall ($\frac{TP}{TP+FN}$), False Positive Rate ($\frac{FP}{FP+TN}$).

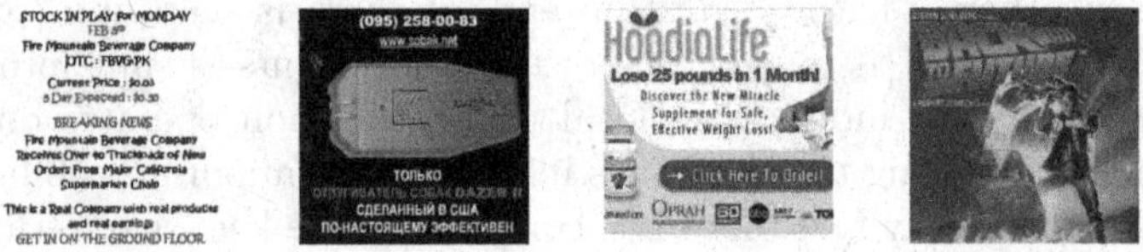

(a) (b) (c) (d)

Fig. 2. Images from (a) Personal Image Spam, (b) SpamArchive, (c) Princeton, (d) Personal Image Ham.

4.1.1 Text Spam E-mails Detection

For textual spam e-mail detection, we chose the Spambase data set [10], in which the histogram of the occurrences of the words is used as a feature. We chose 3626 instances in the data set, half of which was spam and the other half was non-spam. The results in Table 1 shows that our proposed model outperforms others in all aspects.

4.1.2 Image Spam E-mails Detection

Three real life image spam data sets were considered: Personal Image Spam (2995 images) [9], SpamArchive Image Spam (3014 images) [9], and Princeton Spam Image (1063 images)[1]. One common legitimate (ham) email data set Personal Image Ham (1650 images) [9] is used for clustering analysis. Sample images from these data sets are shown in Fig. 2. After several trials, the optimal number of visual vocabulary is 50. The results shown in Table 2 validates varSDMM's performance over other models.

[1] http://www.cs.princeton.edu/cass/spam/.

Table 2. Results on image spam detection using different models

Method	Measure (%)	Dredze	SpamArchive	Princeton
varSDMM	Accuracy	88.63	86.94	86.18
	Precision	96.25	98.98	90.66
	Recall	85.71	80.62	72.15
	False positive rate	6.06	1.52	4.79
varDMM	Accuracy	87.56	80.87	84.11
	Precision	94.58	96.74	81.35
	Recall	85.61	72.86	71.14
	False positive rate	8.91	4.48	11.39
varGMM	Accuracy	86.29	81.56	84.37
	Precision	89.91	96.95	85.38
	Recall	88.68	73.79	72.53
	False positive rate	18.06	4.24	8.36
GMM	Accuracy	87.26	80.83	84.56
	Precision	91.73	95.45	85.86
	Recall	88.18	73.86	72.53
	False positive rate	14.42	6.42	7.70

4.2 Image Categorization

The task to automatically differentiate random objects has always been frequently discussed in computer vision [1]. Indeed, even similar objects could raise significant problems due to different angles, surrounding environments, and various depth of the captured images. Furthermore, recent research works have addressed related challenging clustering analysis, such as sports activities [12] and scenes [17]. Thus, two object clustering applications are discussed in this experiment, and the efficiency of our model is confirmed by comparison with other novel methods.

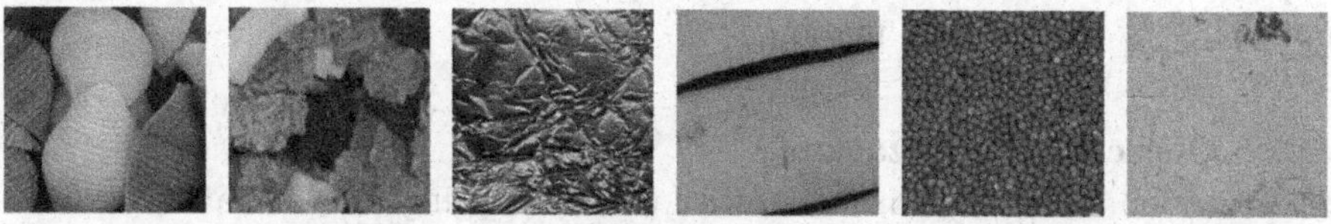

(a) (b) (c) (d) (e) (f)

Fig. 3. Sample images from ALOT. (a) Macaroni, (b) Corn Flakes, (c) Silver foil, (d) Banana peel, (e) Mustard seed, (f) Plaster

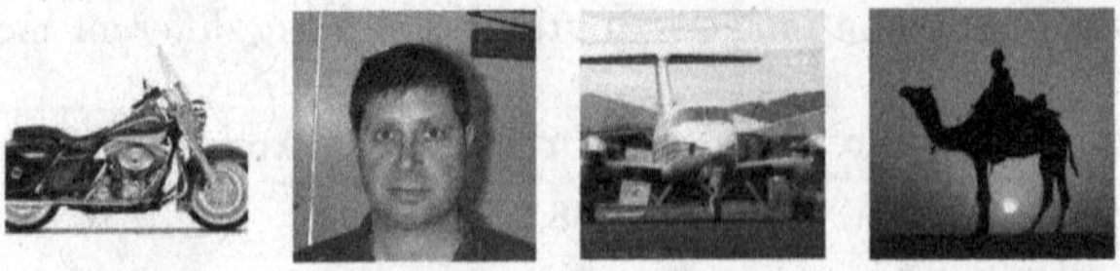

(a) (b) (c) (d)

Fig. 4. Examples from Caltech. (a) Bikes, (b) Faces, (c) Planes, (d) Camels.

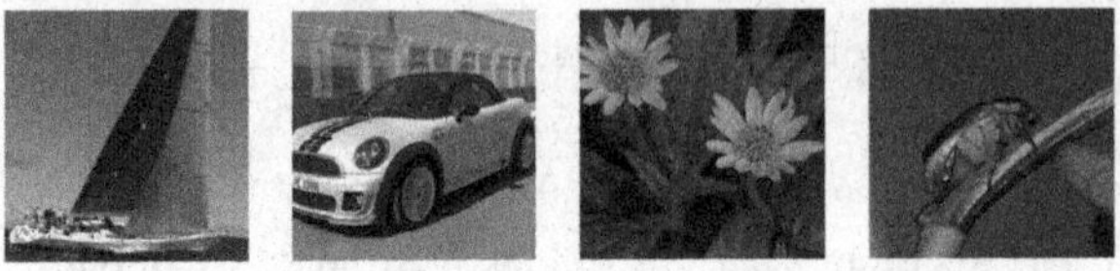

(a) (b) (c) (d)

Fig. 5. Sample images from GHIM10K. (a) Boats, (b) Cars, (c) Flowers, (d) Bugs

Table 3. Results on texture and object clustering data sets using different models

Method	Accuracy (%)		
	ALOT	Caltech	GHIM10K
varSDMM	94.83	83.00	94.25
varDMM	78.83	69.50	83.75
varGMM	76.16	76.00	83.50
GMM	71.50	76.30	83.25

4.2.1 Texture Categorization

In this section, Amsterdam Library of Textures (ALOT), a real life texture data set, is chosen for testing. We tested 600 images evenly divided into six clusters from ALOT: Macaroni, Corn Flakes, Silver foil, Banana peel, Mustard seed, and Plaster; sample images are in Fig. 3. The preprocessing step was similar to that mentioned in Sect. 4.1 with the optimal value for vocabulary was 50. The results are presented in Table 3, showing that the proposed model surpasses other novel approaches by a significant margin.

4.2.2 Object Categorization

In this section, we tested our model with two challenging real life data sets: Caltech256 [15] and GHIM10K[2]. In other words, we had a 600-image data set from Caltech256 evenly divided into four classes: Bikes, Faces, Planes, and Camels and a 400-image data set from GHIM10K whose clusters included Boats, Cars, Flowers, and Bugs with 100 images in each cluster. The objects were captured from different angles, distances, lighting conditions, and background environments to

[2] http://www.ci.gxnu.edu.cn/cbir/dataset.aspx.

elevate the demand of the challenge. The examples of the datasets are presented in Figs 4 and 5. The preprocessing step was the same as that described in Sect. 4.1, and the optimal number of vocabulary was also 50. The accuracy of varSDMM is compared with other widely used models in Table 3, confirming its flexibility and capability to efficiently differentiate various objects in different environments.

5 Conclusion

We have proposed a novel model selection framework based on the variational learning of finite Scaled Dirichlet mixture model by automatically splitting the components until reaching convergence with the optimal number of clusters. By replacing the global model selection with a more efficient local one, our model has proven its capability of handling different challenging problems while maintaining a steady performance. Future works could be building an online learning approach for the proposed model.

Acknowledgement. The completion of this research was made possible thanks to the Natural Sciences and Engineering Research Council of Canada (NSERC) and Concordia University Research Chair Tier 2.

References

1. Aggarwal, C.C.: Data Classification: Algorithms and Applications. Frontiers in Physics. Chapman and Hall/CRC, New York (2014)
2. Bdiri, T., Bouguila, N.: Positive vectors clustering using inverted dirichlet finite mixture models. Expert Syst. Appl. **39**(2), 1869–1882 (2012)
3. Bouguila, N., Ziou, D.: Unsupervised selection of a finite dirichlet mixture model: an mml-based approach. IEEE Trans. Knowl. Data Eng. **18**(8), 993–1009 (2006)
4. Bouguila, N., Elguebaly, T.: A fully bayesian model based on reversible jump mcmc and finite beta mixtures for clustering. Expert Syst. Appl. **39**(5), 5946–5959 (2012)
5. Bouguila, N., Ziou, D.: Using unsupervised learning of a finite dirichlet mixture model to improve pattern recognition applications. Pattern Recogn. Lett. **26**(12), 1916–1925 (2005)
6. Bouguila, N., Ziou, D., Hammoud, R.I.: On bayesian analysis of a finite generalized dirichlet mixture via a metropolis-within-gibbs sampling. Pattern Anal. Appl. **12**(2), 151–166 (2009)
7. Bourouis, S., Bouguila, N., Li, Y., Azam, M.: Visual scene reconstruction using a bayesian learning framework. In: Mansouri, A., El Moataz, A., Nouboud, F., Mammass, D. (eds.) ICISP 2018. LNCS, vol. 10884, pp. 225–232. Springer, Cham (2018). https://doi.org/10.1007/978-3-319-94211-7_25
8. Constantinopoulos, C., Likas, A.: Unsupervised learning of gaussian mixtures based on variational component splitting. IEEE Trans. Neural Netw. **18**(3), 745–755 (2007)
9. Dredze, M., Gevaryahu, R., Elias-Bachrach, A.: Learning fast classifiers for image spam, January 2007
10. Dua, D., Graff, C.: UCI machine learning repository (2017)

11. Everitt, B.S., Landau, S., Leese, M.: Cluster Analysis, 4th edn. Wiley Publishing, New York (2009)
12. Fan, W., Bouguila, N., Ziou, D.: Variational learning for finite dirichlet mixture models and applications. IEEE Trans. Neural Netw. Learn. Syst. **23**(5), 762–774 (2012)
13. Fan, W., Bouguila, N., Ziou, D.: Variational learning of finite dirichlet mixture models using component splitting. Neurocomputing **129**, 3–16 (2014)
14. Fu, S., Bouguila, N.: A Bayesian intrusion detection framework. In: 2018 International Conference on Cyber Security and Protection of Digital Services (Cyber Security), pp. 1–8, June 2018
15. Griffin, G., Holub, A., Perona, P.: Caltech-256 object category dataset. Technical report, 7694, California Institute of Technology (2007)
16. Hong, J.: The state of phishing attacks. Commun. ACM **55**(1), 74–81 (2012)
17. Ihou, K.E., Bouguila, N.: Variational-based latent generalized dirichlet allocation model in the collapsed space and applications. Neurocomputing **332**, 372–395 (2019)
18. Lowe, D.G.: Distinctive image features from scale-invariant keypoints. Int. J. Comput. Vis. **60**(2), 91–110 (2004)
19. McLachlan, G.J., Peel, D.: Finite Mixture Models. Wiley Series in Probability and Statistics. Wiley, New York (2000)
20. Mehdi, M., Bouguila, N., Bentahar, J.: Trustworthy web service selection using probabilistic models. In: 2012 IEEE 19th International Conference on Web Services, Honolulu, HI, USA, 24–29 June 2012, pp. 17–24 (2012)
21. Oboh, B.S., Bouguila, N.: Unsupervised learning of finite mixtures using scaled dirichlet distribution and its application to software modules categorization. In: 2017 IEEE International Conference on Industrial Technology (ICIT), pp. 1085–1090, March 2017
22. Parisi, G.: Statistical Field Theory. Frontiers in Physics. Addison-Wesley Pub. Co., Boston (1988)
23. Siponen, M., Stucke, C.: Effective anti-spam strategies in companies: an international study. In: Proceedings of the 39th Annual Hawaii International Conference on System Sciences (HICSS 2006), vol. 6, p. 127c, January 2006

Sequential Image Synthesis for Human Activity Video Generation

Fahim Hasan Khan(✉), Akila de Silva, Jayanth Yetukuri, and Narges Norouzi

University of California, Santa Cruz, CA 95064, USA
{fkhan4,audesilv,jyetukur,nanorouz}@ucsc.edu

Abstract. In the field of computer graphics and multimedia, automatic synthesis of a new set of image sequences from another different set of image sequences for creating realistic video or animation of some human activity performed is a research challenge. Traditionally, creating such animation or similar visual media contents is done manually, which is a tedious task. Recent advancements in deep learning have made some promising progress for automating this type of media creation process. This work is motivated by the idea to synthesize a temporally coherent sequence of images (e.g., a video) of a person performing some activity by using a video or set of images of a different person performing a similar activity. To achieve that, our approach utilized the cycle-consistent adversarial network (CycleGAN). We present a new approach for learning to transfer a human activity from a source domain to a target domain without using any complicated pose detection or extraction method. Our objective in this work is to learn a mapping between two consecutive sequences of images from two domains representing two different activities and use that mapping to transfer the activity from one domain to another for synthesizing an entirely new consecutive sequence of images, which can be combined to make a video of new human activity. We also present and analyze some qualitative results generated by our method.

Keywords: Image synthesis · Generative adversarial networks

1 Introduction

In the graphics, animation, and media content generation industry, synthesizing a sequence of temporally coherent images is one of the most frequently used and significant tasks. Usually, the image synthesis for producing animation or video is done manually, often by using some of the large selection of software tools available. However, manual creation of such animations is tedious, expensive and time-consuming even for the expert animation artists and multimedia content developers. Recent advancements in the field of Artificial Intelligence (AI) and Deep Learning (DL) has made some much-needed progress for automating this

All the authors shared an equal amount of contribution to this work.

F. Karray et al. (Eds.): ICIAR 2019, LNCS 11663, pp. 129–133, 2019.
https://doi.org/10.1007/978-3-030-27272-2_11

process. Despite a significant amount of work in this area, this is still an active research problem and has room for many improvements.

As video synthesis is a challenging problem, extensive research studies have been done over the last few decades for addressing this. Recently, with the advents of the DL techniques, the research problem has seen a promising new direction. The early methods used traditional image processing techniques for modifying existing video footage to create new contents [4]. Our approach uses machine learning to synthesize new movements of human activity instead of using straightforward image processing. There are quite a few numbers of works which used 3D transfer motion for graphics and animation purposes. One such very recent work utilized DL algorithms to retarget motion into 3D objects without using any existing data [5]. Our research focuses on generating synthetic movements directly in the 2D space without using any 3D information, which is convenient for working with datasets lacking 3D details. Other contemporary works based on DL techniques have been able to learn information from one image and transfer them to another image. One such technique, the Generative adversarial networks (GAN) [3] framework has been used for many purposes, including high-quality image generation with sharp details [4]. With the advancements of GAN, quite a few novel specialized sub-classes are introduced. CycleGAN [6] is one of them, which can learn to do arbitrary image-to-image translations using adversarial training. A very recent work done by Chan et al. made some promising advancements. They were able to transfers dance performance from a source video to a novel target with a few minutes of moves from a target subject [2]. They also investigated some techniques for generating images of human subjects with various new poses in their paper [2]. While their work focuses on extracting motions as an intermediate step using pose stick figures to transfer them to new images, in contrast, our work aims toward a more straightforward generation of sequential images of a new human activity without any such intermediate step for extracting motion explicitly.

This work is motivated by the ongoing research efforts to generate a complete synthetic video of a person performing some action from limited or different input images of that person. The main contribution of our work is to explore the novel idea of generating temporally coherent image sequences of new human activity using CycleGAN [6], which is a fairly new class of machine learning algorithm. In this paper, we present a method based on CycleGAN to learn a mapping between two consecutive sequences of images from two domains representing two different activities. Our method uses this unpaired activity-to-activity mapping to transfer the activity from one domain to another to synthesize a sequence of images of performing a new activity by a person by using another input video of the same person performing another different activity. For demonstrating our method, we present experimental results using the four datasets we created and a qualitative evaluation of the results.

2 Models and Algorithms

We have used CycleGAN [6] for implementing our method. CycleGAN is an extension of the GAN framework, and it trains on two domains of data and learns from both of the actions. The traditional GAN framework has one network called the "Generator" for generating image sequences, and another network called the "Discriminator" for evaluating the generated images [3]. The generator learns to map from the training dataset to a particular data distribution of interest representing the intended movement, while the discriminator distinguishes between instances from the actual data distribution and results produced by the generator. The generator's training objective is to convince the discriminator to pass the generated images as real ones. Training the discriminator involves presenting it with image samples from the input dataset until it reaches some level of accuracy. The discriminator attempts to distinguish between fake samples produced by the generator and real ones sampled from the training data, which trains the generator to create more realistic images.

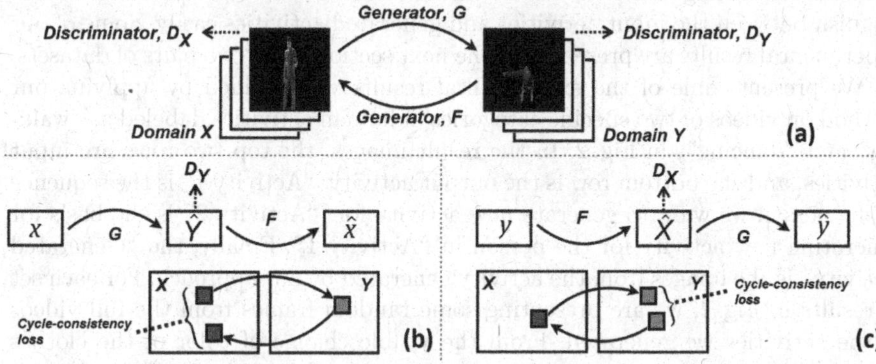

Fig. 1. The architecture of the model used in our approach is based on the CycleGAN [6]. It contains two mapping functions G: $X \rightarrow Y$ and F: $Y \rightarrow X$, and associated adversarial discriminators D_Y and D_X. (b) forward cycle-consistency loss: $x \rightarrow G(x) \rightarrow F(G(x)) \approx x$, and (c) backward cycle-consistency loss: $y \rightarrow F(y) \rightarrow G(F(y)) \approx y$.

CycleGAN, on the other hand, performs unpaired image to image translation using two generators and two discriminators as illustrated in Fig. 1. The goal of CycleGAN is to learn mapping functions between two domains X and Y from given training samples. In our method, the two domains are the two different input activities, and the frames from the image sequences of the two activities are the training examples. Each of the two generators converts images from their own domain to the domain of the other generator. Two functions G: $X \rightarrow Y$ and F: $Y \rightarrow X$ are trained to generate images from one input domain to another domain. The functions have two associated adversarial discriminators, D_Y and D_X respectively. D_Y encourages G to translate X into outputs indistinguishable from domain Y, and vice versa for D_X. CycleGAN introduces two cycle consistency losses to regularize the mapping further. The cycle consistency loss is based on the intuition that if some data is translated back and forth from one domain to the other, the process should return to the starting point. We have used a CycleGAN to train the models to learn two different activities. The model is trained on two unpaired data set of sequence of temporally coherent images of two different actions performed by two different subjects. Once trained, our model can generate new synthetic activity seemingly performed by a person based on the input activities from two different domains. The CycleGAN used in our method is implemented using Python with the machine learning libraries, Keras and Tensorflow.

3 Results and Analysis

We have created our datasets from the publicly available videos from the image database website shutterstock.com [1]. For simplicity, most of the image sequences we selected are with a single-colored background. We selected human subjects performing activities while wearing clothing with different colors to distinguish between the input activities and generated activities easily. Some of our experimental results are presented in the next section using two pairs of datasets.

We present some of the experimental results we obtained by applying our method on videos of two specific categories of human activities, labeled as "walking" and "dancing", in Fig. 2. In the result images, the top two rows are input activities, and the bottom row is the output activity. "Activity 1" is the sequence of the person we want to generate new activity for. "Activity 2" is the basis for generating new activity for the person in "Activity 1". Finally, the "Generated Activity" is the images from the activity generated by our approach. For each set of results in Fig. 2, we are presenting some random frames from the full videos of the activities we generated. From the visible change of color of the clothes of the subjects in the presented images, the successful synthesis of new human

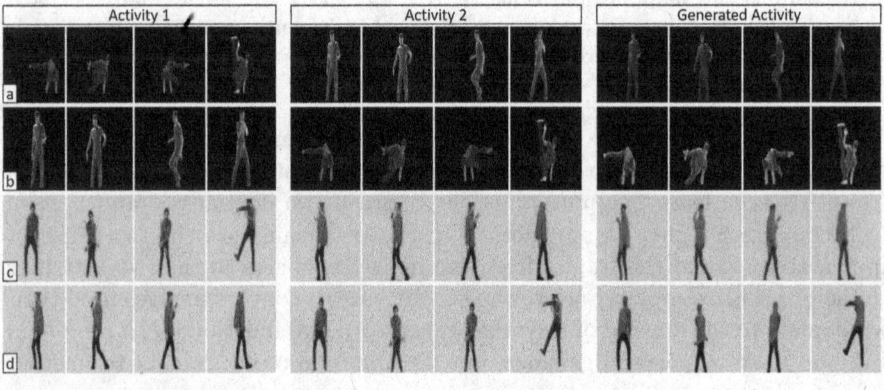

Fig. 2. Four sets of results obtained by applying CycleGAN for generating human activities labeled as "Dancing" (a and b) and "Walking" (c and d).

activities is evident. These results are presented as the progress of our ongoing development and proof-of-concept demo of our new method.

We also performed a qualitative evaluation in a survey format on our generated results. In the study, fifteen (15) independent observers rated the quality of the generated images on a scale of 1 to 5 for two different types of activities individually, as well as the overall quality of the synthesized images. We present the average results of the qualitative evaluations in Table 1 after converted to percentage scores. Our metric of "success" is the generation of realistic images judged by the eyes of the independent human observers.

Table 1. Results of qualitative evaluation

Activity domain of synthesized images	Walking	Dancing	Overall quality
Average qualitative score, in percentage	73.3	61.3	68.0

4 Conclusion and Future Works

In this paper, we present a novel method for synthesizing temporally coherent images of new human activity using CycleGAN. As the initial results are promising, our approach has the potential to be used in the animation and media content generation industry. This method can be extended to generate labeled human activities the model is already trained on, e.g., using a short video of a person performing an activity and be able to generate many possible other activities performed by the same person. Using our method, multiple learning models specific to different activity domains can be trained to generate videos of all the different activities. The limitation of our method is that it works well for large movements, e.g., walking, jumping, dancing, etc., while it does not work well for smaller movements, such as hand waving, nodding, etc. Also, the two training sequences should be unpaired and not too similar. We plan to address these limitations and potential extensions to our methodology in our future works.

References

1. Stock images, photos, vectors, video, and music. https://www.shutterstock.com/
2. Chan, C., Ginosar, S., Zhou, T., Efros, A.A.: Everybody dance now. arXiv preprint arXiv:1808.07371 (2018)
3. Goodfellow, I., et al.: Generative adversarial nets. In: Advances in Neural Information Processing Systems, pp. 2672–2680 (2014)
4. Liu, J., Kuipers, B., Savarese, S.: Recognizing human actions by attributes. In: CVPR 2011, pp. 3337–3344. IEEE (2011)
5. Villegas, R., Yang, J., Ceylan, D., Lee, H.: Neural kinematic networks for unsupervised motion retargetting. In: Proceedings of the IEEE Conference on Computer Vision and Pattern Recognition, pp. 8639–8648 (2018)
6. Zhu, J.Y., Park, T., Isola, P., Efros, A.A.: Unpaired image-to-image translation using cycle-consistent adversarial networks. In: Proceedings of the IEEE International Conference on Computer Vision, pp. 2223–2232 (2017)

A Deep Learning-Based Noise-Resilient Keyword Spotting Engine for Embedded Platforms

Ramzi Abdelmoula(✉), Alaa Khamis(✉), and Fakhri Karray

Centre for Pattern Analysis and Machine Intelligence (CPAMI),
University of Waterloo, Waterloo, ON, Canada
{r2abdelm,karray}@uwaterloo.ca, akhamis@pami.uwaterloo.ca

Abstract. Keyword spotting (KWS) is important in numerous trigger, trigger-command and command and control applications of embedded platforms. However, the embedded platforms used currently in the fast growing market of the Internet of Things (IoT) and in standalone systems have still considerable processing power, memory and battery constraints. In IoT and smart devices applications, speakers are usually far from the microphone resulting in severe distortions and considerable amounts of noise and noticeable reverberation. Speech enhancement can be used as a front-end or pre-processing module to improve the performance of the KWS. However, denoisers and dereverberators as front-end processing modules add to the complexity of the keyword spotting system and the computing, memory and battery requirements of the embedded platforms. In this paper, a noise robust keyword spotting engine with small memory footprint is presented. Multi-condition utterances training of a deep neural networks model is developed to increase the keyword spotting noise robustness. A comparative study is conducted to compare the deep learning approach with Gaussian mixture model. Experimental results show that deep learning outperforms the Gaussian approach in both clean and noisy conditions. Moreover, deep learning model trained using partially noisy data saves the need for using speech enhancement module or denoiser for front-end processing.

Keywords: Keyword spotting · Phoneme classification · Deep learning · Deep belief network · Embedded platform · Noisy speech

1 Introduction

Speech recognition is still a complex task and needs powerful computational engines that do not fit usually into small embedded systems. Therefore, the computation has to take place in the cloud. This means, that every speech utterance is being sent through the Internet posing serious privacy threats and time delays and jitters due to the non-deterministic nature of Internet performance. In addition, the smart small devices such as, locks, lights, A/C or irrigation sprinklers

F. Karray et al. (Eds.): ICIAR 2019, LNCS 11663, pp. 134–146, 2019.
https://doi.org/10.1007/978-3-030-27272-2_12

do not require the full potential of the modern speech recognition with its natural language understanding. Yet they require accuracy and fast response. Moreover, embedded platforms have considerable processing power, memory and battery constraints. This calls for the need of a smaller and simpler, yet effective technology to recognize several commands capable of controlling these small, yet smart devices. Such technology is known as keyword spotting.

Keyword spotting (KWS) is the process of detecting predefined keywords in spoken utterances. Continuous Speech Keyword Spotting is the problem of spotting keywords in recorded conversations, when a small number of instances of keywords are available in training data [1]. KWS is important in numerous trigger, trigger-command and command and control applications of embedded platforms. These applications include, but are not limited to, triggering smart devices, command and control of domestic appliances, verbal human-robot interaction, audio texting and voice dialing for hand-free and wearable devices, telephone routing, call-content analytics and real-time speech analytics for customer services to name just a few. For example, a keyword spotter can be used to trigger normal operation of an electronic device and terminating sleep, standby or hibernation mode.

In this paper, a noise robust keyword spotting engine with small footprint is presented. The remainder of the paper is organized as follows: Sect. 2 introduces keyword spotting problem and the various standard approaches for tackling it. Noise robustness of the keyword spotting process is highlighted in Sect. 3 followed by presenting the proposed keyword spotting engine in Sect. 4. Experimental results are presented and discussed in Sect. 5. Finally, conclusion and future directions are summarized in Sect. 6.

2 Keyword Spotting

Keyword spotting methods [2] can be classified into Large Vocabulary Continuous Speech Recognition (LVCSR)-based keyword spotting, acoustic KWS and phonetic search KWS and Phonetic search KWS [3]. A LVCSR transcribes the speech input into text format using Automatic Speech Recognizer (ASR) and feeds it the KWS module. The recognized text is then processed by Keyword detection module or Keyword spotting (KWS) engine. This KWS engine searches the recognized text to determine the existence and the positions of a specific keywords encoded in a keyword list. In [4], LVCSR keyword spotting method was tested giving unsatisfactory results of only 61.2% accuracy. Unlike the LVCSR, the acoustic KWS system does not estimate the whole text of the audio, yet it uses the same search algorithm. Instead of having one large acoustic model trained using representative data of the English language, this technique performs speech recognition based on a small subset of specific words alongside a general non-keyword model. Having a model for keywords and another for other words that are usually referred to as "garbage", the acoustic KWS can execute its search in one single step [5]. In fact, Google [6] uses a similar method to train their trigger word "Okey Google" using Deep Neural Network (DNN). Instead of having multiple models, they train their neural network using multiple occurrences of the trigger word with another training set classified as filler [7].

Phonetic search KWS consists of finding the keyword based on their phonetic transcript which is performed over two steps. The input represents acoustic utterances from a live source such as microphone or microphone array or recorded audio. The first step performs phoneme decoding that transforms the audio input to an array of phonemes in contrast of the LVCSR that produces a list of words. The second consists of a phonetic search calculating the distance between the produced phonetic sequence from the previous stage with the list defining the keywords [8]. It is noted that the engine requires a keyword list with their phonetic description alongside a general phoneme database. The latter is used by the decoder to produce an estimate of the phoneme sequence present in the input audio file [7].

The major comparison metrics for the above mentioned KWS techniques are accuracy, processing time, keyword level flexibility and training data availability [9]. There is no single best approach with high efficiency for all three metrics. However, for the work presented in this paper, more emphasis is put on keyword flexibility as embedded systems are known to be versatile and are produced in big numbers for different target domains, hence retraining for each keyword change would make the KWS engine less practical and less desirable. In addition, the data availability plays an important role as it excludes the acoustic KWS technique due to the lack of training data. Therefore the phonetic search based approach is adopted in this paper as our platform for KWS.

3 Noise Resilience in KWS

In IoT and smart devices applications, speakers are usually located far from the microphone resulting in severe distortions and large amounts of noise and noticeable reverberation. Moreover, tests for speech recognition engines are usually carried out in ideal environments within laboratories, hence their accuracy level is substantially degraded when tested in real world conditions. The different noises and disturbances accompanying the highly variant testing environments create a considerable mismatch between the training and the testing set, hence the accuracy degradation [10]. The latter mismatch has been the motivator behind the design of more robust speech engines. Increasing robustness of the automatic speech recognizer (ASR) can be achieved in the following three levels: (i) Improving the signal to noise ration (SNR) in the acoustic level by different speech enhancement approaches [11–13]; (ii) Choosing a parametric representation that is more robust to noise [14,15] and (iii) Including both the noisy and clean signal in the modeling stage allowing the new model to recognize the speech under specific noisy environments [16]. Dealing with the mismatch is a crucial step in the speech recognition development and its introduction to real world environments. Most of speech enhancement approaches under a multitude of assumptions have had limited success [11,17,18].

Several methods have been used to incorporate noise robustness into the Deep Neural Network (DNN) training in the speech recognition area [19]. These methods include multi-condition utterances training, denoising the utterances before the training and noise estimation incorporated into the network. These approaches are similar to noise robustness techniques in the traditional Hidden Markov Model-Gaussian Mixture Modelling (HMM-GMM) engines [20]. The following is a brief description of each method.

- **Multi-condition utterances training:** Using multi-condition data for DNN training permits a higher level features learning by the network. These features are more robust to the noise effect on the overall classification. In this regard, DNN is considered as nonlinear feature extractor and also a nonlinear classifier. The lower layers represent discriminative features that are independent from the various conditions across the many acoustic conditions existing in the training data. Hence in multi-condition utterances training data, the input vector is a combination of the noisy utterances frames. Although the multi-condition technique is theoretically similar for both GMM and DNN, they are substantially different. For GMM, a Gaussian mixture directly models the data, hence the noise introduced variability is captured and modeled. In discriminative training, noisy features are discarded by the GMM while the deep neural network extracts helpful information using the nonlinear processing of the layers [20].
- **Enhanced features for DNN training:** One intuitive solution to noisy data is to filter out the noise from the speech utterances before the training stage. Hence, using a speech enhancement technique reduces the noise effects on the input signal. The classifier learns any flaw introduced by the enhancement algorithm if the latter is used on both, the testing and training data. The HMM-GMM version of this technique is called feature space noise adaptive training [20,21]. The same technique could directly be applied to the DNN training.
- **DNN noise-aware training:** The last technique consists of adapting the model to the environment noise by introducing a noise estimation in the model itself. The noise model adapts the GMM parameters based on a model that determines how the clean speech is corrupted. The DNN is informed of the noise and not adapted to it, therefore this technique is called DNN noise-aware training. According to [20], multi-condition utterances training is the best approach for noise robustness, combined with the dropout technique, the accuracy is improved by 7.5% relative to the best published result in speech recognition. Therefore, the multi-condition training is adopted in this work as the DNN approach to achieve noise robustness.

In this paper, A DNN model was trained using large size speech data under various conditions, encompassing clean speech data and data with stationary and non-stationary noises. The following section provides more details about the proposed approach.

4 Proposed Approach

In order to fulfill the need of the fast growing market of the IoT, the main goal of this work is to develop a keyword spotting engine that is robust to noisy environments and that could also sit on a platform with considerable memory and processing power constraints. This is accomplished by applying multi-condition utterances training of the recognizer. The targeted noises are injected into the training data enabling the model to simulate the noisy environments as it is trained with the clean and noisy data. Therefore, dismissing the need for a denoiser as the robustness will be incorporated in the deep learning model. As mentioned in Sect. 2, the keyword spotting method used here is the phoneme search based method. Indeed, this approach presents the best combination of excellent keyword flexibility with the ability to frequently change the list of keywords as desired and with relative ease. Moreover, it ensures real-time response and satisfactory accuracy which are most important when it comes to any classification problem. Finally, the training data for the phoneme search based KWS is widely available. Figure 1 illustrates the different modules of a KWS engine based on phoneme search and depicts the data flow and what format the data takes going from one module to another [3]. The first module being the Mel-frequency cepstral coefficients (MFCC) pre-processing, takes in the raw speech signal generating features that represent the most important information of the speech data. The second module is very crucial as it decodes the speech features into phonemes producing the input for the next module. Finally, the keyword mapper module generates the list of detected keywords if they exist in the input signal [5].

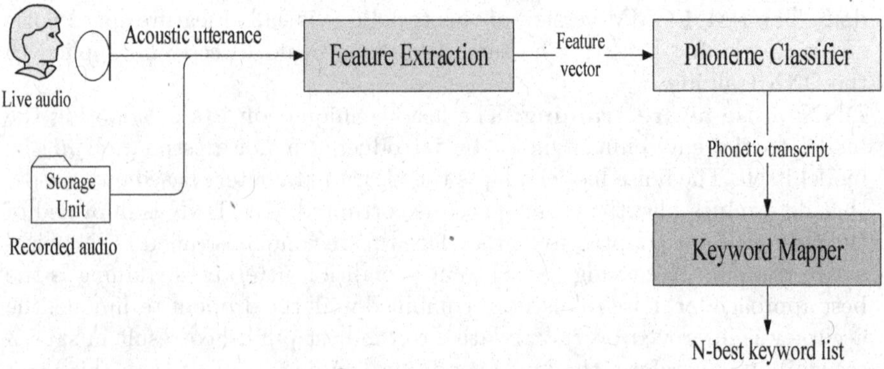

Fig. 1. Keyword spotting engine

The scope of the work presented in this paper only focuses on optimizing the phoneme decoder, in terms of small memory foot-print and faster response time while maintaining good robustness and accuracy.

Deep learning performs a pre-training step followed by a network fine-tuning step based on the standard backpropagation algorithm. The pre-training itself has been used in two different ways in the literature. The first method is to generate a new set of features using either restricted Boltzmann machine (RBM) or Stacked Autoencoder (SdA) from the input training data. The new features are considered more abstract and are more representative than the original features. However, for speech recognition, MFCC is considered the standard representation and is used by most of the speech recognition engines in the market [22]. In this paper, we use the second method of deep learning which consists of using the pre-training stage to initialize the weights of the neural networks in preparation for the next fine-tuning process [23].

The first stage of designing a DNN is the most important part in the training process. Therefore, choosing the correct pre-training algorithm would greatly influence the trained network accuracy. For speech recognition, the two main methods used in the literature are RBM and SdA [22,24]. To ensure that the best technique is used, both methods have been tested and the results are reported in the next section.

5 Experimental Results and Discussion

Different experiments have been conducted to assess the proposed approach. The following subsections summarize data preparation process, experiment setup, deep neural network tuning, experimental results and discussion.

5.1 Data Preparation

The different parameters of the proposed techniques in the phoneme classification process are discussed. Starting from the pre-processing features extraction and ending with the classification task, the reasoning behind the selected scenarios is presented in the following subsections.

Noise Contamination in the scope of this work, the WSJ database is selected. In fact, the WSJ is composed of over 82,700 audio files with a sampling frequency of 100 samples per second. The database offers around 60 million data points. However, WSJ dataset only contains clean speech. Noise contamination is performed to include noisy data in the training of the DNN. Clean speech data is contaminated with two types of noises: fan noise as stationary noise sample and restaurant noise as non-stationary noise sample. Different levels of SNR are used ranging from −10 dB to 20 dB.

Feature Extraction. The pre-processing stage is important as it is the first step in the phoneme recognition process, thus any poor choice in the parameters will propagate and will greatly influence the final classification results. In addition, to fairly compare the proposed approach using DNN to the HMM/GMM based phoneme recognizer, similar feature extraction parameters have to be selected. Therefore, no changes are made to tune the pre-processing stage parameters. Instead, the optimal values that produce the best phoneme classification results for the hybrid HMM/GMM based recognizer are selected. These parameters are number of MFCC features (13 coefficients plus the differential Δ and the acceleration $\Delta\Delta$ coefficients), 10 ms frame size and a 25 ms Hamming window.

Phoneme Classification. Phonemes classification probability output is also the input to the keyword recognition algorithm, making the phoneme recognition process accuracy crucial to the final keyword detection result. Given the multitude and sensitivity of parameters to be tuned in the neural networks structure, cross validation is performed for each of the test scenarios. The selected parameters for the DNN phoneme classifier are 3, 4 and 5 context padding, 2-fold cross-validation, 3, 4 and 5 layers, 450, 500, 550 and 600 neurons, adaptive learning rate with starting value of 0.08 and dropout ratios of 0.2, 0.3 and 0.4. If the validation error reduction between two consecutive epochs is less than 0.001, the learning rate is scaled by 0.02 during each of the remaining epochs. Training terminates when the validation error reduction between a number of consecutive epochs (e.g. 5 epochs) falls below 0.0001. The minimum number of epoch is selected to be 20, after which scaling can be performed. The number of epochs in the pre-training stage are selected to be 8, 10 and 12 as RBM and SdA do not require many epochs to converge.

One of the drawbacks of DNN is the difficulty of selecting the network parameters, making the network tuning one of the major steps in any machine learning application that uses connectionist modeling. Different experiments have been conducted to tune the neural networks [9]. These experiments are very helpful in directing us forward. The final network parameters are 4-layers with number of neurons of 500, 350, 200 and 100 for first, second, third and fourth layer respectively. Dropout ratio is 0.2 and context padding is 4 frames on each side of the current frame.

5.2 Test Scenarios Results

In the scope of this paper, the reference model is a mono-phone 3-state HMM for 40 phonemes with the probability distribution on each state being 5 mixture GMM. For the following tests, the use of noisy data is considered. As previously mentioned, noisy data are a combination of clean (25%), "Fan" (25%), "Restaurant" (25%) and Fan convoluted with "Restaurant" contaminated data. The DNN is tested with both, context dependent (CD) and context independent (CI) for fair comparison with GMM and to see the impact of context padding on the testing error of the DNN.

Clean Data Modeling. The first test sets used only the clean data of the WSJ database for model training.

- **Clean data testing:** This test is performed to compare the efficiency of the DNN based model with the GMM based model to determine if the DNN is more accurate than GMM for phoneme classification under clean data for training and testing. This test showed the superiority of the DNN approach over the GMM with a substantial improvement of 7% in the testing Word Error Rate (WER). Using context dependent input to the DNN with "4" frames on each side further improves the accuracy by 4%. This proves that DNN is better than GMM in the phoneme classification of clean data.
- **Noisy data testing:** The following test is performed as a reference to prove that a clean model performs poorly when tested with noisy data. High WER rate is obtained when using both approaches with noisy data on clean models (GMM: 65% and DNN: 62%). This is an expected outcome. Still the DNN model performs slightly better.

Noisy Data Modeling. In this section noisy data is used to model GMM and DNN models and a conclusion is drawn from comparing their respective results.

- **Noisy data testing:** The purpose of training noisy models is to improve the performance of the phoneme decoder when tested under noisy condition, thus the noisy DNN model. The latter model is then compared to the GMM model that is also trained with noisy data and the best approach under both clean and noisy environment is selected to carry the phoneme classification for the KWS process. The GMM modeled with noisy data has poor performance (61% WER) of the as it only decreased the testing error by 4% when tested with noisy data. On the other hand, DNN efficiently modeled the noisy training data, as the testing error decreased by 19% for the context independent bringing the classification error to 43% which is only 15% away from the clean model with clean testing data. The Context dependent DNN also decreased the testing error by 8% which still outperforms the GMM model by 7%.
- **Denoised data testing:** The previous tests proved that using a DNN model with noisy training outperforms the GMM counterpart with the same training data. But it could be argued that the use of a denoiser could replace the DNN noisy training. Thus, this test is performed to monitor the behaviour of the clean model with denoised testing data. The illustrated results in Table 1 prove that using a denoiser prior to feeding the testing data to the clean DNN model improved the performance by 4%. Whereas the DNN noisy trained model gives a testing error of 54% which is substantially better considering that there is no use of a denoiser. Performing the context padding improved accuracy by an extra 4% when using denoised data. Context dependent noisy DNN training outperforms the denoised clean model DNN by a considerable 11%. Removing the denoiser from the system and reaching a better accuracy for noisy data is one of the contributions of this paper. Better performance under noisy condition only implies that the system will have two models one for noisy and the other for clean data. Context dependent input features reduced the testing error considerably in the various above tests. Therefore,

the rest of the DNN experiments are performed using context padding with "4" frames on each side of the current frame.

Table 1. GMM vs. DNN WER (%) - Denoised testing

Modeling approach	Training data	Testing data	Testing error
DNN (CI)	Clean	Denoised	58%
DNN (CD)	Clean	Denoised	54%
DNN (CI)	Noisy	Noisy	54%
DNN (CD)	Noisy	Noisy	**43%**

- **Clean data testing:** To prove that the noisy trained DNN noisy model could be the sole replacement of multiple models without the need for a denoiser, which is usually expensive to deploy in real world applications, testing the noisy model in clean conditions and comparing it to GMM is required. A degradation in the performance of DNN noisy model is observed when compared to the DNN clean model using clean testing. The degradation is about 10% (from 28% to 38% WER) but the noisy model still outperforms the clean model in noisy conditions by 19%. This is considered as a good compromise when it comes to the overall behaviour of the classifier. However, a better compromise could be reached by increasing the clean data component currently at 25% in the noisy data set.

Increased Clean Data Ratio. Increasing the clean data ratio in the mixed training error from 25% to 50% may bring an increase of the testing error under noisy conditions while it also promises an increase of the performance when tested with clean data. In fact, the model is less familiar with the noisy data and more familiar with clean data as the proportions shift toward a half and half ratio. Table 2 depicts the expected degradation of the noisy DNN model with the noisy testing data from 43% to 46%. However, the testing error is improved from 38% to 31%. The same test is performed using GMM generating a testing error of 45% which is quite higher than the DNN. This confirms the superiority of the DNN over GMM when testing the noisy model with clean data. This presents a better compromise for both condition.

The above results indicate that using DNN instead of GMM to train the phoneme classifier model substantially improves the performance of the decoder. Indeed, using clean data for both testing and training, DNN model outperformed the GMM-based model by 13% in accuracy. Furthermore, using a mix of noisy and clean data to model the DNN classifier prove to be a better alternative than using a denoiser in noisy conditions. It also avoids catastrophic speech

Table 2. GMM vs. Context-dependent DNN WER (%) for different clean data ratios

Modeling approach	Training data	Testing data	Testing error
GMM (25% Clean)	Noisy	Clean	45%
DNN (25% Clean)	Noisy	Noisy	43%
DNN (50% Clean)	Noisy	Noisy	46%
DNN (25% Clean)	Noisy	Clean	38%
DNN (50% Clean)	Noisy	Clean	**31%**

enhancement, which is the case when the clean data is mistakenly considered as noisy data, leading the denoiser to disturb the clean utterance and producing corrupt data that is wrongly classified.

Speed and Memory Consumption. DNNs reach the top of their potential when they are deep (many layers) and having many neurons per layer [25]. Training them on a traditional CPU would require very long periods. The high data transfer latency limits the multi-threading programming making it not suitable for this situation. Nonetheless, recent parallel neural networks for graphics cards GPUs have solved the training speed limitation of the DNN [26]. GPU designed code for classification should be up to two orders of magnitude faster than the CPU [27]. In our case, only one NVIDIA Tesla GPU was available and has been used to train the different models needed for this paper. The actual speed up was not calculated as the CPU took a seemingly very long time to train the model, which makes the speed up seem very high, as the GPU only takes a dozen hours to train the model. The DNN training speed is not the only issue as the decoding of a DNN is also slower than the GMM decoding due to the high number of float multiplications required for a classification especially for deep networks. According to [29], using a GMM model on embedded systems is twice as fast as using a DNN for a speech recognition decoding task. However, there are a number of techniques that speed up the decoding of DNN to reach a speed equal to that of GMM. Theses techniques are the following: using fixed point operations and frame skipping technique [29]. In this paper, none of the mentioned techniques has been used, but they will be used once the network is tuned and tested on embedded systems as the decoding speed is also crucial in real-time embedded applications such as keyword spotting.

Although the DNN decoding process is more complex than the GMM decoding, the memory footprint does not follow the same pattern. Indeed, according to [29], a DNN model with 1.48 M parameters outperforms the GMM in accuracy, with a disk size of only 17% of the GMMs. This is considered a major advantage for deep neural networks as small memory consumption enable smaller embedded platform to be speech enabled. The trained DNN model has been tested on ArmV7 processor with Ubuntu operating system. The obtained memory footprint is 2 MB.

6 Conclusion

This paper presented a noise resilient keyword spotting engine with small footprint for embedded platforms. Using DNN mixed data training approach promised to enhance the system robustness to background noises without the need for a hardware or a software denoiser. This technique also allows replacing the two model approach, one for noisy and the other for clean environment, by a single model with a small penalty in terms of accuracy but with large gain in terms of less model complexity. The trained DNN model is just a few hundreds of kilobytes large which is smaller than the GMM model size. The absence of the denoiser and the noise sensing tool means less memory and less processing time as only the DNN multiplications are needed to reach a phoneme classification with no need for a denoiser. However, the DNN decoding is slower than GMM decoding which will be rectified when introducing the mentioned speedup techniques for DNN such as fixed-point operations and frame skipping.

Future work will include testing more noise samples and different levels of reverberation as audible effects that result from interacting the sound with the environment. The following step involves developing a small and fast phoneme mapping algorithm that would be the module taking the phoneme classifier output and deciding if a keyword is spoken in the given speech utterance.

References

1. Seth, H., Kumar, P., Srivastava, M.M.: Prototypical metric transfer learning for continuous speech keyword spotting with limited training data. arXiv preprint arXiv:1901.03860 (2019)
2. Mary, L., G, D.: Keyword spotting techniques. In: Searching Speech Databases. SST, pp. 45–60. Springer, Cham (2019). https://doi.org/10.1007/978-3-319-97761-4_4
3. Moyal, A., Aharonson, V., Tetariy, E., Gishri, M.: Keyword spotting methods. In: Phonetic Search Methods for Large Speech Databases. SpringerBriefs in Electrical and Computer Engineering, pp. 7–11. Springer, New York (2013). https://doi.org/10.1007/978-1-4614-6489-1_2
4. Chen, I.-F., Ni, C., Lim, B.P., Chen, N.F., Lee, C.-H.: A novel keyword+LVCSR-filler based grammar network representation for spoken keyword search. In: 9th International Symposium on Chinese Spoken Language Processing (ISCSLP), pp. 192–196. IEEE (2014)
5. Szoke, I., et al.: Comparison of keyword spotting approaches for informal continuous speech. In: Interspeech, pp. 633–636 (2005)
6. Chen, G., Parada, C., Heigold, G.: Small-footprint keyword spotting using deep neural networks. In: 2014 IEEE International Conference on Acoustics, Speech and Signal Processing (ICASSP), pp. 4087–4091. IEEE (2014)
7. Moyal, A., Aharonson, V., Tetariy, E., Gishri, M.: Phonetic Search Methods for Large Speech Databases. Springer Science and Business Media, New York (2013)
8. Alon, G.: Key-word spotting the base technology for speech analytics. Natural Speech Communications (2005)
9. Abdelmoula, R.: Noise robust keyword spotting using deep neural networks for embedded platforms. Master's thesis, University of Waterloo (2016)

10. Ortega-Garcia, J., Gonzalez-Rodrguez, J.: Overview of speech enhancement techniques for automatic speaker recognition. In: Proceedings of the Fourth International Conference on Spoken Language, ICSLP 1996, vol. 2, pp. 929–932. IEEE (1996)
11. Loizou, P.: Speech Enhancement: Theory and Practice. CRC Press, Boca Raton (2013)
12. Yousefian, N., Loizou, P.C.: A dual-microphone speech enhancement algorithm based on the coherence function. IEEE Trans. Audio Speech Lang. Process. **20**(2), 599–609 (2012)
13. Xu, Y., Du, J., Dai, L.-R., Lee, C.-H.: An experimental study on speech enhancement based on deep neural networks. IEEE Signal Process. Lett. **21**(1), 65–68 (2014)
14. Gemmeke, J.F., Virtanen, T., Hurmalainen, A.: Exemplar-based speech enhancement and its application to noise-robust automatic speech recognition. In: International Workshop on Machine Listening in Multisource Environments, pp. 53–75 (2011)
15. Liu, D., Smaragdis, P., Kim, M.: Experiments on deep learning for speech denoising. In: Proceedings of the Annual Conference of the International Speech Communication Association (INTERSPEECH) (2014)
16. Lu, X., Tsao, Y., Matsuda, S., Hori, C.: Speech enhancement based on deep denoising autoencoder. In: INTERSPEECH, pp. 436–440 (2013)
17. Cohen, I., Gannot, S.: Spectral enhancement methods. In: Benesty, J., Sondhi, M.M., Huang, Y.A. (eds.) Springer Handbook of Speech Processing. SH, pp. 873–902. Springer, Heidelberg (2008). https://doi.org/10.1007/978-3-540-49127-9_44
18. Ephraim, Y., Malah, D.: Speech enhancement using a minimum mean-square error log-spectral amplitude estimator. IEEE Trans. Acoust. Speech Signal Process. **33**(2), 443–445 (1985)
19. Seltzer, M.L., Yu, D., Wang, Y.: An investigation of deep neural networks for noise robust speech recognition. In: 2013 IEEE International Conference on Acoustics, Speech and Signal Processing (ICASSP), pp. 7398–7402. IEEE (2013)
20. Virtanen, T., Singh, R., Raj, B.: Techniques for Noise Robustness in Automatic Speech Recognition. Wiley, Hoboken (2012)
21. Deng, L., Acero, L., Plumpe, M., Huang, X.: Large-vocabulary speech recognition under adverse acoustic environments. In: INTERSPEECH, pp. 806–809 (2000)
22. Hinton, G.E., Osindero, S., Teh, Y.-W.: A fast learning algorithm for deep belief nets. Neural Comput. **18**(7), 1527–1554 (2006)
23. Janni, D.: Introduction to deep neural network (2015). http://derekjanni.github.io/Easy-Neural-Nets/
24. Vincent, P., Larochelle, H., Lajoie, I., Bengio, Y., Manzagol, P.-A.: Stacked denoising autoencoders: learning useful representations in a deep network with a local denoising criterion. J. Mach. Learn. Res. **11**, 3371–3408 (2010)
25. Ciresan, D.C., Meier, U., Masci, J., Maria Gambardella, L., Schmidhuber, J.: Flexible, high performance convolutional neural networks for image classification. In: IJCAI Proceedings-International Joint Conference on Artificial Intelligence, vol. 22, no. 1, p. 1237 (2011)
26. Ciresan, D., Meier, U., Schmidhuber, J.: Multi-column deep neural networks for image classification. In: 2012 IEEE Conference on Computer Vision and Pattern Recognition (CVPR), pp. 3642–3649. IEEE (2012)

27. Strigl, D., Kofler, K., Podlipnig, S.: Performance and scalability of GPU-based convolutional neural networks. In: 2010 18th Euromicro International Conference on Parallel, Distributed and Network-Based Processing (PDP), pp. 317–324. IEEE (2010)
28. Uetz, R., Behnke, S.: Large-scale object recognition with cudaaccelerated hierarchical neural networks. In: IEEE International Conference on Intelligent Computing and Intelligent Systems, ICIS 2009, vol. 1, pp. 536–541. IEEE (2009)
29. Lei, X., Senior, A., Gruenstein, A., Sorensen, J.: Accurate and compact large vocabulary speech recognition on mobile devices. In: INTERSPEECH, pp. 662–665 (2013)

A Compact Representation of Histopathology Images Using Digital Stain Separation and Frequency-Based Encoded Local Projections

Alison K. Cheeseman[1], Hamid Tizhoosh[2], and Edward R. Vrscay[1](✉)

[1] Department of Applied Mathematics, Faculty of Mathematics, University of Waterloo, Waterloo, Ontario N2L 3G1, Canada
{alison.cheeseman,ervrscay}@uwaterloo.ca

[2] Kimia Lab, University of Waterloo, Waterloo, Ontario N2L 3G1, Canada
hamid.tizhoosh@uwaterloo.ca

Abstract. In recent years, histopathology images have been increasingly used as a diagnostic tool in the medical field. The process of accurately diagnosing a biopsy sample requires significant expertise in the field, and as such can be time-consuming and is prone to uncertainty and error. With the advent of digital pathology, using image recognition systems to highlight problem areas or locate similar images can aid pathologists in making quick and accurate diagnoses. In this paper, we specifically consider the encoded local projections (ELP) algorithm, which has previously shown some success as a tool for classification and recognition of histopathology images. We build on the success of the ELP algorithm as a means for image classification and recognition by proposing a modified algorithm which captures the local frequency information of the image. The proposed algorithm estimates local frequencies by quantifying the changes in multiple projections in local windows of greyscale images. By doing so we remove the need to store the full projections, thus significantly reducing the histogram size, and decreasing computation time for image retrieval and classification tasks. Furthermore, we investigate the effectiveness of applying our method to histopathology images which have been digitally separated into their hematoxylin and eosin stain components. The proposed algorithm is tested on the publicly available invasive ductal carcinoma (IDC) data set. The histograms are used to train an SVM to classify the data. The experiments showed that the proposed method outperforms the original ELP algorithm in image retrieval tasks. On classification tasks, the results are found to be comparable to state-of-the-art deep learning methods and better than many handcrafted features from the literature.

This research has been supported in part by a Natural Sciences and Engineering Research Council of Canada (NSERC) Doctoral Scholarship (AKC).

F. Karray et al. (Eds.): ICIAR 2019, LNCS 11663, pp. 147–158, 2019.
https://doi.org/10.1007/978-3-030-27272-2_13

Keywords: Digital histopathology · Encoded local projections (ELP) · Radon transform · Digital stain separation · Digital image retrieval and classification

1 Introduction

Histopathology, the examination of tissue under a microscope to study biological structures as they relate to disease manifestation, has recently attracted a lot of interest from the medical imaging research community. With the introduction of whole slide digital scanners, histopathology slides can now be digitized and stored in a digital form. As a result, it is now possible to apply computer-aided diagnosis and image analysis algorithms to the emerging field of digital histopathology [4]. Content-based image retrieval (CBIR) and image classification are two important components of computer-aided image analysis which we consider in this paper. In a classification approach, the objective is to classify each image as belonging to a disease category. Image retrieval involves finding images which share the same visual characteristics as the query image. The identification and analysis of similar images can assist pathologists in quickly and accurately obtaining a diagnosis by providing a baseline for comparison.

As a result of the extremely large size of digital histopathology images, it is desirable to generate compact image descriptors for both retrieval and classification tasks. A large number of well-known image descriptors already exist, however the different requirements of a new application make constant innovation necessary. This becomes particularly important in a field where trained feature extraction algorithms, such as deep networks, may not always be feasible. Deep networks require massive volumes of labelled data for optimal training, yet large (and balanced) data sets are not always available in the medical field. This is especially true when we consider digital histopathology, as obtaining ground truth annotations is time-consuming and requires expert knowledge. Handcrafted image descriptors, such as the well-known local binary patterns (LBP) [6], scale-invariant feature transform (SIFT) [1], and histogram of oriented gradients (HOG) [3] get around this issue by incorporating expert knowledge directly into their design without requiring any training data.. Such descriptors and their successors have been quite successful in a range of diverse imaging applications [12]. More recently, a projection-based histogram descriptor was proposed in [12] specifically for the application of CBIR and classification of medical images. The ELP image descriptor has been very successful thus far on histopathology images, outperforming many well-known handcrafted features, and even outperforming some deep features generated using a convolutional neural network (CNN) when applied to medical imaging applications [12].

In this paper we build upon the ELP descriptor, a dense-sampling method introduced in [12] and propose a frequency-based ELP (F-ELP) descriptor which captures the local frequency information of the image. Instead of storing entire projections, as in the ELP method, our proposed method quantifies the number of changes in each projection and uses this as an estimate of local frequency.

While the original ELP method results in large histograms, the size of our F-ELP histograms has linear dependence on the local window size. The compact nature of our descriptor is desirable from the perspective of both memory usage for storage of descriptors and computation requirements when applied to image retrieval and classification type tasks. In addition to the introduction of our novel histogram representation, we also discuss the use of digital stain separation to improve the performance of our descriptor.

We test the performance of the proposed F-ELP descriptor on both image retrieval and image classification tasks. The publicly available invasive ductal carcinoma (IDC) dataset is used to evaluate the performance of our method and for comparison to state-of-the-art results from the literature.

2 The Proposed Method

Our proposed method involves two main innovations, which are described in more detail here. First, we introduce our proposed image descriptor and discuss how it differs from the ELP descriptor in [12]. We then introduce the idea of separating the histopathology images into their histochemical stain components to generate more meaningful image descriptors.

2.1 Frequency-Based ELP (F-ELP)

The ELP image descriptor is a dense-sampling method which encodes the gradient changes of multiple Radon projections in small local windows of the image. To maintain some level of robustness to rotation, a dominant angle is determined for each local neighbourhood using the image gradient. The dominant, or anchor, angle is then used to anchor the projections in that window so that the end result does not depend on image orientation. Projection gradients are encoded using the *MinMax* [12] method to generate a binary number which is then used to build a histogram. It should be noted here that in [12] an alternate method of computing the anchor angle based on the overall Radon sinogram is initially proposed. However, when applying their method to a pathology data set, the authors choose to save time by approximating the anchor angle computation by the median of the image gradient directions. In order to have a fair comparison, we consider this particular implementation of the ELP descriptor in this work.

The computation of our proposed F-ELP descriptor follows the same overall steps as the ELP descriptor, with some modifications along the way to improve rotational invariance, reduce sensitivity to shifts in the image and reduce redundancy by encoding only the frequency information from each projection. We describe each step in detail as follows, highlighting where our method differs from the ELP method.

Identify Local Windows: The first step is to identify a set of small local windows for processing. Here, our method does not differ at all from the original ELP method. Since we are interested in finding projections which uniquely describe the patterns/textures in local neighbourhoods, we only consider regions which are sufficiently non-homogeneous so as to ensure projections contain something of interest. We let $\mathbf{W}$ denote a local window of size $n \times n$ and calculate the homogeneity, H of each window according to

$$H = 1 - \frac{1}{2^{n_{bits}}} \sqrt{\sum_i \sum_j (\mathbf{W}_{ij} - m)^2}, \tag{1}$$

where m denotes the median pixel value of $\mathbf{W}$ and n_{bits} is the number of bits used to encode the image. A threshold is used to eliminate any windows with high homogeneity.

Determine the Anchor Angle, $\boldsymbol{\theta^*}$: In order for our descriptor to be rotationally invariant, we seek a unique angle in each window by which to "anchor" our projections. We do so by computing the image gradient, binning the gradient directions into one degree intervals and selecting θ^* to be the mode (most frequently occurring) of the gradient directions. Our approach differs just slightly from the original method, in that we choose to use the mode instead of the median to find the average angle. We do so as the median is not invariant under circular shifts (i.e. angular rotations), whereas the mode is, so long as there is one unique angle which occurs at the highest frequency (i.e. a clearly dominant direction in the window).

Compute the Projection Along $\boldsymbol{\theta^*}$: As in the ELP method we compute projections using the Radon transform, which is given by

$$R(\rho, \theta) = \int_{-\infty}^{\infty} \int_{-\infty}^{\infty} f(x, y) \delta(\rho - x \cos\theta - y \sin\theta) dx dy, \tag{2}$$

where $\delta(\cdot)$ is the Dirac delta function. We extract the projection $\mathbf{p}_{\theta^*}$ by taking the Radon transform along parallel lines ρ for the fixed anchor angle θ^*.

Encode Projections and Create Histogram: It is in the encoding of the projections where our algorithm differs the most notably from the ELP method. Instead of encoding the entire gradient of each projection, we quantify the gradient changes in the projection vector and use this to build our histogram. The benefits of this modification are two-fold. Primarily, we remove the storage overhead of encoding entire projections, and instead just capture the general trend (low or high frequency) of the projections along each direction, resulting in much smaller histograms which still perform very well. Our proposed method also avoids the use of a binary encoding to capture the projections. This is beneficial as the binary encoding used by the ELP is very sensitive to small shifts in the projection, i.e. a change in one binary bit can lead to a very large difference in the resulting histogram. On the other hand, when the local projection frequency changes, the resulting change in the F-ELP histogram reflects the size of the frequency change.

Given a projection vector $\mathbf{p}$ of length n and its derivative $\mathbf{p}'$, we compute the following quantized encoding of the derivative,

$$\mathbf{q}(i) = \begin{cases} 0 & \text{if } \mathbf{p}'(i) \leq -T \\ 1 & \text{if } |\mathbf{p}'(i)| < T \\ 2 & \text{if } \mathbf{p}'(i) \geq T. \end{cases} \tag{3}$$

The three levels given in (3) indicate regions where the projection, $\mathbf{p}$, is decreasing, nearly constant (we use a small threshold, T, here to ignore small fluctuations), and increasing, respectively. Next, we count the number of transitions in $\mathbf{q}$ to get our estimate of local frequency which will be an integer value, d which satisfies $0 \leq d \leq n-2$. Once we have d we can increment the histogram $\mathbf{h}(d)$.

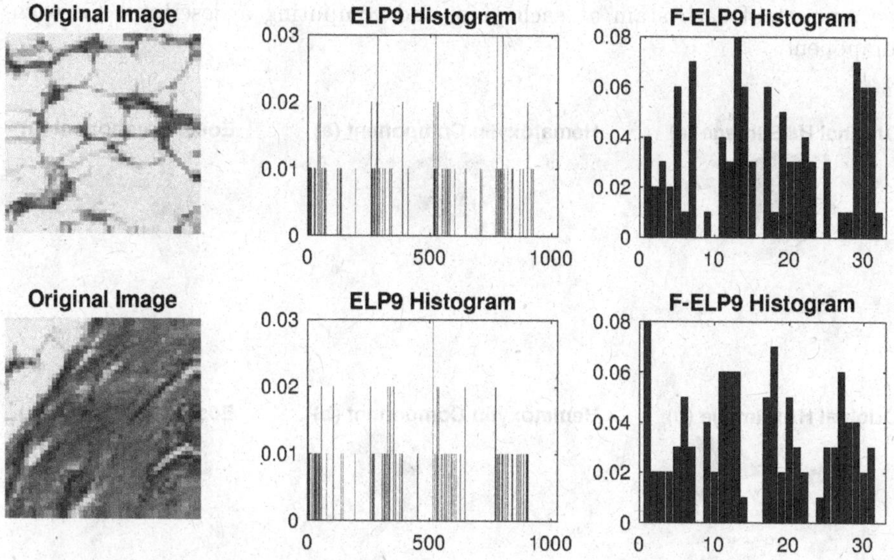

Fig. 1. Sample histograms generated using the ELP and F-ELP methods with a window size of $n = 9$.

Similar to the original ELP descriptor, we obtain more information by computing three additional projections relative to our anchor angle θ^*. These are equidistant projections, given by $\Theta = \{\theta^*, \theta^* + \pi/4, \theta^* + \pi/2, \theta^* + 3\pi/4\}$. For each additional angle, the projections are computed and encoded in the same manner. The final histogram is generated by concatenating all four histograms into one longer histogram.

Figure 1 shows an example of both the ELP and F-ELP descriptors for two sample images from the IDC dataset which contain somewhat different textures. In both cases, the histograms have been normalized according to the $L1$-norm. We see that the F-ELP descriptor, although it has less bins, appears to show a more varied distribution. When looking at the ELP histograms, we observe that the distribution is similar for both images, with many bins empty. This indicates that there is some redundancy in this image representation which we try to remove using the F-ELP method.

2.2 Digital Stain Separation

Prior to imaging, histology slides are stained to enhance the detail in tissues and cells. The most common stain protocol used in practice is hematoxylin and eosin (H&E), where hematoxylin components stain cell nuclei blue, and eosin stains other structures varying shades of red and pink [11]. The colours which appear in a slide and the size, shape and frequency at which they appear are all relevant factors a pathologist might assess when making a diagnosis. For this reason, we consider separating the input images into two components which give the amount of each stain at each pixel and computing a descriptor for each component.

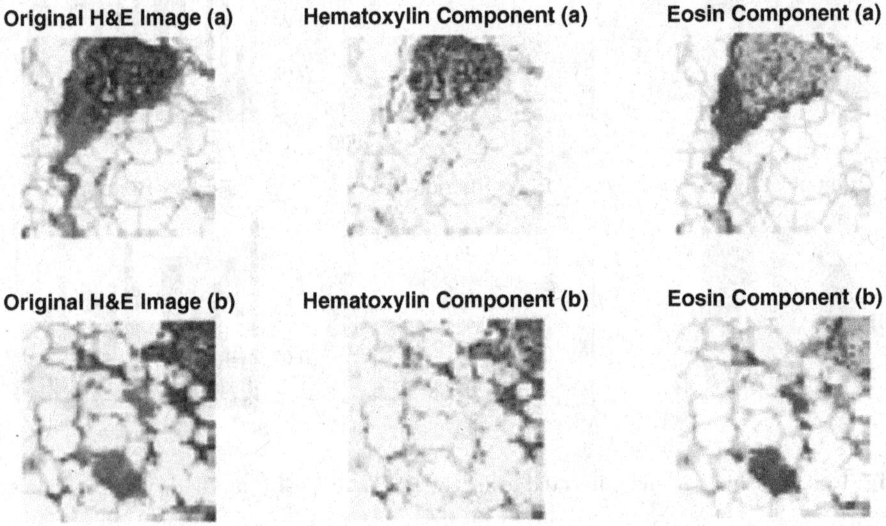

Fig. 2. Sample images from the IDC dataset showing the hematoxylin and eosin stane components after applying the stain separation algorithm from [8]. (Color figure online)

A number of methods already exist in the literature for digital stain separation of H&E slides that perform quite well. Although their intended usage is for stain normalization to control for variation in stain intensities and colours, these same methods are suitable for our purposes. In this paper we adopt the method proposed in [8], an extension of the wedge finding method from [7]. Unlike some previous methods for stain separation [11], this method does not require any calibration or knowledge of the exact stain colours, instead it works by using the available image data to estimate an H&E basis. Given that our image descriptor should ultimately be applied to data from multiple sources, this is an important feature of the stain separation algorithm. Figure 2 shows two examples of image patches before and after stain separation is applied. We can see that the algorithm does a good job of isolating the hematoxylin (blue/purple) component from the eosin (pink/red) component, even in regions where both stains contribute to the overall pixel colour.

Given the resulting stain separated image components, we proceed as described above to compute our F-ELP image descriptor, simply computing the F-ELP histogram for each component of the image separately. This results in two histograms, $\mathbf{h}_H$ and $\mathbf{h}_E$ which are concatenated to form the final longer histogram $\mathbf{h} = [\mathbf{h}_H \ \mathbf{h}_E]$.

3 Dataset and Image Preprocessing

We have used the publicly available IDC data set to test our method in both image retrieval and image classification. The dataset consists of digitized breast cancer slides from 162 patients diagnosed with IDC at the University of Pennsylvania Hospital and the Cancer Institute of New Jersey [2]. Each slide was digitized at 40x magnification and downsampled to a resolution of 4 µm/pixel. The supplied data was randomly split into three different subsets of 84 patients for training, 29 for validation and 49 test cases for final evaluation. The dataset provides each WSI split into image patches which are 50px × 50px in size. Ground truth annotation regarding the presence of IDC in each patch was obtained by manual delineation of cancer regions performed by expert pathologists.

For each image patch, we computed the F-ELP descriptor using the method described in the previous section. For these experiments we implement the algorithm with a threshold $T = 0.08$, determined by observation of the data, and a homogeneity threshold of 1, rejecting only completely homogeneous windows within each patch. In a future work, it would be beneficial to optimize these parameters and carry out some form of sensitivity analysis.

Since the image patches are quite small, each patch may not contain the presence of both hematoxylin and eosin. For better results, we use the entire whole slide image (WSI) to perform the stain separation and then split the image back into 50×50 patches to compute individual histograms. The stain separation algorithm we used assumes two stain components (H&E in our case) exist in the image, however some images are observed to have significant discoloration, such as large dark blue patches, and the introduction of other colours not caused by H&E staining. The prevalence of such artefacts negatively impacts the ability of the stain separation algorithm to provide good results for some patients, so we remove them by searching for images which have minimal variation in the RGB channels across the entire image. A total of 686 images were flagged and removed from the total data set, all of which contain significant artefacts/discoloration.

To evaluate the performance of our method in both image retrieval and classification tasks we have used the provided test data set consisting of 49 patients as our input data. For consistency with previous works we use both the balanced accuracy (BAC) and F-measure (F1) as performance metrics, which are defined as follows [2]:

$$\mathrm{BAC} = \frac{\mathrm{Sen} + \mathrm{Spc}}{2} \tag{4}$$

$$F1 = \frac{2 \cdot \mathrm{Pr} \cdot \mathrm{Rc}}{\mathrm{Pr} + \mathrm{Rc}}, \tag{5}$$

where Sen is sensitivity, Spc is specificity, Pr is precision and Rc, recall.

4 Experimental Results

In this section we present the results of using our proposed F-ELP descriptor for both image retrieval and classification of the IDC dataset. For each task we compare our method to relevant methods from the literature.

4.1 Image Retrieval

In order to evaluate the image retrieval performance of our descriptor we implement the k-Nearest Neighbours (kNN) algorithm in MATLAB with the F-ELP histograms as inputs. The kNN algorithm searches through the training data partition and classifies each image based on the class of its k nearest neighbours. Since there is no exact metric to quantitatively test image retrieval performance, we evaluate the expressiveness of the ELP-based descriptors for image retrieval tasks based on the accuracy of classification using kNN. In this work, we test the kNN algorithm using three different values for k ($k = 1, 3$ and 5). Four different distance metrics were used to determine the nearest neighbours, including the commonly used L_1, L_2 and cosine distances. We also used the Hutchinson (or Monge-Kantorovich) distance [9], a metric between two probability measures, as it is considered to be a good measure of distance between histograms. In the finite one-dimensional case, the Hutchinson distance can be computed in linear-time using the method from [10].

Table 1. F1 & BAC results for image retrieval ($k = 1$) on the IDC dataset

Method	L1		L2		Cosine		Hutchinson	
	F1	BAC	F1	BAC	F1	BAC	F1	BAC
ELP9	0.3072	0.5616	0.3728	0.5842	0.2965	0.5594	**0.3985**	**0.5904**
ELP9 + SS	0.3004	0.5654	0.4339	0.6167	0.2688	0.5574	**0.4527**	**0.6236**
F-ELP9	0.4177	0.6008	0.4179	0.6015	**0.4200**	**0.6022**	0.4189	0.6025
F-ELP9 + SS	0.5489	0.6881	0.5486	0.6879	**0.5504**	**0.6891**	0.5472	0.6869
F-ELP11	**0.3969**	**0.5865**	0.3947	0.5855	0.3954	0.5863	0.3792	0.5774
F-ELP11 + SS	0.5237	0.6707	0.5173	0.6666	0.5185	0.6673	**0.5347**	**0.6784**

Table 2. F1 & BAC results for image retrieval ($k = 3$) on the IDC dataset

Method	L1		L2		Cosine		Hutchinson	
	F1	BAC	F1	BAC	F1	BAC	F1	BAC
ELP9	0.4009	0.6092	0.4837	0.6432	0.3807	0.6015	**0.5117**	**0.6523**
ELP9 + SS	0.3662	0.5976	0.5372	0.6743	0.3240	0.5830	**0.5609**	**0.6833**
F-ELP9	0.5106	0.6514	0.5100	0.6515	**0.5122**	**0.6526**	0.5056	0.6490
F-ELP9 +SS	0.6267	0.7350	0.6251	0.7339	0.6257	0.7345	**0.6309**	**0.7375**
F-ELP11	0.5010	0.6420	0.5034	0.6443	**0.5043**	**0.6450**	0.4879	0.6355
F-ELP11 + SS	0.6117	0.7223	0.6003	0.7149	0.6053	0.7184	**0.6190**	**0.7279**

Table 3. F1 & BAC results for image retrieval ($k = 5$) on the IDC dataset

Method	L1		L2		Cosine		Hutchinson	
	F1	BAC	F1	BAC	F1	BAC	F1	BAC
ELP9	0.4138	0.6159	0.5057	0.6559	0.3904	0.6064	**0.5405**	**0.6699**
ELP9 + SS	0.3599	0.5948	0.5563	0.6861	0.3142	0.5786	**0.5897**	**0.7016**
F-ELP9	0.5345	0.6659	0.5314	0.6645	**0.5364**	**0.6675**	0.5284	0.6629
F-ELP9 +SS	0.6492	0.7505	0.6485	0.7498	0.6474	0.7494	**0.6521**	**0.7519**
F-ELP11	0.5294	0.6591	**0.5303**	**0.6603**	0.5282	0.6595	0.5155	0.6519
F-ELP11 + SS	0.6381	0.7398	0.6306	0.7349	0.6309	0.7351	**0.6427**	**0.7437**

For comparison purposes, we implement the image retrieval algorithm with both the original ELP descriptor and our F-ELP descriptor as inputs. Both descriptors are implemented with and without stain separation (SS) of the image data. The ELP descriptor was designed using a window size of $n = 9$, which is what we implement here using code obtained from the authors of [12]. This results in histograms of length 1024 (without SS) and 2048 (with SS). Since the F-ELP descriptor is much shorter in length, in addition to $n = 9$, we also test a larger window size, $n = 11$. Even with this larger window size, the maximum histogram length for the F-ELP is just 80 bins. Tables 1, 2 and 3 summarize the results of our comparison for the three values of k implemented. For each method, the best performance across all distance metrics is highlighted in bold. We observe that as k is increased the F-measure and balanced accuracy improve for all methods. Based on these results we expect that implementations of the kNN algorithm with even larger values of k may yield even further improvements in accuracy measures, however in this work we are primarily concerned with the comparison between descriptors.

From the above results we observe that for both descriptors, the use of stain separation to generate histograms improves performance. In particular, we see a significant improvement in accuracy scores when we apply stain separation to the F-ELP descriptor. With stain separation, our proposed method significantly outperforms the ELP descriptor, all with much shorter histograms. In general, we find that the choice of distance function used does not seem to have a significant effect on the performance of the image retrieval algorithm, with accuracy scores being fairly similar across all distance functions.

4.2 Image Classification

To evaluate image classification performance we used our F-ELP descriptor as input to train a support vector machine (SVM), a popular classification algorithm. We used the provided training data partition and the `fitcsvm` function in MATLAB to train an SVM to classify each image as containing IDC cells or not. The SVM hyperparameters were optimized using a Bayesian optimization routine in MATLAB and two kernel functions, linear and Gaussian, were tested. As in the previous section, we implemented our method with two different window sizes and with/without stain separation. In Table 4 the classification results obtained with the optimal hyperparameters are recorded for each implementation of the F-ELP.

From the results in Table 4 we can see that using stain separation to generate our descriptor provides a significant improvement in classification performance for both window sizes that were tested.

Table 4. F1 & BAC results for classification of the IDC dataset using F-ELP with and without stain separation

Method	F1	BAC
F-ELP9	0.4048	0.6174
F-ELP9 + SS	**0.7182**	**0.8076**
F-ELP11	0.3385	0.5911
F-ELP11 + SS	0.6715	0.7665

From Table 4 we can also observe that classification performance is significantly better when we use the smaller window size. The optimal window size for a given task is likely determined by a number of factors, including image magnification and scale of the textures and patterns which are relevant to the particular classification task at hand. We did not test other window sizes at this time, however one could perform further testing to determine an optimal window size for the given application.

We now compare the performance of our best proposed method to the most recent results from the literature for classification of the IDC data, including handcrafted features and deep learning approaches. In Table 5 we see that our F-ELP descriptor outperforms many of the state-of-the-art handcrafted features, achieving accuracy levels that are more comparable to those of recent deep learning approaches, such as a CNN from [2] and Alexnet, as implemented in [5].

Table 5. F1 & BAC results for classification of the IDC dataset

Method	F1	BAC
Alexnet, resize [5]	0.7648	0.8468
CNN [2]	0.7180	0.8423
F-ELP9 + SS	**0.7182**	**0.8076**
Fuzzy Color Histogram [2]	0.6753	0.7874
RGB Histogram [2]	0.6664	0.7724
Gray Histogram [2]	0.6031	0.7337
JPEG Coefficient Histogram [2]	0.5758	0.7126
M7 Edge Histogram [2]	0.485	0.6979
Nuclear Textural [2]	0.3915	0.6199
LBP [2]	0.3518	0.6048
Nuclear Architectural [2]	0.3472	0.6009
HSV Color Histogram [2]	0.3446	0.6022

Although we do not achieve quite the same accuracy level of deep-learning approaches at this time, we find these results very encouraging. Using our F-ELP method with digital stain separation, we are able to achieve comparable accuracy with a much simpler approach. Our proposed method does not require any training data to generate the descriptors as they are handcrafted, meaning that a data set can be encoded using our method fairly quickly.

5 Conclusion

In this paper, we have introduced a new frequency-based descriptor for digital histopathology images. The proposed descriptor, F-ELP, is a histogram descriptor which estimates directional frequency information from local image patches. The F-ELP method outperforms its successor, the ELP descriptor, in image retrieval tasks, while requiring less storage overhead and shorter computation times due to its compact nature.

When compared to the state-of-the-art from the literature, our method outperforms a number of popular handcrafted features as an image classifier. We achieve classification results which are comparable to those of deep-learning methods. Our method achieves these results with a very compact representation that does not require large amounts of training data to generate. Our descriptor is also physically meaningful, being based on estimates of local frequency, and thus has the potential to be interpreted by medical experts.

References

1. Ahonen, T., Hadid, A., Pietikainen, M.: Face description with local binary patterns. IEEE Trans. Pattern Anal. Mach. Intell. **28**(12), 2037–2041 (2006)

2. Cruz-Roa, A., et al.: Automatic detection of invasive ductal carcinoma in whole slide images with Convolutional Neural Networks. In: Progress in Biomedical Optics and Imaging - Proceedings of SPIE, vol. 9041 (2014)
3. Dalal, N., Triggs, B.: Histograms of oriented gradients for human detection. In: 2005 IEEE Computer Society Conference on Computer Vision and Pattern Recognition, San Diego, CA, USA, pp. 886–893 (2005)
4. Gurcan, M.N., Boucheron, L.E., Can, A., Madabhushi, A., Rajpoot, N.M., Yener, B.: Histopathological image analysis: a review. IEEE Rev. Biomed. Eng. **2**(2), 147–171 (2009)
5. Janowczyk, A., Madabhushi, A.: Deep learning for digital pathology image analysis: a comprehensive tutorial with selected use cases. J. Pathol. Inform. **7**(29) (2016)
6. Lowe, D.G.: Distinctive image features from scale-invariant keypoints. Int. J. Comput. Vision **60**(2), 91–110 (2004)
7. Macenko, M., et al.: A method for normalizing histology slides for quantitative analysis. In: Proceedings of IEEE International Symposium on Biomedical Imaging, Chicago, IL, pp. 1107–1110 (2009)
8. McCann, M.T., Majumdar, J., Peng, C., Castro, C.A., Kovacevic, J.: Algorithm and benchmark dataset for stain separation in histology images. In: Proceedings of 2014 IEEE International Conference on Image Processing (ICIP), Paris, France, pp. 3953–3957 (2014)
9. Mendivil, F.: Computing the monge-kantorovich distance. Comput. Appl. Math. **36**(3), 1389–1402 (2017)
10. Molter, U., Brandt, J., Cabrelli, C.: An algorithm for the computation of the hutchinson distance. Inform. Process. Lett. **40**(2), 113–117 (1991)
11. Ruifrok, A.C., Johnston, D.A.: Quantification of histochemical staining by color deconvolution. Anal. Quant. Cytol. Histol. **23**(4), 291–299 (2001)
12. Tizhoosh, H.R., Babaie, M.: Representing medical images with encoded local projections. IEEE Trans. Biomed. Eng. **65**(10), 2267–2277 (2018)

Computer-Aided Tumor Segmentation from T2-Weighted MR Images of Patient-Derived Tumor Xenografts

Sudipta Roy and Kooresh Isaac Shoghi(✉)

Department of Radiology, Washington University School of Medicine,
St. Louis, MO 63110, USA
{sudiptaroy, shoghik}@wustl.edu

Abstract. Magnetic resonance imaging (MRI) is typically used to detect and assess therapeutic response in preclinical imaging of patient-derived tumor xenografts (PDX). The overarching objective of the work is to develop an automated methodology to detect and segment tumors in PDX for subsequent analyses. Automated segmentation also has the benefit that it will minimize user bias. A hybrid method combining fast k-means, morphology, and level set is used to localize and segment tumor volume from volumetric MR images. Initial centroids of k-means are selected by local density peak estimation method. A new variational model is implemented to exploit the region information by minimizing energy functional in level set. The mask specific initialization approach is used to create a genuine boundary of level set. Performance of tumor segmentation is compared with manually segmented image and to established algorithms. Segmentation results obtained from six metrics are Jaccard score (>80%), Dice score (>85%), F score (>85%), G-mean (>90%), volume similarity matrix (>95%) and relative volume error (<8%). The proposed method reliably localizes and segments PDX tumors and has the potential to facilitate high-throughput analysis of MR imaging in co-clinical trials involving PDX.

Keywords: Computer aided detection · Magnetic resonance imaging · Tumor segmentation · Level set

1 Introduction

Computer aided detection and analysis of medical images plays an essential role in co-clinical imaging research. In particular, Magnetic Resonance Imaging (MRI) of Patient-Derived Tumor Xenografts (PDX) can be used to detect tumors as well as assess or predict response to therapy in co-clinical imaging investigations [1]. However, automatic tumor segmentation in small animal MRI is difficult due to the presence of artifacts, noise and variability within images [2]. The goal of this work is to develop an automated tumor segmentation method that can be applied to PDX of triple negative breast cancer to assess response to therapy.

F. Karray et al. (Eds.): ICIAR 2019, LNCS 11663, pp. 159–171, 2019.
https://doi.org/10.1007/978-3-030-27272-2_14

In past few years, several tumor segmentation techniques have been developed [3] but no single method has been developed that can suitable for all image types. The methods typically need user defined constraints for specific type of images such as T1w, T2w, proton density (PD), diffusion-contrast enhanced (DCE)-MR, diffusion-weighted imaging (DWI)-MR, and FLAIR images. A surface based [4] approach including deformable and region based active contour is very useful for tumor segmentation from MRI. Usually, active contours models use energy minimization by gradient descent approach. The energy minimization converges to local minima and gives segmentation results. But active contour models may fail due to convergence in undesirable local minima and produce some erroneous segmentation [5]. Level set approaches overcome the problem of convergence to an undesirable minima, however, convergence may be slow due to inadequate initialization. An extension of active contour and level set methods [6] has been proposed to solve initialization problem. The segmentation may leak out and region overlapping may occur due to improper handling of initialization criterion.

Composite or hybrid segmentation [7, 8] is a strategy to segment the tumor with the permute combination of thresholding, C-means, fuzzy C-means, morphology, active contour and geometric active contour to segment different anatomical regions of small animal imaging. But the increase with volume and variability of the data, increases the complexity of hybrid method, if proper care not taken. This means lower computing time with higher number of different initialization and parameter needed to tune for specific segmentation. Thus, hybrid method needs to take care to produce effective and efficient segmentation results.

To address the limitations described above, we propose a method that is based on the combination of fast k-means, morphology and modified level set. The local density peaks search in k-means is used to reduce the time computation of clustering algorithm. The appropriate use of regularization operation using binary mask generated from k-means and morphology makes the growth function genuine to start from a true boundaries in level set. The addition of local mean intensity in region fitting energy function and modification in second-order central differences of curvature divergence is solved the problem of convergence towards local minima. This method does not require weighted coefficients in level set energy function. This method requires a minimum set of constants and inputs, and runs mostly on homogeneous data. Homogeneity of the tumor is recognized as low intensity variability, necrotic cores and high textures similarity within the tumor. We compared the performance of the proposed method to established methodologies such as Fuzzy C means (FCM) and active contour. Overall, the proposed method performs better than those two comparable methods in terms of accuracy and error metrics. High similarity metric and low error metric of proposed method results in very low false positive detection, false negative detection and spurious lesion generation compare to other methods.

The paper is organized as follows: Sect. 2, describes the proposed method for tumor segmentation; Sect. 3, describes the results and discussion; Sect. 4, describes the performance analysis with mathematical metrics and comparison with gold standard methods. Finally, we conclude our paper in Sect. 5.

2 Methodology

MR images were acquired on Varian 4.7T MR scanner with 25 slices, 25.6 × 25.6 × 1 mm^3, in-plane matrix 128 × 128, TE 60 ms, and TR 1.5 s. K-means algorithm requires initial seed points of each clusters to start the clustering process. Automatic k (>1) number of good seed point's selection is called initialization of cluster centers. Appropriate initialization reduces the overall computing time in clustering. Initialization using local density peaks (LDP) [9] searching method leads to very fast convergence towards means when clusters are separable. Thus, the initial clusters seeds obtained from LDP searching method is defined as $\left\{x^{(i)} | i \in I_{in}^{ldp}\right\}$. Here, x is observation obtained from input image I_{in}. According to computational geometry, initial seed points found by LDP [10] have reasonably high local intensity densities information's. LDP avoid the outliers due to the high local densities and lying very close to each other's. Let, k number of initial cluster centers have selected to compute the distance between each observation x_i to the each cluster centers $m_1, \ldots, m_k$, where distance is calculated by the squared Euclidean distance formulae taken on parameters p.

$$d(x_i, m_K) = \sum_{j=1}^{p} (x_{ij} - m_k)^2 = ||x_{ij} - m_k)||^2 \quad (1)$$

Then each observation x_i is assigned to the kth cluster that defined m_k by minimizing differences between $d(x_i, \ldots, m_k)$. Now, all observations x_i have to assign to a cluster and then compute the average of the assigned points $x'(k)$.

$$x'(k) = \left\{x'_{i1}, x'_{i2}, x'_{i3}, \ldots, x'_{ip}\right\} \quad (2)$$

Now, $x'(k)$ has the new cluster centers m_k. Repeat above two (Eqs. 1 to 2) steps until the cluster converges or assignments to the cluster centers are stable. Four clusters are segmented from gray images and the segmented clusters are stored into separate binary images BIC1, BIC2, BIC3, and BIC4. Then three times morphological dilation is applied on BIC1, BIC2, BIC3, and BIC4 to disconnect the weakly connected components. This morphological separation of tumor to the neighboring similar structures is directed by distance map between tumor and non-tumor intensity similarity. Sum up all single largest connected component of BIC3 from selected number of slices (NS) to apply conditional voting. Then conditional voting (>(NS/2-1)) scheme is applied to find out the tumor location. The same number of morphological erosions is applied on selected largest 3D connected area to balance morphological opening and closing. Select the tumor lesion from BIC1, BIC2, BIC3, and BIC4 that overlap the tumor location. Three times morphological closing on previous/next slice can be applied if no lesion found on any selected slice. These binary lesions (BI1) are used as initial mask of level set. Then BI1 tumor lesions is added to generate 'extreme maxima' as maximum tumor boundary (BI2).

Level set requires appropriate initialization with stable evaluation curve, it does not affect much about the information applied to determination the level set function. Re-initializations of level set is required after first iteration. Although, re-initiation may increase computation cost with little increase of numerical inaccuracy. A good signed partial differential equation (PDE) initialization was appeared in [11] with initial contour $\phi_t(x, y, 0) = \phi_0(x)$ as:

$$\phi_t = sign(\phi_0)(1 - |\nabla\phi|) \tag{3}$$

Where ϕ_0 is contour at zero interface that implicitly defined by $\{x \epsilon \Omega : \phi_0(x, y) = 0\}$. The Hamilton-Jacobi equations enforces to become zero for highly irregular level set function. Thus, flexible initialization is very good advantage of level set method. The initial function $\phi_0(x, y)$ is defined as follows:

$$\phi_0(x, y) = \begin{cases} -d & if\ (x, y) \in \Omega_{in} \\ 0 & if\ (x, y) \in \Omega_0 \\ +d & if\ (x, y) \in \Omega_{out} \end{cases} \tag{4}$$

Where Ω_0 represent the level zero boundary and a subset in the image domain Ω. Ω_{in} and Ω_{out} are the inside and outside region of Ω_0, and distance d > 0 is a constant. According to Eq. 4, an initial contour starts from a specified binary region BI. The binary image BI obtained from the clustering is considered as the initial level set function in Eq. 4. Then, a regulation operation is conducted as follows:

$$\phi_0(x, y) = (|E_{dist}(BI) - E_{dist}(1 - BI)|) * (BI - 0.5) \tag{5}$$

Equation 5 means that, if BI = 1 then ϕ_0 will be positive and if BI = 0 then ϕ_0 will be negative. This satisfies the preliminary demands of level set. This, simple initialization scheme makes the evolution start from a genuine boundary. For a given image I, closed curve C, and variable v at position (i, j), the following energy function [5] minimization is as follows:

$$E^R\left(\phi^n_{i,j}\right) = \lambda_1 \int_{in(C)} |I_v(i, j) - c_1|^2 dp + \lambda_2 \int_{out(C)} |I_v(i, j) - c_2|^2 dp \tag{6}$$

Where, out(C) and in(C) represent the regions outside and inside of contour C respectively. Two constant c_1, and c_2 denote the average intensities of inside and outside of C. The parameters λ_1, and λ_2 are constants, and the values $\lambda_1 = \lambda_2 = 1$.

Our new variational model uses the region oriented information to find out the segmentation outline using the energy function $E(\phi)$ minimization. We defined a region fitting energy E derived from the Chan and Vese [5] model, and minimized when the evolution curve C is on the boundaries of the objects. The proposed energy functional is defined as:

$$E\left(\phi^n_{i,j}\right) = E^R\left(\phi^n_{i,j}\right) + E^C\left(\phi^n_{i,j}\right) \tag{7}$$

The time-based partial derivative $\partial\varphi/\partial t$ is estimated by the forward difference. Thus, level set growth function [12] can be represented by the following forward differential equation:

$$\frac{\phi_{i,j}^{n+1} - \phi_{i,j}^{n}}{dt} = E\left(\phi_{i,j}^{n}\right) \tag{8}$$

Where, dt is the time step and $E\left(\phi_{i,j}^{n}\right)$ is the numerical estimated energy value from above Eq. 7. Time step dt is given as follows in Eq. 9.

$$dt = \frac{T_c}{\max\left(E\left(\phi_{i,j}^{n}\right) + eps\right)} \tag{9}$$

Constant time T_c is set to 0.45 and the constant eps is set to very close to zero (here, eps is $2.2204e^{-16}$). Constant eps is used to avoid denominator value as zero. The corresponding curvature $div(\nabla\phi/|\nabla\phi|)$ in the $E^C\left(\phi_{i,j}^{n}\right)$ is calculated by

$$\begin{aligned} C_d &= \frac{\phi_{pp}\phi_q^2 - 2\phi_p\phi_q\phi_{pq} + \phi_{qq}\phi_p^2}{(\phi_p^2 + \phi_q^2)^{\frac{3}{2}} \times (\phi_p^2 + \phi_q^2)^{\frac{1}{2}}} \\ E^C\left(\phi_{i,j}^{n}\right) &= \alpha \times C_d \end{aligned} \tag{10}$$

Here, α is a small diffusion parameter to control the degree of smoothing of contour and set to 0.1. The second-order central differences [12] are defined as follows:

$$\begin{aligned} \phi_p &= \left(\phi_{i+1,j}^{n} - \phi_{i-1,j}^{n}\right), \phi_q = \left(\phi_{i,j+1}^{n} - \phi_{i,j-1}^{n}\right) \\ \phi_{pp} &= \left(\phi_{i+1,j}^{n} - 2 \times \phi_{i,j}^{n} + \phi_{i-1,j}^{n}\right), \phi_{qq} = \left(\phi_{i,j+1}^{n} - 2 \times \phi_{i,j}^{n} + \phi_{i,j-1}^{n}\right) \\ \phi_{pq} &= \frac{\left(\phi_{i+1,j+1}^{n} + \phi_{i-1,j-1}^{n} - \phi_{i-1,j}^{n} - \phi_{i+1,j-1}^{n}\right)}{4} \end{aligned} \tag{11}$$

Level set applied using mask BI1 and BI2 to produce R1 and R2 region of every slice. R2 can be considered only when there are no tumor lesion found on R1. Segmented tumor region is extracted by multiplying binary R1/R2 with the original input image.

3 Result and Discussion

The automatic segmentation algorithm is applied to 2D multi-slice, T2-weighted MR images of TNBC PDX. Input MR slices where tumor is present in index three to ten shown in Fig. 1(A). Four clusters from input image (Fig. 1(A)) using fast k-means is

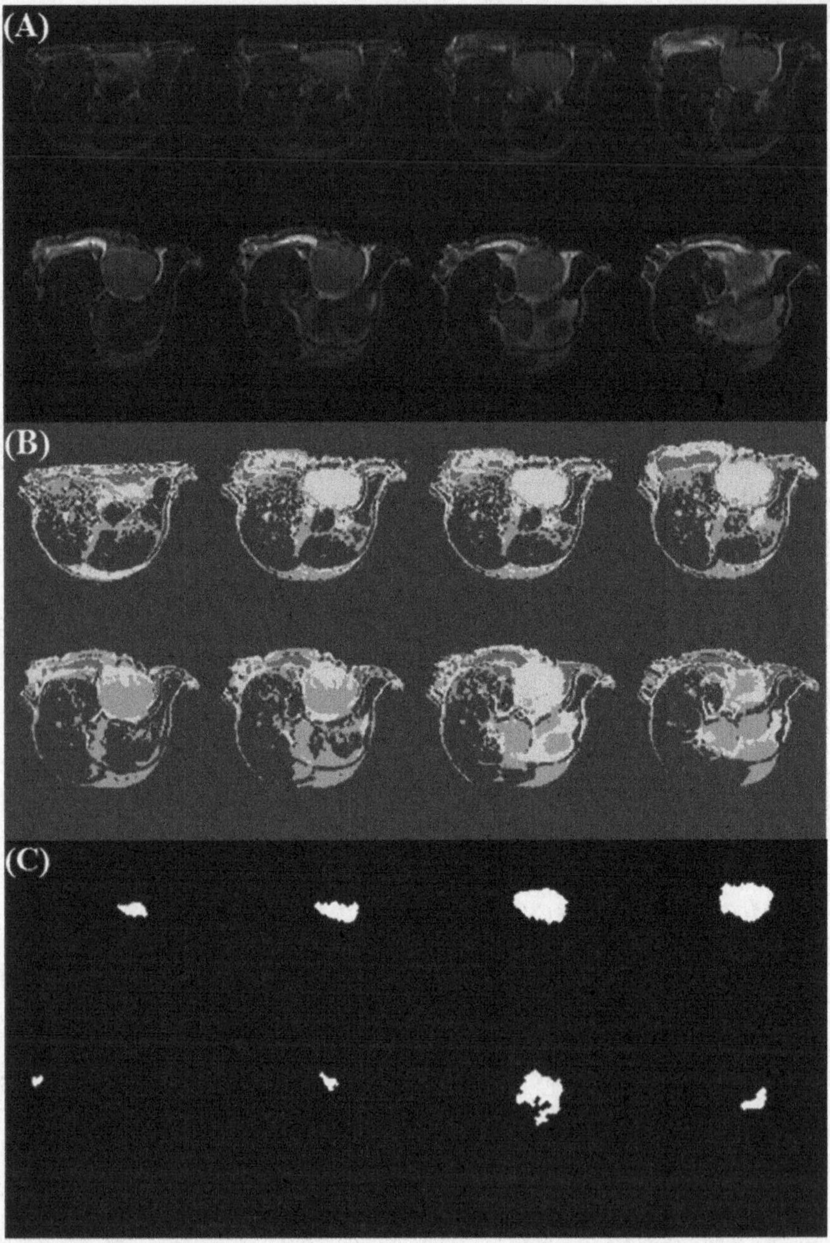

Fig. 1. (A) T2 weighted MR slices as input; tumor present in slice index 3 to slice 10. (B) Fast k-means applied on slice index 3 to 10 from top left to bottom right with number of cluster is four. Tumor location visible on Yellow and Sky color cluster. (C) Binary image of cluster number three for tumor location finding on 3D image. (Color figure online)

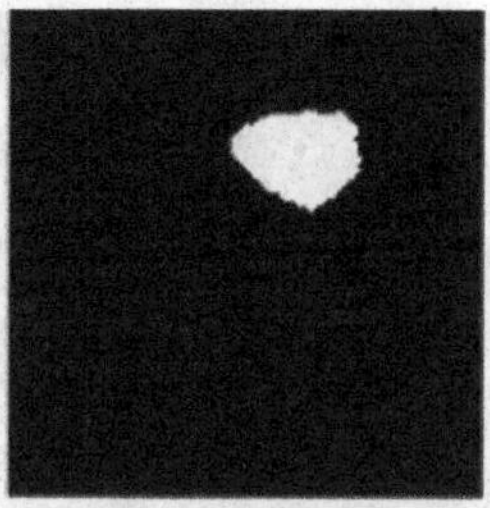

Fig. 2. Largest connected area is selected based on voting (>total number of tumor slice in Z direction/2-1)) on Cluster 3 (yellow) and then morphological erosion is applied to balance morphological dilation and erosion. (Color figure online)

shown in Fig. 1(B). After preprocessed by morphological operation, the largest connected area selection of cluster three is shown in Fig. 1(B).

Voting scheme is applied to the Fig. 1(C) to find the tumor location succeded by morphological operation. The output after finding tumor loaction is shown in Fig. 2.

Now, the largest connected lesion is selected from clusters 2, cluster 3 and cluster 4. Then the selected lesion is compared with the tumor position. The nearest lesion from tumor position is considered as binary mask of each MR slice. Final mask for level set initialization is generated by applying three times morphological dilation on binary mask. This mask is shown in Fig. 3(A) with yellow contour and in parallel extreme maxima is generated by summing up all the masked binary images followed by morphological operation is shown in Fig. 3(B). This extreme maximum is used as the stopping criteria of level set method. The final segmented results using both mask in Fig. 3(A) and (B) is shown in Fig. 3(C).

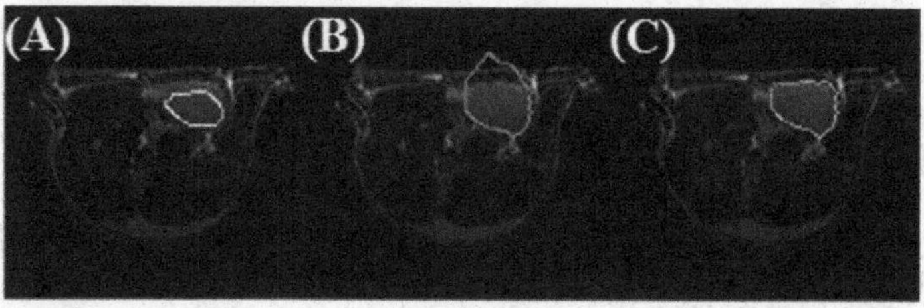

Fig. 3. (A) Mask initialization generated from different cluster and used in level set. (B) Mask initialization generated from extreme maxima. (C) Segmented tumor contour shown in green color within the input image by level set after performing some intermediate steps. (Color figure online)

The results give a new direction of automatic 3D segmentation on T2 weighted MR images. The proposed method also solved the shortcomings of traditional methods. The method tested on several preclinical MR images and found to be effective as seen visually from Fig. 3(C). An additional tumor segmentation result is shown in Fig. 4.

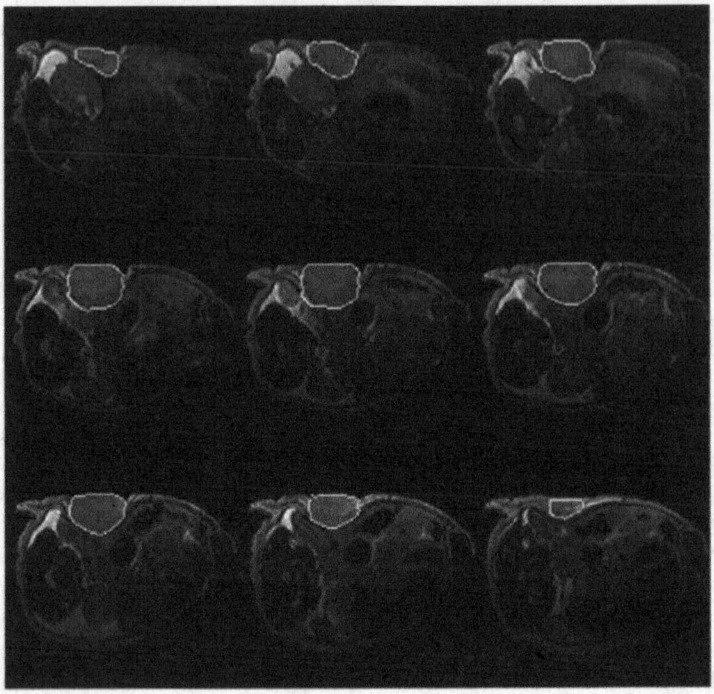

Fig. 4. Segmented tumor shown in green contour line. (Color figure online)

4 Performance Analysis

Quantitative analysis of automatic segmentation needs to be validated by comparing gold standard or ground truth. The ground truth can be defined by one or more experts to segment the tumor manually. Six metrics are used to evaluate performance between proposed segmentation and manual ground truth. Four most popular metrics [13] such as Dice coefficient, Jaccard coefficient, F score, and G-Mean are applied on 2D images and average of 2D slice metric is considered as metric value in 3D. Other two metrics such as volume similarity index and relative volume error are directly applied on 3D volume data.

Dice coefficient (DC) [13] measure the voxels overlapping between the segmented binary image and binary ground truth image. The DC ranges from 0 (poor overlapping) to 1 (perfect overlapping). The DC is referred as follows:

$$DC(i) = \frac{2 \times TP}{(AS + GT)} \tag{12}$$

Where, i ranges from 1 to number of slice (NS). TP (also called true positive) is intersection between binary automatic segmentation (AS) and binary ground truth (GT). DC of 3D MR images is considered by taking average of DC(i).

Jaccard coefficient (JC) [13] measures the voxels overlapping between segmented binary image and binary ground truth images divided by the size of the union of two labels AS and GT. JC ranges from 0 (poor segmentation) and 1 (perfect segmentation). JC is referred as follows:

$$JC(i) = \frac{AS \cap GT}{AS \cup GT} \tag{13}$$

DC and JC of proposed segmentation is shown in Fig. 5 below. Proposed methods give more than 85% DC and more than 80% JC for most the input images. These comparison metrics suggest that proposed segmentation method achieves a robust automatic segmentation tool for segmentation of preclinical MR image for subsequent quantification and analysis.

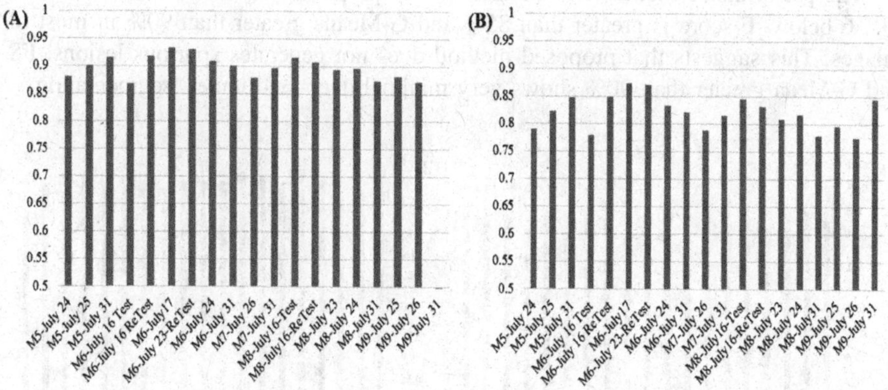

Fig. 5. (A) Column chart representation of Dice score and (B) column chart representation of Jaccard coefficient. Both metric compared with manual segmented images. Average values of 2D segmented slices considered as metric value of each 3D MR images. Dice score is good for most of the images and gives more than 85% score. Jaccard score gives more than 80% in most of the cases and these are good indication of good segmentation.

F score (FS) [13] is measured by the harmonic average of the precision and recall. The FS ranges from 0 (poor overlapping) to 1 (perfect overlapping).

$$FS(i) = \frac{2 \times (Precision \times Recall)}{(Precision + Recall)} \tag{14}$$

Precision is defined as the fraction of TP to the segmented tumor and Recall is defined by the fraction of TP to the grand truth (GT).

$$Precision = \frac{TP}{AS} \text{ and } Recall = \frac{TP}{GT} \tag{15}$$

G-Mean [14] is the measure by the square root of multiplication between positive class accuracy and negative class accuracy. The G-Mean ranges from 0 (poor overlapping) to 1 (perfect overlapping).

$$G - Mean(i) = \sqrt{\left(\frac{TP}{TP + FN} \times \frac{TN}{TN + FP}\right)} \tag{16}$$

Where, FP (false positive) is number of voxels falsely segmented as foreground, TN (true negative) is the number voxels correctly segmented as background, FN (false negative) is the number of voxels falsely segmented as background.

The performance metrics FS and G-Mean of proposed segmentation is shown in Fig. 6 below. F score is greater than 85% and G-Means greater than 90% in most of images. This suggests that proposed method does not generates spurious lesions. FS and G-Mean greater than 90% shows very minimal over- and under- segmentation.

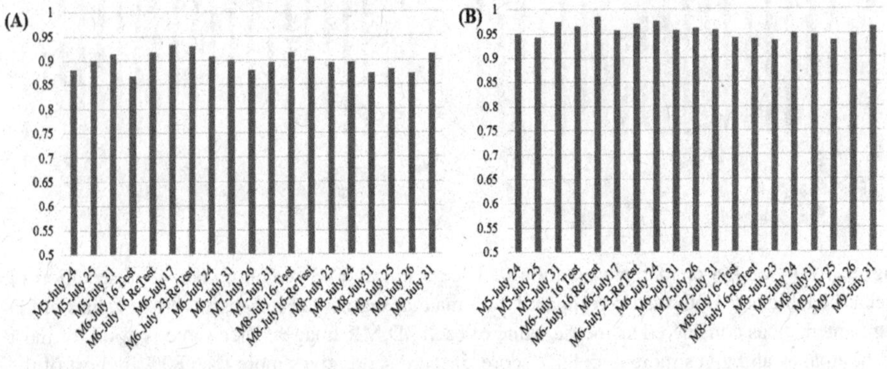

Fig. 6. (A) Column chart representation of F score and (B) column chart representation of G-Mean. Both metric compared with manual segmented images. Average of 2D segmented slices considered as metric value of each 3D MR images. F score is good for most of the images and gives more than 85% score. G-Mean gives more than 90% in all cases.

The volume similarity index (VSI) is measured by one minus absolute difference of volume to the sum of compared volume. Thus, VSI can be defined by:

$$VSI = 1 - \frac{|ASV - GTV|}{(ASV + GTV)} \tag{17}$$

Where, ASV is automated segmented volume and GTV is the ground truth volume.

The relative volume error (RVE) is measured by the ratio of the absolute volume difference between automated segmentation and ground truth divided by ground truth volume. Thus, RVE can be defined as:

$$RVE = \frac{|CSV - GTV|}{GTV} \tag{18}$$

The column chart representation of VSI and RVE are shown in Fig. 7. VSI ranges from 0 (poor segmentation) to 1 (perfect segmentation) and RVE ranges from 0 (perfect segmentation) and 1 (poor segmentation). VSI and RVE both metric are gives very good segmentation results. Average RVE is less than 0.10 and average VSI is greater than 0.95 means proposed method have very low over and under segmentation problems.

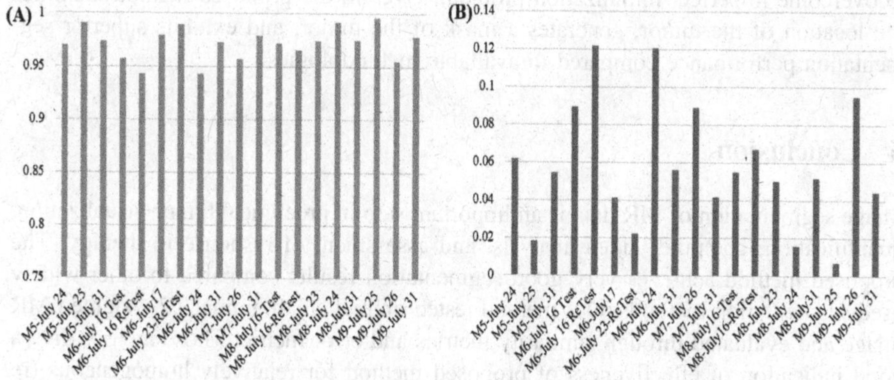

Fig. 7. (A) Column chart representation of volumetric similarity index and (B) relative volume error. In most of images volumetric similarity index is greater than 95% and relative volume error is less than 8%.

For comparison task, we have chosen two popular segmentation algorithms: Fuzzy C means (FCM) [8] and active contour [12]. A comparison table of proposed method with other two comparable methods are shown in Table 1 below.

Table 1. Comparative study with performance metrics

Method used	VSI	RVE
Fuzzy C-means [8]	72.1%	27.61%
Active contour [12]	84.2	13.56
Proposed method	97.1%	5.77%

Our method exhibits great improvement in VSI and RVE performance metrics. Average VSI above 95% and average RVE below 6% reflect a significant improvement compared to other two Fuzzy C-means [8] and active contour [12] as shown in Table 1. Fuzzy C-means [8] and active contour [12] methods have a tendency of over segmentation or under-segmentation of tumor. FCM is sensitive to very little noise and very small variability of texture. FCM does not provide an effective segmentation due to the presence of inevitable noise and low variability. The active contour [12] make an automatic search of minimum energy positions, but sometimes convergence at a local minimum makes them ineffective segmentation. The active contour also depends on initialization of function. Fast k-means alone cannot deliver good segmentation with smooth boundary as well level set alone cannot deliver good segmentation without proper initialization and energy function adjustment. Thus, the combination of fast k-means, morphology and level set provides better segmentation. Finding tumor location and generating mask using fast k-means clustering is used to initialize level set to overcome imperfect initialization problem. Overall, the proposed method identifies the location of the tumor, generates a mask of the tumor, and exhibits superior segmentation performance compared to available methodologies.

5 Conclusion

Image segmentation of MR data is an important step in preclinical tumor visualization, quantification, computer aided analysis, and assessment of response to therapy. The proposed method achieves very good segmentation results compared to other widely used segmentation methods. Our method tested on real small animal T2 weighted MR image and evaluated through similarity metrics and error metric. Those metrics give a good indication of effectiveness of proposed method for relatively homogeneous (re T2 W) PDX. Future work will be targeted at more heterogeneous PDX, e.g., those with enhancing or non-enhancing or necrotic cores. Our goal is to eventually be capable of handling large data with computationally efficient through optimization.

Acknowledgments. Preclinical MRI data were acquired by Xia Ge and John Engelbach. Funding was provided by NCI grant U24 CA209837, Washington University Co-Clinical Imaging Research Resource, and the Small-Animal Cancer Imaging Shared Resource of the Alvin J. Siteman Cancer Center, an NCI-Designated Comprehensive Cancer Center (Cancer Center Support Grant P30 CA91842).

References

1. AM O'Flynn, E., Collins, D., D'Arcy, J., Schmidt, M., de Souza, N.M.: Multi-parametric MRI in the early prediction of response to neo-adjuvant chemotherapy in breast cancer: value of non-modelled parameters. Eur. J. Radiol. **85**(4), 837–842 (2016)
2. Despotovi, I., Goossens, B., Philips, W.: MRI segmentation of the human brain: challenges, methods, and applications. Comput. Math. Methods Med. **2015**, 1–24 (2015). Article ID 450341

3. Pal, N.R., Pal, S.K.: A review on image segmentation techniques. Pattern Recogn. **26**(9), 1277–1294 (1993)
4. Meng, X., Gu, W., Chen, Y., Zhang, J.: Brain MR image segmentation based on an improved active contour model. PLoS ONE **12**(8), e0183943 (2017)
5. Vese, L.A., Chan, T.F.: A multiphase level set framework for image segmentation using the Mumford and Shah model. Int. J. Comput. Vis. **50**(3), 271–293 (2002)
6. Chambolle, A., Cremers, D., Pock, T.: A convex approach to minimal partitions. SIAM J. Imaging Sci. **5**(4), 1113–1158 (2012)
7. Singh, G., Ansari, M.A.: Efficient detection of brain tumor from MRIs using K-means segmentation and normalized histogram. In: 2016 1st India International Conference on Information Processing (IICIP), Delhi, pp. 1–6 (2016)
8. Singh, P.A.: Detection of brain tumor in MRI images, using fuzzy C-means segmented images and artificial neural network. In: Afzalpulkar, N., Srivastava, V., Singh, G., Bhatnagar, D. (eds) Proceedings of the International Conference on Recent Cognizance in Wireless Communication & Image Processing. Springer, New Delhi (2016). https://doi.org/10.1007/978-81-322-2638-3_14
9. Li, F., Qiao, H., Zhang, B.: Effective Deterministic Initialization for k-Means-Like Methods via Local Density Peaks Searching. arXiv preprint arXiv:1611.06777 (2016)
10. Rodriguez, A., Laio, A.: Clustering by fast search and find of density peaks. Science **344** (6191), 1492–1496 (2014)
11. Keck, R.: Reinitialization for level set methods. In: ECMI 1998, Germany, pp. 1–2 (1998)
12. Yu, C.-Y., Zhang, W.-S., Yu, Y.-Y., Li, Y.: A novel active contour model for image segmentation using distance regularization term. Comput. Math. Appl. **65**(11), 1746–1759 (2013)
13. Vania, M., Mureja, D., Lee, D.: Automatic spine segmentation from CT images using convolutional neural network via redundant generation of class labels. J. Comput. Des. Eng. **6**(2), 224–232 (2018)
14. Win, K.Y., Choomchuay, S., Hamamoto, K., Raveesunthornkiat, M.: Detection and classification of overlapping cell nuclei in cytology effusion images using a double-strategy random forest. Appl. Sci. **8**(1608), 1–20 (2018)

Applications

Sit-to-Stand Analysis in the Wild Using Silhouettes for Longitudinal Health Monitoring

Alessandro Masullo(✉), Tilo Burghardt, Toby Perrett, Dima Damen, and Majid Mirmehdi

University of Bristol, Bristol, UK
a.masullo@bristol.ac.uk

Abstract. We present the first fully automated Sit-to-Stand or Stand-to-Sit (StS) analysis framework for long-term monitoring of patients in free-living environments using video silhouettes. Our method adopts a coarse-to-fine time localisation approach, where a deep learning classifier identifies possible StS sequences from silhouettes, and a smart peak detection stage provides fine localisation based on 3D bounding boxes. We tested our method on data from real homes of participants and monitored patients undergoing total hip or knee replacement. Our results show 94.4% overall accuracy in the coarse localisation and an error of 0.026 m/s in the speed of ascent measurement, highlighting important trends in the recuperation of patients who underwent surgery.

Keywords: Sit-to-Stand · Human motion analysis · Long term monitoring

1 Introduction

Novel concepts and technologies like the Internet of Things (IoT) for Ambient Assisted Living (AAL) or specific health monitoring enable people to live independently, to be aided in their recuperation, and improve their quality of life. Such systems often include multiple sensors and monitoring devices, producing large amounts of data that need to be analysed and summarised in a few, clinically relevant parameters [22]. The transition from a sitting position to a standing one (StS[1]) is one of the most essential movements in daily activities [6], especially for older patients suffering from musculoskeletal illnesses. StS has been linked to recurrent falls [4], sedentary behaviour [7] and fall histories [20]. Continuous monitoring of the StS action over a long period of time can therefore highlight important trends, particularly for subjects undergoing physical rehabilitation.

To the best of our knowledge, the automatic analysis of StS has not been attempted for long term monitoring and trend analysis. Some previous

[1] In this work, by StS we do in fact mean both 'Sit-to-Stand' and 'Stand-to-Sit', but will specify which of the two, if and when necessary.

F. Karray et al. (Eds.): ICIAR 2019, LNCS 11663, pp. 175–185, 2019.
https://doi.org/10.1007/978-3-030-27272-2_15

works have focused on automating the Sit-to-Stand clinical test, performed under supervised conditions and often in the presence of a clinician, e.g. [3]. Shia et *al.* [16] suggested modelling the physics of the human body during stand-up transitions by using a motion capture suite. Their method was tested in the lab on 10 healthy individuals but this approach is clearly impractical for long-term monitoring. In [9], Galna et *al.* investigated the suitability of skeleton data extracted by the Kinect sensor to assess clinically relevant movements, showing that the StS timing can be accurately captured with errors comparable to the VICON motion capture system. Their method was applied in the lab on 9 individuals with Parkinson's Disease and 10 control subjects. Skeleton data was also used in [8] to estimate the StS timing by using the vertical displacement of the head joint and a manual threshold. Their method was tested in the laboratory for 94 subjects and in participants' own homes for 20 individuals.

The detection of StS transitions can be seen as an action classification problem, and a large body of research has investigated the application of deep convolutional neural networks (CNN) for this task, for example [5,17]. However, while these works enable high accuracy in action classification, they always make use of RGB or depth data, which is not compatible with the privacy requirements of home monitoring systems, for instance [2,23]. As already addressed in [13], silhouettes constitute a valid alternative form of data that allows action recognition to be performed whilst respecting privacy requirements.

The aim of this work is to propose a novel approach to continuously monitor StS transitions in the wild and, while addressing privacy issues, to generate automatic trend analysis. For each StS transition, we measure the speed of ascent/descent as an indicator of physical function. We installed RGBD cameras (PrimeSense) in participants' own houses and recorded silhouette video data from 9 subjects in 4 different habitations, for a minimum period of 4 months, up to 1 year, under the auspices of the SPHERE and HemiSPHERE projects [10,22]. Two of the participants, aged between 65 and 90, underwent total hip or knee replacement and we monitored them before and after their intervention. The remaining 7 participants, aged between 40 and 60, did not record any particular health condition that could affect their mobility. We show that our method can identify StS transitions into the wild with 94.4% overall accuracy and our measurement of the speed of ascent is comparable with the VICON motion capture gold standard in a supervised setting. Moreover, our analyses highlight important trends linked to the rehabilitation process, potentially allowing for surgeons to follow the progress of their patients remotely and anticipate possible complications.

2 Methodology

Monitoring people in their homes poses stringent ethical restrictions on the type of data that can be recorded, analysed and shared, e.g. prohibiting the use of RGB data [14,21]. To provide a privacy-compatible monitoring system (based on a user study [22]), we generate silhouettes and 3D bounding boxes from the

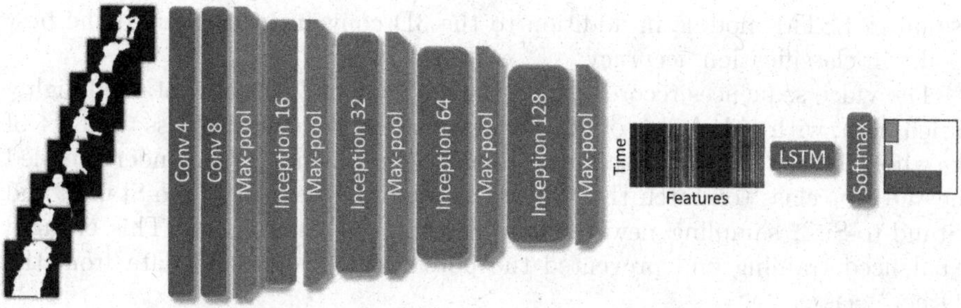

Fig. 1. Network architecture of the proposed method.

RGB data and discard the raw pixel values immediately thereafter. We deployed one camera in each house (in the living room) and set it up at a similar height to have a comparable field of view.

Our proposed pipeline can be divided into three steps: pre-processing of videos, classification and StS measurement. First, the incoming silhouettes are cropped at the detected bounding boxes and resized, producing one video per individual. These videos are subdivided into short clips of 10 seconds each[2], which are then classified with a deep CNN (detailed in Sect. 2.1) into one of three categories: "Sit-to-Stand", "Stand-to-Sit" or "Other". The StS video clips only are then further analysed to measure the speed of ascent/descent using the 3D bounding boxes, as described in Sect. 2.2.

Contrary to previous works that have focused on StS duration [3,16], our method measures the speed of ascent/descent, defined as the maximal transferring velocity of the centre of gravity (CG) between the start and the completion of the StS movement [15]. The speed of ascent/descent does not depend on a specific beginning or end of the movement, but rather on the maximum velocity. Thanks to this property, the speed of ascent/descent shows no significant difference between the Sit-to-Stand and the Sit-to-Walk movements [12], or the Stand-to-Sit and the Walk-to-Sit movements, making it a more suitable measurement for free-living monitoring.

2.1 Classification

Inspired by the work from Carreira et *al.* [5], we built our classifier network using Inception modules with 3D convolutions, as presented in Fig. 1. It was shown in our previous work [13] that using very deep networks on silhouette data increases the computational cost without inducing any advantages. We therefore adopted a shallow architecture composed of 4 stacks of Inception modules, followed by a Long Short-Term Memory (LSTM) layer located between the last convolutional layer and the final fully connected layer. In our experiments, we found that the

[2] The frame-rate of the silhouette recorder varied according to different conditions and produced 10 fps on average.

use of an LSTM module in addition to the 3D convolution produced the best results in classification accuracy.

The video sequences recorded from the participants' homes contained highly varied data, with video clips of StS transitions only constituting less than 1% of the whole dataset. To tackle this class imbalance problem [11], we under-sampled the "Other" class to match the size of the minority classes "Sit-to-Stand" and "Stand-to-Sit", sampling new random elements for each epoch. This ensured a balanced training and prevented the potential loss of useful data from the "Other" class.

2.2 Speed of Ascent Measurement

The 10-seconds clip classifier provides a coarse time localisation of the StS transitions. To narrow the exact frame of the transition and measure the speed of ascent[3], we employ data from the 3D bounding boxes, in particular the evolution in time of the upper edge. Let the 3D bounding box B for the time interval $[t_{\text{start}},\ t_{\text{end}}]$ of a clip be $B\,(t) = [x_1(t), y_1(t), z_1(t); x_2(t), y_2(t), z_2(t)]$, where the indices 1 and 2 respectively represent the 'right', 'top', 'front', and 'left', 'bottom', 'back' vertices of the 3D box. Let us call $y_1 \equiv y_{\text{top}}$ the y component of the top vertex, and the vertical speed of the subject can then be estimated as:

$$V_y(t) = \pm \frac{dy_{\text{top}}}{dt}\,, \tag{1}$$

where the sign is + for "Sit-to-Stand" and − for "Stand-to-Sit" classes. Using the definition of speed of ascent as the maximum vertical velocity during the StS movement, we can then compute the speed of ascent V_{SOA} as:

$$V_{\text{SOA}} = \max_{[t_{\text{start}},\ t_{\text{end}}]} \{V_y(t)\}\,. \tag{2}$$

It is important to note that the computation of Eq. (2) is only performed on those clips classified earlier as StS. In fact, its simplicity is built upon the accuracy of the classifier, which filters out all the other possible movements that might contain a vertical motion and are not StS transitions. A visualisation of this computation can be seen in Fig. 2, showing a strong correlation between the vertical speed of the bounding box and the Sit-to-Stand action.

In order to reduce noise of the 3D bounding boxes, we adopted a Savitzky-Golay filter (`savgol`) as implemented in SciPy. The advantage of the `savgol` filter is that it replaces each data-point by the least-squares polynomial fit of its neighbours, allowing noise reduction and a simple analytical derivative of the polynomial. We used a kernel window size of 11 points and a polynomial of 3rd order. The vertical velocity can then be computed as the ratio between the filtered y_{top} and the filtered time vector:

$$V_y = \frac{\text{savgol}(y_{\text{top}}, \text{deriv} = 1)}{\text{savgol}(t, \text{deriv} = 1)} \tag{3}$$

[3] Although here we refer to the computation of the speed of ascent, the methodology applies identically for the speed of descent by simply using the negative sign in Eq. 1.

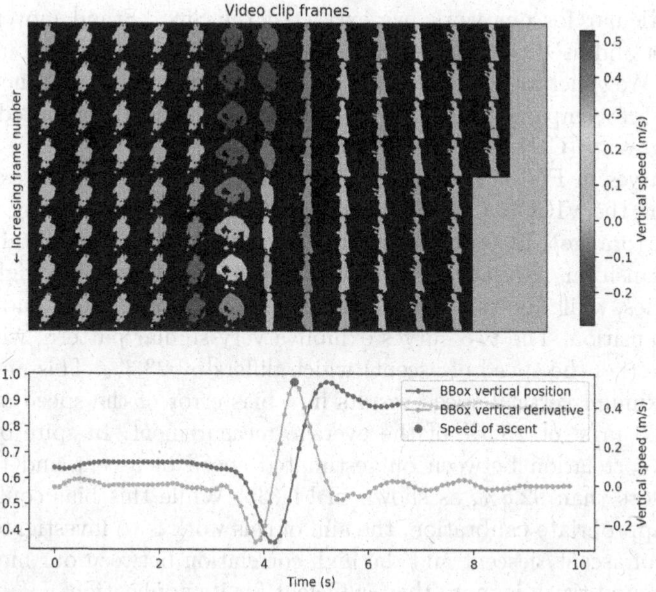

Fig. 2. Example computation of the speed of ascent: (top) video frames of a Sit-to-Stand sequence from the SPHERE data, colour coded with intensity of the vertical derivative; (bottom) 3D bounding box vertical coordinate and derivative. The maximum intensity of the vertical speed corresponds to the speed of ascent. (Color figure online)

3 Experiments

The architecture was built with 4 Inception modules [18], each composed of a sequence of (1) 3D convolutions, (2) batch normalisation and (3) activation ReLu, using respectively 16, 32, 64 and 128 filters. The last layer produces a set of convolutional features which are, once reshaped, 512 dimensional for 25 pseudo-time steps. The resulting features are fed into an LSTM module with 128 units, whose output is then fed into a 3D fully connected layer with *softmax* activation. The input comprises video clips of 100 frames, each 100 by 100 pixels, while the output is a 3 by 1 classifier.

We demonstrate the validity of our algorithm by assessing the StS video classifier and the speed of ascent/descent computation independently on two different datasets.

3.1 Physical Rehabilitation Movements Data Set

The UI-PRMD dataset includes skeleton data from typical exercises and movements which are performed by patients during therapy and rehabilitation programs [19]. It consists of 10 healthy subjects, performing 10 different movements 10 times each, and recorded simultaneously using a Kinect and a VICON (gold standard) motion-capture system.

In particular for our work, we extracted the Sit-to-Stand movement from the dataset and used the VICON motion capture data to validate our proposed approach. We generated 3D bounding boxes using the extent of Kinect skeleton joints and we compared the speed of ascent with the one computed using the centre of gravity (CG) from the VICON data[4].

The curves in Fig. 3a show a comparison of the true speed of ascent, computed using the VICON CG (blue curve), and our estimation using the Kinect head joint (orange). In both cases, the vertical derivative was obtained for all the StS transitions available ($N_{\text{StS}} = 100$) and averaged to highlight possible discrepancies, while the time was normalised using the beginning and the end of the StS transition. The two curves exhibit a very similar pattern, with a maximum value (i.e. the speed of ascent) which differs by 23.3%. This amplification of the maximum vertical speed results in a bias error of the speed of ascent of about 0.026 m/s, or 28.3% of the average measurement. In spite of this bias error, the correlation between our estimated speed of ascent and the ground truth is more than 92.8%, as shown in Fig. 3b. While this bias could be mitigated by appropriate calibration, the aim of this work is to investigate trends in the speed of ascent/descent and the high correlation between our measurement and the ground truth is more than sufficient for its application.

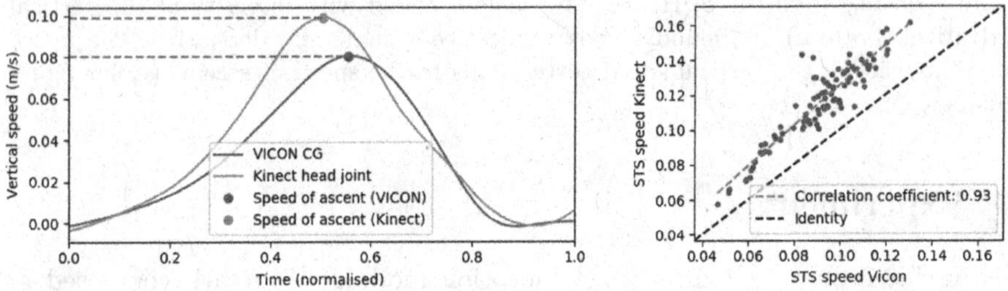

(a) (b)

Fig. 3. Comparison of speed of ascent computed with our algorithm using the Kinect data and the VICON system

3.2 SPHERE Data

The SPHERE project (Sensor Platform for Healthcare in a Residential Environment) [22] developed a multi-modal sensing platform aimed to record data from up to 100 houses in the Bristol (UK) area for healthcare monitoring. Each house was equipped with a variety of sensors, including RGBD cameras, which were used to generate human silhouettes and 2D/3D bounding boxes via the OpenNI API [1], from different communal spaces: living room, kitchen and hall.

[4] The CG was estimated using the average of the Left, Right, Anterior and Posterior Superior Illiac skeletal joints.

The HEmiSPHERE (Hip and knEe study of SPHERE) project [10] is an UK National Health Service application of SPHERE sensors within the homes of patients undergoing a total hip or knee replacement.

In this work, we present data collected from the living room of 4 different houses, described in Table 1, two belonging to the HEmiSPHERE cohort and two belonging to the SPHERE one. This subset includes a total of 1,177,082 video clips, of which 5,645 are StS transitions and the rest belong to the "Other" class. The videos were manually labelled by the authors using the MuViLab annotator tool[5] and were used for cross-validation as per Table 2. The discrepancy between the number of Sit-to-Stand and Stand-to-Sit transitions can be explained by the type of silhouette detector adopted (OpenNI), that was optimised for standing poses. This increases the chances of detecting a person walking and sitting down and hence the number of Stand-to-Sit transitions recorded.

Table 1. Description of the data from the 4 houses: 2 cohorts of SPHERE (bottom two rows) and HemiSPHERE (top two rows).

Id	Duration	Occup.	#Other	#Sit-to-Stand	#Stand-to-Sit
House *A*	4 months	2	107404	339	491
House *B*	3 months	2	266853	1289	2051
House *C*	9 months	4	416628	297	1054
House *D*	6 months	1	380552	54	70

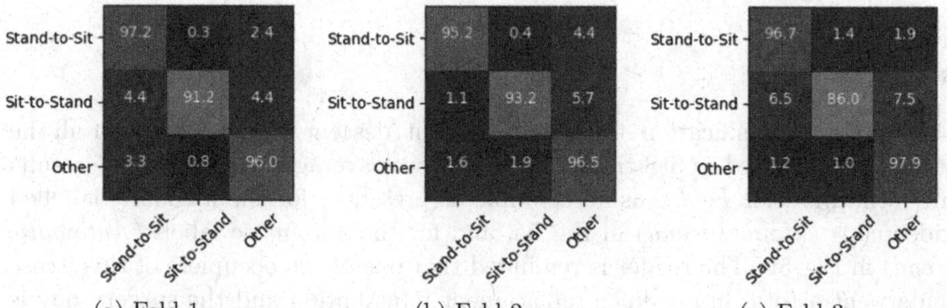

(a) Fold 1 (b) Fold 2 (c) Fold 3

Fig. 4. Confusion matrix for each validation fold.

3.3 Classification

Data from homes *A*, *B* and *C* was used to train and validate the network (described in Sect. 2.1) using a cross-validation strategy, as depicted in Table 2. Data from *House D* was left out of this procedure and was only used to generate the trend plot. Results are presented in Table 2 and show an overall accuracy of

[5] Available on GitHub: https://github.com/ale152/muvilab.

94.8%, 95.0% and 93.5% for the three validation folds, computed by averaging the accuracy of the three classes. The average accuracy across the three folds is 94.4%. Details of the classification results are presented in Fig. 4, showing the confusion matrices for each validation fold.

Particular attention must be paid to the false positive scores. The number of "Other" videos mis-classified as StS was found to be 1.63%, producing 28119 false positive against the 6548 correctly identified StS transitions. While these values might potentially damage our score, a manual inspection of the false positives concluded that many of the mis-classification videos are, indeed, visually similar to StS transitions. This included subjects interacting with the environment for long periods of time while standing up, raising from the floor, kneeling while doing exercises or housekeeping chores. Although these movements are not strictly StS transitions, they still involve a vertical motion that requires physical effort. As we will show in the next Section, although the presence of these false detection increases the uncertainty of our measurements, it does not hamper the calculation of the trend plots.

Table 2. Cross-validation accuracy results, with 94.4% overall average accuracy.

Fold	Train	Validate	Stand-to-Sit	Sit-to-Stand	Other	Overall
1	House C, B	House A	97.2%	91.2%	96.0%	94.8%
2	House C, A	House B	95.2%	93.2%	96.5%	95.0%
3	House A, B	House C	96.7%	86.0%	97.9%	93.5%
					Average	94.4%

3.4 Trend Plots

Following the classification, the speed of ascent/descent was computed for all the video clips detected as StS transitions and it was averaged per week. The resulting trend plot, for *Fold 2* as an example, is presented for the manually labelled video clips (*Manual trend*) in Fig. 5a, and for the automatic labels (*Automatic trend*) in Fig. 5b. The reader is reminded that one of the occupiers of this house underwent a total hip or knee replacement intervention and the surgery day is marked with a solid black line. Before surgery, the speed of ascent is between 0.35 and 0.45 m/s, which is followed by a sudden drop soon after the operation. This is due to the pain and the discomfort following the surgery, which impair the physical ability of the patient and hence their speed of ascent. In the following weeks, the speed of ascent shows a slow but steady increase with a slope of around 0.04 m/s per month. Finally, 14 weeks after the surgery, the speed of ascent reaches a value which is just shy of 0.5 m/s, confirming a full recovery. The presence of the trend is also corroborated by a high coefficient of determination $R^2 = 0.86$.

The comparison between the *Manual trend* and the *Automatic trend* from Fig. 5 shows a very similar pattern, with a correlation coefficient between the two plots of 0.88. In spite of the higher error bars, due to false positives, the main characteristic aspects of the plot are preserved, including the drop in the speed of ascent following the surgery and the full recovery after 14 weeks.

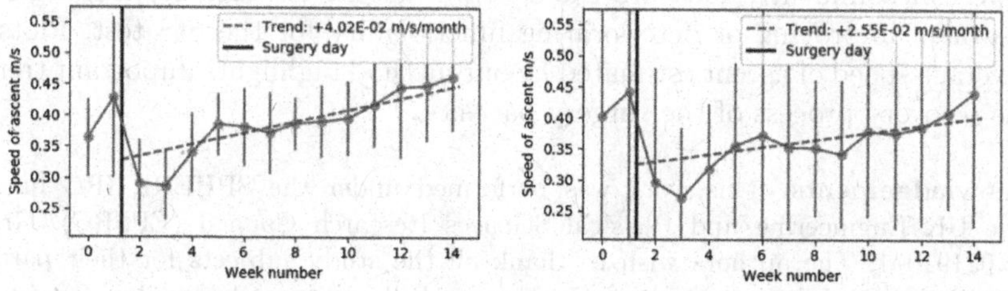

(a) Manual (b) Automatic

Fig. 5. Comparison of speed of ascent trend for Fold 2, extracted from (a) the manually labelled StS transitions and (b) the video clips automatically labelled as StS. The correlation between the plots is 0.88.

For comparison, we present *Automatic trends* generated for *House C* and *D* in Fig. 6, occupied by healthy participants. As expected, no particular trend can be noticed for these houses, as confirmed by the low coefficients of determination R^2 of -0.21 and -0.45 respectively.

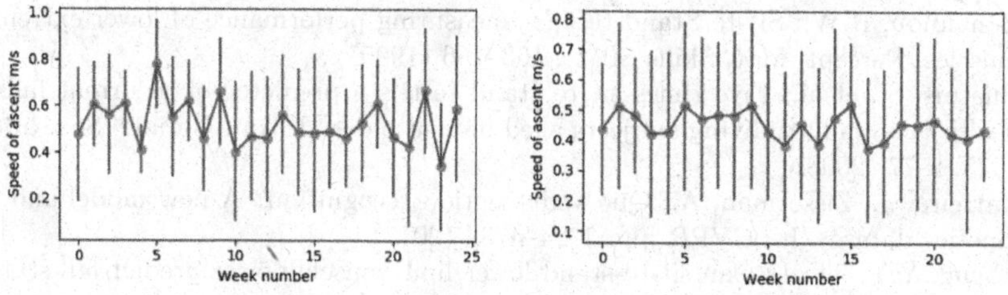

(a) House C (b) House D

Fig. 6. Comparison of speed of ascent trend for *House C* and *D* from the SPHERE cohort.

Although the trend plots presented in this section only refer to the speed of ascent (i.e. Sit-to-Stand), the trend plot computed using the speed of descent (i.e. Stand-to-Sit) showed a very similar behaviour and were omitted from this paper for brevity.

4 Conclusions

The demand of AAL technologies for home monitoring is continuously increasing. We presented a simple and efficient approach for the detection and analysis of

StS transitions for home monitoring in completely unsupervised environments. We implemented and tested our method in 4 different houses, 2 of which were occupied by patients with total hip or knee replacement. We showed that we are able to reliably identify StS transitions in video clips of binary silhouettes and we can confidently measure the speed of ascent for each transition as an indicator of improving or deteriorating functionality for the StS test. Plots of the average speed of ascent estimated by our method highlights important trends in the recovery process of the surgery patients.

Acknowledgements. This work was performed under the SPHERE IRC funded by the UK Engineering and Physical Sciences Research Council (EPSRC), Grant EP/K031910/1. The authors wish to thank all the study subjects for their participation in this project and Rachael Gooberman-Hill, Andrew Judge, Ian Craddock, Ashley Blom, Michael Whitehouse and Sabrina Grant for their support with the HEmiSPHERE project. The HEmiSPHERE project was approved by the Research Ethics Committee (reference number: 17/SW/0121).

References

1. OpenNI. https://structure.io/openni
2. Birchley, G., Huxtable, R., Murtagh, M., Ter Meulen, R., Flach, P., Gooberman-Hill, R.: Smart homes, private homes? An empirical study of technology researchers' perceptions of ethical issues in developing smart-home health technologies. BMC Med. Ethics **18**(1), 1–13 (2017)
3. Bohannon, R.W.: Sit-to-Stand test for measuring performance of lower extremity muscles. Percept. Mot. Skills **80**(1), 163–166 (1995)
4. Buatois, S., et al.: Five times sit to stand test is a predictor of recurrent falls in healthy community-living subjects aged 65 and older. J. Am. Geriatr. Soc. **56**(8), 1575–1577 (2008)
5. Carreira, J., Zisserman, A.: Quo vadis, action recognition? A new model and the kinetics dataset. In: CVPR, pp. 4724–4733 (2017)
6. Cheng, Y.Y., et al.: Can sit-to-stand lower limb muscle power predict fall status? Gait Posture **40**(3), 403–407 (2014)
7. Dall, P.M., Kerr, A.: Frequency of the sit to stand task: an observational study of free-living adults. Appl. Ergon. **41**(1), 58–61 (2010)
8. Ejupi, A., Brodie, M., Gschwind, Y.J., Lord, S.R., Zagler, W.L., Delbaere, K.: Kinect-based five-times-sit-to-stand test for clinical and in-home assessment of fall risk in older people. Gerontology **62**(1), 118–124 (2015)
9. Galna, B., Barry, G., Jackson, D., Mhiripiri, D., Olivier, P., Rochester, L.: Accuracy of the Microsoft Kinect sensor for measuring movement in people with Parkinson's disease. Gait Posture **39**(4), 1062–1068 (2014)
10. Grant, S., et al.: Using home sensing technology to assess outcome and recovery after hip and knee replacement in the UK: the HEmiSPHERE study protocol. BMJ Open **8**(7), 1–11 (2018)
11. Japkowicz, N., Stephen, S.: The class imbalance problem: a systematic study. Intell. Data Anal. **6**(5), 429–449 (2002)
12. Kouta, M., Shinkoda, K., Kanemura, N.: Sit-to-Walk versus Sit-to-Stand or gait initiation: biomechanical analysis of young men. J. Phys. Ther. Sci. **18**(2), 201–206 (2006)

13. Masullo, A., Burghardt, T., Damen, D., Hannuna, S., Ponce-Lopez, V., Mirmehdi, M.: CaloriNet: from silhouettes to calorie estimation in private environments. In: Britic Machine Vision Conference, pp. 1–14 (2018)
14. Sánchez, V.G., Taylor, I., Bing-Jonsson, P.C.: Ethics of smart house welfare technology for older adults: a systematic literature review. Int. J. Technol. Assess. Health Care **33**(06), 691–699 (2017)
15. Schot, P.K., Knutzen, K.M., Poole, S.M., Mrotek, L.A.: Sit-to-Stand performance of older adults following strength training. Res. Q. Exerc. Sport **74**(1), 1–8 (2003)
16. Shia, V., Bajcsy, R.: Vision-based event detection of the Sit-to-Stand transition. In: International Conference on Wireless Mobile Communication and Healthcare. ICST (2015)
17. Simonyan, K., Zisserman, A.: Two-stream convolutional networks for action recognition in videos, pp. 1–9 (2014)
18. Szegedy, C., et al.: Going deeper with convolutions. In: CVPR, vol. 91, pp. 1–9. IEEE (2015)
19. Vakanski, A., Jun, H.P., Paul, D., Baker, R.: A data set of human body movements for physical rehabilitation exercises. Data **3**(1), 2 (2018)
20. Yamada, T., Demura, S., Takahashi, K.: Center of gravity transfer velocity during Sit-to-Stand is closely related to physical functions regarding fall experience of the elderly living in community dwelling. Health **05**(12), 2097–2103 (2013)
21. Zagler, W., Panek, P., Rauhala, M.: Ambient Assisted Living Systems - The Conflicts between Technology, Acceptance, Ethics and Privacy. Assisted Living Systems - Models Architectures and Engineering Approaches, pp. 1–4. Dagstuhl, Wadern (2008)
22. Zhu, N., et al.: Bridging e-Health and the internet of things: the SPHERE project. IEEE Intell. Syst. **30**(4), 39–46 (2015)
23. Ziefle, M., Röcker, C., Holzinger, A.: Medical technology in smart homes: exploring the user's perspective on privacy, intimacy and trust. In: International Computer Software and Applications Conference, pp. 410–415 (2011)

Target Aware Visual Object Tracking

Caner Ozer(✉), Filiz Gurkan, and Bilge Gunsel

Multimedia Signal Processing and Pattern Recognation Group,
Istanbul Technical University, Istanbul, Turkey
{ozerc,gurkanf,gunselb}@itu.edu.tr

Abstract. We propose a visual object tracker that improves accuracy while significantly decreasing false alarm rate. This is achieved by a late fusion scheme that integrates the motion model of particle sampling with the region proposal network of Mask R-CNN during inference. The qualified bounding boxes selected by the late fusion are fed into the Mask R-CNN's head layer for the detection of the tracked object. We refer the introduced scheme, TAVOT, as target aware visual object tracker since it is capable of minimizing false detections with the guidance of variable rate particle sampling initialized by the target region of interest. It is shown that TAVOT is capable of modeling temporal video content with a simple motion model thus constitutes a promising video object tracker. Performance evaluation performed on VOT2016 video sequences demonstrates that TAVOT 22% increases the success rate, while 73% decreasing the false alarm rate compared to the baseline Mask R-CNN. Compared to the top tracker of VOT2016 around 5% increase at the success rate is reported where intersection over union is greater than 0.5.

Keywords: Visual object tracking · Region proposal network · Particle filtering

1 Introduction

Although the recently developed visual object trackers highly robust to scale changes that yields perfectly localized object bounding boxes, specification of the tracked object bounding box (BB) among a number of detected BBs constitutes a challenging problem. The problem becomes harder in video object tracking where we have several moving objects in the scene. In order to alleviate these drawbacks, new deep architectures that enable to include the temporal information into the tracking model are introduced. These networks mostly propose enforced solutions to video object tracking with the expense of high computational load but elimination of the false detections is still an open problem.

There are numerous ways to aggregate temporal information with spatial information for video processing. One of the most common practice is using long short term memory (LSTM) along with CNNs. LSTMs use hidden and cell states to make a prediction for the current video frame using the predictions of previous frames and stores the temporal context into its memory. Current practices involve several improvements on RNNs that ConvLSTMs [21] add

F. Karray et al. (Eds.): ICIAR 2019, LNCS 11663, pp. 186–198, 2019.
https://doi.org/10.1007/978-3-030-27272-2_16

convolutional kernels instead of weight vectors and ST-LSTMs [14] introduce a new memory mechanism, different from the generic LSTM cells. A different methodology for spatiotemporal video processing is using 3D-CNNs by stacking multiple video frames for the input. For instance, two-stream inflated 3D-CNNs [1] perform fusion on two models designed for processing RGB and optical flow information for activity recognition. Recently, E3D-LSTMs [23] merged these two methodologies and added a different type of gating mechanism to provide self-attention. Yet in the context of object tracking, only few methods use the RNN based architectures for capturing the temporal information. ROLO proposed in [18] performs single object tracking by placing an LSTM layer on the top of the YOLO object detector. There are several other works [6,15], which use the RNN-like architectures for multiple object tracking as well. Still, they all diverge from being a simple model since the utilities used to capture the temporal information are complex and an additional training is needed to tune the parameters of the sequential layers. In addition, neither of the settings above can be directly applied on an object tracking objective such that, learning from tracking datasets are prohibited. In this regard, using other cues as motion information is a stronger candidate to aggregate temporal information for video processing. There are also visual object trackers with motion guidance which carries out online learning for learning the target representations. For example, MDNet [17] proposes a domain-specific online learning scheme and MGNet [5] extends this approach by stacking optical flow information on the RGB video frames and selecting candidate region of interests via a particle filter. Yet, the motion guidance is less reliable comparing variable rate particle sampler (VRPS) that we are using, seeing that they have increased the number of input channels from 3 to 5 by stacking optical flow channels on the RGB channel. Moreover, MGNet requires a training from scratch due to the change in the number of input channels, in contrast to our work which can be trained by using an object detection dataset with segmentation annotations such as COCO [13].

Differ from the existing models we propose a motion guided deep object tracking method referred as Target Aware Visual Object Tracker (TAVOT) based on Mask R-CNN, a state-of-the-art deep object detector. Inspiring from [7] in which accuracy of the variable-rate color particle filter is significantly improved by fusing the region proposals of Mask R-CNN and particle proposals, in this work we adopt the baseline architecture of Mask R-CNN to video object tracking by including the state transition model of particle filtering into the inference scheme. TAVOT applies a late fusion on the proposals generated by Mask R-CNN's Region Proposal Network (RPN) and VRPS that enables integrating a simple motion model into the system. The qualified BBs selected by the late fusion are fed into the Mask R-CNN's head layer for the detection of the tracked object. We refer TAVOT as target aware visual object tracker since it is capable of minimizing false detections with the guidance of VRPS initialized by the target RoI.

The rest of the paper is organized as follows. Section 2 summarizes the baseline methods that we used as the object detector and particle sampler. Section 3 describes the proposed target aware visual object tracker. Experimental results are reported in Sect. 4 and Sect. 5 presents the conclusions.

2 Theoretical Background

This section presents a brief overview on Mask R-CNN in Sect. 2.1 and variable rate color particle filter (VRCPF) in Sect. 2.2, where we used as the baseline models for the proposed tracker.

2.1 Mask R-CNN

Mask R-CNN [8] is a state-of-the-art object detector that simultaneously performs classification and segmentation on the detected objects. It extends its predecessor, Faster R-CNN [20], by integrating the concept of instance segmentation into the detector that segments the individual objects while detecting the object bounding boxes. Moreover, Mask R-CNN uses RoIAlign for enhancing the detection performance, thus we used it as a baseline for the proposed visual object tracker. Figure 1(a) illustrates pipeline of Mask R-CNN and in the following we describe the main blocks.

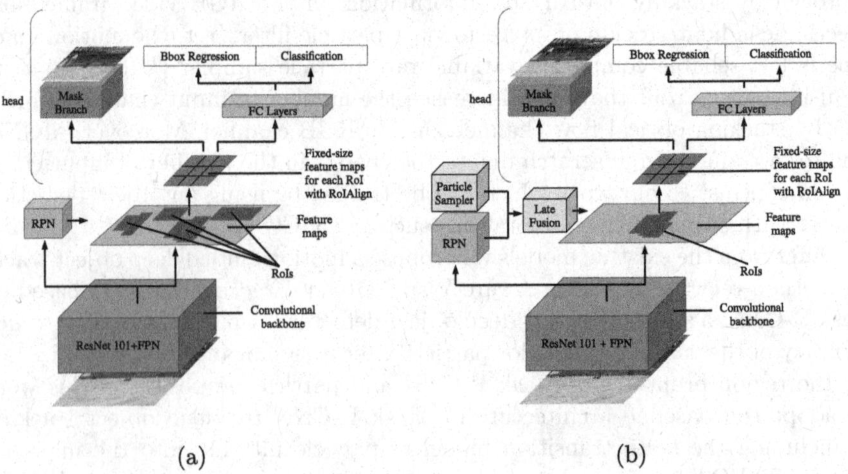

Fig. 1. (a) Mask R-CNN architecture. (b) Architecture of the proposed TAVOT tracker.

Feature Extraction. ResNet-101 [9] and feature pyramid networks (FPN) [12] are used for extracting the backbone features from the image, which creates 5 different shaped feature maps with spatial dimensions of $256^2, 128^2, 64^2, 32^2$ and 16^2 after resizing the image to 1024×1024 resolution, while preserving the

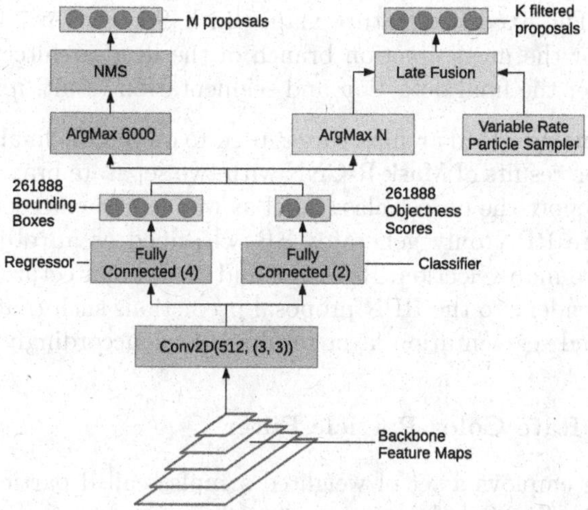

Fig. 2. Region Proposal Network of mask R-CNN (blue path), and qualified BB selection proposed by TAVOT (blue+gray path). (Color figure online)

image's original aspect ratio by padding zeros. These feature maps, namely, the backbone feature maps are notated as P_2, P_3, P_4, P_5 and P_6, respectively.

Region Proposal Network (RPN). RPN generates proposal BBs with their corresponding objectness scores which are defined as the probability of the regions containing an object. Figure 2 demonstrates the steps of proposal generation. First all of the backbone feature maps are fed into the RPN layer by passing 512 convolutional filters each with 3×3 kernel on these feature maps in order to construct a shared feature map. Using the shared feature map, objectness scores and object bounding boxes for each anchor scale and anchor aspect ratio (0.5, 1, 2) are obtained by employing a binary classifier using SoftMax and a regression layer, respectively. This process generates the proposed object BBs collected in a set B_{RPN}, and corresponding objectness scores, p_{RPN}, for 261,888 distinct regions. After that, ArgMax 6000 block selects the 6,000 BBs with the highest objectness scores and non-maximum suppression (NMS) with an IoU threshold of 0.7 is applied for selecting less overlapping M region proposals. Filtered object proposal BBs and their corresponding feature maps are transmitted to the RoIAlign layer in order to create a fixed-size feature map.

RoIAlign. RoIAlign is a transformation applied on the selected backbone feature map using the BB coordinates collected in the set $\mathbf{B}_{RPN}$, which are denormalized to the feature map's spatial dimension $H \times W$. The motivation behind using RoIAlign is to create a fixed-size feature map having a spatial dimension of $S \times S$ which can be passed through fully connected layers and to reduce the misalignment problem between the input and output feature maps which was occurring in its predecessor, RoIPool [20]. It is shown that RoIAlign improves the BB localization accuracy [8] and for details about RoIAlign, we refer the readers to [10] and [8]. The fixed-size feature map, which S is chosen 7 for the classification and 14 for the mask creation branch of the head architecture, is passed through to gather the final detection and segmentation result, respectively.

Head Architecture. Head architecture is used to obtain the final BB detections and segmentation results of Mask R-CNN with two separate branches. Note that both branches report the object class label as well as the corresponding objectness score, where RPN only generates BBs classified as an object candidate. Backbone feature map selection, RoIAlign and head architecture steps of Mask R-CNN are dependent to the RPN proposal predictions such that classification, BB regression and segmentation layer results change accordingly.

2.2 Variable Rate Color Particle Filter

Particle filtering employs a set of weighted samples called particles to approximate the posterior density of the target state. In our notation $\mathbf{s}_t = \{s_t^1, s_t^2 ..., s_t^P\}$ and $\mathbf{w}_t = \{w_t^1, ..., w_t^P\}$ respectively denote the set of state vectors of particles and corresponding weights where the number of particles is P. Each particle state s_t^i refers to an object proposal BB thus the set of the BBs proposed by the particle sampler is denoted by $\mathbf{B}_{PS,t} = \{B_{PS,t}^1, B_{PS,t}^2 ..., B_{PS,t}^P\}$ where $B_{PS,t}^i$ denotes the BB proposed by the particle i at time t.

$$s_t^i \sim p(s_t^i | s_{t-1}^i) \tag{1}$$

where s_t^i denotes the sampled state vector of particle i at frame t given its estimation at frame $(t-1)$.

In our work, we use particle sampler of VRCPF which is formulated in Eq. 1. The target RoI is initialized in the first frame as in a standard tracking setup. Let $B_{PS,t}^{tar}$ denotes the target RoI specified in the form of a BB and $m(B_{PS,t}^{tar})$ denotes a kernel density estimate of the color distribution of the target BB at time t. Similarly, $B_{PS,t}^i$ refers to the candidate object BB pointed by the ith particle where the corresponding kernel density estimate of the color distribution is $m(B_{PS,t}^i)$. As in [4], we use Bhattacharya distance $d[m(B_{PS,t}^{tar}), m(B_{PS,t}^i)]$ to measure similarity between the target and candidate distributions. Thus the likelihood distribution which constitutes observation model of VRCPF is formulated by Eq. 2,

$$p(\mathrm{y}_t | s_t^i) \propto e^{-\lambda(d^2[m(B_{PS,t}^{tar}), m(B_{PS,t}^i)]} \tag{2}$$

where y_t is the observed video frame and λ is a smoothing parameter. Finally the update rule of particle weights can be formulated as;

$$w_t^i \propto w_{t-1}^i . p(y_t | s_t^i). \tag{3}$$

The final state of the tracked object is estimated at each frame as weighted average of particle states.

3 TAVOT: The Proposed Visual Object Tracker

Despite the decent object detection performance on individual video frames, Mask R-CNN is lacking robustness to blur, occlusion and illumination changes as a visual object tracker. In addition, as a deep detector Mask R-CNN outputs all detected object BBs hence itself is not able to identify the desired target object of interest. Choosing the BB with the highest objectness score among Mask R-CNN predictions causes instabilities in tracking that it mostly results in selecting the wrong target BB. In this case, adopting Mask R-CNN to a video object tracker including motion information enables us to deal with such problems. In this section, we present our proposed method for video object tracking where we adopt a pre-trained Mask R-CNN to a video object tracker. This is achieved by integrating a variable rate color particle sampler into the region proposal generation stage that guides a late fusion mechanism during inference as shown in Fig. 1(b). The steps for the proposed scheme that yields the final visual object tracker, TAVOT, are explained in the following.

Proposal Generation by TAVOT RPN. All processing steps up to generation of BBs and corresponding objectness scores for 261888 distinct regions are exactly the same as the original Mask R-CNN (Fig. 2). We activate the late fusion for the rest of the proposal generation scheme. Main drawback of the described NMS scheme in RPN is a BB having the highest objectness score may not be the one that provides the best object localization. Therefore during the inference there may not be any detected object at the output of the head layer or a badly localized object may be detected. This happens since RoIAlign layer of the deep object detector is very sensitive to small localization shifts. In order to alleviate this drawback, we do not use the original NMS during the BB proposal creation, instead among 261888 BBs with objectness scores proposed by RPN, top-N bounding boxes with the highest objectness scores are selected without checking their overlapping ratio. Let $B_{RPN_{LF}}$ denotes the set of selected N proposal BBs that we fed into the late fusion block. VRCPF learns the initial target object appearance model with one positive sample specified by the initial RoI at the first frame of tracking. Then, the particle sampler samples P object proposals $\mathbf{B}_{PS} = \{B^1_{PS}, B^2_{PS}..., B^P_{PS}\}$ from the state transition distribution formulated by Eq. 1 and assigns the corresponding particle weights $\mathbf{w}$. Note that the time variable t is dropped to simplify the notation. Particle weights imply the probability of a sampled BB to contain a target object or not thus can be interpreted as the objectness scores of the BBs.

Late Fusion. The particle sampler enforces localization of the proposed BBs around the target object of interest with its state transition model and RPN has a great ability of generating object instances with high confidence scores. In this regard, uniting these two proposal generators improves the localization of the target object of interest while reducing the false detection rate. Therefore we formulate a late fusion scheme to get benefit from both proposal generators. Let $\mathbf{B}_P$ denotes the union of two sets, $\mathbf{B}_{RPN_{LF}}$ and $\mathbf{B}_{PS}$, and it is obtained by appending $\mathbf{B}_{PS}$ on $\mathbf{B}_{RPN_{LF}}$. For any RPN bounding box having an IoU over γ with PS BBs or vice versa, Eq. 4 identifies the qualified BBs of $\mathbf{B}_P$;

$$I^j = \begin{cases} 1 & \text{if} \quad \beta(B_P^j, \mathbf{B}_P^{N:(P+N-1)}) > \gamma \quad \text{and} \quad 0 \le j < N \\ 1 & \text{if} \quad \beta(B_P^j, \mathbf{B}_P^{0:(N-1)}) > \gamma \quad \text{and} \quad N \le j < P+N \\ 0 & \text{otherwise} \end{cases} \tag{4}$$

where j denotes the integer indexes of the BBs ranged between 0 and $P+N-1$ and $I^j = 1$ shows that B_P^j to be used in the next step as a qualified BB. β is the operator that calculates the maximum IoU between a BB and a set of BBs and γ is the IoU threshold.

Then in order to retrieve the set of K qualified BBs, $\mathbf{B}_{Qual}$, a multiplication is performed between $\mathbf{I}$ and $\mathbf{B}_P$ as in Eq. 5,

$$\mathbf{B}_{Qual} = \mathbf{I} \odot \mathbf{B}_P \tag{5}$$

where $\odot$ is the element-wise multiplication operation. $\mathbf{B}_{Qual}$ is then transmitted to the RoIAlign layer which is used for creating a fixed-size feature map. Note that K varies from frame to frame since the number of detected object BBs as well as their overlapping ratios would differ.

Regression and Classification. Feature maps describing $\mathbf{B}_{Qual}$ at the end of RoIAlign layer are being used for retrieving TAVOT predictions by using the head architecture of Mask R-CNN with a small but important modification. In particular, knowing that the target of interest is initialized at the first frame, we perform BB classification and regression for only the known object class label. This enables TAVOT not to provide any output in case the tracked output has a different object class label. Note that the tracked object class label information is not being used in RPN or late fusion schemes since they apply a two class classification.

Mask R-CNN's RoIAlign and head architecture are sensitive to the small perturbations in BB locations that the detection results, specifically the objectness score of a RoI being an object, can be drastically changed even with a small change depending on the RoI locations provided by RoIAlign. In fact this is a common problem in deep object detectors arising mainly from interpolations. Target aware nature of TAVOT alleviates this problem by providing more RoIs with different sizes and aspect ratios with particle sampling. For instance as it is reported at Fig. 3(a), the target RoI is classified by Mask R-CNN as a *kite* with objectness score 0.91 but none of the RoIs are classified as *person*. However the target RoI is detected as *person* by TAVOT even though the assigned objectness score for *person* is as low as 0.48 (Fig. 3(b)). This clearly indicates that Mask R-CNN is vulnerable to the position changes and in order to overcome this problem, RPN has to be supported by qualified particles for boosting head architecture. Furthermore, target aware nature of TAVOT enables us to track *person* with such a low objectness score since 0.48 is the highest score for the class *person*.

4 Test Results

The proposed visual tracker is evaluated on commonly used benchmarking dataset VOT2016 and performance reported compared to the top trackers of VOT2016 benchmarking. We used 36 of the VOT2016 [11] videos that include object classes learned by the released model of Mask R-CNN trained on COCO dataset [13] which consists of 118,287 video frames from 80 categories. We modified the code available at https://github.com/matterport/Mask_RCNN to interfere RPN proposals and head architecture. Experiments and evaluations are conducted with Intel Core i7 4790 CPU 3.6 GHz and GeForce GTX TITAN X GPU. Tracking performance is reported by success rate which is the ratio of the number of successfully tracked frames over total number of frames in a video sequence for a given IoU threshold where IoU is defined as the area of intersection over union between ground truth and the tracker result. Also we have evaluated accuracy and robustness that measures the average IoU calculated over all successfully tracked video frames and how many times the tracker drifts off the target, respectively. Besides false alarm rate is reported for each video sequences to demonstrate the improvement achieved by TAVOT in minimizing false detection rate. While performing these experiments, we set $P = 400$, $N = 1,000$ and $\gamma = 0.3$.

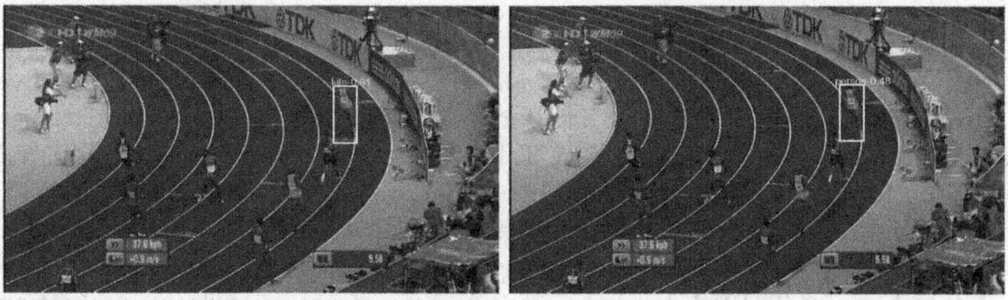

(a) (b)

Fig. 3. Bolt 1, frame no: 321. (a) Target tracked by Mask R-CNN. (b) Target tracked by TAVOT.

Overall tracking performance of TAVOT compared to the top trackers of VOT2016, CCOT [3], DDC [11], DNT [2], EBT [24], MLDF [22], SRBT [11], SSAT [19] and TCNN [16], is reported at Fig. 6 and Table 1 in terms of success rate and accuracy/robustness. Performance improvement on VOT2016 dataset achieved by TAVOT compared to SSAT,. the top tracker, is 1% for accuracy, while it is 2% for success rate at IoU-th = 0.5. Also it is shown in Fig. 6, all other trackers are lacking of localization thus the tracking accuracy significantly decreases at higher IoU-th values, while our method TAVOT is much more robust at high IoU thresholds (Performance increment at IoU-th = 0.6 is about 6%) because of the improved localization accuracy. It is also observed that we have better performance in terms of accuracy but poor robustness which indicates that miss detection rate is high. We also compared our proposed tracker with Mask R-CNN and report that the accuracy increases about 5%, while robustness decreases 27% that clearly demonstrate the improvement gained by including the temporal model of VRCPF sampler into the visual object tracking (Fig. 4).

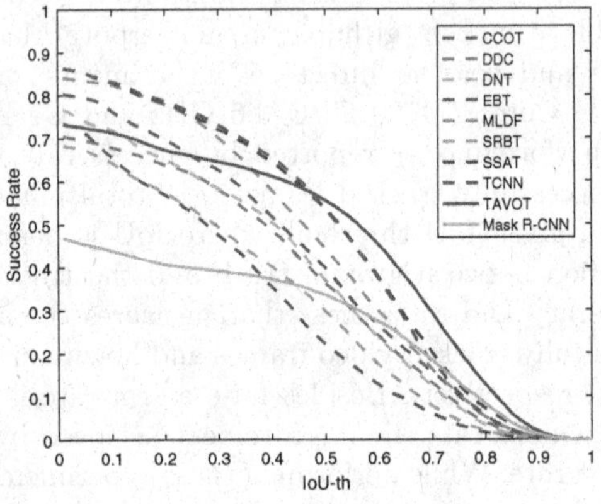

Fig. 4. Success rates achieved by TAVOT on VOT2016 compared to the state of the art trackers and Mask R-CNN.

We have also evaluated performance of TAVOT according to the five attributes labeled in VOT2016 as illumination change, motion change, size change, occlusion and camera motion. Table 2 reports our performance compared to the top four trackers of VOT2016 benchmarking and Mask R-CNN. TAVOT provides higher success rates particularly for illumination and size change where the improvement is 13% and 6% compared to the best tracker, respectively. This is mainly because TAVOT keeps tracking in case of occlusion by using motion model of particle sampler where deep detectors fail to track under blur and abrupt illumination changes.

Table 1. Accuracy and robustness achieved by TAVOT on VOT2016 dataset compared to the top trackers.

Tracker	Accuracy	Robustness	Tracker	Accuracy	Robustness
TAVOT	**0.605**	0.307	CCOT	0.553	0.263
Mask R-CNN	0.556	0.572	MLDF	0.551	0.179
SSAT	0.594	0.169	SRBT	0.524	0.395
TCNN	0.590	**0.164**	DNT	0.521	0.311
DDC	0.570	0.320	EBT	0.444	0.398

Table 2. Attribute based success rates achieved by TAVOT and the top four trackers on VOT2016 dataset. (IoU-th = 0.5).

Attribute	TAVOT	Mask RCNN	SSAT	TCNN	MLDF	CCOT
Illumination change	0.702	0.369	0.550	0.568	0.538	0.350
Occlusion	0.554	0.304	0.523	0.552	0.494	0.441
Motion change	0.565	0.343	0.516	0.531	0.404	0.353
Camera motion	0.609	0.384	0.605	0.600	0.522	0.437
Size change	0.610	0.391	0.550	0.547	0.476	0.393

In order to visually demonstrate the improvement achieved by TAVOT, in Fig. 5 we illustrate some tracking results that allow us to compare TAVOT with Mask R-CNN. Figure 5(a) clearly shows that TAVOT provides better localization under blur where the blurred parts of object of interest are tracked with BBs provided by the particle sampler. Figure 5(b) shows three video frames where Mask R-CNN does not track any object but TAVOT does. This is mainly because RPN does not fed an accurate object BB proposal to Mask R-CNN. However TAVOT provides accurate results, this is because either the particle sampler generates better BBs at aspect ratios differ from the anchors or target aware decision maker at the head layer of TAVOT can classify the object of interest. Interested readers can access to the tracking results at https://mspritu.github.io/research/tavot.

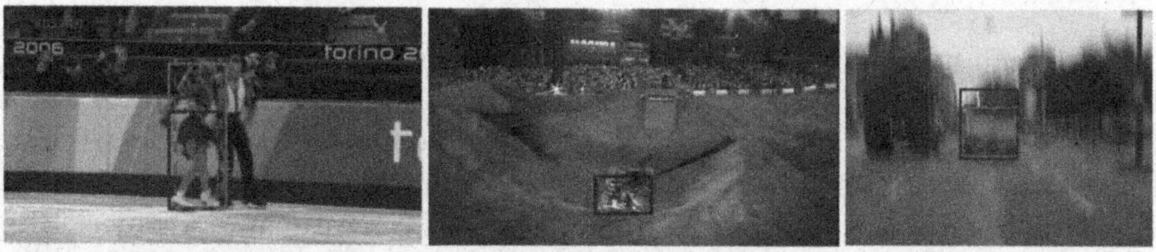

(a)

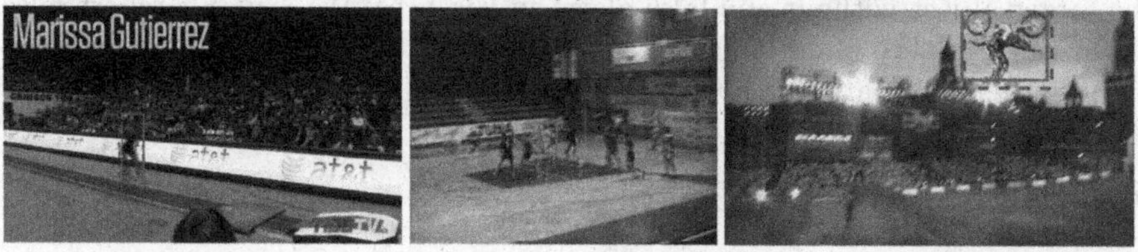

(b)

Fig. 5. Tracked object BB by mask R-CNN (blue), GT (red-dashed) and TAVOT (magenta). (a) iceskater2, motocross1, car1 (frame no:13,62,257), (b) gymnastics3, handball2, motocross1 (frame no:17,306,85). (Color figure online)

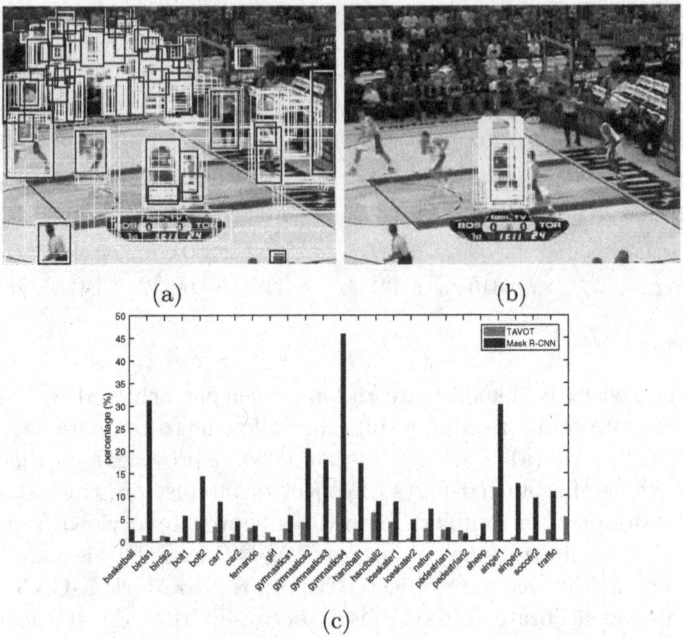

Fig. 6. Basketball, frame no:35. (a) Proposal BBs generated by RPN (green), the tracked object BBs (blue) by Mask R-CNN. (b) Proposal BBs after late fusion (green), the tracked object BB (magenta) by TAVOT. (c) False alarm ratios of Mask R-CNN and TAVOT obtained on VOT2016 videos. (Color figure online)

Since high false alarm rate is a common problem of deep detectors we report the false alarm rate for each video sequence at Fig. 6(c). False alarm rate of Mask R-CNN significantly higher than TAVOT because the introduced late fusion scheme reduces the false alarms by eliminating unqualified proposals. Figure 6(a) visually illustrates the false alarms where Mask R-CNN estimates 38 object BBs using BBs proposed by RPN where 37 of them are false detection, TAVOT tracks the target object without any false alarm in Fig. 6(b). We couldn't report false alarm rates for the state-of-the-art methods used for success rate comparison because this information is not available.

5 Conclusion

This work aims to improve the tracking accuracy of visual object tracking by including a simple motion model that inserts the temporal information of video into the scheme. To achieve this, we proposed a visual object tracker which uses a late fusion scheme for merging region proposal network and particle sampling. We demonstrated that the late fusion scheme guides the detection results such by eliminating the disqualifying proposals based on the motion model of particle sampling. We observed a reduction for both the miss detection and false detection rates that yields a higher tracking accuracy. Numerical results demonstrate that since TAVOT uses more proposals with aspect ratios differ from RPN anchors, this assists the head architecture to assign the correct class label.

References

1. Carreira, J., Zisserman, A.: Quo vadis, action recognition? A new model and the kinetics dataset. In: IEEE CVPR, pp. 4724–4733 (2017)
2. Chi, Z., Li, H., Lu, H., Yang, M.: Dual deep network for visual tracking. IEEE Trans. Image Process. **26**(4), 2005–2015 (2017)
3. Danelljan, M., Robinson, A., Shahbaz Khan, F., Felsberg, M.: Beyond correlation filters: learning continuous convolution operators for visual tracking. In: Leibe, B., Matas, J., Sebe, N., Welling, M. (eds.) ECCV 2016. LNCS, vol. 9909, pp. 472–488. Springer, Cham (2016). https://doi.org/10.1007/978-3-319-46454-1_29
4. Kumlu, D., Gunsel, B.: Variable rate adaptive color-based particle filter tracking. In: IEEE ICIP, pp. 1679–1683 (2016)
5. Gan, W., Lee, M.S., Wu, C.h., Kuo, C.C.J.: Online object tracking via motion-guided convolutional neural network (MGNet). J. Vis. Commun. Image Represent. **53**, 180–191 (2018)
6. Gordon, D., Farhadi, A., Fox, D.: Re^3: Real-time recurrent regression networks for visual tracking of generic objects. IEEE Robot. Autom. Lett. **3**(2), 788–795 (2018)
7. Gurkan, F., Gunsel, B., Ozer, C.: Robust object tracking via integration of particle filtering with deep detection. Digit. Signal Process. **87**, 112–124 (2019)
8. He, K., Gkioxari, G., Dollar, P., Girshick, R.: Mask R-CNN. In: IEEE ICCV, pp. 2980–2988 (2017)
9. He, K., Zhang, X., Ren, S., Sun, J.: Deep residual learning for image recognition. In: IEEE CVPR, pp. 770–778 (2016)
10. Jaderberg, M., Simonyan, K., Zisserman, A., Kavukcuoglu, K.: Spatial transformer networks. In: NIPS, pp. 2017–2025 (2015)
11. Kristan, M., et al.: The visual object tracking VOT2016 challenge results. In: Hua, G., Jégou, H. (eds.) ECCV 2016. LNCS, vol. 9914, pp. 777–823. Springer, Cham (2016). https://doi.org/10.1007/978-3-319-48881-3_54
12. Lin, T., Dollar, P., Girshick, R., He, K., Hariharan, B., Belongie, S.: Feature pyramid networks for object detection. In: IEEE CVPR, pp. 936–944, July 2017
13. Lin, T.-Y., et al.: Microsoft COCO: common objects in context. In: Fleet, D., Pajdla, T., Schiele, B., Tuytelaars, T. (eds.) ECCV 2014. LNCS, vol. 8693, pp. 740–755. Springer, Cham (2014). https://doi.org/10.1007/978-3-319-10602-1_48
14. Liu, J., Shahroudy, A., Xu, D., Wang, G.: Spatio-temporal LSTM with trust gates for 3D human action recognition. In: Leibe, B., Matas, J., Sebe, N., Welling, M. (eds.) ECCV 2016. LNCS, vol. 9907, pp. 816–833. Springer, Cham (2016). https://doi.org/10.1007/978-3-319-46487-9_50
15. Milan, A., Rezatofighi, S.H., Dick, A.R., Reid, I.D., Schindler, K.: Online multi-target tracking using recurrent neural networks. In: AAAI, pp. 4225–4232 (2017)
16. Nam, H., Baek, M., Han, B.: Modeling and propagating CNNs in a tree structure for visual tracking. CoRR abs/1608.07242 (2016)
17. Nam, H., Han, B.: Learning multi-domain convolutional neural networks for visual tracking. In: IEEE CVPR, pp. 4293–4302 (2016)
18. Ning, G., et al.: Spatially supervised recurrent convolutional neural networks for visual object tracking. In: IEEE International Symposium on Circuits and Systems, pp. 1–4, May 2017

19. Qi, Y., Qin, L., Zhang, S., Huang, Q., Yao, H.: Robust visual tracking via scale-and-state-awareness. Neurocomputing **329**, 75–85 (2019)
20. Ren, S., He, K., Girshick, R., Sun, J.: Faster R-CNN: towards real-time object detection with region proposal networks. IEEE Trans. PAMI **39**(6), 1137–1149 (2017)
21. Shi, X., Chen, Z., Wang, H., Yeung, D.Y., Wong, W.K., Woo, W.C.: Convolutional LSTM network: a machine learning approach for precipitation nowcasting. In: NIPS, pp. 802–810 (2015)
22. Wang, L., Ouyang, W., Wang, X., Lu, H.: Visual tracking with fully convolutional networks. In: IEEE ICCV, pp. 3119–3127, December 2015
23. Wang, Y., Jiang, L., Yang, M.H., Li, J., Long, M., Li, F.F.: Eidetic 3D LSTM: a model for video prediction and beyond. In: ICLR (2019)
24. Zhu, G., Porikli, F., Li, H.: Beyond local search: Tracking objects everywhere with instance-specific proposals. In: IEEE CVPR, pp. 943–951 (2016)

Design of an End-to-End Dual Mode Driver Distraction Detection System

Chaojie Ou(✉), Qiang Zhao, Fakhri Karray, and Alaa El Khatib

Center for Pattern Analysis and Machine Intelligence, Department of Electrical and Computer Engineering, University of Waterloo, Ontario, Canada
{c9ou,q74zhao,karray,alaa.elkhatib}@uwaterloo.ca

Abstract. This paper provides initial results on developing a deep neural network-based system for driver distraction detection which is operational at daytime as well as nightime. Unlike other existing methods that rely on only RGB images for daytime detection, the proposed system consists of two operating modes. The daytime mode uses a convolutional neural network to classify drivers' states based on their body poses in RGB images. The nighttime mode classifies Near Infrared images using a different neural network-based model and trained under different circumstances. To the best of our knowledge, this is the first work that explicitly addresses driver behavior detection at night using end-to-end convolutional neural networks. With initial experimental results, we empirically demonstrate that, with a relatively modest model complexity, the proposed system achieves high performance on driver distraction detection for both modes. Furthermore, we discuss the feasibility of developing a system with a small footprint and design structure but accurate enough to be deployed on a memory-restricted computing platform environment.

Keywords: Driver distraction · Deep learning · Nighttime driving

1 Introduction

Driving distraction represents a significant source of driving risks, and many governments are taking legal steps to mitigate this situation. However, distraction detection of drivers through human inspection (through law enforcement) is time-consuming and inefficient. The automotive industry has been developing in-vehicle distraction detection and alert systems through computer vision methods and machine learning methods for several years. The research work in this area can be categorized into two areas. In the first category, researchers work on designing features that can effectively represent drivers' distraction states. Through computer vision methods and with cameras facing drivers, these systems extract features to analyze drivers' physiological changes, such as the percentage of eye closure [1], eyelid activity [2], and head movements [3]. These features are then combined with diverse machine learning classification algorithms, such as Support Vector Machine (SVM), Artificial Neural Networks (ANNs), and

F. Karray et al. (Eds.): ICIAR 2019, LNCS 11663, pp. 199–207, 2019.
https://doi.org/10.1007/978-3-030-27272-2_17

Random Forest, to form classification systems. In the other category of studies, representation learning is employed and frequently achieves high accuracy for distraction detection [4–7]. In some of these deep learning-based systems, RGB images are collected through cameras facing drivers and classified by convolutional neural networks (CNN) according to drivers' body poses. In the system proposed in [8], a CNN detects the positions of phones in RGB images then infers whether drivers are distracted based on the positions of the phones with respect to the drivers' heads.

One major drawback for most computer vision-based existing methods is that they only work during daytime since they require RGB images as inputs for classification or phone detection. However, luminance condition at night limits the collection of RGB images. One system that addresses distraction detection but does not rely on visible light is in [9]. This system works on Near Infrared (NIR) images; after the localization of a driver's face in an image, features from image patches around his/her ears are extracted for image classification. Inspired by this work, we propose to detect drivers' distraction at nighttime based on in-vehicle NIR images of drivers' side views.

In this paper, we explore a driver distraction detection system that works at both daytime and nighttime by two modes, respectively. To the best of our knowledge, this is the first work on an end-to-end method for driver distraction detection at nighttime. In each mode, a camera collects corresponding images and sends them to a CNN for classification. A light sensor in this system detects the light condition in the vehicle and enables this system to switch between two modes when necessary. More than just detecting whether a driver is distracted, the proposed system also detects the distraction activity that driver is performing for further more targeted assistance or alerts. We evaluate our approach on an image data set of distracted driving collected in a simulator environment with different drivers. Three distraction activities are included in this data set: talking on a cell phone, texting on a cell phone, and interacting with a (Global Positioning System) GPS device [10]. We demonstrate that the proposed system detects driver distraction with a high performance on both modes, 95.98% of images of daytime are classified correctly while 92.24% of images of nighttime are classified correctly.

The rest of this paper is organized as follows. The proposed approach is detailed in Sect. 2. In Sect. 3, a description of our data set, experimental setup and fine-tuning approaches are described. Analysis of our results is in Sect. 4 and finally the conclusion is presented in Sect. 5.

2 Proposed Approach

To handle distraction detection in both daytime and nighttime, we propose using two detection modes: an RGB mode and an NIR mode. The RGB mode is activated in daytime and uses images collected from an RGB camera to identify distraction. The NIR mode, on the other hand, is activated in nighttime and uses an NIR camera. In each mode, the system identifies distraction by passing the images captured from the camera to a CNN classifier. To know which mode to activate at any given time, the system uses a light sensor to estimate the in-vehicle luminance. If the luminance is above a certain threshold, the RGB mode is triggered. Otherwise, the NIR mode is activated. Figure 1 shows a schematic of the proposed system.

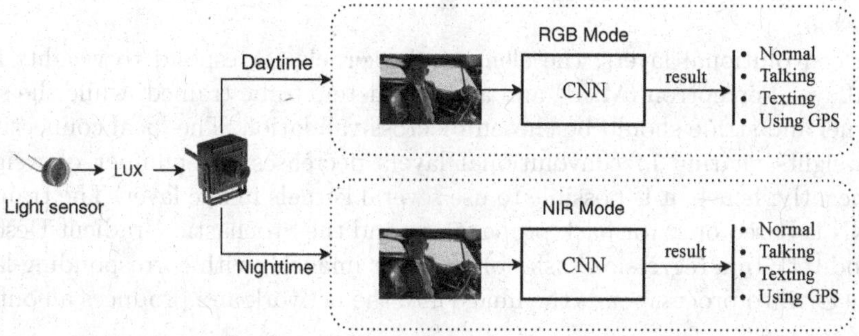

Fig. 1. A schematic representation of the proposed system.

We approach driver distraction detection as a 4-class classification problem, one class for "normal driving" and 3 classes for various distraction activities. The detection system receives an image I_i at every time stamp i then classifies it according to the driver body pose in it, and results in a probability distribution

$$Act_i = [Act_{i1},\ Act_{i2},\ \ldots,\ Act_{i4}], \tag{1}$$

where Act_{ij} represents the probability that at time point i the driver is performing a distraction activity j. Moreover, $\sum_{j=1}^{4} Act_{ij} = 1$ since Act_i is a probability distribution. In other words, the classifier models the conditional probability

$$Act_{ij} = P(Act_j | I_i). \tag{2}$$

Our system employs end-to-end CNNs as image classifiers. There are usually four kinds of layers in a CNN: input layers, convolutional layers, pooling layers, and fully connected layers. An input layer is an image I_i (charactered by its height and width) with several channels, and in some literature, the number of channels is also referred to as the depth. The first convolutional layer implements a convolution operation on the image with a convolution kernel of size $height \times width \times depth$. During the forward pass computation, the network convolves each kernel across the input image and computes dot products between elements of the kernel and the input patch at every position. Here the kernel is a 3-dimensional tensor, and the dot product is calculated on all input channels. The result of convolution operations with one kernel is a 2-dimensional feature map that gives the responses of that kernel at every spatial position. The resulting feature map should pass a nonlinear activation layer to form a nonlinear activation map.

With several different kernels, the convolutional layer will produce several different feature maps. Then, in next layer, these feature maps are stacked and treated as channels in input images. After a nonlinear activation layer, there is usually a pooling layer which aims at reducing the dimensions of the feature map. Two common pooling layers are the max-pooling layer and the average-pooling layer. After a stack of several convolutional layers and pooling layers, there are several fully connected layers which achieve the final classification or regression.

In convolutional layers, the elements in kernels correspond to weights in a MultiLayer Perceptron (MLP) and are parameters to be trained, while the sizes of kernel and stride should be chosen by cross-validation. The local connectivity and weights sharing in convolutional layers decreases the number of weights significantly; hence, it is possible to use several kernels in one layer. The training of CNN is based on error back propagation and the Stochastic Gradient Descent method [11]. In a regression task, for an input image I_i with corresponding label $\hat{y}_i$, the forward process sends the image into the network and produces an output

$$y_i = f_\Theta(I_i), \tag{3}$$

where f is the function implemented by the network, and Θ denotes its parameter set. A error function will measure the difference between the ground truth label $\hat{y}_i$ and the output y_i, and a popular error function is the mean squared error over N samples

$$error = \frac{1}{N}\sum_{i=1}^{N}(\hat{y}_i - y_i)^2. \tag{4}$$

Using the chain rule in error back propagation, the gradient of the error to each weight $\frac{\partial error}{\partial \Theta}$ can be calculated. The weight update process performs the following iteration

$$\Theta_t = \Theta_{t-1} - \eta\frac{\partial error}{\partial \Theta}, \tag{5}$$

where η is the step length in the Stochastic Gradient Descent. For a classification task, we can form a label as a one-hot vector in which every element represents the probability that the image belongs to that class.

3 Data Collection and Experimental Setup

In this section, we describe the data collection process and present the experimental setup to evaluate the performance of the proposed system.

3.1 Data Collection

To evaluate the proposed system, we collected an image data set of several distraction activities in a driving simulator. A camera is located at the right frontal side of drivers to capture a complete view of drivers' upper body movements.

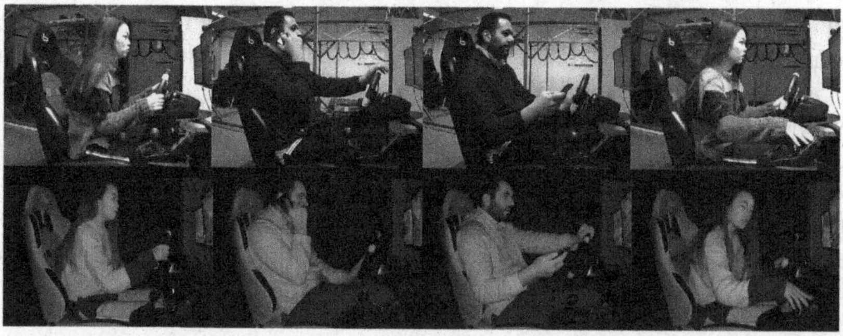

Fig. 2. Images sample from a simulator environment. The first row shows images taken at daytime, the second row shows images taken at nighttime. The first column represents images of normal driving, and the rest columns represent talking, texting, and programming GPS while driving, respectively.

Images were collected on 14 participants of different ages, genders, and ethnicities. Before experiments, each participant was asked to drive the simulator for a short time to get familiar with the experimental environment. Then, each driver was instructed to perform the following driving activities: normal/safe driving, driving while typing messages with his/her right hand, driving while talking on a cell phone, and driving while operating a device near the gear stick of the simulator to mimic programming a GPS device. Images were extracted from a video stream of 5 frames per second. With this low frame rate, images of adjacent time stamps present different body poses. Figure 2 gives some sample images of different activities. The number of images for each class is given in Table 1.

Table 1. Number of samples in image data sets.

Class	Daytime	Nighttime
Normal driving	2800	2800
Talking while driving	5513	5600
Texting while driving	5600	5570
Operating GPS while driving	2800	2800

3.2 Experimental Settings

The kernal part of this work is to train CNN classifiers for detection, and we explored and compared several CNNs that were proposed for Imagenet competition [12]. Since a potential future direction is to deploy this system on a small portable computing platform, we selected four CNNs (ResNet18, ResNet34, ResNet50, and SqueezeNet) with relatively small sizes but powerful representation abilities. The last fully connected layer in the original ResNet models was replaced by two fully connected layers of 128 and 4 nodes, respectively. We also added a dropout layer between feature extraction layers and fully connected layers to reduce overfitting. For the SqueezeNet model, we added these three new layers after the last pooling layer.

All models that were pretrained on ImageNet dataset were retrained with an Adam optimizer with a learning rate of 1e-4 and a batch size of 32 [13]. Each model was trained on images of 10 drivers and tested on the other 4 drivers, we run these experiments with 10 different random driver combinations and report average values in the results. The performances of all models are measured based on their classification accuracy.

4 Results and Analysis

4.1 Experimental Results for Both Modes

Table 2 shows the performances achieved by different models under different modes. The sizes of models are also shown in this table.

Table 2. Testing accuracy of 4 different models.

Models	Params (MB)	Mode	
		RGBM	NIRM
SqueezeNet	5	83.05 ± 5.66	77.21 ± 6.97
ResNet18	45	92.37 ± 6.10	92.24 ± 4.42
ResNet34	83	95.98 ± 3.64	90.33 ± 5.27
ResNet50	98	94.43 ± 4.55	90.36 ± 3.73

As can been seen in the third column, SqueezeNet achieves an accuracy of 83.05% on RGB Mode with a model size of 5 MB while ResNet18, which has a more sophisticated structure and a large model size, achieves an accuracy of 92.37% on RGB Mode. As the model size increases to 83 MB, ResNet34 gives an accuracy of 95.98%. However, a further increment of model size does not always lead to a better performance, as the accuracy by ResNet50 is 1.55% less than the one by ResNet34 on the RGB Mode.

The confusion matrices of testing results on RGB Mode by SqueezeNet and ResNet34 are shown in Fig. 3. In testing results for SqueezeNet, many samples of normal driving and driving while texting are mis-classified as driving while talking, and the class of driving while talking has the best accuracy. In testing results by ResNet34, detecting driving while texting is the most difficult task, and more than half of mis-classified samples are classified as talking, as body positions in images of these two classes are similar to each other.

Even in day time, the luminance of in-vehicle environments varies frequently on different time and weather conditions. To explore the performance of the detection system (trained on images from similar luminance conditions) under

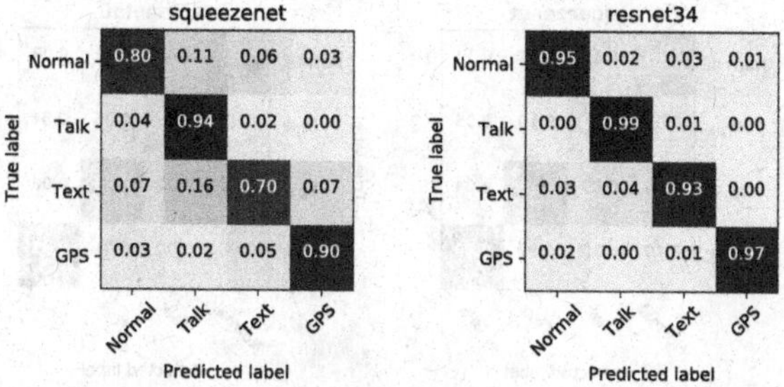

Fig. 3. Confusion matrix of testing results by SqueezeNet and ResNet34 model on RGB Mode.

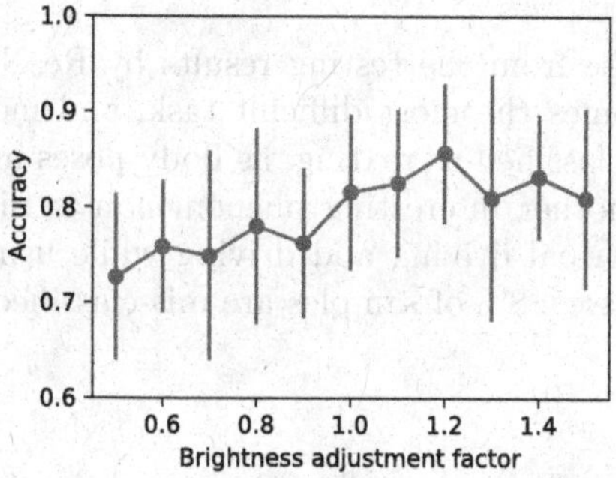

Fig. 4. Testing performances with different brightness adjustment factors.

changing luminance conditions, we adjust the brightness of testing images to simulate different luminance conditions. Figure 4 presents testing performances with different brightness adjustment factors. A brightness adjustment factor of 1 means images are not changed, while a factor that is larger than 1 means the brightness of images is increased. There is a clear trend that, if the brightness of images is increased, the system can maintain its performance and the testing accuracy fluctuates around the one achieved on not adjusted images. On the other side, if images are changed to dark, the performance drops obviously and darker images lead to worse accuracy (from 0.8156 by a brightness adjustment factor of 1 to 0.7268 by a brightness adjustment factor of 0.5). These results show that, the limitation that image data are collected under the same luminance hinders the system from generalizing to different brightness conditions and further work is required to mitigate this negative effect.

The forth column of Table 2 shows that, on NIR Mode, SqueezeNet achieves the worst accuracy while ResNet18 achieves the best accuracy which is 92.24%. Large models do not lead to better testing performance under night mode. The confusion matrices of testing results on NIR Mode by SqueezeNet and ResNet50 are shown in Fig. 5. In testing results by SqueezeNet, like on RGB Mode, many samples of normal driving and driving while texting are mis-classified as driving while talking, and the class of driving while talking has the best accuracy.

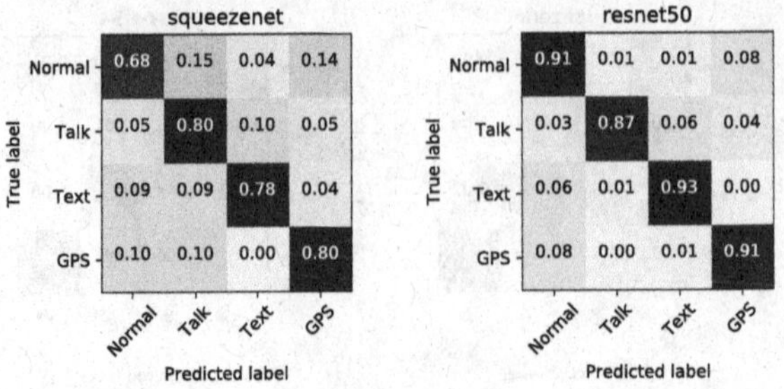

Fig. 5. Confusion matrix of testing results by SqueezeNet and ResNet50 model on NIR Mode.

By contrast, we can see from the testing results by ResNet50, detecting driving while talking becomes the most difficult task, and more than half of mis-classified samples are classified as texting, as body poses in images of these two classes are similar. Another interesting phenomenon is that the proportion of mis-classification of normal driving and driving while using GPS is the same. Moreover, for both classes, 8% of samples are mis-classified.

4.2 Discussion

These results show that, for both modes, the accuracy achieved by SqueezeNet is not enough for a real-time distraction detection. Using ResNet, on the other hand, we achieved a high accuracy of 90%. However, in terms of computational complexity, the speed of inferences by SqueezeNet (with the smallest model size) on Raspberry Pi is about 1 frame per second. This speed is insufficient for the design of an adequate real-time detection system. Thus, all these models are not suitable to be deployed on embedded processors, such as Raspberry Pi. The future work will tackle two aspects: improving accuracy and improving inference speed. The results in this work have shown that these two objectives cannot be achieved simultaneously. One promising direction is to design a better CNN structure that is specific for driver distraction detection.

5 Conclusion

In this paper, we proposed a driver distraction detection system which works at both daytime and nighttime. Several adjusted versions of well-known image classification networks are trained. The testing results show that the proposed system classifies images on nighttime mode with an accuracy of 92.24% and classifies images on daytime mode with an accuracy of 95.98%. We also explored the possibility of deploying deep learning models on small computing platforms and found that developing a specific network structure with a small model size (but with a better representation ability) is critical for a real-time distraction detection system. Moreover, for both modes, more work should be focused towards identifying the differences between talking and texting while driving.

References

1. Dinges, D.F., Perclos, R.G.: A valid psychophysiological measure of alertness as assessed by psychomotor vigilance. US Department of Transportation, Federal Highway Administration, Publication Number FHWA-MCRT-98-006 (1998)
2. Damousis, I.G., Tzovaras, D.: Fuzzy fusion of eyelid activity indicators for hypovigilance-related accident prediction. IEEE Trans. Intell. Transp. Syst. **9**(3), 491–500 (2008)
3. Smith, P., Shah, M., da Vitoria Lobo, N.: Determining driver visual attention with one camera. IEEE Trans. Intell. Transp. Syst. **4**(4), 205–218 (2003)
4. Hssayeni, M.D., Saxena, S., Ptucha, R., Savakis, A.: Distracted driver detection: deep learning vs handcrafted features. Electron. Imaging **2017**(10), 20–26 (2017)
5. Koesdwiady, A., Bedawi, S.M., Ou, C., Karray, F.: End-to-end deep learning for driver distraction recognition. In: Karray, F., Campilho, A., Cheriet, F. (eds.) ICIAR 2017. LNCS, vol. 10317, pp. 11–18. Springer, Cham (2017). https://doi.org/10.1007/978-3-319-59876-5_2
6. Ou, C., Ouali, C., Bedawi, S.M., Karray, F.: Driver behavior monitoring using tools of deep learning and fuzzy inferencing. In: IEEE International Conference on Fuzzy Systems, pp. 1–7 (2018)
7. Ou, C., Ouali, C., Karray, F.: Transfer learning based strategy for improving driver distraction recognition. In: Campilho, A., Karray, F., ter Haar Romeny, B. (eds.) ICIAR 2018. LNCS, vol. 10882, pp. 443–452. Springer, Cham (2018). https://doi.org/10.1007/978-3-319-93000-8_50
8. Ngan Le, T.H., Zheng, Y., Zhu, C., Luu, K., Savvides, M.: Multiple scale faster-RCNN approach to driver's cell-phone usage and hands on steering wheel detection. In: IEEE Conference on Computer Vision and Pattern Recognition Workshops, pp. 46–53 (2016)
9. Artan, Y., Bulan, O., Loce, R.P., Paul, P.: Driver cell phone usage detection from HOV/HOT NIR images. In: IEEE Conference on Computer Vision and Pattern Recognition Workshops, pp. 225–230 (2014)
10. What counts as distracted driving. https://www.ontario.ca/page/distracted-driving. Accessed at 3 Dec 2019
11. LeCun, Y., Bengio, Y., Hinton, G.: Deep learning. Nature **521**(7553), 436–444 (2015)
12. Deng, J., Dong, W., Socher, R., Li, L.-J., Li, K., Li, F.-F.: A large-scale hierarchical image database, Imagenet (2009)
13. Kingma, D.P., Ba, J.: Adam: a method for stochastic optimization. arXiv preprint. arXiv:1412.6980 (2014)

Key-Track: A Lightweight Scalable LSTM-based Pedestrian Tracker for Surveillance Systems

Pratik Kulkarni(✉), Shrey Mohan, Samuel Rogers, and Hamed Tabkhi

University of North Carolina at Charlotte, Charlotte, USA
pkulkar7@uncc.edu

Abstract. There has been a growing interest in leveraging state of the art deep learning techniques for tracking objects in recent years. Most of this work focuses on using redundant appearance models for predicting object tracklets for the next frame. Moreover, not much work has been done to explore the sequence learning properties of Long Short Term Memory (LSTM) Neural Networks for object tracking in video sequences. In this work we propose a novel LSTM tracker, Key-Track, which effectively learns the spatial and temporal behavior of pedestrians after analyzing movement patterns of human key-points provided to it by OpenPose [3]. We train Key-Track on single person sequences that we curated from the Duke Multi-target Multi-Camera (Duke-MTMC) [26] dataset and scale it to track multiple people at run-time, further testing its scalability. We report our results on the Duke-MTMC dataset for different time-series sequence lengths we feed to Key-Track and find three as the optimum time-step sequence length producing the highest Average Overlap Score (AOS). We further present our qualitative analysis on these different time-series sequence lengths producing different results depending on the type of video sequence. The total observed size of Key-Track is under 1 megabytes which paves its way into mobile devices for the purpose of tracking in real-time.

Keywords: LSTM · OpenPose · Multi-object tracking

1 Introduction

Visual object tracking poses an interesting challenge in the Computer Vision community. It is commonly required in domains like autonomous vehicles [2,13], surveillance systems, and robot navigation. Object tracking is broadly performed either as detection-free tracking (DFT) or detection-based tracking (DBT) [17]. Real-world scenarios are often comprised of challenging characteristics such as occlusion, illumination variation, target deformation, and background clutter

This research was supported by the National Science Foundation (NSF) under Award No. 1831795.

F. Karray et al. (Eds.): ICIAR 2019, LNCS 11663, pp. 208–219, 2019.
https://doi.org/10.1007/978-3-030-27272-2_18

[22]. To improve robustness against these types of scenarios trackers have recently adopted many of the deep learning techniques used in other vision tasks such as object detection and classification [6] where they achieve human-like or even beyond-human accuracy in their respective domain [29], albeit at high computational cost. When working on a domain with real-time constraints, such as surveillance or autonomous driving, it is necessary to balance these computational loads with real-time constraints. Unfortunately many of the deep trackers evaluated on the MOT benchmark [20] and other multi-object benchmarks are unable to achieve real-time throughput (FPS) and latency due to their reliance on large Convolution neural networks (CNNs) [1]. More recent works have begun to explore hybrid networks that combine CNNs with recurrent elements such as LSTM and GRU cells to reduce computational overhead and improve performance [5,12,22].

With the growing interest in deep learning, more recent works like [4,10,11,14] use Convolution Neural Network (CNN) based appearance model to track objects. The task of tracking inherently has a strong temporal component, which is very costly to implement in CNNs. This has prompted interest in other solutions using recurrent neural networks (RNN). Some works like [9,10,22,28] use Long Short Term Memory (LSTM) but overload them with unnecessary background noise, increasing model complexity without significantly improving accuracy. These shortcomings have prompted us to explore more compact feature representations that prioritize the spatio-temporal characteristics of tracking targets. In this work we focus specifically on pose keypoints as a means of understanding and predicting the movement of human targets over time.

We propose a hybrid tracking by detection framework Key-Track, that employs OpenPose (explained in Sect. 3.1) for human key-point detection and an LSTM for future frame prediction in surveillance systems. The key idea here is to use only prominent human key-points instead of the whole appearance model to understand movement behaviors and patterns in humans using LSTM. We do this by training our LSTM model on different kinds of movement patterns individually (single object) and then scale it to multiple objects at run time with the help of batching. Our results show that our model scales well as we only use key-point information for predictions, improving the scalability of the system as the number of tracking targets increases. Furthermore the LSTM layer can be trained on single target examples, but evaluated on multi-object scenarios of varying complexity simply by batching. We achieve this training and evaluation paradigm via the following contributions:

- Training on single object and testing on multiple objects by scaling the LSTM with effective batching
- Curation of a single-object dataset for training by introducing a Data wrangling technique and associating keypoint/feature information per object to their ground truth
- Lightweight tracker model less than a size of 1 MB capable for deployment over edge

2 Related Work

In this section we will discuss some prior work done using LSTMs for tracking and some other applications.

2.1 LSTM for Tracking

Early works in object tracking, such as [25], relied on Kalman Filters to try and stabilise predictions of object movement but they are not very reliable as they do not account for any historic patterns for their predictions.Some early works that incorporated LSTM for application in tracking like [19] demonstrate promising results. Works like [7] also confirms their effectiveness in understanding patterns in data. Recently, works like [4,22] employed LSTM for the purpose of tracking. [22] uses the YOLOv1 object detection framework for generating labeled bounding boxes as well as a reduce image feature map of 4096 $\times$ 1 features. These 4k features are appended to the bounding box dimensions and passed to an LSTM layer for predicting the position of the bounding in future frames. The large feature map is necessary for providing context about the object beyond its mere position and scale, but also contains a large amount of irrelevant features that increase computational overhead while also degrading overall tracker accuracy. A similar work [28] uses a 500-dimensional feature vector with VGG-16 as the feature detector rendering merely 1 Hz of FPS. Another method uses an online object tracking strategy [21] that implements LSTM inspired from Bayesian Filtering idea which makes data association, state updates and initiation and termination of tracks and train their model on a synthetic dataset. The authors end up with a model which learns to track and gives good real time performance on the expense of accuracy. Furthermore, another Detection based tracking approach [9] uses Faster RCNN in the backend as an object detector along with an RNN for tacking the targets. The RNN is less capable of addressing the long-term dependencies in lengthy video sequences. Further, the work focuses on a single object tracking mechanism rather than a Multi-object.

2.2 LSTM for Pattern Recognition

Recent works like [15,24] have demonstrated the effectiveness of LSTMs on understanding patterns from unstructured data. Authors in [16] employed LSTMs for understanding texts and putting it to semantic context. On similar lines in [31] the authors improved the character recognition properties of CNNs by adding a recurrent layer in their model structure. Similarly in [23] LSTMs were used to predict end points in the Chinese language. Authors in [18] used LSTMs to model human motion detection to predict time dependent motion representation for human poses. All these aforementioned developments signify the importance to explore the role of LSTMs in understanding human behavior and leverage its pattern recognition properties.

3 Background

In this section we are going to briefly discuss the front-end detection framework and the dataset we used.

3.1 OpenPose Framework

Human pose estimation frameworks can also be effectively used as human (pedestrian) detectors in applications such as pedestrian tracking. One such framework is OpenPose [3] which provides fast, accurate pose estimations that scales independently of the number of poses to estimate in a scene. It is more capable of realizing real-time performance when compared to other pose estimation frameworks. It is built upon the VGG-19 classification network [30] and convolution blocks to calculate predict body keypoints and their part affinity fields (PAF) in order to generate a pose estimate. To overcome associating maps of different people among one another, the PAFs preserve both location and orientation information across the region of support of the limb. The authors in [3] demonstrate their state of the art results on the recent key-point detection datasets. We leverage the robust spatio-temporal information encapsulated in the keypoints and PAFs as inputs to our tracking model.

3.2 Duke Dataset (DukeMTMC)

Ergys et al. [26] introduce a new large scale dataset (possibly the largest) for multi-object tracking in multiple cameras called Duke-MTMC. Figure 1 shows the 8 camera angles from the dataset and the environment settings. It has 2834 different people annotated across 8 different cameras with total video footage of 1 h 25 min per camera recorded at about 60 frames per second (FPS) inside the Duke University Campus between lectures when the foot traffic is expected to be the highest. The camera resolution is high (1080p) with a total of about 2 million frames which have around 1800 self occlusion scenarios and semi-automatically generated object bounding boxes. People carry different kinds of accessories like backpacks, umbrellas, bags and bicycles. The movements are also irregular, some abrupt, slow, non-linear posing many challenges to the tracking algorithm. Such properties emulate perfect real world surveillance scenarios that we want for our model testing.

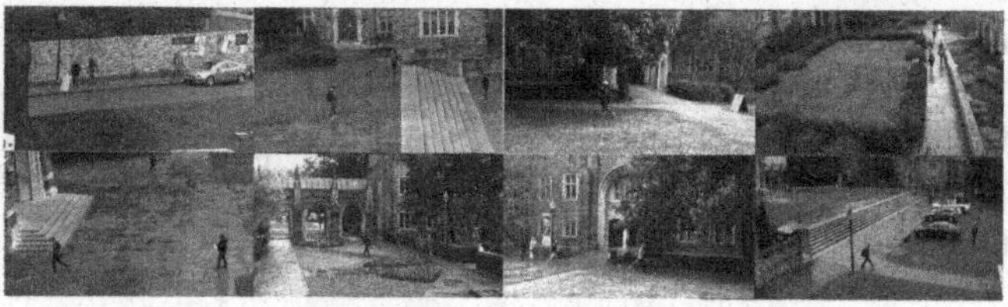

Fig. 1. Eight different camera angles from the dataset

4 Approach

In the following section, first we introduce our system architecture and its components,then we talk about the training method followed by the Data wrangling technique for dataset curation. Finally we talk about the scalabilty aspect of LSTM and Multi-Object tracking.

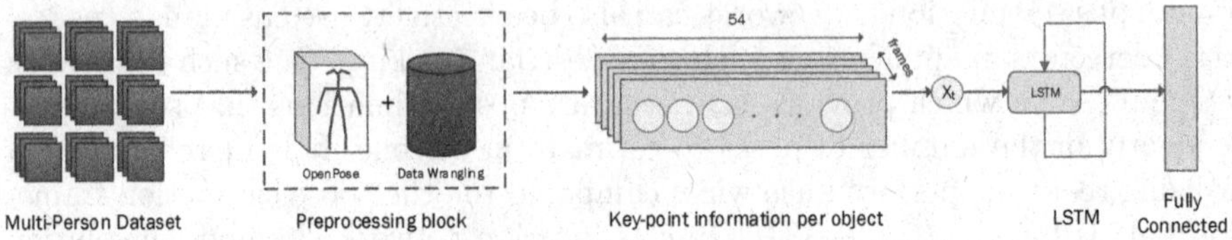

Fig. 2. Overview of the system architecture pipeline depicting blocks and flow of data

4.1 Architecture

Our framework, like DeepCC [27], starts with detection generated in the form of person keypoints through OpenPose [3]. A pre-processing framework, shown in Fig. 2 and described below in Sect. 4.2, re-identifies and isolates the keypoints for individual tracking targets. These keypoints, consisting of the the X and Y coordinates as well as confidence for 18 different body parts are then aggregated across frames and passed into a LSTM as seen in Fig. 2. The LSTM layer then uses these keypoints from frames N to $N + timesteps$ to predict the keypoint values for the next frame. This prediction is then passed to a fully connected which transforms the predicted keypoints to a bounding box prediction. The advantage of basing an LSTM tracking system on keypoint detections is that they provide ample context about an object that can be used to understand its motion, while also keeping the overall model size down. Whereas other works like ROLO and Re3 [12] utilize deep features to represent the spatial context of an a object resulting in large model sizes (100 MB+) and training times, our trained LSTM model can achieve comparable performance with a much smaller model (<1 MB).

4.2 Data Preprocessing

Scenes in the Duke MTMC [26] dataset generally contain multiple tracking targets in any given frame. Since the scope of our work is to improve the back-end tracking of these objects, we utilize data wrangling techniques to isolate individuals and their keypoints within the camera sequences. To achieve this we localise the object present in the frame by matching the object's keypoints generated by OpenPose framework to the ground truth provided by the dataset. The data wrangling technique can generate nearly 2700 individual object sequences (the maximum objects present in the dataset) improving model generalization.

For the purpose of evaluation on the Duke MTMC dataset we choose a starting frame from the labeled dataset and an end frame to prepare a continuous video sequence. Every new object appearing in the scene is assigned its own index in the 3D tensor (Fig. 4) with its respective keypoint-feature vector for that image frame. This is necessary to maintain its trajectory and movement properties in the subsequent frames. If an object moves out of the screen, the rest of the sequence is padded with zeros. Similarly the entire index is padded with zeros to denote no object is present or if the object is yet to enter the scene. Hence, we try to maintain exclusivity for however many objects enter or exit throughout the sequences.

4.3 Training Method

We use the OpenPose [3] detection for each object in each frame. A 54-dimensional feature vector consisting of keypoint positions and confidences is then fed to the LSTM. The keypoints are pixel values and represent different parts of the body of the person. Keypoints are of the format (x1, y1, c1, ..., x18, y18, c18) where x and y denote the location of the keypoint with respect to the image and c denotes confidence of the detection. These keypoints are then fed to the LSTM cell at every time step. As seen in Fig. 3, the vector is fed at each time step and the prediction for the final time step is then mapped to (x, y, w, h) using a fully connected layer. The fully connected layer behaves like a decoder where x, y denote centroid of the object and w and h denote the height and width of bounding box. Training on the centroid makes the input to the LSTM less susceptible to abrupt bounding box changes. The LSTM is trained on root mean square error where B refers to the bounding box values (x, y, w, h)

$$L_{MSE} = 1/n \sum_{i=1}^{n} ||B_{target} - B_{pred}||^2 \tag{1}$$

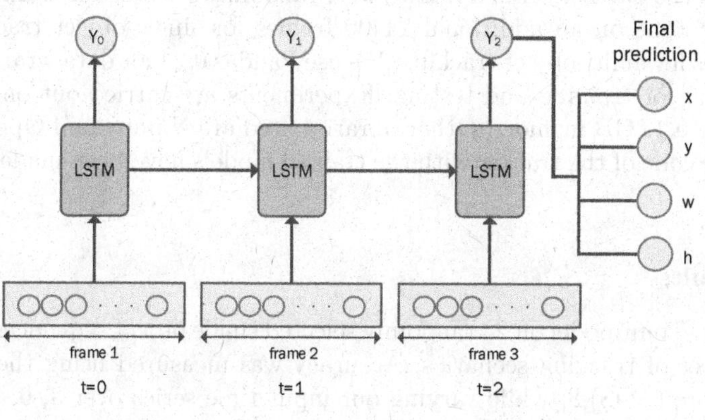

Fig. 3. Training instance for a single iteration

4.4 Scalability

We are able to scale our trained model to run inference on multi-object scenarios with an arbitrary number of targets via batching. Batching in the deep learning context functions in a similar fashion to SIMT operation, in that each data lane in the batch shares the same set of weights and operations, but is otherwise independent of the other inferences. In this way, we can train our model on a single object, and dynamically scale the number of objects we are tracking by dynamically adjusting the batch size of inference. Figure 4 shows the shape of the tensor we feed to the LSTM layer. By carefully observing the scene we adjust the maximum batch size depending on maximum objects to be tracked.

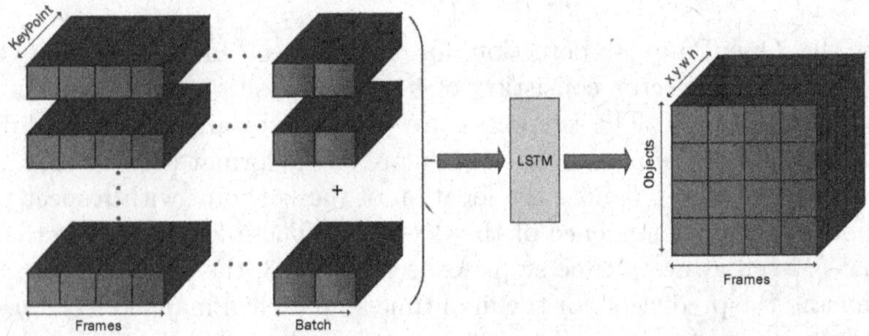

Fig. 4. The figure shows the scalability aspect of the approach. The input tensor is of shape [objects, numframes, features] while the output is [objects, frames, boundingbox]

5 Experimental Setup

The dataset we used consists of a total of 64 video sequences curated from the Data Wrangling technique explained in Sect. 4.2. Of the over 5 million frames available in the dataset, 41,268 frames were randomly selected for training. Evaluation was done on an additional 14400 frames for single-object tracking and 3600 frames for multi-object tracking. We use Pandas 0.24 for data wrangling and PyTorch 1.0 for training and testing. Experiments are carried out on NVIDIA Titan V with 12 GB memory. Other libraries used are Numpy and OpenCV 4.0. The source code of the tracker with the trained models have been made available online.[1]

5.1 Results

We evaluated our model on 24 randomly selected single object sequences covering a diverse set of tracking scenarios. Accuracy was measured using the Average overlap score (AOS)[8] while varying our input time series over 3, 6, 8, and 10 input frames, per iteration. The AOS can be calculated using the Intersection

[1] Project page: https://github.com/TeCSAR-UNCC/key-track.

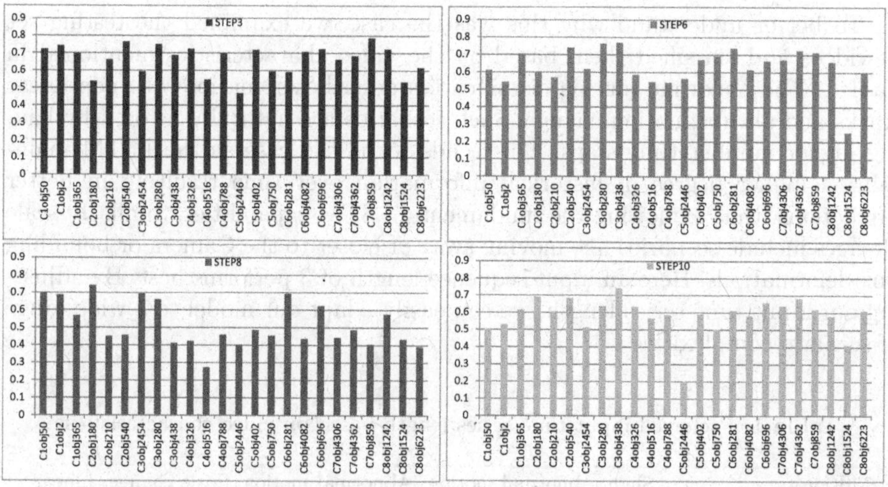

Fig. 5. Step comparison and average overlap score per sequence (C:CameraID, Obj:ObjectID)

over Union (IoU) method. It is a ratio of the area of overlap between the predicted bounding box and the ground-truth bounding box and the area of union. An IoU score of 50% or more is considered a successful detection. Figure 5 shows that a 3-step input series performed the best, with a 78% overlap of the predicted bounding box with the ground truth box. Figure 6(a) shows the impact of input sequence length on AOS *averaged over all 24 sequences.* We found that there was only a weak correlation between the length of the input time series and the resulting accuracy.

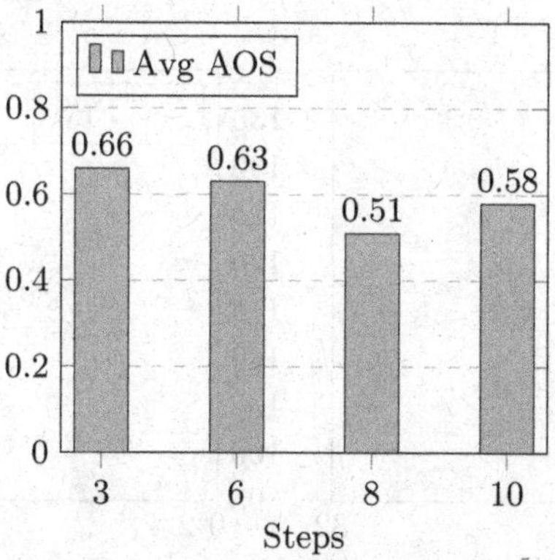

Fig. 6. Step comparison with average AOS in single-object sequences

To better understand why this was the case, we examined the testing set of videos and classified them based on the video characteristics mentioned in Table 1. The abnormal motion classification describes scenarios with non-linear tracks and abrupt motion change. Such scenarios are naturally favored by having higher number time steps. This tends to be the case as the LSTM maintains a higher degree of historical information over time resulting in better predictions, thus exploiting the fundamental LSTM capabilities. Similarly scale changes include scenarios like moving away or closer to the Camera or bounding box deformations. Here an input sequence length of 3 performs best. By adjusting our input time series length, we can easily adapt our model to a wide range of scenario complexities.

Table 1. Preferred input time series length based on video characteristics

Motion type	Slight abnormal motion	Abnormal motion	Scale change	Linear
Time-steps	3	6,8	3	6
Number of sequences	13	4	3	4

To evaluate our model on Multi-Object sequences, we employed a technique using data wrangling to study and report different metrics for Scalability. We curated an entirely new test set of 32 single object sequences and concatenated these sequences to simulate a scene with 32 objects per frame. This allowed us to test the effect of scaling on inference time. As shown in Fig. 7(a) we vary batch size, corresponding to the number of objects present in scene. Here we considered a sequence of 2343 frames. It can be seen from the graph that an exponential increase in batch size has linear effect on inference time making the model robust to any scale.

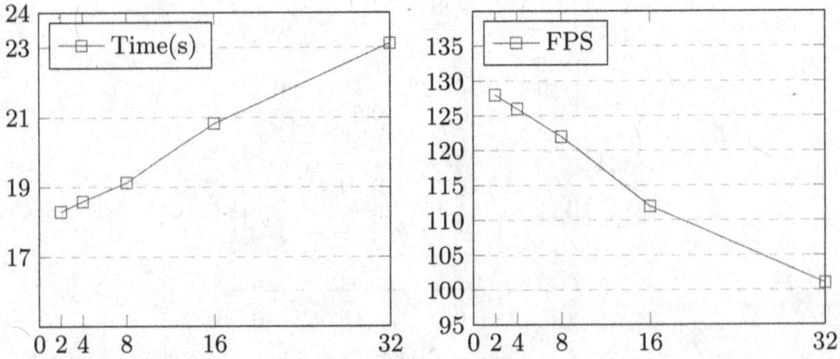

(a) Number of Objects vs Time (b) Number of Objects vs FPS

Fig. 7. Scalability test showing the effect of varying objects in scene with respect to inference time and frame rate

A similar comparison was done to test the throughput in terms of FPS. As shown in Fig. 7(b), the FPS decreases to certain extent as computation increases, still keeping the overall FPS for offline tracking comparatively high and stable. The number of objects in a scene has no impact on the accuracy of our tracker, since all objects are tracked individually, and simply batched as inputs to the tracker.

6 Conclusion and Future Work

This work presents a novel approach for Multi-object tracking for Surveillance cameras without compromising much on throughput and maintaining the accuracy of detections irrespective of the number of objects to be tracked, showcasing the pattern learning property of LSTM for object tracking. Sequences with varying complexities were successfully tracked using different time-steps. We do see further opportunities to enhance the performance of the system by predicting many more future frames for a better predictive analysis. This would essentially mean being detached from the heavily reliable detection framework and also could result in better tracking accuracy over long-term sequences. While we've succeeded in keeping the model size less than 1 MB, making it super lightweight, we envisage to deploy the system over edge for real time inference for various applications.

References

1. Bertinetto, L., Valmadre, J., Henriques, J.F., Vedaldi, A., Torr, P.H.S.: Fully-convolutional siamese networks for object tracking. CoRR abs/1606.09549 (2016). http://arxiv.org/abs/1606.09549
2. Bontemps, L., Cao, V.L., McDermott, J., Le-Khac, N.-A.: Collective anomaly detection based on long short-term memory recurrent neural networks. In: Dang, T.K., Wagner, R., Küng, J., Thoai, N., Takizawa, M., Neuhold, E. (eds.) FDSE 2016. LNCS, vol. 10018, pp. 141–152. Springer, Cham (2016). https://doi.org/10.1007/978-3-319-48057-2_9
3. Cao, Z., Hidalgo, G., Simon, T., Wei, S.E., Sheikh, Y.: OpenPose: realtime multi-person 2D pose estimation using part affinity fields. arXiv preprint. arXiv:1812.08008 (2018)
4. Chu, Q., Ouyang, W., Li, H., Wang, X., Liu, B., Yu, N.: Online multi-object tracking using cnn-based single object tracker with spatial-temporal attention mechanism. In: IEEE International Conference on Computer Vision, ICCV 2017, Venice, Italy, 22–29 October 2017, pp. 4846–4855 (2017). https://doi.org/10.1109/ICCV.2017.518
5. Cui, Z., Ke, R., Wang, Y.: Deep bidirectional and unidirectional LSTM recurrent neural network for network-wide traffic speed prediction. CoRR abs/1801.02143 (2018). http://arxiv.org/abs/1801.02143
6. Deng, J., Dong, W., Socher, R., Li, L.J., Li, K., Fei-Fei, L.: ImageNet: a large-scale hierarchical image database. In: CVPR09 (2009)

7. Dequaire, J., Ondruska, P., Rao, D., Wang, D.Z., Posner, I.: Deep tracking in the wild: end-to-end tracking using recurrent neural networks. Int. J. Robot. Res. **37**(4–5), 492–512 (2018). https://doi.org/10.1177/0278364917710543
8. Everingham, M., Van Gool, L., Williams, C.K., Winn, J., Zisserman, A.: The pascal visual object classes (VOC) challenge. Int. J. Comput. Vision **88**(2), 303–338 (2010)
9. Fang, K.: Track-RNN: joint detection and tracking using recurrent neural networks
10. Feichtenhofer, C., Pinz, A., Zisserman, A.: Detect to track and track to detect. In: IEEE International Conference on Computer Vision (2017)
11. Girdhar, R., Gkioxari, G., Torresani, L., Paluri, M., Tran, D.: Detect-and-track: efficient pose estimation in videos. In: 2018 IEEE/CVF Conference on Computer Vision and Pattern Recognition, pp. 350–359, June 2018. https://doi.org/10.1109/CVPR.2018.00044
12. Gordon, D., Farhadi, A., Fox, D.: Re3 : Real-time recurrent regression networks for object tracking. CoRR abs/1705.06368 (2017). http://arxiv.org/abs/1705.06368
13. Hochreiter, S., Schmidhuber, J.: Long short-term memory. Neural Comput. **9**(8), 1735–1780 (1997)
14. Kokul, T., Fookes, C., Sridharan, S., Ramanan, A., Pinidiyaarachchi, U.A.J.: Gate connected convolutional neural network for object tracking. In: 2017 IEEE International Conference on Image Processing (ICIP), pp. 2602–2606, September 2017. https://doi.org/10.1109/ICIP.2017.8296753
15. Lin, P., Mo, X., Lin, G., Ling, L., Wei, T., Luo, W.: A news-driven recurrent neural network for market volatility prediction. In: 2017 4th IAPR Asian Conference on Pattern Recognition (ACPR), pp. 776–781, November 2017. https://doi.org/10.1109/ACPR.2017.35
16. Liu, P., Qiu, X., Huang, X.: Recurrent neural network for text classification with multi-task learning. In: Proceedings of the Twenty-Fifth International Joint Conference on Artificial Intelligence, IJCAI 2016, New York, NY, USA, 9–15 July 2016, pp. 2873–2879 (2016). http://www.ijcai.org/Abstract/16/408
17. Luo, W., et al.: Multiple object tracking: a literature review. arXiv preprint. arXiv:1409.7618 (2014)
18. Martinez, J., Black, M.J., Romero, J.: On human motion prediction using recurrent neural networks. In: 2017 IEEE Conference on Computer Vision and Pattern Recognition (CVPR), pp. 4674–4683, July 2017. https://doi.org/10.1109/CVPR.2017.497
19. Masala, G.L., Golosio, B., Tistarelli, M., Grosso, E.: 2D recurrent neural networks for robust visual tracking of non-rigid bodies. In: Proceedings of Engineering Applications of Neural Networks - 17th International Conference, EANN 2016, Aberdeen, UK, 2–5 September 2016, pp. 18–34 (2016). https://doi.org/10.1007/978-3-319-44188-7_2
20. Milan, A., Leal-Taixé, L., Reid, I.D., Roth, S., Schindler, K.: MOT16: a benchmark for multi-object tracking. CoRR abs/1603.00831 (2016). http://arxiv.org/abs/1603.00831
21. Milan, A., Rezatofighi, S.H., Dick, A., Reid, I., Schindler, K.: Online multi-target tracking using recurrent neural networks. In: Thirty-First AAAI Conference on Artificial Intelligence (2017)
22. Ning, G., Zhang, Z., Huang, C., He, Z., Ren, X., Wang, H.: Spatially supervised recurrent convolutional neural networks for visual object tracking. CoRR abs/1607.05781 (2016). http://arxiv.org/abs/1607.05781
23. Oh, D.H., Shah, Z., Jang, G.: Line-break prediction of hanmun text using recurrent neural networks. In: 2017 International Conference on Information and Communi-

cation Technology Convergence (ICTC), pp. 720–724, Oct 2017. https://doi.org/10.1109/ICTC.2017.8190763
24. Ray, A., Rajeswar, S., Chaudhury, S.: Text recognition using deep BLSTM networks. In: 2015 Eighth International Conference on Advances in Pattern Recognition (ICAPR), pp. 1–6, January 2015. https://doi.org/10.1109/ICAPR.2015.7050699
25. Reid, D.: An algorithm for tracking multiple targets. IEEE Trans. Autom. Control **24**(6), 843–854 (1979)
26. Ristani, E., Solera, F., Zou, R., Cucchiara, R., Tomasi, C.: Performance measures and a data set for multi-target, multi-camera tracking. In: European Conference on Computer Vision Workshop on Benchmarking Multi-Target Tracking (2016)
27. Ristani, E., Tomasi, C.: Features for multi-target multi-camera tracking and re-identification. In: Conference on Computer Vision and Pattern Recognition (2018)
28. Sadeghian, A., Alahi, A., Savarese, S.: Tracking the untrackable: learning to track multiple cues with long-term dependencies. In: The IEEE International Conference on Computer Vision (ICCV), October 2017
29. Schulter, S., Vernaza, P., Choi, W., Chandraker, M.: Deep network flow for multi-object tracking. In: 2017 IEEE Conference on Computer Vision and Pattern Recognition (CVPR), pp. 2730–2739, July 2017. https://doi.org/10.1109/CVPR.2017.292
30. Simonyan, K., Zisserman, A.: Very deep convolutional networks for large-scale image recognition. In: International Conference on Learning Representations (2015)
31. Wang, Q., Huang, H.: Learning of recurrent convolutional neural networks with applications in pattern recognition. In: 2017 36th Chinese Control Conference (CCC), pp. 4135–4139, July 2017. https://doi.org/10.23919/ChiCC.2017.8028007

KPTransfer: Improved Performance and Faster Convergence from Keypoint Subset-Wise Domain Transfer in Human Pose Estimation

Kanav Vats(✉), Helmut Neher(✉), Alexander Wong(✉), David A. Clausi(✉), and John Zelek(✉)

Department of Systems Design Engineering, University of Waterloo, Waterloo, Canada
{k2vats,hneher,a28wong,dclausi,jzelek}@uwaterloo.ca

Abstract. In this paper, we present a novel approach called KPTransfer for improving modeling performance for keypoint detection deep neural networks via domain transfer between different keypoint subsets. This approach is motivated by the notion that rich contextual knowledge can be transferred between different keypoint subsets representing separate domains. In particular, the proposed method takes into account various keypoint subsets/domains by sequentially adding and removing keypoints. Contextual knowledge is transferred between two separate domains via domain transfer. Experiments to demonstrate the efficacy of the proposed KPTransfer approach were performed for the task of human pose estimation on the MPII dataset, with comparisons against random initialization and frozen weight extraction configurations. Experimental results demonstrate the efficacy of performing domain transfer between two different joint subsets resulting in a PCKh improvement of up to 1.1 over random initialization on joints such as wrists and knee in certain joint splits with an overall PCKh improvement of 0.5. Domain transfer from a different set of joints not only results in improved accuracy but also results in faster convergence because of mutual co-adaptations of weights resulting from the contextual knowledge of the pose from a different set of joints.

Keywords: Domain transfer · Pose estimation · Convolutional neural networks

1 Introduction

In any keypoint estimation problem, the location of a particular keypoint holds contextual information about the location of another. In pose estimation, for example, the position of the elbows and wrists are naturally constrained, being part of the same limb. Deep keypoint estimation algorithms take advantage of this fact by learning different keypoint locations simultaneously. For

F. Karray et al. (Eds.): ICIAR 2019, LNCS 11663, pp. 220–231, 2019.
https://doi.org/10.1007/978-3-030-27272-2_19

instance, deep pose estimation algorithms predict human joint locations together [3,14,17,22] or use a two-pipeline framework for body part detection and association [18,20]. However, domain transfer between keypoints remains an unexplored area. We hypothesize that domain transfer can be used for utilizing the contextual relationships between keypoint locations for improving convergence and generalization. Since a large number of keypoint detection datasets [1,13,15] are available which differ in keypoint location annotations, one obvious question arises: *Can domain transfer between separate keypoint sets help in improving generalization performance and convergence?*

In this paper, we introduce a novel approach termed KPTransfer for performing domain transfer between keypoint subsets representing separate domains. We apply our approach on the problem of 2D human pose estimation. However, our approach is completely task and model agnostic and can be used to evaluate domain transfer using any deep pose estimation model in any other keypoint detection problem such as facial landmark detection and 3D pose estimation. We use the stacked hourglass pose estimation network [17] to demonstrate that contextual cues can be transferred between different sets of human joints through transfer learning to improve convergence and performance.

We perform domain transfer with the help of transfer learning and compare it with frozen weights and random initialization settings. Concretely, for domain transfer, a pose estimation network is first trained on a subset of total joints, after which, a second, bigger network is trained on a different subset of joints, half of which is initialized by the weights of the previous network. Two more settings are investigated: random weight initialization and frozen weights. Random weight initialization is done by initializing **all** the weights of the second, bigger network randomly. In the frozen weights setting, the second, bigger network is trained after freezing/not updating the weights of the first network. The three settings are illustrated in Fig. 1. We compare the three settings with four different subset splits of human joints (Fig. 2) of the MPII dataset [1] and demonstrate that the transfer learning setting results in improved generalization performance and faster convergence.

The paper begins by detailing background information related to domain transfer, pose estimation, and the basis for our approach are discussed briefly in Sect. 2. The Methodology, Sect. 3, describes the pose estimation network employed for the experiments, the experimental settings and training details. The results and discussion forms Sect. 4 with Sect. 5 concluding the paper.

2 Background

Domain transfer utilizes information in one domain to help learn tasks in another domain. The two domains involved may represent separate datasets [7], classes in the same dataset [26] or different data modalities [9,11,28]. Effectiveness of domain transfer techniques has been tested in various problems like image classification [26], object detection [12] and semantic segmentation [5]. Transfer learning [26] and knowledge distillation [10,27] are two popular ways of performing domain transfer. Yosinki *et al.* [26] demonstrate that performing transfer learning

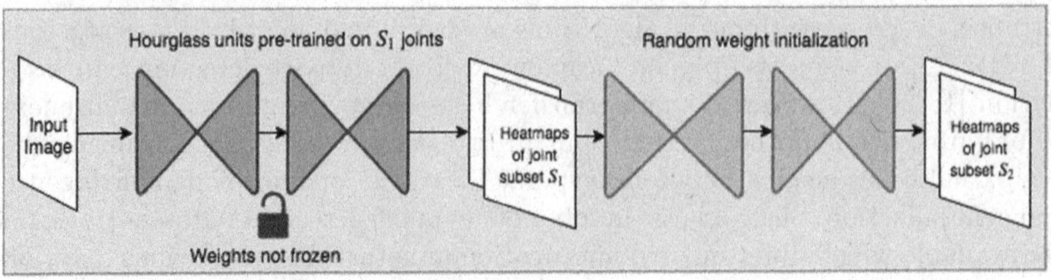

(a) Transfer learning

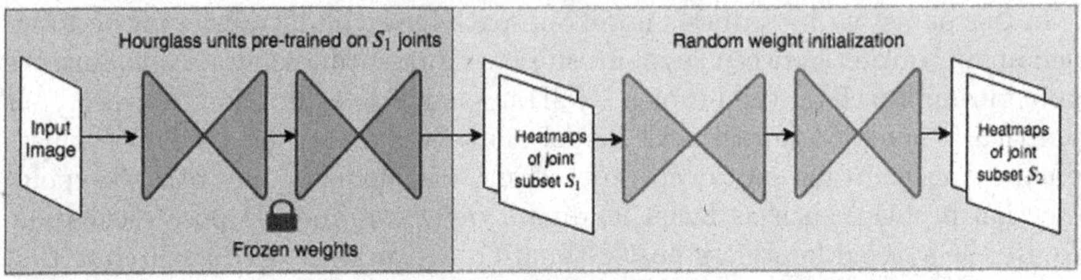

(b) Frozen weights

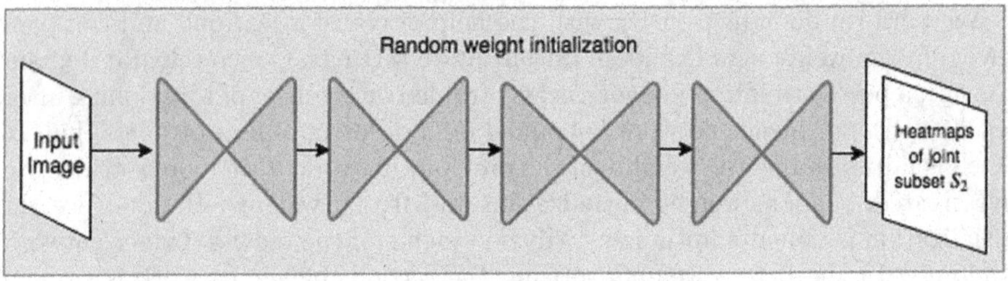

(c) Random initialization

Fig. 1. The figure shows the three experimental configurations used. (a) The transfer learning configuration wherein the two-stack hourglass trained on the subset S_1 of joints is used to transfer knowledge to the subset S_2 through transfer learning. (b) The frozen weights configuration which is similar to (a), the difference being that the weights of the two-stack hourglass trained on the subset S_1 of joints are frozen. (c) The random initialization configuration where four stacked hourglass units, initialized with random weights are trained on the subset S_2 of joints.

by initializing first n layers of a base network with weights learned on approximately half of Imagenet [8] classes with the remaining layers randomly initialized improves generalization performance on the other half of Imagenet classes. Hinton *et al.* [10] introduced knowledge distillation by producing soft probability distribution over targets by modifying the softmax function and introducing an objective function consisting of those soft targets to train a student network. Techniques such as using weight regularizers to make weights of source and target domain networks similar [19] and adversarial learning [16,24] are also employed for domain transfer.

With the advent of deep networks, there has been a significant progress in the field of human pose estimation. Toshev *et al.* [21] was among one of the earliest works incorporating deep neural networks (DNN) for pose estimation. Heatmap based pose estimation [3,6,17,22] is the most widely used pose estimation technique. In heatmap based methods, joint heatmaps, equal to the number of joint locations present in the images are generated. Each heatmap represents a two dimensional probability distribution where each heatmap pixel represents the probability with which a joint is present in a particular pixel location. Intermediate supervision is commonly used in heatmap based methods, wherein loss is calculated at subsequent stages of the pose estimation network to refine heatmap predictions. Regression based approaches [2,4,21] are also prevalent in human pose estimation literature, however, their limitation is that the regression function is often sub-optimal. The work presented in this paper makes use of a heatmap based approach [17].

Domain transfer between separate keypoints subsets in deep human pose estimation is an unexplored avenue. Multimodal pose transfer methods exist in pose estimation literature. Zhao *et al.* [28] predict human pose from RF signals by transferring visual knowledge from an RGB images based pose estimation model [3] in a multimodal setting. Yang *et al.* [24] perform adversarial learning to transfer knowledge between annotated 3D human pose datasets and 2D in-the-wild images. Zhou *et al.* [29] use a weakly supervised approach and propose a geometric constrained to regularize depth predictions from 2D in-the-wild images. Zhang *et al.* [27] use knowledge distillation [10] to transfer knowledge from a teacher pose estimation network to a smaller network. In contrast, we are concerned with the task of domain transfer between separate body keypoint/joint subsets. Human body joints possess information about the location of one another through various constraints imposed by the overall body pose and structure. We present an approach to transfer rich contextual information between human body joints. Our work differs from approaches such as [26] in the way that instead of splitting a dataset based on classes, we have used subsets of human joint locations as separate domains and demonstrate that contextual knowledge can be transferred from one domain to the other using transfer learning. Our approach can be readily extended to other keypoint estimation problems such as facial landmark detection and 3D human pose estimation.

3 Methodology

In this section, the stacked hourglass network, experimental approach and training details are discussed. The MPII [1] dataset is used in the experiments which consists of around 28k training images and 11k testing images annotated with 16 body joints. Since the experiments involve evaluation on subsets of 16 annotated joints, a validation set of 3000 images is used for evaluation since the test annotations are not public.

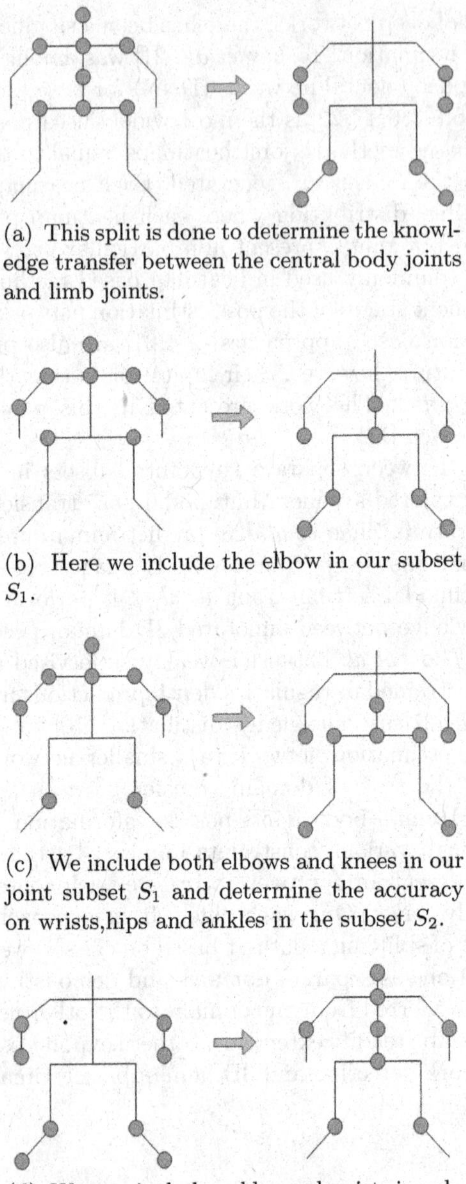

(a) This split is done to determine the knowledge transfer between the central body joints and limb joints.

(b) Here we include the elbow in our subset S_1.

(c) We include both elbows and knees in our joint subset S_1 and determine the accuracy on wrists,hips and ankles in the subset S_2.

(d) We now include ankles and wrists in subset S_1 and determine the performance on elbows and knees

Fig. 2. The joint subsets S_1 and S_2 used in the experiments shown as $S_1 \rightarrow S_2$.

Table 1. The subsets considered for experiments

	Subset S_1	Subset S_2
(a)	Head, Neck, Shoulders, Pelvis, Thorax, Hip	Knees, Ankles, Wrists, Elbows
(b)	Head, Neck, Shoulders, Elbows, Hip	Knees, Ankles, Wrists, Pelvis, Thorax
(c)	Head, Neck, Shoulders, Elbows, Knees	Wrist, Ankles, Hip, Pelvis, Thorax
(d)	Knees, Ankles, Wrists, Elbows	Head, Neck, Elbows, Knee, Pelvis, Thorax

3.1 Stacked Hourglass Network

Being the backbone of many state-of-the-art pose estimation algorithms [14,23] on the MPII dataset [1], the stacked hourglass network [17] is used in our experiments. The hourglass architecture consists of repeated bottom-up and top-down processing in order to utilize features at various scales. Convolution and max pooling layers bring down the input resolution from 64×64 pixels to 4×4 pixels. After downsampling to a resolution of 4×4 pixels, the features are upsampled with nearest neighbour upsampling and are combined with features of the same resolution. Several hourglass units are stacked together such that the output of one hourglass unit serves an input to the next hourglass unit. Intermediate supervision is applied such that mean squared loss is evaluated between the predicted heatmaps and ground truth heatmaps and gradients are back-propagated at every hourglass unit. The output of the network is a set of heatmaps equal to the number of joints with each pixel in the heatmap representing the probability with which the joint is present at that point.

3.2 Experiments

Domain transfer in keypoint estimation in performed by splitting the dataset joints into two subsets, S_1 and S_2 containing the same number of joints/keypoints. Both the subsets represent two separate domains. Note that $S_1 \cap S_2$ may or may not be an empty set, such that the two domains differ in atleast one keypoint location. Domain transfer is experimentally determined using three different configurations illustrated in Fig. 1. The network performance is evaluated on the joint subset S_2 using the three experiment configurations discussed below:

Transfer Learning. Since we are interested in determining the domain transfer from domain to another, a two-stack hourglass network initially trained on the subset S_1 of joints is jointly trained in conjugation with another two-stack hourglass network on the subset S_2 of joints (Fig. 1(a)). The joint training is done such that supervision is performed for all the four hourglass units.

Frozen Weights. This configuration is similar to transfer learning except that the weights of the first two-stack hourglass network trained on the subset S_1 of joints are frozen. Another two-stack hourglass network is trained on the remaining subset of eight joints S_2 such that the features obtained from the frozen network are used as an input for the network trained on subset S_2 (Fig. 1(b)). The loss is calculated only for the last two hourglass units. This is done to avoid the possibility of mutual co-adaptation of weights between the two domains.

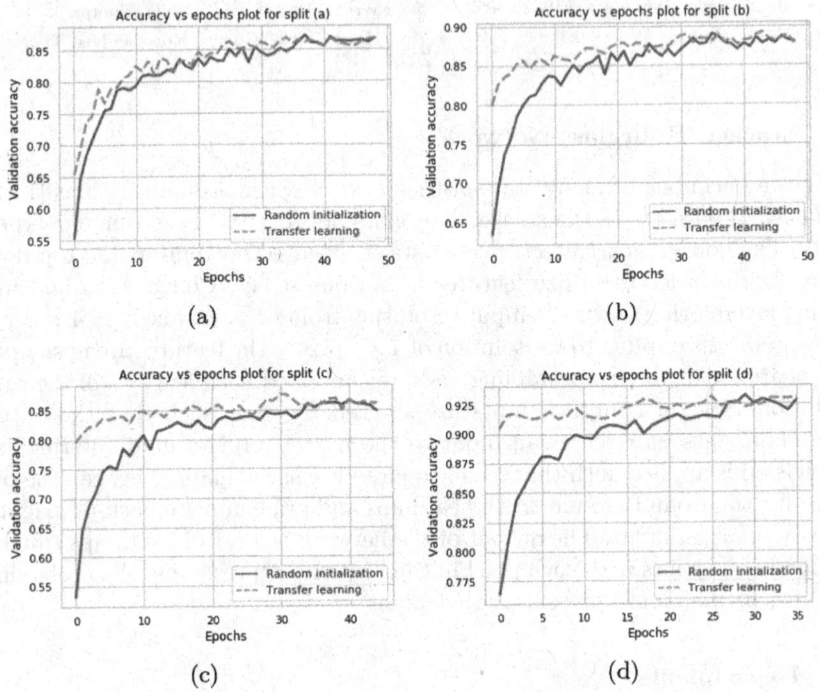

Fig. 3. The figure shows the comparison between the convergence rates of validation accuracy in case of transfer learning and random weight initialization. An important observation is that the convergence and accuracy obtained are complementary to each other such that in split (a) where there is no significant improvement in accuracy, the convergence between random initialization and transfer learning comparable. But, the opposite is observed in split (d), where both convergence and accuracy achieved is better than random initialization.

Random Initialization. A stacked hourglass network with four hourglass units with weights initialized randomly is trained on the subset S_2 of joints (Fig. 1(c)).

The performance of the three configurations are evaluated with four different splits of subsets S_1 of joints and corresponding subset S_2 (split (a)–(d)) listed in the Table 1. Since, a very large number of subsets are possible, the joint subsets are chosen such that the result of knowledge transfer between adjacent limb joints when compared to random initialization can be evaluated as shown in Fig. 2. Note that all the three configurations have roughly the same number of parameters. The goal of the experiments is not to improve the state-of-the-art pose estimation benchmark, but to evaluate keypoint domain transfer.

3.3 Training Details

The input image resolution for the network is 256 × 256 pixels and the heatmap resolution is 64 × 64 pixels. For all the experiments, rmsprop optimizer is used. The learning rate is divided by 5 each time the accuracy plateaus. Early stopping is implemented such that the model is said to be converged if there is no improvement in validation accuracy in 10 epochs with each epoch consisting of 8000 iterations. Data augmentation is carried out with .75 – 1.25 scale augmentation and +/− 30° of rotation augmentation. The training is carried on an NVIDIA Geforce Titan X GPU.

4 Results

The PCKh metric [1] is used to evaluate pose estimation performance. A joint is correctly predicted if the distance between the ground truth and predicted joint location is less than half the length of the head segment. The PCKh values for the joint subset S_2 corresponding to the four joint subset splits with respect to the three experiment configurations i.e., transfer learning, frozen weights and random weight initialization is shown in Tables 2, 3, 4 and 5 respectively. Note that the **pelvis and thorax torso joints are not considered in average PCKh computation** since, being at the centre of the body, they are almost perfectly localized in all scenarios and just increase the average values. Figure 3 show the validation accuracy vs epochs curves comparisons between random initialization and transfer learning configurations. Apparently, transfer learning from pre-learned weights from other joints not only helps in achieving better accuracy values but also results in much faster convergence when compared to random initialization. The accuracy values shown in the validation accuracy vs epochs plots (Fig. 3) use the PCK metric [25].

Table 2. PCKh comparison for joint split **a**

Configuration	Elbow	Wrist	Knee	Ankle	Average
Transfer learning	87.9	**84.2**	82.9	**80.6**	83.9
Frozen weights	74.7	56	72.7	66.8	67.5
Random initialization	87.9	83.9	**83.4**	80.5	83.9

Table 3. PCKh comparison for joint split **b**

Configuration	Wrist	Knee	Ankle	Average
Transfer learning	**84.1**	84.5	81.5	83.4
Frozen weights	69.7	73.0	62.6	68.43
Random initialization	83.6	**85**	**81.6**	83.4

Table 4. PCKh comparison for joint split **c**

Configuration	Wrist	Hip	Ankle	Average
Transfer learning	**84**	**87.1**	**80.1**	**83.7**
Frozen weights	71.2	83.7	69.9	74.9
Random initialization	82.9	87.0	79.7	83.2

4.1 Discussion

A number of interesting observations can be made:

1. Firstly, it can be observed from the splits (a)–(d) that features transferred from frozen weights of one domain i.e., subset S_1 do not achieve good accuracy on the second domain i.e subset S_2, when compared to random initialization and transfer learning. This is because, in the frozen weights configuration, since the loss is not computed on the first two hourglass units, there is no mutual co-adaptation of weights between the two domains.
2. From Table 2, in the case of split (a), it can be seen that transfer learning from torso joints improves accuracy on the wrists when compared to random initialization (83.9 vs 84.2), but does not have a considerable impact on the other limb joints. However, as elbows (split (b)) and ankles (split (c)) are included in subset S_1, we find that the performance on joints such as wrist (Table 3 and 4) and ankle (Table 4) becomes much better, such that, in split (c) the average PCKh over all joints (83.7) becomes better than random initialization (83.2). The effectiveness of domain transfer is further demonstrated in split (d) where wrists and ankles present in domain S_1 provide contextual knowledge to domain S_2. From Table 5, a higher average PCKh value (89.8) for transfer learning demonstrates the success of keypoint-wise domain transfer. The weights learned from one domain co-adapt with the other domain.

Table 5. PCKh comparison for joint split **d**

Configuration	Head	Elbow	Knee	Average
Transfer learning	96.8	**88.3**	**84.4**	**89.8**
Frozen weights	91.1	87.9	82.9	87.3
Random initialization	**97.1**	87.9	83.3	89.4

3. From Fig. 3 it is observed that the convergence and performance is complementary; i.e., in case of split (a) where, domain transfer does not result in any significant accuracy improvement, the convergence between random initialization and transfer learning configurations is comparable (Fig. 3a). On the other hand, in case of split (d), where domain transfer performs better

than random initialization, the convergence of transfer learning case is much better when compared to random initialization (Fig. 3d). Whereas, in the two other cases the convergence is "between" the two extreme situations of split (a) and (d). This is the result of the mutual co-adaptation of the network weights in learning adjacent limb joints. This shows that the weights learned on the one domain helps in better initialization of the cost function of the other domain which leads to faster convergence.

5 Conclusion

This paper introduces the KPTransfer approach for evaluating keypoint subset-wise domain transfer. We demonstrate that knowledge can be transferred between keypoint subsets in pose estimation such that the contextual cues present across domains helps in better generalization and faster convergence. This work also opens the door for cross-dataset domain transfer in keypoint estimation. Future work include: (1) Determining the exact joint subsets/domain between which domain transfer is most effective. (2) Extending this work to other problems like facial landmark detection and 3D human pose estimation. (3) Evaluation of the proposed keypoint domain transfer strategy with other pose estimation networks.

References

1. Andriluka, M., Pishchulin, L., Gehler, P., Schiele, B.: 2D human pose estimation: new benchmark and state of the art analysis. In: IEEE Conference on Computer Vision and Pattern Recognition (CVPR), June 2014
2. Bulat, A., Tzimiropoulos, G.: Human pose estimation via convolutional part heatmap regression. In: Leibe, B., Matas, J., Sebe, N., Welling, M. (eds.) ECCV 2016. LNCS, vol. 9911, pp. 717–732. Springer, Cham (2016). https://doi.org/10.1007/978-3-319-46478-7_44
3. Cao, Z., Simon, T., Wei, S.E., Sheikh, Y.: Realtime multi-person 2D pose estimation using part affinity fields. In: 2017 IEEE Conference on Computer Vision and Pattern Recognition (CVPR), pp. 1302–1310 (2017)
4. Carreira, J., Agrawal, P., Fragkiadaki, K., Malik, J.: Human pose estimation with iterative error feedback. In: 2016 IEEE Conference on Computer Vision and Pattern Recognition (CVPR), pp. 4733–4742 (2016)
5. Chen, Y.H., Chen, W.Y., Chen, Y.T., Tsai, B.C., Wang, Y.C.F., Sun, M.: No more discrimination: cross city adaptation of road scene segmenters. In: 2017 IEEE International Conference on Computer Vision (ICCV), pp. 2011–2020 (2017)
6. Chen, Y., Wang, Z., Peng, Y., Zhang, Z., Yu, G., Sun, J.: Cascaded pyramid network for multi-person pose estimation. In: 2018 IEEE/CVF Conference on Computer Vision and Pattern Recognition, pp. 7103–7112 (2018)
7. Chu, B., Madhavan, V., Beijbom, O., Hoffman, J., Darrell, T.: Best Practices for fine-tuning visual classifiers to new domains. In: Hua, G., Jégou, H. (eds.) ECCV 2016. LNCS, vol. 9915, pp. 435–442. Springer, Cham (2016). https://doi.org/10.1007/978-3-319-49409-8_34

8. Deng, J., Dong, W., Socher, R., Li, L.J., Li, K., Fei-Fei, L.: ImageNet: a large-scale hierarchical image database. In: CVPR (2009)
9. Gupta, S., Hoffman, J., Malik, J.: Cross modal distillation for supervision transfer. In: 2016 IEEE Conference on Computer Vision and Pattern Recognition (CVPR), pp. 2827–2836 (2016)
10. Hinton, G., Vinyals, O., Dean, J.: Distilling the knowledge in a neural network. In: NIPS Deep Learning and Representation Learning Workshop (2015). http://arxiv.org/abs/1503.02531
11. Hoffman, J., Gupta, S., Leong, J., Guadarrama, S., Darrell, T.: Cross-modal adaptation for RGB-D detection. In: 2016 IEEE International Conference on Robotics and Automation (ICRA), pp. 5032–5039, May 2016. https://doi.org/10.1109/ICRA.2016.7487708
12. Hoffman, J., et al.: LSDA: large scale detection through adaptation. In: NIPS (2014)
13. Ionescu, C., Papava, D., Olaru, V., Sminchisescu, C.: Human3.6M: large scale datasets and predictive methods for 3D human sensing in natural environments. IEEE Trans. Pattern Anal. Mach. Intell. **36**(7), 1325–1339 (2014)
14. Ke, L., Chang, M.-C., Qi, H., Lyu, S.: Multi-scale structure-aware network for human pose estimation. In: Ferrari, V., Hebert, M., Sminchisescu, C., Weiss, Y. (eds.) ECCV 2018. LNCS, vol. 11206, pp. 731–746. Springer, Cham (2018). https://doi.org/10.1007/978-3-030-01216-8_44
15. Lin, T.-Y., et al.: Microsoft COCO: common objects in context. In: Fleet, D., Pajdla, T., Schiele, B., Tuytelaars, T. (eds.) ECCV 2014. LNCS, vol. 8693, pp. 740–755. Springer, Cham (2014). https://doi.org/10.1007/978-3-319-10602-1_48
16. Liu, M.Y., Tuzel, O.: Coupled generative adversarial networks. In: NIPS (2016)
17. Newell, A., Yang, K., Deng, J.: Stacked hourglass networks for human pose estimation. In: Leibe, B., Matas, J., Sebe, N., Welling, M. (eds.) ECCV 2016. LNCS, vol. 9912, pp. 483–499. Springer, Cham (2016). https://doi.org/10.1007/978-3-319-46484-8_29
18. Pishchulin, L., et al.: DeepCut: joint subset partition and labeling for multi person pose estimation. In: 2016 IEEE Conference on Computer Vision and Pattern Recognition (CVPR), pp. 4929–4937 (2016)
19. Rozantsev, A., Salzmann, M., Fua, P.: Beyond sharing weights for deep domain adaptation. IEEE Trans. Pattern Anal. Mach. Intell. **41**, 801–814 (2018)
20. Tompson, J., Jain, A., LeCun, Y., Bregler, C.: Joint training of a convolutional network and a graphical model for human pose estimation. In: Proceedings of the 27th International Conference on Neural Information Processing Systems, NIPS 2014, vol. 1, pp. 1799–1807. MIT Press, Cambridge (2014). http://dl.acm.org/citation.cfm?id=2968826.2969027
21. Toshev, A., Szegedy, C.: DeepPose: human pose estimation via deep neural networks. In: 2014 IEEE Conference on Computer Vision and Pattern Recognition, pp. 1653–1660, June 2014. https://doi.org/10.1109/CVPR.2014.214
22. Wei, S.E., Ramakrishna, V., Kanade, T., Sheikh, Y.: Convolutional pose machines. In: 2016 IEEE Conference on Computer Vision and Pattern Recognition (CVPR), pp. 4724–4732 (2016)
23. Yang, W., Li, S., Ouyang, W., Li, H., Wang, X.: Learning feature pyramids for human pose estimation. In: 2017 IEEE International Conference on Computer Vision (ICCV), pp. 1290–1299 (2017)
24. Yang, W., Ouyang, W., Wang, X., Ren, J.S.J., Li, H., Wang, X.: 3D human pose estimation in the wild by adversarial learning. In: 2018 IEEE/CVF Conference on Computer Vision and Pattern Recognition, pp. 5255–5264 (2018)

25. Yang, Y., Ramanan, D.: Articulated human detection with flexible mixtures of parts. IEEE Trans. Pattern Anal. Mach. Intell. **35**(12), 2878–2890 (2013). https://doi.org/10.1109/TPAMI.2012.261
26. Yosinski, J., Clune, J., Bengio, Y., Lipson, H.: How transferable are features in deep neural networks? In: Advances in Neural Information Processing Systems, pp. 3320–3328 (2014)
27. Zhang, F., Zhu, X., Ye, M.: Fast human pose estimation. CoRR abs/1811.05419 (2018)
28. Zhao, M.Y., Katabi, D.: Through-wall human pose estimation using radio signals. In: 2018 IEEE/CVF Conference on Computer Vision and Pattern Recognition, pp. 7356–7365 (2018)
29. Zhou, X., Huang, Q.X., Sun, X., Xue, X., Wei, Y.: Towards 3D human pose estimation in the wild: a weakly-supervised approach. In: 2017 IEEE International Conference on Computer Vision (ICCV), pp. 398–407 (2017)

Deep Learning Model for Skin Lesion Segmentation: Fully Convolutional Network

Adekanmi Adegun and Serestina Viriri(✉)

School of Mathematics, Statistics and Computer Science,
University of KwaZulu-Natal, Durban, South Africa
218082884@stu.ukzn.ac.za, viriris@ukzn.ac.za

Abstract. Segmentation of skin lesions is a crucial task in detecting and diagnosing melanoma cancer. Incidence of melanoma skin cancer which is the most deadly form of skin cancer has been on steady increase. Early detection of the melanoma cancer is necessary to improve the survival rate of the patients. Segmentation is an important task in analysing skin lesion images. Skin lesion segmentation has come with some challenges such as low contrast and fine grained nature of skin lesions. This has necessitated the need for automated analysis and segmentation of skin lesions using state-of-the-arts techniques. In this paper, a deep learning model has been adapted for the segmentation of skin lesions. This work demonstrates the segmentation of skin lesions using fully convolutional networks (FCNs) that train skin lesion images from end-to-end using only the images pixels and disease ground truth labels as inputs. The fully convolutional network adapted is based on U-Net architecture. The model is enhanced by employing multi-stage segmentation approach with batch normalisation and data augmentation. Performance metrics such as dice coefficient, accuracy, sensitivity and specificity were used for evaluating the performance of the model. Experimental results show that the proposed model achieved better performance compared with the other state-of-the arts methods for skin lesion image segmentation with a dice coefficient of 90% and sensitivity of 96%.

Keywords: Melanoma · Skin lesions · Deep learning · Segmentation · FCNs · U-Net

1 Introduction

Melanoma is a form of skin cancer with a very high mortality rate. Early detection of melanoma in dermoscopy images has been shown to significantly increase the survival rate [1]. Segmentation is an important task in analyzing skin lesion images. Over the years computing techniques have been applied to carry out this task. Accurate recognition of melanoma is challenging and difficult due to some notable reasons. Firstly, there is always low contrast between lesions and the skin.

F. Karray et al. (Eds.): ICIAR 2019, LNCS 11663, pp. 232–242, 2019.
https://doi.org/10.1007/978-3-030-27272-2_20

Secondly, there is close visual similarity between melanoma and non-melanoma lesions [1]. Thirdly, artifacts presence such as presence of hair, reflections, air and oil bubbles [2] on these images also contributes to the challenges. Thus, there is a need for a reliable system that can perform proper and accurate analysis of skin lesions images for lesion segmentation.

The need for more reliable and accurate system towards melanoma detection has led to the application of state-of-the-arts methods such as deep learning techniques for segmentation of skin lesions images. Some of these methods have not been efficient due to their tendency to over-or under-segment the lesions most especially when the lesions images have low contrast, characterize with artifacts or inhomogeneous textures [3]. In this work, fully convolutional networks (FCNs) based on U-Net architecture is explored for the segmentation of skin lesions. This architecture has been enhanced by adapting standard and rich-feature models for image classification tasks into fully convolutional networks for segmentation purpose. The proposed model is made up of an encoder network followed by a decoder network. In this case, the encoder adapts a pre-trained classification network of Visual Geometry Group (VGG) network followed by a decoder network. The decoder maps the low resolution discriminative features from the encoder to higher and full input resolution features [4,5]. The up-sampling networks in the decoding phase reduce the number of the parameters for training the networks thereby minimizing the training time and refining the networks for better performance. The proposed Fully convolutional networks (FCNs) model trains skin lesion images in an end-to-end manner using image pixels and disease ground truth labels as inputs [4]. The proposed FCN model uses a multi-stage segmentation approach to overcome the challenges of low contrast and fuzzy boundaries composing of early stage learning of coarse appearance and localisation information and late stage learning of the features of lesion boundaries [3]. The proposed model is also improved with batch normalization.

This model was evaluated on skin lesions image dataset of ISIC 2018 and it was noted that the enhanced U-NET architecture outperforms some existing models. The performance of the model was evaluated using metrics such as dice coefficient, accuracy, sensitivity and specificity.

2 Related Works

In the last decade, some research works have been particularly carried out in the segmentation process of skin lesion analysis using state-of-the arts techniques. Recently, some models of deep learning have been used for image segmentation. Chen et al. [6] carried out investigation on the segmentation of skin lesions using different U-Net models based on three architectures that used different ensemble strategies such as weighted average, unweighted average and hierarchical average. A U-Net-GAN based architecture comprising generator and discriminator was proposed by Xu et al. [7] for skin lesions segmentation. The system used further post processing technique such as binary holes filling and removing of artifacts and small objects to improve the final output. Venkatesh et al. [8] proposed a methodology for automatic skin lesion region segmentation based on U-Net and residual network. Krashenyi et al. extended a U-Net network architecture by adding dilated convolutions to the central segment known as bottleneck block [9]. The encoder of the model was built of the blocks that have a structure of stacked convolutional layers. Most of these U-Net models have become huge in size and will require more computing resources to perform efficiently.

Badrinarayanan et al. [10] applied deep fully convolutional neural network architecture for semantic pixel-wise segmentation on images. The architecture termed SegNet consists of an encoder network, a corresponding decoder network followed by a pixel-wise classification layer. Jafari et al. [11] performed preprocessing of input image to reduce noisy artifacts and then applied deep convolutional neural network (CNN). The model combined both local and global contextual information and outputted a label for each pixel to produce segmentation mask. A fully convolutional network(FCN) based on U-Net to identify cell nuclei in certain images was proposed by Bartolome et al. [12]. It is a modified U-Net architecture that retained feature maps from the encoding phase and transferred them to the decoding phase. Generative Adversarial Networks (GANs) was used for data augmentation in an image segmentation process [13] and Convolutional-DE convolutional Neural Networks (CDNNs) was later used to automatically generate lesion segmentation mask from dermoscopic images.

Al-masni et al. [14] applied a modified Fusion Net which consists of three modules of encoder, decoder and bridge on skin lesion segmentation. The system produced result with low sensitivity score. A Deep learning framework consisting of two fully-convolutional residual networks (FCRN) that simultaneously produced segmentation result was developed by Li et al. [1]. A Full Resolution Convolution Network (FrCN) method which can learn high-level features and improve segmentation performance was developed by Yuming et al. [15]. Nasr-Esfahani et al. proposed a Dense Fully Convolutional Network (DFCN) for segmentation of lesion regions in non-dermoscopic images [15]. The system was not actually tested on dermoscopic images that require dealing with much noise.

Three boundary enhancement block (BEB) and a pooling pyramid embedded the general VGG16 network [16] to build a network architecture for segmentation process. The system yielded an average Jaccard index of 0.769. A system based on two coupled modules which trained end-to-end over the augmented dataset of clinical cases was presented [17] for image segmentation. The modules included an FCN that was used to provide a pixel-wise segmentation for the images and a Region-Proposal Network (RPN) that specified elliptical regions over a low-resolution segmentation map. The system gave three different output loss of pixel-wise loss of the FCN, the loss of RPN predictor and the classification loss of the RPN simultaneously which may reduce the accuracy.

Mask R-CNN model with ResNet50 backbone architecture that was pre trained on COCO datasets for Lesion Boundary Segmentation was proposed by Yang et al. [18] for skin lesion segmentation. Another version of Mask R-CNN model which extended Faster R-CNN by adding FCN for predicting object masks was applied by Moutselos et al. [19]. Lastly, transposed convolutional layers that increased spatial resolution and reduced the number of channels by half to up-sample feature maps was used in [20] for image segmentation.

Most of the methods discussed above employed large number of trainable parameter. This increased their complexity and consequently made them inefficient with tendency to perform over-or under-segmentation of skin lesions with low contrast. They also consume lot of computational resources such as processor time and memory. Our proposed framework is designed to be efficient both in terms of memory and computational time during inference. The system will through its multi-stage approach apply smaller number of trainable parameters than other competing architectures.

3 Methods and Techniques

3.1 Fully Convolutional Networks (FCN) for Skin Lesion Segmentation

In this work, a contemporary classification network of VGG net has been adapted into fully convolutional networks. The normal process of learning in classification task is transferred into segmentation task by fine-tuning. The system operates by learning and mapping skin lesion image from pixels to pixels in an end-to-end manner. The supervised end-to-end training of the FCN produces pixel-wise prediction. Both learning and inference are performed on the skin lesions image input by the feed forward and back propagation networks of the FCN simultaneously. The up-sampling layers gives pixel wise prediction while learning takes place at the down-sampling (pooling)stage. The segmentation networks usually have 2 paths:

Downsampling path: This is the encoder stage and it captures and interprets semantic and contextual information of skin lesions image for model learning. The encoder is adapted from the VGG classification network by replacing the last two layers with full convolutional layers. The convolution layers perform features extraction from the input image through the downsampling path. The pooling layers also reduce the resolution of the image feature maps by two times.

Upsampling path: This is the decoder stage. This path recovers spatial information for output prediction. The decoder works on the discriminative features with lower resolution learnt from the encoder. The up-sampling layer increases and recovers the resolution of feature map. This is followed by a softmax classifier that predicts pixel-wise labels for an output. The output has the same resolution as the input image.

The general layout of the FCN segmentation method is illustrated with Fig. 1 below.

3.2 The Proposed U-Net Based FCN Model

The proposed model in this research work is a fully convolutional network (FCN) based on U-Net architecture. It was trained on a set of skin lesion images

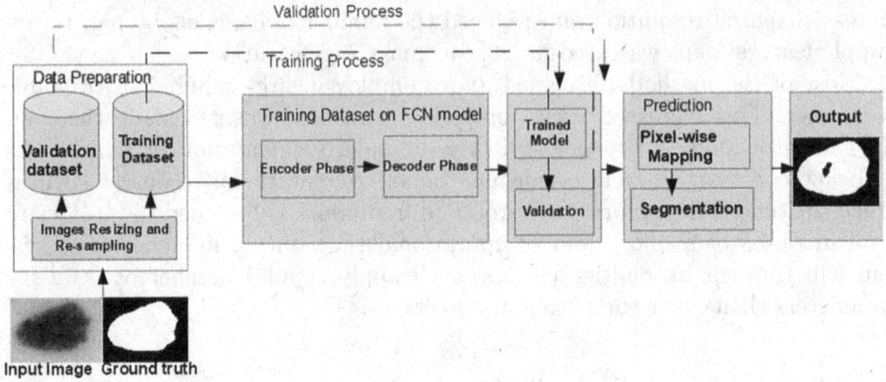

Fig. 1. General architecture of a fully convolutional networks for skin lesion segmentation

and ground truth labels. The model is not only computationally inexpensive, but also achieved outstanding results on the dermoscopic dataset. The model was designed using a highly optimized deep network architecture for accuracy and speed for segmentation task. This was done by adopting multi-stage approach to segmentation. It also applies batch processing and data augmentation. Using multistage networks for segmentation allowed us to design faster and more portable models for each task in the segmentation process.

The proposed model shown by Fig. 1 accepts skin lesion image as input and produces a segmented image as the output. At the input section, resizing and resampling of the images takes place in the repository as shown in Fig. 1. This is sent into the encoding phase and then to the decoder phase. Learning and training take place through the model from the input section. Validation also takes place simultaneously. The model is mainly categorised into encoder and decoder stages. The segmentation output is finally produced through the pixel-wise mapping that takes place during the training process.

The encoder stage is composed of four set of convolution layers composing 32, 64, 128 and 256 channels respectively as shown in Fig. 2. Each of the layers applies Rectified Linear Units (ReLU) activation function and a pooling(max-pooling) layer. Features extraction is carried out at each stage of the convolution layer with the pooling layer reducing the resolution of the feature maps. The decoder part is also made up of four convolution layers that matches the four convolution layers in the encoding part directly. It also makes use of the ReLU activation function at each layer. The model further got enhanced by using a robust up-sampling layer that adopts 3 by 3 convolutional layers which increases the feature size during the decoding phase. The decoder network up-samples and also convolutes its input feature maps using the memorized max-pooling indices from the corresponding encoder feature maps. The system concatenates and merges the encoder feature maps to the up-sampled feature maps from the decoder at every stage. This architecture has the capacity that allows the decoder at each stage to learn back relevant features that were lost when pooled in the encoder through concatenation connections.

The system uses refinement techniques such as batch normalization and data augmentation to improve the performance. Data augmentation is required to increase the amount of our training image data set for better performance. The system applied elastic deformations through random displacements for augmenting data. Batch Normalization is introduced in the input and convolutional layers to alleviate over-fitting. Batch Normalization makes training more resilient to the parameter scale. During training, the layer keeps track of statistics for each input variable and use them to standardize the data. The statistics used to perform the standardization, e.g. the mean and standard deviation of each variable, are updated for each mini batch and a running average is maintained. Batch normalisation also improves the performance and stability of the fully convolutional networks by allowing the model to use much higher learning rates. Finally, the rectified linear unit (ReLU) employed in the convolutional layers also accelerates training.

4 Experimental Results and Analysis

4.1 DataSet

The dataset used in this work comes from the ISIC Dermoscopic Archive. The ISIC Archive contains over 13,000 dermoscopic images, which were collected from leading clinical centers internationally and acquired from a variety of devices within each center. The training images are set of 2000 images for both the training and the ground truth respectively. The input data are dermoscopic lesion images in JPEG format while the ground truth are mask image provided for training and used internally for scoring validation and test phases data using several techniques. Ground truth segmentations are normally generated through fully-automated algorithm, reviewed and accepted by a human expert or manual polygon tracing by a human expert. The dataset samples are shown in Fig. 3.

4.2 Performance Evaluation

The performance of the U-Net model was evaluated on ISIC dataset comprising of 2000 image sets. The results displayed as shown in Table 1. The dice coefficient performs similarity measure between the predicted output and expected output. The improved U-Net model gives the dice coefficient of 90% which is higher. This shows higher similarity between the predicted results and the expected results in the improved U-Net model as shown. The resultant segmentation accuracy was also assessed by comparing the automatically obtained melanoma-detected areas with the manual version. The results of the test segmentation were compared with the ground truth as displayed in Fig. 4. The results of the proposed UNET model was compared with some recently developed methods as shown in Table 2.

Evaluation was also done using Dice's coefficient and some other metrics, which are calculated as:

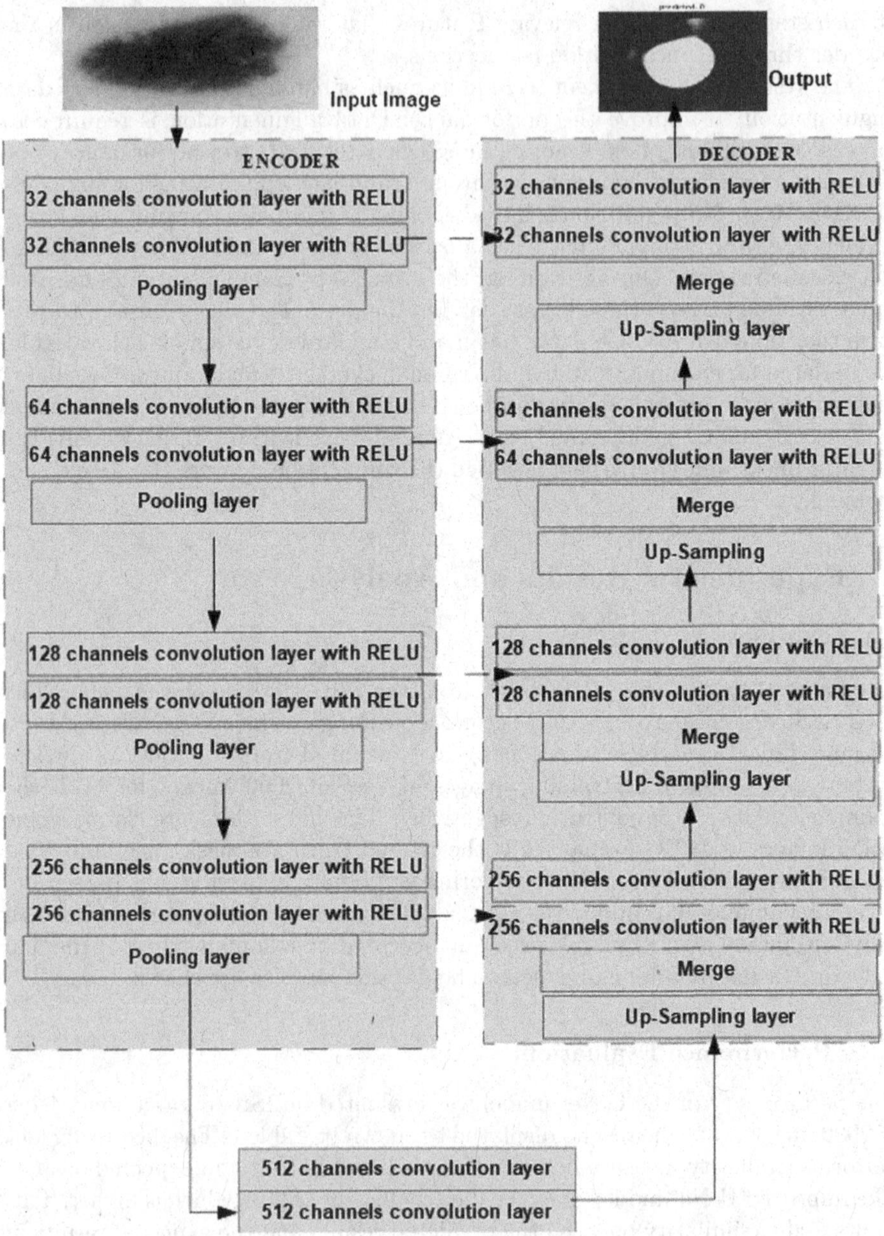

Fig. 2. Architectural diagram for the proposed U-Net model

Dice Similarity Coefficient: It measures the similarity or overlap between the ground truth and the automatic segmentation. It is defined as

$$\mathbf{DSC} = \frac{2TP}{FP + 2TP + FN} \tag{1}$$

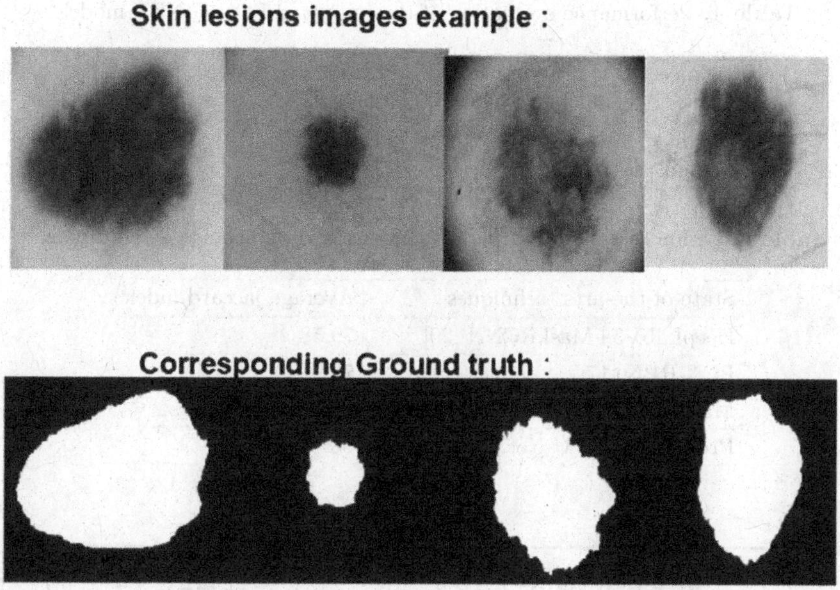

Fig. 3. A sample skin lesions image data set and the corresponding ground truth

Sensitivity: It measures the proportion of those who test positive(diagnosed) for the disease among those who actually have the disease.

$$\textbf{Sensitivity} = \frac{TP}{TP + FN} \tag{2}$$

Specificity: This is the proportion of healthy patients known not to have the disease, who will test negative for it among those who actually do not have the disease.

$$\textbf{Specificity} = \frac{TN}{TN + FP} \tag{3}$$

Accuracy: It measures the proportion of true results (both true positives and true negatives) among the total number of cases examined.

$$\textbf{Accuracy} = \frac{TP + TN}{TP + TN + FP + FN} \tag{4}$$

Where FP is the number of false positive pixels, FN is the number of false negative pixels, TP is the number of true positive pixels and TN is the number of true negative pixels.

The evaluation results shows that the proposed model when compared against some recently used techniques presents better performance. Each of the images was compared with the corresponding ground truth segmentation using the dice similarity coefficient as shown in Fig. 5. Table 2 shows that the proposed model outperforms the other state-of-the-art techniques. The performance is calculated in percentage against 1. The results show the dice coefficient of 90% which

Table 1. Performance evaluation of the improved FCN U-NET model

Performance metrics	Dice coefficient	Jaccard index	Positive predictive value	Sensitivity
FCN U-Net based model	90	83	96	96

Table 2. Lesion segmentation performances based on average jaccard index

State-of-the-arts techniques	Average jaccard index
DeepLabV3+MaskRCNN [20]	79.58
FCN-RPN [17]	79.9
MaskRcnn2 [22]	82.0
Proposed FCN U-Net based model	83

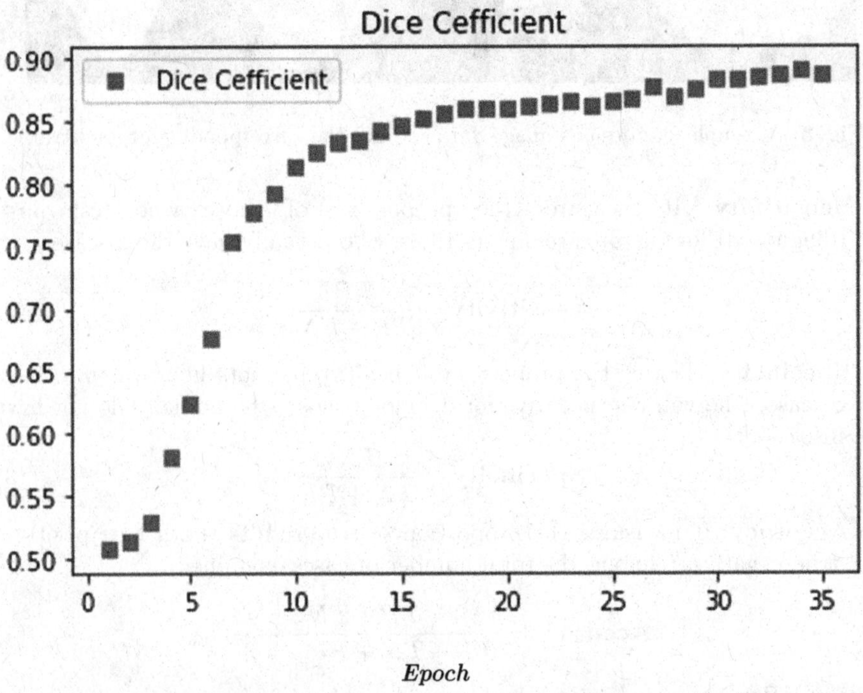

Fig. 4. A curve showing increase in dice coefficient rate of the proposed model

indicates high similarity between the ground truth labels and the segmentation output of the proposed model. This can also be seen when compared the images in Fig. 5. This can also be inferred from Fig. 4 showing the curve for the dice coefficient.

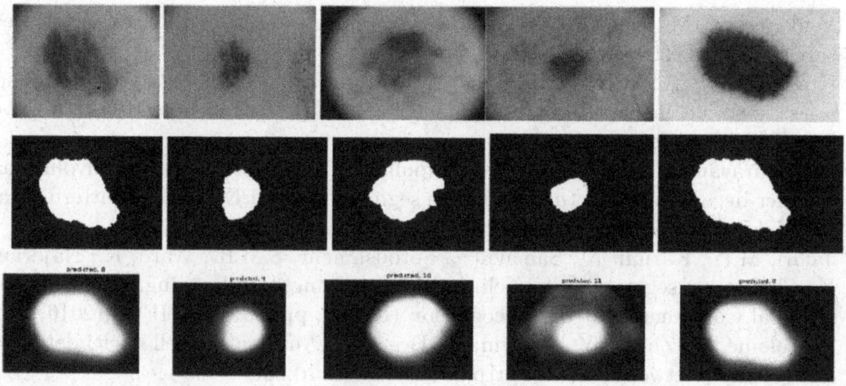

Fig. 5. The 5 melanoma image segmentation sample results from the FCN U-NET based model. *The first row shows the lesion images that was segmented; the second row displays segmentation experts' manual segmentation known as ground truth mask while the third row shows the predicted mask of the test image.*

5 Conclusion

This work performed analysis and segmentation of skin lesion images using the FCN UNET-based segmentation methods. This work shows that the proposed enhanced U-Net model outperforms some of the existing model with little difference in average jaccard index. This is due to the robust architecture adapted by the FCN U-Net based model. The proposed model also performed well with small image data set. Ensemble methods of the improved U-Net model with some other state-of-the arts techniques will be worked on in the future.

References

1. Li, Y., Shen, L.: Skin lesion analysis towards melanoma detection using deep learning network. Sensors **18**(2), 1–16 (2018). (Switzerland)
2. Bi, L., Kim, J., Ahn, E., Kumar, A., Fulham, M., Feng, D.: Dermoscopic image segmentation via multi-stage fully convolutional networks. IEEE Trans. Biomed. Eng. **64**(9), 2065–2074 (2017)
3. Gelfand, A.: Deep learning and the future of biomedical image analysis. Biomed. Comput. Rev. (2017)
4. Badrinarayanan, V., Kendall, A., Cipolla, R.: Segnet: A deep convolutional encoder-decoder architecture for image segmentation. arXiv preprint arXiv:1511.00561 (2015)
5. Shelhamer, E., Long, J., Darrell, T.: Fully Convolutional Networks for Semantic Segmentation preprint arXiv:1605.06211, pp. 1–12 (2016)
6. Chen, D., et al.: U-Net Ensemble for Skin Lesion Analysis towards Melanoma Detection. arXiv preprint, pp. 3–6 (2016)
7. Xu, X., Liu, X., Li, X.: U-Net-GAN based skin lesion segmentation (2018). https://challenge2018.isic-archive.com/leaderboards

8. Venkatesh, G.M., Naresh, Y.G., Little, S., Connor, N.O.: Deep Residual Architecture for Skin Lesion Segmentation, pp. 1–5
9. Krashenyi, I., Voloshyna, A., Popov, A., Panichev, O.: CNN-based lesion boundaries detection in dermoscopic images (2018). https://challenge2018.isic-archive.com/leaderboards
10. Badrinarayanan, V., Kendall, A., Cipolla, R.: SegNet: a deep convolutional encoder-decoder architecture for image segmentation. IEEE Trans. Pattern Anal. Mach. Intell. **39**(12), 2481–2495 (2017)
11. Jafari, M.H., Karimi, N., Samavi, S., Soroushmehr, S.M.R., Ward, K., Najarian, K.: Skin lesion segmentation in clinical images using deep learning. In: 23rd International Conference Pattern Recognition (ICPR), pp. 337–342. IEEE (2016)
12. Bartolome, C., Zhang, Y., Ashwin, R.: DeepCell: Automating cell nuclei detection with Neural Networks (2018). http://cs230.stanford.edu
13. Pollastri, F., Cancilla, M., Bolelli, F., Grana, C.: A ImageLab at ISIC Challenge 2018 (2018)
14. Al-masni, M.A., Al-antari, M.A., Choi, M.T., Han, S.M., Kim, T.S.: Skin lesion segmentation in dermoscopy images via deep full resolution convolutional networks. Comput. Methods Programs Biomed. **162**, 221–231 (2018)
15. Nasr-Esfahani, E., et al.: Dense Fully Convolutional Network for Skin Lesion Segmentation. arXiv Preprint arXiv:1712.10207 (2017)
16. Tan, X., Chen, M.: "Saliency-based Skin Lesion Segmentation by Deep Network": Participation in ISIC 2018 Skin Lesion Analysis Towards Melanoma Detection Challenge (2018). https://challenge2018.isic-archive.com/leaderboards/
17. Vesal, S., Malakarjun Patil, S., Ravikumar, N., Maier, A.K.: A multi-task framework for skin lesion detection and segmentation. In: Stoyanov, D., et al. (eds.) CARE/CLIP/OR 2.0/ISIC -2018. LNCS, vol. 11041, pp. 285–293. Springer, Cham (2018). https://doi.org/10.1007/978-3-030-01201-4_31
18. Yang, J., Chen, W.: "Skin Lesion Analysis Using Deep Neural Networks": Participation in ISIC 2018 Skin Lesion Analysis Towards Melanoma Detection Challenge (2018). https://challenge2018.isic-archive.com/leaderboards/
19. Molina-moreno, M., González-díaz, I., Díaz-de-maría, F.: "An Elliptical Shape-Regularized Convolutional Neural Network for Skin Lesion Segmentation": Participation in ISIC 2018 Skin Lesion Analysis Towards Melanoma Detection Challenge (2018). https://challenge2018.isic-archive.com/leaderboards/
20. Goyal, M., Yap, M.H.: Automatic Deep Learning Ensemble Methods for Skin Lesion Boundary Segmentation, preprint arXiv: 1711.10449, vol. 5, no. 1, pp. 2–6
21. Zhang, X.: Melanoma segmentation based on deep learning. Comput. Assist. Surg. **22**, 267–277 (2017)
22. Qian, C., et al.: "ISIC 2018 - Skin Lesion Analysis": Participation in ISIC 2018 Skin Lesion Analysis Towards Melanoma Detection Challenge (2018). https://challenge2018.isic-archive.com/leaderboards/

Deep Learning Using Bayesian Optimization for Facial Age Estimation

Marwa Ahmed[1] and Serestina Viriri[2(✉)]

[1] College of Computer Science and Information Technology, Sudan University of Science and Technology, Khartoum, Sudan
jamal.marwa@gmail.com

[2] School of Mathematics, Statistics and Computer Science, University of KwaZulu-Natal, Durban, South Africa
viriris@ukzn.ac.za

Abstract. Age Estimation plays a significant role in many real-world applications. Age estimation is a process of determining the exact age or age group of a person depending on his biometric features. Recent research demonstrates that the deeply learned features for age estimation from large-scale data result in significant improvement of the age estimation performance for facial images. This paper propose a Convolutional Neural Network (CNN) - approach using Bayesian Optimization for facial age estimation. Bayesian Optimization is applied to minimize the classification error on the validation set for CNN model. Extensive experiments are done for evaluating Deep Learning using Bayesian Optimization (DLOB) on three datasets: MORPH, FG-NET and FERET. The results show that using Bayesian Optimization for CNN outperforms the state of the arts on FG-NET and FERET datasets with a Mean Absolute Error (MAE) of 2.88 and 1.3, and achieves comparable results compared to the most of the state-of-the-art methods on MORPH dataset with a 3.01 MAE.

Keywords: Age estimation · Feature learning · Convolutional Neural Networks · Bayesian optimization

1 Introduction

Facial images of humans contain rich information around personal characteristics, comprising emotional identity, age, expression, gender, etc. Generally, human images can be taken as a complex signal which covers a number of facial attributes such as skin color and geometric facial feature. These facial attributes play a critical role in real applications for facial image analysis. The estimated attributes from face image in such applications can deduce additional system reactions. Particularly, age is further significant surrounded by these attributes [1].

Age estimation is a significant task in facial image classification. It plays an important role in numerous applications such as multimedia communication,

F. Karray et al. (Eds.): ICIAR 2019, LNCS 11663, pp. 243–254, 2019.
https://doi.org/10.1007/978-3-030-27272-2_21

security control, surveillance and human computer interaction. Age estimation is the procedure of determining the person's age depending on his biometric features by computers [2]. The major aim of age estimation is to estimate age closely to appearance age as possible.

Machine learning algorithms are rarely parameter-free: parameters controlling the rate of learning or the capacity of the underlying model must often be specified. These parameters are frequently considered annoyances, making it interesting to develop machine learning algorithms with fewer of them.

Another good solution is to optimize such parameters as a procedure to be automated. Specifically, viewing such tuning as optimizing an unknown black-box function and appeal algorithms developed for such problems. Bayesian optimization [3] is a good choice, which outperforms other state of the art global optimization algorithms on many challenging optimization benchmark functions [4]. The parameters of the machine learning algorithms that control the capacity and learning rate of the underlying model must be identified. These parameters are frequently considered annoyances, making it interesting to develop machine learning algorithms with fewer of them.

In this paper, Bayesian Optimization is used to improve the performance of age estimation. The variables that required to be optimized are specified firstly. These selected variables are the parameters of the network architecture, as well as options of the training algorithm. Then the objective function is defined, which receipts the values of these specified variables as inputs. This function specifies the training options and network architecture, training the network on training set and validating it on the test set. Then the Bayesian Optimization is performed with several objectives by minimizing the classification error on the validation set.

2 Literature Review and Related Works

2.1 Deep Learning

Deep learning is a class of machine learning techniques, in a way that several layers of information processing stages are exploited in hierarchical architectures for pattern classification and for representation or feature learning. It lies in the connections of numerous research areas, including graphical modeling, neural networks, signal processing, pattern recognition, and optimization. Deep learning's basic concept is created from research of artificial neural network [5].

Convolutional Neural Networks (CNNs) are one of the most important deep learning approaches whose multiple layers are trained in a robust manner [6]. A CNN in convolutional layers convolve the whole image by exploiting different kernels as well as the intermediate feature maps, generating various feature maps, CNN in general is a hierarchical neural network, where its convolutional layers alternate with pooling layers [7]. The Pooling layer follows the convolutional layer and it minimizes the feature maps' dimensions and network parameters. Due to taking computations of neighboring pixels into account, these layers are translation invariant [6]. Fully-connected layer follows the last pooling layer in the network. There are numerous fully connected layers which convert the 2D feature maps into a 1D feature vector, for additional feature representation. Fully-connected layers achieve like a traditional neural network and consist of about 90% of the parameters in a CNN [6].

Recently, deep learning algorithms have been applied by a number of researchers to face related tasks like face verification, gender identification and age estimation. A Deep ID structure is proposed to extract discriminative features from the face for face verification process [8]. To improve the Deep ID algorithm, a verification constraint is added in loss function to obtain better performance [9]. For detecting landmark points of the face, a cascaded Deep ConvNets structure is proposed [10]. Also [11] proposed a new algorithm to detect landmark points, which named deep multi-task learning algorithm.

A new framework is built for age feature extraction which is based on the deep learning model. CNN is used to estimate ages [12]. Comparing to previous models, feature maps resulted from different layers are used as an alternative of using a feature extracted from the top layer. Furthermore, the proposed scheme incorporates the manifold learning algorithm. This significantly increases the performance. From the other hand, the deep learned aging pattern (DLA) is used to evaluate different classification and regression schemes for age estimation. Experimental results evaluated on two datasets indicate that the approach is better than the state-of the-art significantly. A framework for age estimation based on deep learning is proposed. Transfer learning is used due to the lack of labeled images. Due to the ordered labels in age estimation, a new loss function for age classification is defined through distance loss addition to cross-entropy loss for relationships description between labels. Results obtained prove the excellent algorithm performance against the state-of- the-art methods [13].

A robust and a fast age modeling algorithm is used with the deep learning to propose age estimation system. They indicate that the local regressors performance for most groups are better than the global regressor. Samples are firstly classified into overlapping age groups. Local regressors estimates the apparent age for each group. The outputs are used for the final estimate. The system is evaluated on the ChaLearn Looking at People 2016 – Apparent Age Estimation challenge dataset, and results in 3.85 MAE on the test set [14]. The largest public IMDB-WIKI dataset with gender and age labels is introduced by [15]. VGG-16 architecture for convolutional neural networks is used which are pre-trained on ImageNet dataset. A robust face alignment is done. They study the perceived age by other humans and the apparent age estimation. The methods are evaluated on standard benchmarks and results achieve state-of-the-art for both apparent and real age estimation.

Both final label encoding and the structure innovation are explored [16]. For the performance evaluation, a novel hierarchical aggregation is proposed based on deep network to study features of aging and their encoding method is applied to transmit the discrete aging labels to a possibility label, this allows the CNN to conduct a classification task rather than regression task. Their deep aging feature can capture both global and local cues in aging. Experimental results of

Algorithm: Bayesian Optimization

1: **for** n= 1,2,..., **do**
2: select new x_{n+1} by optimizing acquisition function α
$x_{n+1} = arg_{max x}\alpha(x; D^n)$
3: query objective function to obtain y_{n+1}
4: augment data $D_{n+1} = D_n(x_{n+1}, y_{n+1})$
5: update statistical model
6: **end for**

age prediction on the FG-NET and the MORPH-II databases indicate that the proposed deep aging feature outperforms state-of-the-art aging features.

2.2 Bayesian Optimization

Bayesian optimization concerned in finding the minimum of a function f(x) as in other kinds of optimization on some bounded set X. It builds a probabilistic model for f(x) and this model is exploited to give decisions about where will be the next evaluation of the function in X, while integrating out uncertainty. The fundamental philosophy is to utilize all of the available information from previous evaluations of f(x) and not only rely on Hessian Approximations and local gradient. This results in a technique that can gain the minimum of difficult non-convex functions with proportion to little evaluations, at the cost of carrying out more computation to decide which the next point to try. Once evaluations of f(x) are costly to accomplish—as is the situation when it needs training a machine learning algorithm—consequently it is easy to warrant some additional computation to make better decisions. For more overview of the Bayesian optimization and a review of previous work, refer to [17]. Mathematically, in view of the problem of discovering a global maximizer (or minimizer) of an unrecognized objective function f

$$X^* = argmax_{x \epsilon X} f(x) \tag{1}$$

Where X is selected design area of interest; within global optimization, X is frequently a compact subset of R_d nevertheless the framework of Bayesian optimization can be stratified to more unusual search spaces that encompass conditional or categorical inputs, or even combinatorial search areas with various categorical inputs [18].

When performing Bayesian optimization, there are two main selections that must be made. Firstly a prior over functions must be selected that prompt assumptions about the function needed to be optimized. Gaussian process prior, is flexible and tractable. Then an acquisition function must be chosen. This function is used to build a utility function from the model posterior, letting us to determine which the next point to be evaluated is [19].

2.2.1 Gaussian Processes

The Gaussian Process (GP) is an appropriate and strength-full on the functions before distribution, the functions will be taken here to the form $f : X \longrightarrow R$ The GP is described by the characteristics or quality which is limited in size of N points $\{x_n \in X\}_{n=1}^{N}$ Persuade of a multifarious Gaussian distributed on R_n. The nth of these points is occupied to be operated value $f(x_n)$, and the properties of elegant marginalization for the Gaussian distribution permit us to calculate conditionals and marginals in closed form [19]. The properties and support of the distribution that resulted on functions are specified by a positive definite covariance function and a mean function.The properties and support of the resulting distribution on functions are specified by a mean function $m : X \longrightarrow R$ and a positive definite covariance function $K : X \times X \longrightarrow R$. For an overview of Gaussian processes, refer to [20]. The predictive covariance and mean under a GP can be respectively stated as:

$$\mu(x; \{x_n, y_n\}, \theta) = K(X, x)^T K(X, X)^{-1}(y - m(X)) \tag{2}$$

$$\sum(x, x'; \{x_n, y_n\}, \theta) = K(x, x') - K(X, x)^T K(X, X)^{-1} K(X, x') \tag{3}$$

At this point $K(X, x)$ is the vector of N-dimensional column of cross-covariances amongst x and the set X. The $N\chi N$ matrix $K(X, X)$ is the Gram matrix aimed at the set X [21].

2.2.2 Acquisition Functions for Bayesian Optimization

Assuming that the function $f(x)$ is drawn from a Gaussian process prior besides that the observations are formed with $\{x_n, y_n\}_{n=1}^{N}$, where $y_n \sim N(f(x_n, v)$ and v is the variance of noise announced into the observations of the function. These data and prior produce a posterior over functions; the acquisition function, which we symbolize by $a : X \longrightarrow R^+$, defines which point in X should be evaluated next through a proxy optimization $x_{next} = argmax_x a(x)$, where numerous diverse functions have been proposed. Generally, these acquisition functions rely on the GP hyperparameters as well as the previous observations; this dependence is denoted as $\sigma(x; \{x_n, y_n\}, \theta)$. There are a number of popular options of acquisition function. Under the Gaussian process prior, these functions rely on the model solely over predictive variance function $\mu(x; \{x_n, y_n\}, \theta)$ and its predictive mean function $\sigma^2(x; \{x_n, y_n\}, \theta))$. In the proceeding, the best current value is denoted as $x_{best} = argmin_{x_n} f(x_n)$ as well as the cumulative distribution function of the standard normal as $\Phi(.)$ [19].

Acquisition Function specifies the non-negative predictable refinement through the best observed objective value previously (symbolized f_{best})

$$EI(x|D) = \int_{f_{best}}^{\infty} (y - f_{best}) p(y|x, D) d_y \tag{4}$$

While Gaussian is the predictive distribution p $(y|x, D)$, $EI(x)$ has an appropriate closed form. A perfect Bayesian treatment of EI comprises integrating through parameters of the probabilistic regression model.

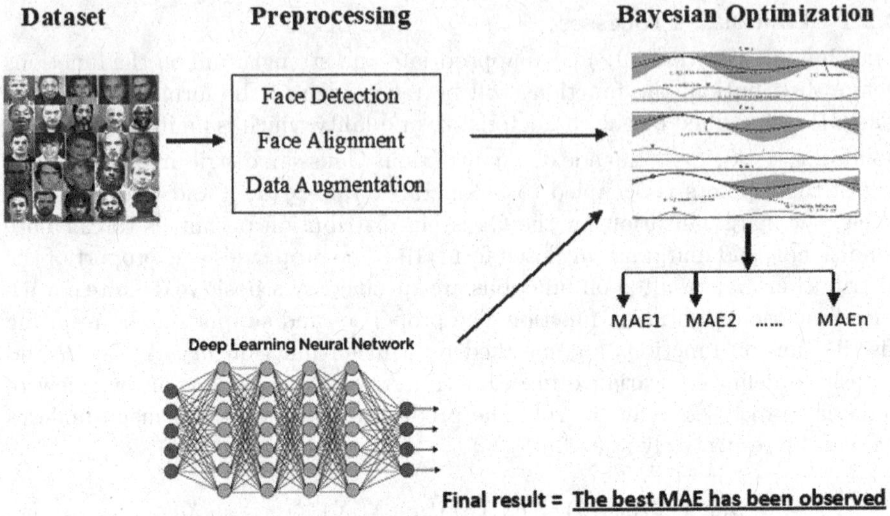

Fig. 1. Framework for the proposed system.

3 Bayesian Optimization with Deep Learning

In order to train CNN, the CNN architecture and options of the training algorithm must be specified firstly. The process of choosing and tuning these parameters is difficult and take long time. The algorithm of Bayesian Optimization (BO) is compatible to optimize internal parameters of regression and classification models. BO algorithm can be used to optimize functions that are discontinuous, non-differentiable, and time-consuming to evaluate. It maintains a Gaussian process model internally of the objective function. This objective functions is used to evaluate training this model. Bayesian optimization is applied to deep learning to find optimal training options and network parameters for CNNs. Figure 1 displays the framework of our proposed system, starting by preprocessing images, which includes Face detection, Face alignment and Data augmentation. Then BO uses the preprocessed data for training and testing through the CNN. This obtained in a number of results (n) which equals to the number of objectives that specified in the BO. Finally the best result that has been obtained from these n results is selected as the final result. The following steps present the details of the proposed system.

To apply Bayesian Optimization with deep learning there are some steps to follow:

1. Dataset Preprocessing for Network Training.
2. Specify the variables to be optimized using Bayesian optimization.
3. Define the objective function and the network architecture.
4. Perform Bayesian optimization.
5. Load the best network.

3.1 Dataset Preprocessing

At the beginning, all the images are aligned. For the alignment stage, the input coordinates which are the facial landmarks are used to warp and transform the image to an output coordinate space. The alignment depends on the position of the two eyes for all images. The alignment is done for MORPH only and failed for FG-NET and FERET datasets. After the face alignment, a face detection process is done using face++ Detector [22] to extract the face only without hair and other features that could be a noise. The MORPH dataset has three images the original image, aligned image, and detected image respectively. While the FG-NET and FERET datasets have two images the original image and the detected one. Finally all the detected faces are resized to 32 × 32 to fit the network for training. Except for MORPH dataset, the data have been resized to 110 × 110. Also, data augmentation is done for FG-NET and FERET dataset, because the data are limited. Data augmentation is used to acquire more data, by making minor alterations to the existing dataset. These minor changes are such as translations or flips or rotations. The augmented data is used for training to improve the results of deep learning.

Table 1. Selected variables for optimization.

Network depth	Momentum	Initial learn rate	L2 regularization
[1–3]	[0.8–0.95]	[1e-3 1e-1]	[1e-10 1e-2]

3.2 Select Variables for Optimization

The variables selected to be optimized are: The Network Depth, Momentum, Initial Learn Rate, and L2 Regularization as shown in Table 1. The Network depth controls the depth of the network. L2 regularization strength is used to prevent over-fitting. L2 is one of the most common types of regularization for Deep learning, that help in reducing overfitting to improve the results. Batch normalization and data augmentation also help regularize the network. The best initial learning rate can depend on the data and the network used. These variables are the parameters of the network architecture as well as options of the training algorithm.

3.3 Objective Function for Optimization

The objective function is defined. Its inputs are the values of the optimization variables that illustrates in Table 1 as well as the training and testing data. This function states the network architecture that will be used for training and specifies the training options. Our Network consists of six convolution layers, which depends on Network variable of Bayesian. Then training and validating this network is involved in this objective function. For every time that the training is done, the objective function saves the trained network to disk.

3.4 Bayesian Optimization

Bayesian optimization is performed, which minimizes the classification error on the validation set. The objective function trains a convolutional neural network and returns the classification error on the validation set. It uses the error rate to choose the best model. The final selected model is tested on the test set to estimate the MAE. The maximum number of objective function evaluations is specified by 25, and the maximum total optimization time is set to eight hours for FG-NET and FERET datasets. All networks are trained on a single GPU (NIVIDIA GeForce 840M) with 2 GB RAM.

3.5 Final Network Evaluation

To evaluate the final network, the best network has been loaded and evaluated on the test set to obtain the MAE result.

4 Results and Discussions

Performance of Bayesian optimization with deep learning was evaluated by testing its ability to estimate ages.

4.1 Datasets

Three facial benchmark datasets are used is this experiment. MORPH [23] is the most commonly used benchmark dataset for deep learning in age estimation. It is a group of mugshot images, containing metadata for race, date of birth, gender, and date of acquisition. It consists of 55K facial images which ranges from 16 to 76 for 13,000 subjects. FG-NET [24] is the second benchmark dataset for facial age estimation. It contains 1002 images with ages between 0–69. Nevertheless over 50% of the subjects are aged between 0 and 13. FERET [25] dataset is used by many researchers for age estimation. It consists of 2366 facial images of 994 subjects. The age range is between 10 and 70.

4.2 Evaluation Metrics

Mean Absolute Error:
This paper uses MAE to evaluate the performance of the age estimation model. MAE is used to measure the error between the groundtruth and predicted age, which is computed as in Eq. (5). Where y and y' mean predicted and groundtruth age value, respectively, and N indicates the number of the testing samples

$$\epsilon = \frac{1}{N} \sum_{i=1}^{N} \mid y'_i - y_i \mid \tag{5}$$

4.3 Results Comparisons

For evaluation on the MORPH dataset, according to the settings in selected previous works on age estimation [26–28], this paper randomly take 54,362 samples of ages from 16 to 66. Then these selected samples are split into two groups: 80% of the samples used for training the network and the 20% for testing. For these two sets, there is no overlapping. This paper repeat five runs independently, and the performance of the five runs has been averaged to obtain the final performance evaluation during experiments. The quantitative results is summarized in Table 2. We compare DLOB with other deep learning models for age estimation. Since the experiments done on the MORPH dataset and the same setting is followed in this paper for data partition, a direct comparison of the MAE of DLOB with the ones resulted by these deep learner can be done. As displayed in this table, DLOB achieves comparable results compared to most of the current state-of-the-art results with 3.01 MAE.

Table 2. Comparison of maes with different state-of-the-art approaches on the morph dataset.

Deep learning-based methods	MAE
OR-CNN [27]	3.34
MR-CNN [27]	3.27
DEX [15]	3.25
GoogLeNet [29]	3.13
Ranking-CNN (without pretraining) [30]	3.03
Ranking-CNN [30]	2.96
Proposed	**3.01**

For FG-NET leave one person out (LOPO) is employed for evaluation protocol as in previous works. This paper selected facial images of one person randomly for testing purpose, and the facial images of the remaining subjects for training. This procedure is repeated for 82 folds to evaluate BO. Eventually the average of the 82 folds results is approved as the final age estimation results. The quantitative results is summarized in Table 3. As shown in the table, DLOB achieves superior results compared to all the current state-of-the-arts. And this is the first time that a MAE error below 3.0 is obtained on FG-NET dataset.

For FERET dataset a 10-Fold cross-validation is performed as in [32]. Specifically, the whole dataset is divided into ten folds with equal size for each fold. Nine folds are used for training and the remaining fold for testing. This process is repeated ten times and the final age estimation result is the average of the ten results. The quantitative results is summarized in Table 4. As presented in the table, DLOB achieves superior results compared to all the previous state-of-the-art results on FERET. Note that, it is the only paper used deep learning with FERET and has a MAE error below 2.0 on FERET dataset.

Table 3. Comparison of maes with different state-of-the-art approaches on the FG-NET dataset.

Deep learning-based methods	MAE
DEX [15]	4.63
Ranking-CNN [30]	4.13
GA-DFL [31]	3.93
DRFs [32]	3.85
ODL + OHRanker [32]	3.89
ODL [32]	3.71
Proposed	**2.88**

Table 4. Comparison of maes with different state-of-the-art approaches on the FG-NET dataset.

Deep learning-based methods	MAE
MAP [33]	4.87
HAP [34]	3.02
MAR [35]	3.0
Proposed	**1.3**

5 Conclusions and Future Work

In this paper Bayesian optimization is applied to deep learning for the first time in age estimation field. It is used to select the optimal training options and network parameters for CNNs. The experimental results show that Bayesian Optimization with deep learning obtains better results compared with the state-of-the-arts, using the FG-NET and FERET datasets with a MAE of 2.88 and 1.3 respectively. Furthermore, achieves comparable results to the state-of-the-art methods on MORPH dataset with MAE of 3.01. Future works involve using images with larger size and pre-trained the network in WIKI-datasets before applying the DLOB on the benchmarks datasets. Also to ensemble this classifier with other CNNs classifiers that obtains good results to improve the performance of age estimation system.

References

1. Lin, C.-T., Li, D.-L., Lai, J.-H., Han, M.-F., Chang, J.-Y.: Automatic age estimation system for face images. Int. J. Adv. Robot. Syst. **9**(5), 216 (2012)
2. Grd, P.: Introduction to human age estimation using face images. Research Papers Faculty of Materials Science and Technology Slovak University of Technology, vol. 21, no. Special Issue, pp. 24–30 (2013)
3. Moćkus, J., Tiesis, V., Źilinskas, A.: The application of Bayesian methods for seeking the extremum, vol. 2 (1978)

4. Jones, D.R.: A taxonomy of global optimization methods based on response surfaces. J. Glob. Optim. **21**(4), 345–383 (2001)
5. Wan, J., et al.: Deep learning for content-based image retrieval: a comprehensive study. In: Proceedings of the 22nd ACM international conference on Multimedia, pp. 157–166. ACM (2014)
6. LeCun, Y., Bottou, L., Bengio, Y., Haffner, P.: Gradient-based learning applied to document recognition. Proc. IEEE **86**(11), 2278–2324 (1998)
7. Zeiler, M.D.: Hierarchical convolutional deep learning in computer vision. Ph.D. thesis, New York University (2013)
8. Sun, Y., Wang, X., Tang, X.: Deep learning face representation from predicting 10,000 classes. In: Proceedings of the IEEE Conference on Computer Vision and Pattern Recognition, pp. 1891–1898 (2014)
9. Sun, Y., Chen, Y., Wang, X., Tang, X.: Deep learning face representation by joint identification-verification. In: Advances in Neural Information Processing Systems, pp. 1988–1996 (2014)
10. Sun, Y., Wang, X., Tang, X.: Deep convolutional network cascade for facial point detection. In: Proceedings of the IEEE Conference on Computer Vision and Pattern Recognition, pp. 3476–3483 (2013)
11. Zhang, Z., Luo, P., Loy, C.C., Tang, X.: Facial landmark detection by deep multi-task learning. In: Fleet, D., Pajdla, T., Schiele, B., Tuytelaars, T. (eds.) ECCV 2014. LNCS, vol. 8694, pp. 94–108. Springer, Cham (2014). https://doi.org/10.1007/978-3-319-10599-4_7
12. Wang, X., Guo, R., Kambhamettu, C.: Deeply-learned feature for age estimation. In: 2015 IEEE Winter Conference on Applications of Computer Vision (WACV), pp. 534–541. IEEE (2015)
13. Dong, Y., Liu, Y., Lian, S.: Automatic age estimation based on deep learning algorithm. Neurocomputing **187**, 4–10 (2016)
14. Gurpinar, F., Kaya, H., Dibeklioglu, H., Salah, A.: Kernel elm and CNN based facial age estimation. In: Proceedings of the IEEE Conference on Computer Vision and Pattern Recognition Workshops, pp. 80–86 (2016)
15. Rothe, R., Timofte, R., Van Gool, L.: Deep expectation of real and apparent age from a single image without facial landmarks. Int. J. Comput. Vis. **126**(2–4), 144–157 (2018)
16. Qiu, J., et al.: Convolutional neural network based age estimation from facial image and depth prediction from single image (2016)
17. Brochu, E., Cora, V.M., De Freitas, N.: A tutorial on bayesian optimization of expensive cost functions, with application to active user modeling and hierarchical reinforcement learning. arXiv preprint arXiv:1012.2599 (2010)
18. Shahriari, B., Swersky, K., Wang, Z., Adams, R.P., De Freitas, N.: Taking the human out of the loop: a review of Bayesian optimization. Proc. IEEE **104**(1), 148–175 (2016)
19. Snoek, J., Larochelle, H., Adams, R.P.: Practical Bayesian optimization of machine learning algorithms. In: Advances in Neural Information Processing Systems, pp. 2951–2959 (2012)
20. Williams, C.K., Rasmussen, C.E.: Gaussian processes for machine learning, vol. 2. The MIT Press, Cambridge (2006). no. 3, p. 4
21. Swersky, K., Snoek, J., Adams, R.P.: Multi-task Bayesian optimization. In: Advances in Neural Information Processing Systems, pp. 2004–2012 (2013)
22. Zhou, E., Fan, H., Cao, Z., Jiang, Y., Yin, Q.: Extensive facial landmark localization with coarse-to-fine convolutional network cascade. In: Proceedings of the IEEE International Conference on Computer Vision Workshops, pp. 386–391 (2013)

23. Ricanek, K., Tesafaye, T.: MORPH: a longitudinal image database of normal adult age-progression. In: 7th International Conference on Automatic Face and Gesture Recognition, FGR 2006, pp. 341–345. IEEE (2006)
24. Panis, G., Lanitis, A., Tsapatsoulis, N., Cootes, T.F.: Overview of research on facial ageing using the FG-NET ageing database. IET Biometrics **5**(2), 37–46 (2016)
25. Phillips, P.J., Moon, H., Rizvi, S.A., Rauss, P.J.: The feret evaluation methodology for face-recognition algorithms. IEEE Trans. Pattern Anal. Mach. Intell. **22**(10), 1090–1104 (2000)
26. Chen, K., Gong, S., Xiang, T., Change Loy, C.: Cumulative attribute space for age and crowd density estimation. In: Proceedings of the IEEE Conference on Computer Vision and Pattern Recognition, pp. 2467–2474 (2013)
27. Niu, Z., Zhou, M., Wang, L., Gao, X., Hua, G.: Ordinal regression with multiple output CNN for age estimation. In: Proceedings of the IEEE Conference on Computer Vision and Pattern Recognition, pp. 4920–4928 (2016)
28. Shen, W., Guo, Y., Wang, Y., Zhao, K., Wang, B., Yuille, A.: Deep regression forests for age estimation. In: 2018 IEEE/CVF Conference on Computer Vision and Pattern Recognition, pp. 2304–2313. IEEE (2018)
29. Hu, Z., Wen, Y., Wang, J., Wang, M., Hong, R., Yan, S.: Facial age estimation with age difference. IEEE Trans. Image Process. **26**(7), 3087–3097 (2017)
30. Chen, S., Zhang, C., Dong, M.: Deep age estimation: from classification to ranking. IEEE Trans. Multimed. **20**(8), 2209–2222 (2018)
31. Liu, H., Lu, J., Feng, J., Zhou, J.: Group-aware deep feature learning for facial age estimation. Pattern Recogn. **66**, 82–94 (2017)
32. Liu, H., Lu, J., Feng, J., Zhou, J.: Ordinal deep learning for facial age estimation. IEEE Trans. Circ. Syst. Video Technol. **29**, 486–501 (2017)
33. Ng, C.-C., Yap, M.H., Costen, N., Li, B.: Will wrinkle estimate the face age? In: 2015 IEEE International Conference on Systems, Man, and Cybernetics (SMC), pp. 2418–2423. IEEE (2015)
34. Ng, C.-C., Yap, M.H., Cheng, Y.-T., Hsu, G.-S.: Hybrid ageing patterns for face age estimation. Image and Vision Comput. **69**, 92–102 (2018)
35. Ng, C.-C., Cheng, Y.-T., Hsu, G.-S., Yap, M.H.: Multi-layer age regression for face age estimation. In: 2017 Fifteenth IAPR International Conference on Machine Vision Applications (MVA), pp. 294–297. IEEE (2017)

Female Facial Beauty Analysis Using Transfer Learning and Stacking Ensemble Model

Elham Vahdati(✉) and Ching Y. Suen

CENPARMI, Department of Computer Science and Software Engineering, Concordia University, Montreal, QC H3G 1M8, Canada
g_vahdat@encs.concordia.ca, suen@cse.concordia.ca

Abstract. Automatic analysis of facial beauty has become an emerging research topic in recent years and has fascinated many researchers. One of the key challenges of facial attractiveness prediction is to obtain accurate and discriminative face representation. This study provides a new framework to analyze the attractiveness of female faces using transfer learning methodology as well as stacking ensemble model. Specifically, a pre-trained Convolutional Neural Network (CNN) originally trained on relatively similar datasets for face recognition task, namely Ms-Celeb-1M and VGGFace2, is utilized to acquire high-level and robust features of female face images. This is followed by leveraging a stacking ensemble model which combines the predictions of several base models to predict the attractiveness of a face. Extensive experiments conducted on SCUT-FBP and SCUT-FBP 5500 benchmark datasets, confirm the strong robustness of the proposed approach. Interestingly, prediction correlations of 0.89 and 0.91 are achieved by our new method for SCUT-FBP and SCUT-FBP5500 datasets, respectively. This would indicate significant advantages over the other state-of-the-art work. Moreover, our successful results would certainly support the efficacy of transfer learning when applying deep learning techniques to compute facial attractiveness.

Keywords: Facial beauty analysis · Stacking ensemble model · VGGFace2

1 Introduction

The importance of facial beauty has become more evident in recent years, and people tend to spend a considerable amount of money and time on plastic aesthetic surgeries and cosmetic products to attain more attractive faces [1–3]. Facial beauty topic has attracted the attention of researchers from several fields, such as computer science as well as medical and human sciences [1, 2]. With the rapid development of machine learning techniques, there is a great interest in analyzing facial attractiveness objectively. The secrets of facial beauty give researchers an incentive to develop computational algorithms to measure facial attractiveness from face images and their characteristics.

Automatic analysis of facial beauty has many applications, some are related to aesthetic plastic surgery and orthodontics, facial make-up synthesis/recommendation, recommendation systems in social networks and facial image beatification [1–4]. It is

F. Karray et al. (Eds.): ICIAR 2019, LNCS 11663, pp. 255–268, 2019.
https://doi.org/10.1007/978-3-030-27272-2_22

noteworthy that the discriminative face representation is considered as one of the essential problem of facial attractiveness prediction. The face representations presented in the existing works fall into three categories including feature-based, holistic as well as hybrid techniques [2]. With the help of these approaches, the most useful data from a huge amount of information provided by face images can be extracted. In order to represent a face, feature-based approach encompasses a wide range of features, namely geometric, color, texture as well as other local structural features [2]. The widespread use of feature-based approach can be observed in existing works. In particular, geometric features are the most significantly used features in face attractiveness research studies. Nevertheless, it should be noted that accurate manual localization of prominent facial landmarks is essential for the extraction of geometric features. This would definitely result in more manual involvement. Even though in some research studies landmarks were chosen automatically, some landmark coordinates needed to be manually adjusted when the coordinates were not accurate. Moreover, their experimental results indicate that the shallow predictors with these heuristic hand-crafted features would definitely impose restrictions on the attractiveness prediction performance, to some extent. Furthermore, holistic techniques are employed by researchers where features are extracted from the whole face [1, 2]. The keystone of holistic techniques is that the appearance information of faces is automatically acquired without any manual effort [2]. Additionally, hybrid representation which integrates the aforementioned features (i.e. feature-based and holistic) is expected to enhance the performance of facial beauty analysis.

Recently, Convolutional Neural Networks (CNNs) have proven to be a powerful tool for facial attractiveness computation task [5–12]. With the help of deep learning methods, especially CNNs, high-level features of face images are automatically extracted instead of traditional geometric features. This would definitely alleviate the problem of manual intervention. In fact, up-to-date deep learning methods (CNNs) possess the ability to extract hierarchical and high-level features which are of paramount importance for tasks which involve analyzing human faces. Considering that our training data are not extensive, transfer learning methodology would definitely be of significant help in overcoming this challenge. Transfer learning would certainly be a feasible solution when researchers are provided with insufficient ground truth. In this paper, we develop a new framework which has advantages in learning accurate and discriminative face representation to assess face attractiveness. This study employs a very deep architecture pre-trained on large-sized face datasets, as a feature extractor. Interestingly, deep features learned by the pre-trained CNN, are mapped to an attractiveness score using a stacked ensemble model, which is also a combination of different regression models.

There are two innovative points which have made our proposed method successful. First, the state-of-the-art deep learning-based feature extractor, namely ResNet-50 first trained on MS-Celeb-1M dataset and then fine-tuned on VGGFace2 dataset (hereinafter "VGGFace2_ft (ResNet)"), is employed to acquire high-level and robust features of facial images. It is worth mentioning that in an attempt to reduce the difference between the source task and target task (our task) in transfer learning scheme, this study exploits a very deep architecture (with 50 layers) which is pre-trained on massive face datasets spanning 10 M and 3.31 M face images, respectively. This is the first time to employ a very deep CNN pre-trained on massive face datasets merely as a feature extractor in facial attractiveness computation task. Second, inspired by the fact that the performance of an ensemble framework combining multiple models would certainly be superior to that of individual ones, a stacking ensemble model is considered in this paper. Said differently, this study reinforces the importance of stacking ensemble model on CNN features.

The remainder of this paper is organized as follows. Related works are presented in Sect. 2. Section 3 presents transfer learning, feature extraction as well as regression technique which are leveraged in this study. In Sect. 4, the face image datasets employed in the tests and the evaluation of the method are introduced and also the experimental results are analyzed and discussed. Finally, Sect. 5 concludes the paper by summarizing the main findings and perspectives on future works.

2 Related Work

Previous facial attractiveness research studies demonstrate that both face representations and prediction models are of key importance for automatic analysis of facial beauty. Geometric features have been extensively used in facial beauty research studies. Besides geometric features [6, 13–15], other handcrafted features, namely texture [6, 16], skin smoothness indicators [13, 14] as well as color [13, 14] have been utilized in some existing work. Furthermore, some researchers have assessed facial beauty using holistic descriptors such as Eigen faces [13]. Afterwards, these low-level features have been fed to traditional machine learning algorithms to construct a face attractiveness predictor. It is worth noting that both regression and classification techniques can be applied to the facial beauty analysis task.

Interestingly, state-of-the-art deep learning techniques have recently achieved great success in analyzing facial attractiveness owing to the fact that high-level and discriminative features learned from these techniques are of great value for face analysis. The work of Xie et al. [6] developed a CNN with six convolutional layers for facial beauty prediction, and their successful results indicate a good correlation between the human scores and the predictor outputs. The authors in [7] attempted to build a six-layer CNN model using a cascaded fine-tuning methodology. They employed several face input channels, namely face image, detail layer image as well as lighting layer image to enhance the performance of facial beauty predictor. Compared with the work of [6], they witnessed a higher performance. Furthermore, a psychologically inspired convolutional neural network utilized by Xu et al. [8].

Additionally, transfer learning scheme has proven to be significantly useful when applying deep learning techniques to the facial beauty prediction task. A very deep convolutional residual network (ResNet [17]) pre-trained on ImageNet dataset [18] has been utilized by Fan et al. [5]. Interestingly, the ideas of label distribution learning (LDL) and feature fusion have enriched their work. They have succeeded in achieving extremely successful results. Very recently, three CNN models pre-trained on the ImageNet dataset have been employed by Liang et al. [9] Furthermore, a VGG-Face model as well as Bayesian ridge regression technique have been used by Xu et al. [10] to assess facial beauty. Deep features have been extracted using a pre-trained CNN model for face recognition, namely the VGG-Face (VGG-16 Network) [19]. Moreover, ResNet-18 architecture has been utilized in the work of [11] where the network is divided into two branches for regression and classification tasks.

3 Automatic Analysis of Facial Attractiveness

Our approach includes two major steps. In the first step, female face images are fed into the pre-trained CNN, i.e. VGGFace2_ft (ResNet). This pre-trained CNN on two face datasets (i.e. MS-Celeb-1M [20] as well as VGGFace2 [21] datasets with 10 M and 3.31 M face images, respectively), performs as a feature extractor. Following this, the extracted features are passed to a stacking ensemble model. The main framework of our method is shown in Fig. 1.

a

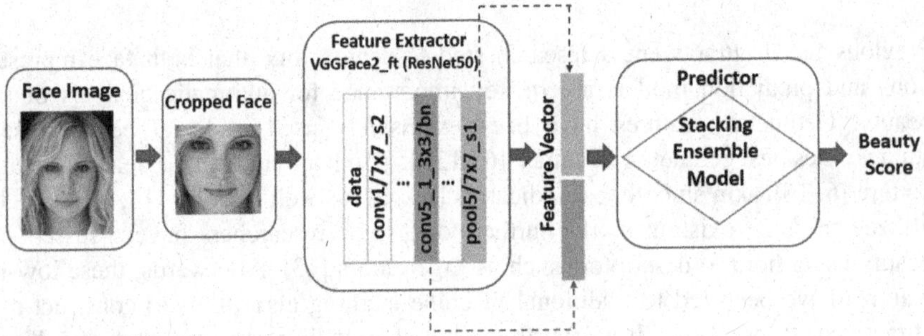

b

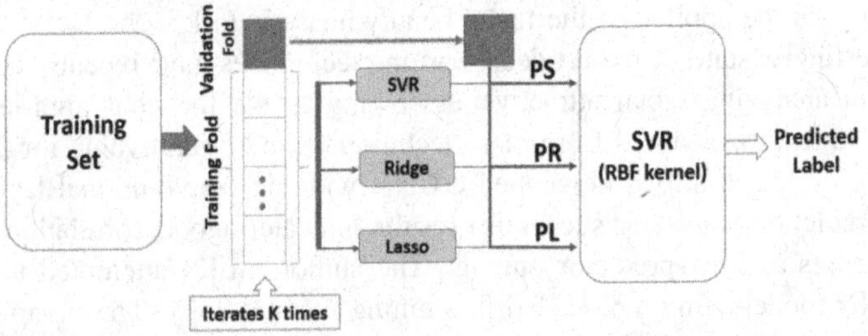

Fig. 1. (a) Framework of our method. (b) Framework of the stacking ensemble model.

It is notable that in Fig. 1(b), “PL”, “PS” and “PR” indicate predictions of Lasso, SVR (linear) and Ridge regression methods, respectively. Additionally, “k” denotes the number of folds in the cross validation scheme.

3.1 Transfer Learning and Deep Feature Extraction

Convolutional Neural Networks have been extensively used by researchers in recent years to create robust computational systems. Two different ways have been presented in recent works to exploit the power of CNNs. In the first method, the training can be performed using a large set of data. Furthermore, the transfer of learning using pre-trained networks has been introduced as the second approach. Therefore, when there are insufficient data to train CNNs from scratch, transfer learning would certainly provide an effective solution. Moreover, transfer learning can be an ideal solution to obviate the need for extensive computational and memory resources by transferring information acquired from the pre-trained CNNs. It is noteworthy that we adapt one of the most popular CNN architectures (i.e. ResNet) to our task through transfer learning. Residual Network developed by Kaiming He et al. [17] was the winner of ILSVRC 2015 classification task. Residual Network is composed of several residual blocks which provide shortcut connections between layers. These shortcut connections will equip researchers with substantially deep networks.

It should be noted that there are two different scenarios for the transfer learning process [22, 23]. In the first scenario, The CNN is leveraged as a fixed feature extractor. In fact, deep features can be extracted after eliminating the output layer. The following scenario involves fine-tuning the weights of the pre-trained network which can be accomplished by continuing backpropagation.

It is noteworthy that the first scenario is employed in this paper. This is because our dataset is small and similar to original dataset. Since our training data is small, it would not be a good idea to fine-tune the CNN (with 50 layers) owing to overfitting concerns. Moreover, our data is similar to the original data, as a result of which higher-level features in the pre-trained CNN would definitely be relevant to our face dataset. Said differently, weights from a face recognition task would certainly encode features specific to the face which are of great value for face attractiveness computation task. It should be noted that the feedforward phase of the VGGFace2_ft (ResNet-50) is performed only once to extract facial features.

As mentioned before, the training of CNNs requires a large set of images, while facial attractiveness computation task is struggling with the scarcity of sufficient training data. Therefore, transfer learning methodology is employed in this paper to alleviate this problem. It is worth mentioning that in order to reduce the difference between source domain and target domain in a transfer learning scheme, this study is equipped with a 50-layer ResNet pre-trained on massive face datasets, i.e. MS-Celeb-1M dataset [20] (including 10 M face images) and VGG-Face2 [21] (spanning 3.31 M face images). In this study the pre-trained ResNet performs as a feature extractor, and the features can be extracted from different layers by experiment.

We fuse semantically rich features from "pool5/7×7_s1" (i.e. global average pooling layer before the output layer of ResNet50) and features from "conv5_1_3×3/bn" layer (i.e. convolutional layer 5_1 followed by batch normalization). Interestingly, intermediate layers would certainly encompass features that are less specific to the original dataset utilized to train the CNN. Since the extracted features are high-dimensional, Principal Component Analysis (PCA) is employed for dimensionality reduction.

3.2 Stacking Ensemble Model

Stacking is a general procedure that involves combining multiple predictive models via a meta-model [24–26]. The first-level learners are created by employing different learning algorithms. First, the original training set is utilized to train first-level base models. Afterwards, the outputs of multiple predictive models (base models) are merged so that they can be considered as input features for the second-level model (meta-model). This means that a new dataset is generated for training the second-level model, where the outputs of the first-level learners and the original labels constitute input features and labels, respectively. Furthermore, in the training process of stacking, a cross-validation scheme is employed to avoid overfitting. Said differently, training examples which are leveraged to generate the new dataset for meta-learner should be eliminated from the training instances for the first-level base models [26].

As illustrated in Fig. 1(b), the training phase of stacking can be described as follows:

Step 1. Split the total training set into two disjointed parts, namely validation and training folds.
Step 2. Train every first-level base model (i.e. linear SVR, Ridge and Lasso) on the training fold and test them on validation fold.
Step 3. Employ predictions on validation fold as input features and also targets (original labels) as outputs to train the second-level learner called meta-model (RBF-SVR here).
Step 4. Repeat steps 1-3 iteratively so that the entire training data can be leveraged to make out-of-fold predictions.

In this study, three popular regression algorithms have been selected in the first level of the stacking model, namely Support Vector Regression (SVR) [27, 28], Lasso [29] as well as Ridge regression [30]. Moreover, SVR with a Radial Basis Function (RBF) kernel is considered as a meta-regressor (see Fig. 1(b)). Lasso regression technique is formulated as the following:

$$\min_{\omega} \|y - X\omega\|_2^2 + \alpha.\|\omega\|_1 \tag{1}$$

where $y \in R^n$ denotes the average scores (the ground-truth score labels) for n faces, and $X \in R^{n \times d}$ is the feature matrix (each row of this matrix represents a single face) [31]. Moreover, ω denotes the model weights to be optimized. The objective is to minimize the above equation where the first term quantifies how the model fits the training data, and the regularization term ($\alpha.\|\omega\|_1$) is used to prevent model from overfitting. It should be noted that Lasso applies the L1 norm of ω, while Ridge applies the L2 norm of ω. Therefore, Lasso and Ridge are also referred to as applying L1 and L2 regularization, respectively. The strength of the regularization term can be controlled by α.

Given the set of n training data $\{(x_i, y_i), 1 \leq i \leq n\}$, where $x_i \in R^m$ denotes the m extracted features and $y_i \in R$ is the ground-truth score label for the ith face. The aim of support vector regression (SVR) algorithm is to solve the following optimization problem:

$$\min_{w,b,\xi,\xi^*} \frac{1}{2}\|w\|^2 + C\sum\nolimits_{i=1}^{n} (\xi_i + \xi_i^*) \tag{2}$$

subject to

$$y_i - \langle w, x_i \rangle - b \le \varepsilon + \xi_i$$

$$\langle w, x_i \rangle + b - y_i \le \varepsilon + \xi_i^*$$

$$\xi_i^*, \xi_i \ge 0, \quad i = 1, 2, \ldots, n$$

where w is the weight vector and b is the bias. Moreover, $\langle .,. \rangle$ denotes the dot product. Slack variables (ξ_i^*, ξ_i) are introduced to measure the deviation of training data from ε-insensitive zone. Furthermore, C is the regularization parameter which determines the trade-off between the model complexity and the empirical error. It should be noted that for nonlinear regression problems, a nonlinear function is used to map the input training data to a higher dimensional space in which a linear model can be learned and solved.

4 Experimental Results

4.1 Experimental Setup and Dataset Description

The Caffe framework [32] is utilized to extract deep features using a publically available pre-trained CNN model for face recognition task (i.e. a ResNet-50 model trained on MS-Celeb-1M and then fine-tuned on VGGFace2 dataset) [33]. Moreover, Scikit-learn [34] and MLxtend [35] libraries in Python are used to implement regression techniques. The hyper-parameter α, which controls the strength of the regularization, is set to 1 and 0.1 for linear Ridge and Lasso regression techniques, respectively. Moreover, K = 5 is selected in the ensemble model.

To assess the performance of our proposed method, female face images of two benchmark datasets, namely SCUT-FBP [6] and SCUT-FBP5500 [9], have been utilized in this study. The former includes only female facial images. Approximately 70 human raters were asked to assign attractiveness scores to 500 images of Asian female faces. The latter recently introduced by Liang et al. [9] contains 5500 facial images of different gender and races. This dataset is composed of four subsets including Asian (2000 females and 2000 males) as well as Caucasian (750 females and 750 males). In this study, only female faces are used. These face images were labelled by 60 human raters. It is noteworthy that in both datasets, each facial image was rated with integer numbers ranging from 1 to 5, which means "1" is most unattractive and "5" is extremely attractive. It should be noted that the ground truth is the average scores for each facial image.

To evaluate our predictor model, a 5-fold cross validation technique is performed where 80% of the facial images are randomly selected as the training set, and the remaining 20% of face images as the testing set. Furthermore, three prediction metrics, i.e. Pearson Correlation (PC), Root Mean Squared Error (RMSE) and Mean Absolute

Error (MAE), are employed to assess the efficacy of the automatic rater. Pearson Correlation of $(x_1, x_2, \ldots, x_n)$ and $(y_1, y_2, \ldots, y_n)$ is defined as [3]:

$$r_{x,y} = \frac{\sum_{i=1}^{n} (x_i - \bar{x})(y_i - \bar{y})}{\left[\sum_{i=1}^{n} (x_i - \bar{x})^2 \sum_{i=1}^{n} (y_i - \bar{y})^2\right]^{\frac{1}{2}}} \quad (3)$$

where $x_1, x_2, \ldots, x_n$ are the ground-truth scores (the average ratings) and $y_1, y_2, \ldots, y_n$ are the predicted scores. Additionally, $\bar{x}$ and $\bar{y}$ denote the mean values of $(x_1, x_2, \ldots, x_n)$ and $(y_1, y_2, \ldots, y_n)$, respectively. Moreover, "r" ranges from −1 to 1, where 1, 0 and −1 represent the strongest positive linear correlation, no correlation and the strongest negative linear correlation, respectively. Moreover, Mean Absolute Error (MAE) and Root Mean Squared Error (RMSE) are given by:

$$\mathrm{MAE} = \frac{1}{n} \sum_{i=1}^{n} |y_i - x_i| \quad (4)$$

$$\mathrm{RMSE} = \sqrt{\frac{1}{n} \sum_{i=1}^{n} (y_i - x_i)^2} \quad (5)$$

Interestingly, higher values of Pearson correlation as well as smaller errors would certainly be derived from more accurate predictions.

4.2 Experiments on the SCUT-FBP Dataset

After face cropping, RGB facial images (224 × 224) are fed into the pre-trained CNN model to extract features from "pool5/7×7_s1" (i.e. layer before the output layer) and "conv5_1_3×3/bn" layers (i.e. convolutional layer 5_1 followed by batch normalization). Table 1 indicates the performance of individual layers as well as their fusion using the SCUT-FBP dataset. In comparison with pooling layer, superior results are achieved by conv5_1. This is because lower layers encompass features that are less specific to the original dataset utilized to train the CNN. Furthermore, it can be observed that feature fusion would lead to a higher performance. As a result, a concatenated vector of these two types of features is generated, following which Principal Component Analysis (PCA) is employed to reduce the vector's dimensionality. In this study, the number of face images in training set is also considered as the dimension of feature vector.

Table 1. Performance of individual layers as well as their fusion.

Dataset	Layer (type, name)	PC	MAE	RMSE
SCUT-FBP	Average pooling "pool5/7×7_s1"	0.8719	0.2573	0.3348
	Conv + BN "conv5_1_3×3/bn"	0.8762	0.2494	0.3245
	Combined	**0.8898**	**0.2409**	**0.3105**

Information in Table 2 would definitely enable us to obtain deeper insights into performance differences among different models for facial beauty prediction. The results of 5-fold cross validation in terms of PC, MAE and RMSE are indicated in Table 2. It can be observed that the stacked ensemble model outperforms other regression methods (with the highest average Pearson Correlation of 0.8898). These experimental results can also support the fact that the performance of the ensemble model which combines multiple predictive models would certainly be superior to that of individual ones.

Table 2. Comparison of different models, in terms of PC, MAE and RMSE using 5-fold cross validation, on the SCUT-FBP dataset.

PC	1	2	3	4	5	**Average**
SVR	0.8642	0.8737	0.8714	0.9023	0.8688	0.8761
Ridge	0.8579	0.8647	0.8649	0.8958	0.8641	0.8695
Lasso	0.8832	0.8836	0.8596	0.9042	0.8617	0.8785
Stacked	0.8993	0.8906	0.8758	0.9062	0.8768	**0.8898**
MAE	1	2	3	4	5	Average
SVR	0.2503	0.2752	0.2611	0.2281	0.2593	0.2548
Ridge	0.2561	0.2864	0.2721	0.2314	0.2663	0.2625
Lasso	0.2382	0.2621	0.2654	0.2213	0.2696	0.2513
Stacked	0.2231	0.2544	0.2487	0.2314	0.2471	**0.2409**
RMSE	1	2	3	4	5	Average
SVR	0.3205	0.3404	0.3274	0.3040	0.3363	0.3257
Ridge	0.3267	0.3545	0.3388	0.3089	0.3447	0.3347
Lasso	0.3035	0.3239	0.3392	0.3153	0.3430	0.3250
Stacked	0.2811	0.3143	0.3217	0.3094	0.3260	**0.3105**

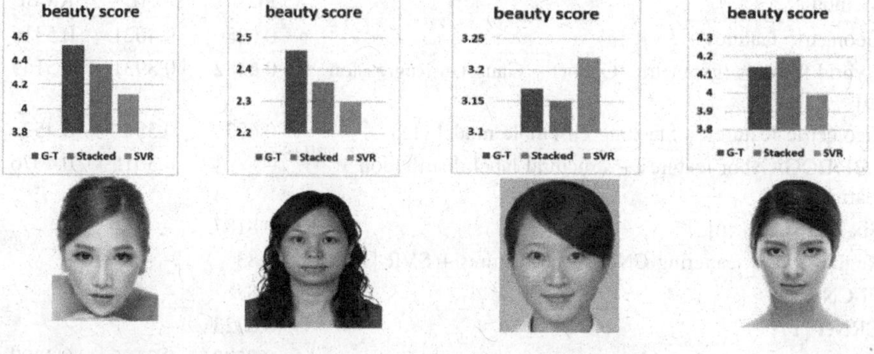

Fig. 2. Comparison of the face attractiveness prediction among ground-truth (G-T), SVR and the proposed stacked model. For each image, ground truth label, predicted score of our proposed stacked model and that of SVR are shown from left to right.

We randomly selected four facial images of the SCUT-FBP benchmark dataset with different levels of beauty. It is noteworthy that the beauty scores range in [1, 5], where beauty score "5" means most attractive. As shown in Fig. 2, it is easy to find that the predicted scores by our proposed method for these face images are highly correlated with the ground truth from human raters. Moreover, the predicted scores of the stacked model is closer to the ground truth scores than those of SVR.

Comparison with the State of the Art on the SCUT-FBP Benchmark Dataset
In order to demonstrate the robustness of our method, the results achieved by our approach are compared with other state-of-the-art methods on the SCUT-FBP benchmark dataset. A summary of the beauty prediction methods as well as their accuracy in existing works in terms of PC, MAE and RMSE are presented in Table 3. It is noteworthy that figures for MAE, RMSE or PC have not been reported by researchers in [6, 8, 11, 12, 16], as a result of which they are denoted with "–" in Table 3. Low-level features have been utilized by the first four works (the first four rows). It is interesting to know that the CNN-based methods have attained a superb performance, among which our model performs the best. It is noteworthy that deeper architectures could extract more discriminative features from face images to some extent.

It can be observed that the prediction accuracy derived from extracted CNN features by our method is significantly higher than those achieved from handcrafted features [6, 15]. It is noticeable that CNN features' superiority over geometric features is more evident, especially when comparing our results with those reported in [15]. Moreover, experimental results indicate that our method achieves the highest correlation of 0.8898, minimum MAE of 0.2409 and RMSE of 0.3105 among all the methods in Table 3. Our work gains benefit from transfer learning methodology as well as stacking ensemble model. In fact, the 50-layer ResNet (very deep architecture) pre-trained on about 13 million face images would definitely be capable of extracting more discriminative facial features.

Table 3. Performance comparison with the related state-of-the-art works on SCUT-FBP dataset.

Method	PC	MAE	RMSE
Geometric features + SVR [6]	0.6080	0.4021	0.5316
Hybrid features (geometric, Gabor) + Gaussian Regression [6]	0.6482	0.3931	0.5149
Geometric features + Stacking ensemble model [15]	0.693	0.334	0.452
LBP/HOG/Gabor features + structural label distribution learning [16]	–	0.3015	0.4076
Six-layer CNN [6]	0.8187	–	–
Region aware scattering CNN-based features + SVR [12]	0.83	–	–
PI-CNN [8]	0.87	–	–
CRNet [11]	0.8723	–	–
VGG-face + Bayesian ridge regression [10]	0.8570	0.2595	0.3397
VGGFace2_ft (ResNet) + Stacking ensemble model	**0.8898**	**0.2409**	**0.3105**

4.3 Experiments on the SCUT-FBP5500 Dataset

In this section, two subsets of different races of the SCUT-FBP5500, namely Asian and Caucasian female faces (with 2000 and 750 face images, respectively), are employed to conduct further experiments. Table 4 shows the results of 5-fold cross validation for both categories (Asian and Caucasian) and two models (SVR and stacked) in terms of PC, MAE and RMSE. Compared with SVR, better results are achieved by the ensemble model (the average Pearson Correlation of 0.9141 and 0.9112 for Asian and Caucasian females, respectively). It is noteworthy that similar results are achieved using 10-fold cross validation technique.

Table 4. Comparison of two models (SVR vs. Stacked), in terms of PC, MAE and RMSE using 5-fold cross validation for both Asian and Caucasian females in the SCUT-FBP5500 dataset.

PC	1	2	3	4	5	Average
Asian (SVR)	0.8944	0.8859	0.8989	0.8958	0.9040	0.8958
Asian (Stacked)	0.9054	0.9017	0.9196	0.9190	0.9248	**0.9141**
Caucasian (SVR)	0.9039	0.9018	0.9031	0.8995	0.9148	0.9046
Caucasian (Stacked)	0.9067	0.9152	0.9093	0.9098	0.9151	**0.9112**
MAE	1	2	3	4	5	Average
Asian (SVR)	0.2496	0.2558	0.2513	0.2497	0.2374	0.2488
Asian (Stacked)	0.2252	0.2280	0.2187	0.2149	0.2113	**0.2196**
Caucasian (SVR)	0.2418	0.2425	0.2443	0.2361	0.2302	0.2390
Caucasian (Stacked)	0.2322	0.2255	0.2365	0.2281	0.2299	**0.2304**
RMSE	1	2	3	4	5	Average
Asian (SVR)	0.3206	0.3259	0.3208	0.3203	0.3104	0.3196
Asian (Stacked)	0.2991	0.2995	0.2852	0.2827	0.2812	**0.2895**
Caucasian (SVR)	0.3111	0.3072	0.3168	0.3133	0.2817	0.3060
Caucasian (Stacked)	0.3063	0.2877	0.3029	0.2972	0.2815	**0.2951**

Moreover, experimental results on these two categories indicate that a significantly higher performance can be achieved using deep CNN features compared with geometric features (see Tables 5 and 6). This would mean that low-level geometric features are not sufficiently discriminative. Said differently, relatively poor results have been reported in the work of [9] for geometric features owing to the insufficient facial representation ability related to attractiveness. In fact, two main reasons why our method achieves a significant improvement over the other methods in Tables 5 and 6, are more-aesthetics-aware face representations and the utilization of stacking ensemble model which is capable of combining the predictions of the different learners to make the final attractiveness prediction.

Table 5. Beauty prediction using geometric and deep CNN features as well as different models for Asian females in the SCUT-FBP5500 dataset.

Method	PC	MAE	RMSE
Geometric features + LR [9]	0.6771	0.402	0.5246
Geometric features + GR [9]	0.7057	0.387	0.5057
Geometric features + SVR [9]	0.7008	0.3876	0.5089
VGGFace2_ft (ResNet) + SVR	0.8958	0.2488	0.3196
VGGFace2_ft (ResNet) + Stacking ensemble model	**0.9141**	**0.2196**	**0.2895**

Table 6. Beauty prediction using geometric and deep CNN features as well as different models for Caucasian females in the SCUT-FBP5500 dataset.

Method	PC	MAE	RMSE
Geometric features + LR [9]	0.6809	0.3986	0.5239
Geometric features + GR [9]	0.7263	0.3862	0.4908
Geometric features + SVR [9]	0.7093	0.4001	0.5087
VGGFace2_ft (ResNet) + SVR	0.9046	0.2390	0.3060
VGGFace2_ft (ResNet) + Stacking ensemble model	**0.9112**	**0.2304**	**0.2951**

5 Conclusion

To sum up, this paper describes an attractiveness computational model using a pre-trained CNN as a feature extractor. It can be concluded that transfer learning, which would definitely be a more time-saving and more effective strategy than training CNN from scratch, can be employed to extract high-level and robust features for facial attractiveness modeling. Furthermore, our superb experimental results demonstrate that it is worthwhile combining multiple regression algorithms using a stacking model for facial beauty assessment task. Remarkable results are obtained using a very deep CNN pre-trained on large-sized face datasets (i.e. MS-Celeb-1M as well as VGGFace2 datasets). It is important to note that using a deep architecture which is pre-trained on two datasets, spanning a wide range of face images, is of great benefit to facial beauty analysis task owing to the fact that the difference between the source task and target task (our task) will be considerably diminished. Since facial expressions and non-permanent features such as makeup exert a significant influence on attractiveness of a face, extending computer analysis of human beauty to these factors will be our next step. Another direction of our future work is to investigate 3D face attractiveness computation task which is of paramount importance for some applications especially for supporting aesthetic plastic surgery.

References

1. Laurentini, A., Bottino, A.: Computer analysis of face beauty: a survey. Comput. Vis. Image Underst. **125**, 184–199 (2014)
2. Liu, S., Fan, Y.-Y., Samal, A., Guo, Z.: Advances in computational facial attractiveness methods. Multimed. Tools Appl. **75**(23), 16633–16663 (2016)
3. Zhang, D., Chen, F., Xu, Y.: Computer Models for Facial Beauty Analysis. Springer International Publishing, Switzerland (2016)
4. Scherbaum, K., Ritschel, T., Hullin, M., Thormählen, T., Blanz, V., Seidel, H.-P.: Computer-suggested facial makeup. Comput. Graph. Forum **30**(2), 485–492 (2011)
5. Fan, Y.-Y., Liu, S., Li, B., Guo, Z., Samal, A., Wan, J.: Label distribution-based facial attractiveness computation by deep residual learning. IEEE Trans. Multimed. **20**(8), 2196–2208 (2018)
6. Xie, D., Liang, L., Jin, L., Xu, J., Li, M.: SCUT-FBP: A benchmark dataset for facial beauty perception. In: 2015 IEEE International Conference on Systems. Man, and Cybernetics, pp. 1821–1826. IEEE, Kowloon (2015)
7. Xu, J., Jin, L., Liang, L., Feng, Z., Xie, D.: A new humanlike facial attractiveness predictor with cascaded fine-tuning deep learning model. arXiv preprint arXiv:1511.02465 (2015)
8. Xu, J., Jin, L., Liang, L., Feng, Z., Xie, D., Mao, H.: Facial attractiveness prediction using psychologically inspired convolutional neural network (PI-CNN). In: 2017 IEEE International Conference on Acoustics, Speech and Signal Processing (ICASSP), pp. 1657–1661. IEEE, New Orleans (2017)
9. Liang, L., Lin, L., Jin, L., Xie, D., Li, M.: SCUT-FBP5500: a diverse benchmark dataset for multi-paradigm facial beauty prediction. In: 2018 24th International Conference on Pattern Recognition (ICPR), pp. 1598–1603. IEEE, Beijing (2018)
10. Xu, L., Xiang, J., Yuan, X.: Transferring rich deep features for facial beauty prediction. arXiv preprint arXiv:1803.07253 (2018)
11. Xu, L., Xiang, J., Yuan, X.: CRNet: classification and regression neural network for facial beauty prediction. In: Hong, R., Cheng, W.-H., Yamasaki, T., Wang, M., Ngo, C.-W. (eds.) PCM 2018. LNCS, vol. 11166, pp. 661–671. Springer, Cham (2018). https://doi.org/10.1007/978-3-030-00764-5_61
12. Liang, L., Xie, D., Jin, L., Xu, J., Li, M., Lin, L.: Region-aware scattering convolution networks for facial beauty prediction. In: 2017 IEEE International Conference on Image Processing (ICIP), pp. 2861–2865. IEEE, Beijing (2017)
13. Eisenthal, Y., Dror, G., Ruppin, E.: Facial attractiveness: beauty and the machine. Neural Comput. **18**(1), 119–142 (2006)
14. Kagian, A., Dror, G., Leyvand, T., Meilijson, I., Cohen-Or, D., Ruppin, E.: A machine learning predictor of facial attractiveness revealing human-like psychophysical biases. Vis. Res. **48**, 235–243 (2008)
15. Vahdati, E., Suen, C.Y.: A novel female facial beauty predictor. In: International Conference on Pattern Recognition and Artificial Intelligence (ICPRAI), Montreal, pp. 378–382 (2018)
16. Ren, Y., Geng, X.: Sense beauty by label distribution learning. In: Twenty-Sixth International Joint Conference on Artificial Intelligence (IJCAI-17), Melbourne, pp. 2648–2654 (2017)
17. He, K., Zhang, X., Ren, S., Sun, J.: Deep residual learning for image recognition. In: 2016 IEEE Conference on Computer Vision and Pattern Recognition (CVPR), pp. 770–778. IEEE, Las Vegas (2016)

18. Deng, J., Dong, W., Socher, R., Li, L.-J., Li, K., Fei-Fei, L.: Imagenet: a large-scale hierarchical image database. In: 2009 IEEE Conference on Computer Vision and Pattern Recognition, pp. 248–255. IEEE, Miami (2009)
19. Parkhi, O.M., Vedaldi, A., Zisserman, A.: Deep face recognition. In: British Conference on Machine Vision (BMVC), p. 6 (2015)
20. Guo, Y., Zhang, L., Hu, Y., He, X., Gao. J.: Ms-celeb-1m: a dataset and benchmark for large-scale face recognition. arXiv preprint arXiv:1607.08221 (2016)
21. Cao, Q., Shen, L., Xie, W., Parkhi, O.M., Zisserman, A.: VGGFace2: a dataset for recognising faces across pose and age. In: 2018 13th IEEE International Conference on Automatic Face & Gesture Recognition (FG 2018), pp. 67–74. IEEE, Xi'an (2018)
22. Zamzmi, G., Goldgof, D., Kasturi, R., Sun, Y.: Neonatal pain expression recognition using transfer learning. arXiv preprint arXiv:1807.01631 (2018)
23. Transfer Learning, CS231n Convolutional Neural Networks for Visual Recognition, Stanford University, http://cs231n.github.io/transfer-learning/. Accessed 17 Mar 2019
24. Wolpert, D.H.: Stacked generalization. Neural Netw. **5**(2), 241–259 (1992)
25. Breiman, L.: Stacked regressions. Mach. Learning **24**(1), 49–64 (1996)
26. Zhou, Z.H.: Ensemble Methods: Foundations and Algorithms. Chapman & Hall/CRC, Boca Raton (2012)
27. Drucker, H., Burges, C.J.C., Kaufman, L., Smola, A.J., Vapnik, V.: Support vector regression machines. Advances Neural Inform. Process. Syst. **9**, 155–161 (1997)
28. Smola, A.J., Schölkopf, B.: A tutorial on support vector regression. Stat. Comput. **14**(3), 199–222 (2004)
29. Tibshirani, R.: Regression shrinkage and selection via the lasso. J. R. Stat. Soc. B **58**(1), 267–288 (1996)
30. Hoerl, A.E., Kennard, R.W.: Ridge regression: biased estimation for nonorthogonal problems. Technometrics **12**(1), 55–67 (1970)
31. Mu, Y.: Computational facial attractiveness prediction by aesthetics-aware features. Neurocomputing **99**, 59–64 (2013)
32. Jia, Y., et al.: Caffe: convolutional architecture for fast feature embedding. In: 22nd ACM International Conference on Multimedia, pp. 675–678. ACM, Orlando (2014)
33. http://www.robots.ox.ac.uk/~vgg/data/vgg_face2/. Accessed 17 Mar 2019
34. Pedregosa, F., Varoquaux, G., Gramfort, A., Michel, V.: Scikit-learn: machine learning in python. J. Mach. Learn. Res. **12**, 2825–2830 (2011)
35. Raschka, S.: MLxtend: providing machine learning and data science utilities and extensions to Python's scientific computing stack. J. Open Source Softw. **3**(24), 638 (2018)

Investigating the Automatic Classification of Algae Using the Spectral and Morphological Characteristics via Deep Residual Learning

Jason L. Deglint[1,2], Chao Jin[1,3], and Alexander Wong[1,2](✉)

[1] Vision and Imaging Processing (VIP) Lab, Department of Systems Design Engineering, University of Waterloo, Waterloo, Ontario, Canada
jdeglint@uwaterloo.ca

[2] Waterloo Artificial Intelligence Institute, Waterloo, Ontario, Canada
a28wong@uwaterloo.ca

[3] School of Environmental Science and Engineering, Sun Yat-sen University, Guangzhou 510275, People's Republic of China

Abstract. Under the impact of global climate changes and human activities, harmful algae blooms (HABs) have become a growing concern due to negative impacts on water related industries, such as tourism, fishing and safe water supply. Many jurisdictions have introduced specific water quality regulations to protect public health and safety. Therefore reliable and cost effective methods of quantifying the type and concentration of algae cells has become critical for ensuring successful water management. In this work we present an innovative system to automatically classify multiple types of algae by combining standard morphological features with their multi-wavelength signals. To accomplish this we use a custom-designed microscopy imaging system which is configured to image water samples at two fluorescent wavelengths and seven absorption wavelengths using discrete-wavelength high-powered light emitting diodes (LEDs). We investigate the effectiveness of automatic classification using a deep residual convolutional neural network and achieve a classification accuracy of 96% in an experiment conducted with six different algae types. This high level of accuracy was achieved using a deep residual convolutional neural network that learns the optimal combination of spectral and morphological features. These findings illustrate the possibility of leveraging a unique fingerprint of algae cell (i.e. spectral wavelengths and morphological features) to automatically distinguish different algae types. Our work herein demonstrates that, when coupled with multi-band fluorescence microscopy, machine learning algorithms can potentially be used as a robust and cost-effective tool for identifying and enumerating algae cells.

Keywords: Algae · Neural networks · Microscopy · Image classification · Multispectral imaging · Supervised learning

F. Karray et al. (Eds.): ICIAR 2019, LNCS 11663, pp. 269–280, 2019.
https://doi.org/10.1007/978-3-030-27272-2_23

1 Introduction

As a result from eutrophication and climate change, harmful algae blooms (HABs) are increasing in frequency, magnitude and duration all around the globe [9]. For instance, Lake Erie, one of the great fresh water lakes in North America had severe blooms in 2011 [10] and 2014 [15]. The 2014 HAB in the Western Basin of Lake Erie resulted in a three-day tap water ban in Toledo, Ohio, affecting approximately half a million people [16]. As seen in Fig. 1, the 2011 bloom was primarily *Microcystis aeruginosa*, a toxic producing type of cyanobacteria [1]. Cyanobacteria can be extremely dangerous for humans and animals, as for example, swallowing *Microcystis* can have serious side effects such as abdominal pain, diarrhea, vomiting, blistered mouths, dry coughs, and headaches. In addition, *Anabaena*, another common cyanobacteria, can produce lethal neurotoxins called anatoxin-a which has shown to cause death by progressive respiratory paralysis [6].

One toxin produced by *Microcystis*, called microcystin-LR, is strictly regulated by the World Health Organization (WHO) as it is lethal for humans [12]. In Canada, the maximum acceptable concentration (MAC) for the cyanobacteria toxin microcystin-LR in drinking water is 0.0015 mg/L (1.5 μg/L) [3,8]. Therefore monitoring of water quality for different cyanobacteria and other micro-algae is essential for the proper management of any water body [4]. The preservation and maintenance of our water directly affects marine wildlife, as well as the recreational, fishing and tourism industries, and most importantly drinking

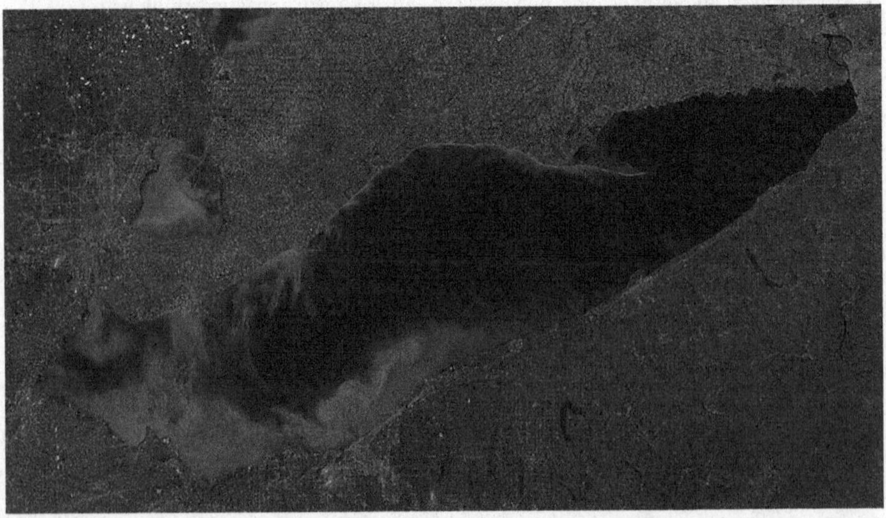

Fig. 1. The Moderate Resolution Imaging Spectroradiometer (MODIS) on the Aqua satellite showing Lake Erie on October 9, 2011. The bloom was primarily *Microcystis Aeruginosa*, according to the Great Lakes Environmental Research Laboratory, which is a common type of cyanobacteria [1].

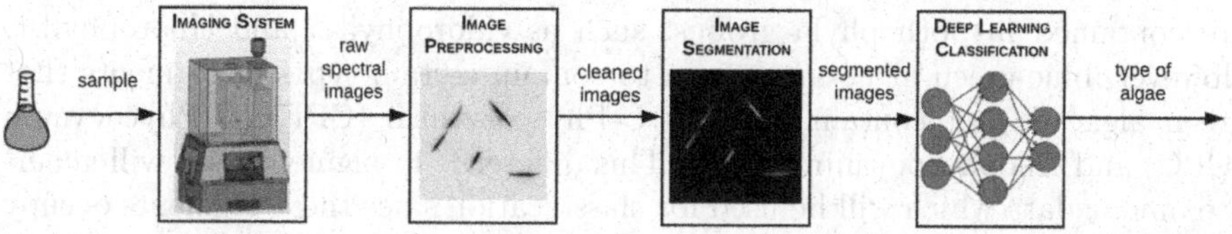

Fig. 2. The SAMSON system is divided into four steps. First, water samples (Sect. 2.1) are imaged using the hardware system (Sect. 2.2). This imaging data is then preprocessed (Sect. 3.1), and each organism is then segmented and cropped (Sect. 3.2). Finally a deep residual learning-based image classification method is used to classify the algae type (Sect. 3.3).

water treatments plants that ensure clean drinking water is distributed to the population.

The standard method of identifying and enumerating microalgae consists of three main steps which are: (1) sample preparation, (2) classification, and (3) enumerating. This current method of manual identification and enumeration by a taxonomist via a microscope is time consuming and can be tedious. Furthermore, each taxonomist requires specialised training and extensive experience to classify algae adequately [4]. Unfortunately the current method of algae identification is quickly becoming unsustainable as algae blooms are increasing in frequency and intensity around the world.

To tackle this challenge, this paper explores and investigates an alternative method for the potential use of on-site water monitoring via the introduction of novel computer vision and deep learning techniques into the **S**pectral **A**bsorption-fluorescence **M**icroscopy **S**ystem for **ON**-site-imaging (SAMSON) imaging system presented by Deglint *et al.* [5]. The proposed method presented here extends the capabilities of the SAMSON system presented in [5]. This proposed method is shown in Fig. 2 and is broken into four steps. First a water sample containing algae (Sect. 2.1) is imaged using the hardware system (Sect. 2.2). Together these two steps, preparing the water sample and imaging it, make up the data collection component (Sect. 2). Once having acquired the data, it can now be processed and analysed (Sect. 3). This can be broken into image preprocessing (Sect. 3.1), image segmentation (Sect. 3.2), and finally a novel deep residual learning-based image classification (Sect. 3.3).

2 Data Collection

The data collection requires two steps. First, pure algae samples must be prepared (Sect. 2.1) and then a given algae type must be imaged using the SAMSON system (Sect. 2.2) in order to build up database of algae images.

2.1 Algae Samples

The two algae groups focused on in this research were the Chlorophyta phylum (green algae) and the Cyanophyta phylum (blue-green algae). Certain pigments are contained in both phyla groups, such as chlorophyll-*a* and chlorophyll-*b*. However, blue-green algae are known to contain certain types of pigments that green algae do not contain, such as C-Phycoerythrin (CPE), C-Phycocyanin (CPC) and Allophycocyanin (APC). This difference in pigmentation will generate unique data which will be used for classification since these pigments occupy different parts of the electromagnetic spectrum and are known to absorb and fluoresce light differently [2].

The six pure samples of algae purchased from the Canadian Phycological Culture Centre (CPCC) were:

I. Cyanophyta (blue-green algae or cyanobacteria)
  1. *Microcystis aeruginosa* (CPCC 300)
  2. *Anabaena flos-aquae* (CPCC 067)
  3. *Pseudanabaena tremula* (CPCC 471)

II. Chlorophyta (green algae)
  4. *Scenedesmus obliquus* (CPCC 005)
  5. *Scenedesmus quadricauda* (CPCC 158)
  6. *Ankistrodesmus falcatus* (CPCC 366)

Microcystis aeruginosa and *Anabaena flos-aquae* where chosen as they are common culprits for producing toxins in a harmful algae bloom. *Pseudanabaena tremula* was chosen since it is filamentous type of algae, just like *Anabaena flos-aquae* and therefore may be difficult to distinguish the two types from each other.

2.2 Imaging System

The SAMSON system [5] was used to capture multispectral images of each algae type. This involved pipetting a subsample of a water sample containing a pure type of algae onto a standard 1" × 3" slide, then placing a coverslip over the subsample, and then placing this prepared slide into the hardware system to be imaged. A 3D render of SAMSON can be seen in Fig. 3. This 3D model houses the scientific camera, the optics required to focus and capture the light, a slide holder for the water sample, as well as LEDs and a custom printed circuit board (PCB) to control the LEDs.

For this research study the hardware system was configured to collect two fluorescent images and seven absorption images, however SAMSON can be configured for a variety of different wavelength combinations. The nine LEDs chosen to image the six previously mentioned algae samples are:

I. Fluorescent LED wavelengths
  1. 385 nm (ultraviolet)
  2. 405 nm (ultraviolet)

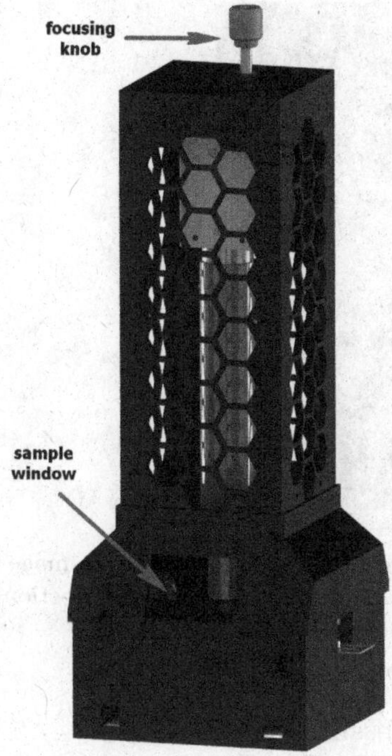

Fig. 3. The SAMSON hardware system, initially presented by Deglint *et al.* [5] is used to collect multispectral images of water samples containing algae. In this work the authors collect two fluorescent images and seven absorption images. The user places the water sample slide in the slide window. Then using custom software the user can view a live image of the sample and adjust the focus of the image using the focusing knob.

II. Absorption LED wavelengths:
 1. 465 nm (blue)
 2. 500 nm (cyan)
 3. 520 nm (green)
 4. 595 nm (amber)
 5. 620 nm (red-orange)
 6. 635 nm (red)
 7. 660 nm (deep-red)

3 Data Analysis

Having collected all the data it must now be preprocessed (Sect. 3.1), and then each organism in each multispectral image must be segmented and cropped (Sect. 3.2). Finally this new data can be used to construct a deep residual learning-based image classification system for classifying algae type (Sect. 3.3).

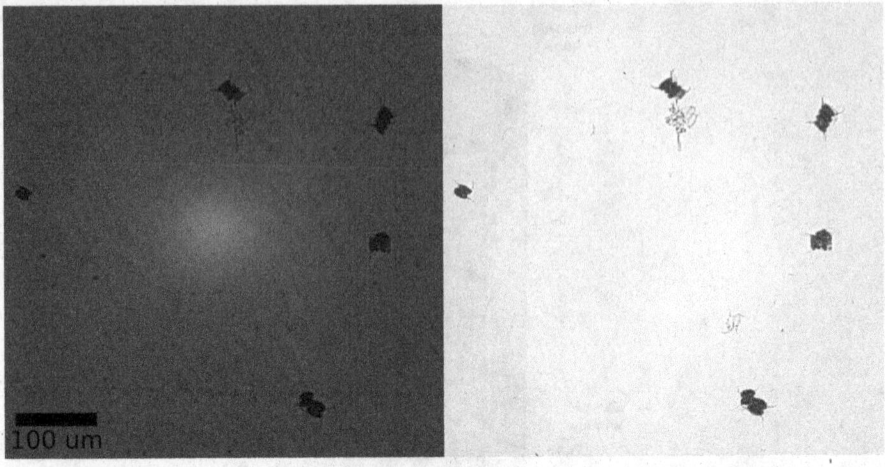

Fig. 4. Using flat field correction (Sect. 3.1), the raw image (left) from the hardware system is corrected (right). The result of flat field correction makes the task of image segmentation (Sect. 3.2) much easier.

3.1 Imaging Preprocessing

The first step in cleaning and preparing the data for a machine learning algorithm is to remove any background illumination inconsistencies, which can be accomplished by a method known as flat field correction [11]. Flat field correction can be mathematically described as

$$I_C = \frac{I_R - I_D}{I_F - I_D} \quad (1)$$

where I_R is the raw image, I_D is an image captured with no light source, that is a dark image, I_F is a image with no sample and only the light source and I_C is the corrected image. In Fig. 4, the raw image I_R can be seen on the left and the corrected image I_C can be seen on the right. From Fig. 4 (left) one can observe the non-uniformity of the light as there is a noticeable bright spot in the centre. After flat-field correction, as in Fig. 4 (right), the corrected image has a complete uniform background. The other major benefit of flat-field correction is that is removes any other background artefacts, such as dust or impurities on the optical elements or camera sensor. This flat-field correction was applied to each absorption wavelength image for a given set of multi-band fluorescence absorption images.

3.2 Imaging Segmentation and Cropping

Given a corrected image the next challenge is to separate the background from the foreground as the algae samples are considered to be foreground objects. Therefore a binary classifier was defined to classify each pixel into either the

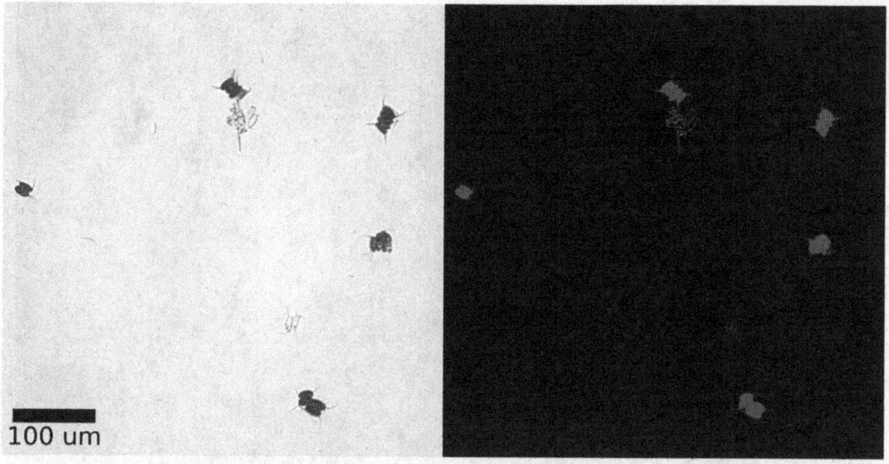

Fig. 5. The preprocessed image (left) can be used to find an optimal threshold between the foreground objects (algae) and the background. This threshold generates the segmented image (right) which can be used to locate and crop certain organisms. In this example the algae (red) have been segmented from the background. (Color figure online)

foreground class, C_f or the background class, C_b. The decision boundary of this classifier, θ, was learned by implementing Otsu's method [13], where the inter-class variability of the image is maximised, which simultaneously minimises the intra-class variability. For any given pixel $\underline{x}$ the class, $C(\underline{x})$, was determined by:

$$C(\underline{x}) = \begin{cases} C_f & \text{if } f(\underline{x}) > \theta \\ C_b & \text{otherwise} \end{cases} \tag{2}$$

where $f(\underline{x})$ is the pixel intensity at pixel $\underline{x}$. As seen in Fig. 5 (left) each pixel in I_C is passed through the classifier, which results in the algae samples being segmented, as seen in Fig. 5 (right).

Once all the organisms in a given multispectral image are segmented, each foreground group of pixels in the image were extracted and cropped to a fixed size. A sample cropped region of interest for each of the six species can be seen in Fig. 6. One initial observation is that all three of the green algae species have a much larger fluorescence signal at 385 nm and 405 nm compared to the blue-green algae, which matches results presented by Poryvkina *et al.* findings [14]. This difference in fluorescent intensity is due to the difference in pigmentation between each phylum, as previously discussed in Sect. 2.1.

Each cropped image was then resized to a fixed dimension as required for input to the deep convolutional neural network. For example, *Microcystis aeruginosa* will appear larger than in the original image and the *Anabaena flos-aquae* will appear smaller. This step results in the images losing their relative scale information, potentially discarding useful information when classifying these

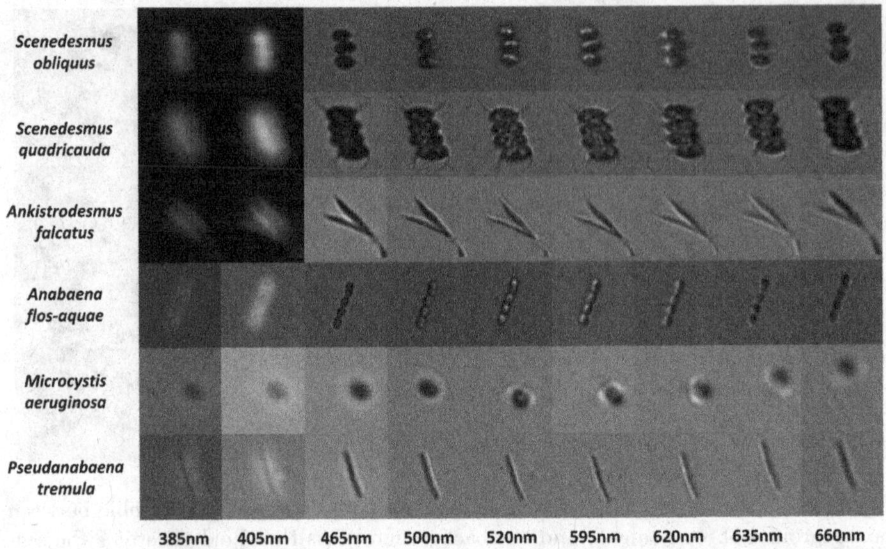

Fig. 6. Six algae types were imaged at two fluorescent wavelengths (385 nm and 405 nm) as well as seven absorption wavelengths (465 nm, 500 nm, 520 nm, 595 nm, 620 nm, 635 nm, and 660 nm). Three of these algae are from the Cyanophyta phylum (blue-green algae) and the remaining three are from the Chlorophyta (green algae) phylum. These images are the result of segmenting and cropping the raw images from the hardware system.

different organisms. Therefore this a potential limitation of the existing method, but is required for the current neural network architecture.

The distribution of how many cropped and resized images for each algae class can be seen in Fig. 7. The total number of multispectral images were 4541, that is, each of these 4541 images are composed of nine sub-images, two of which are fluorescence based, and seven which are absorption based. This set of images makes up the available data to now train and test a deep neural network classifier.

3.3 Deep Residual Learning-Based Classification

The automatic classification of different types of algae was achieved via deep learning, which has been demonstrated in recent years to provide state-of-the-art performance across a wide variety of applications. In particular, we leverage the concept of deep convolutional neural networks, a type of deep neural network in the realm of deep learning that has been demonstrated to be particularly effective for visual perception and understanding. Here, we construct a custom 18-layer deep residual convolutional neural network that takes the cropped multi-spectral image data as input, and outputs the predicted algae type. A deep residual network architecture [7] was leveraged for its modeling capacity with the only

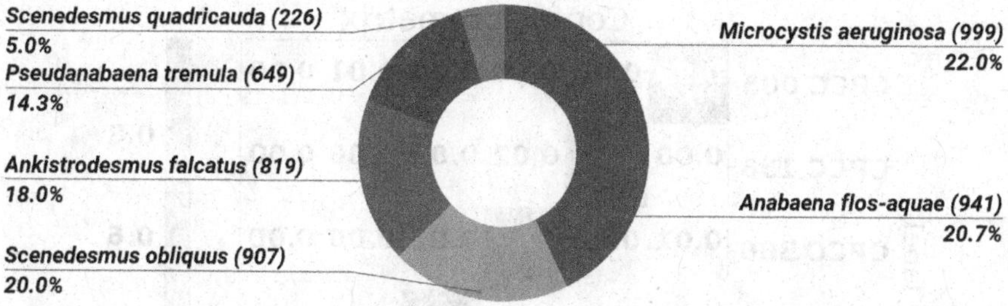

Fig. 7. A total of 4541 segmented and cropped multispectral images were generated from the raw image collected from the imaging system. The class distribution of six types of algae can be seen above.

modification of the input and output dimensions to match the input size of the multispectral image as well as to match the number of output classes.

Due to the relatively small amount of data available, we leverage transfer learning when training this deep residual convolutional neural network, where the network is first trained on a larger dataset from a different domain prior to being finetuned for the task at hand. This enables the network to build a strong model for characterizing image properties before being trained specifically to differentiate between different algae types. More specifically, the deep residual convolutional neural network is first trained using the ImageNet dataset, a dataset of 1000 image classes containing over 14 million images. After this training process, the network was fine-tuned with 70% of our available data. Using the remaining 30% of the available data to test the performance of the constructed network, it was found that the custom deep residual convolutional neural network was able to achieve a classification accuracy of 96%.

A confusion matrix, as seen in Fig. 8, was created to get a more nuanced understanding of the performance of the constructed deep residual convolutional neural network. On the vertical axis of the confusion matrix we can see the true algae type for a given sample, while on the horizontal axis we see the predicted algae type. For example, for CPCC 005 (*Scenedesmus obliquus*), 99% was classified correctly as CPCC 005, while 1% was classified as CPCC 300 (*Microcystis aeruginosa*). Therefore the two highest performing classes were CPCC 005 (*Scenedesmus obliquus*) and CPCC 300 (*Microcystis aeruginosa*) each having a classification accuracy of 99%. The lowest classification accuracy was CPCC 067 (*Anabaena flos-aquae*), as 3% were miss-classified as CPCC 366 (*Ankistrodesmus falcatus*), 3% were miss-classified as CPCC 300 (*Microcystis aeruginosa*), and 3% were miss-classified as CPCC 471 (*Pseudanabaena tremula*). This high performance demonstrates the potential use of such a system such as SAMSON for on-site use of algae identification.

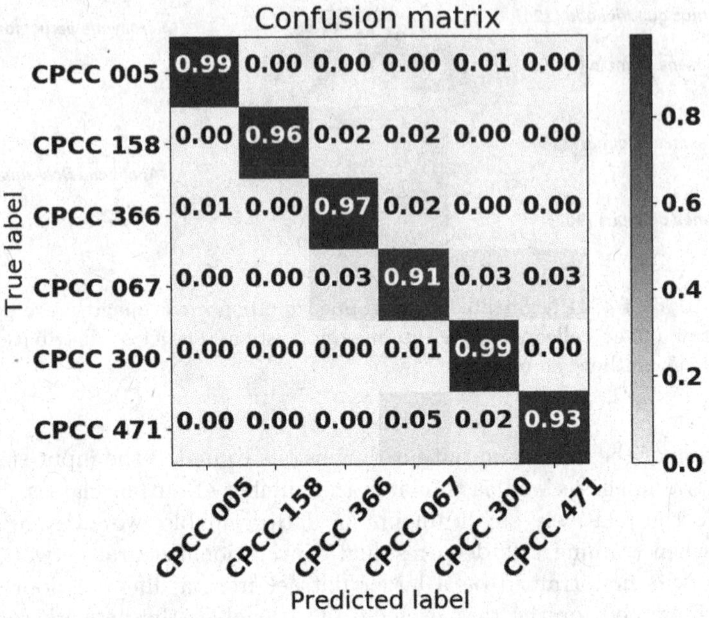

Fig. 8. The confusion matrix is used to investigate the performance of the constructed deep residual convolutional neural network when classifying six types of algae. The overall classification accuracy of the constructed network is 96%. The highest performing classes were *Scenedesmus obliquus* (CPCC 005) and *Microcystis aeruginosa* (CPCC 300).

4 Conclusions

The current method to manually determine which types of algae are present in an harmful algae bloom is time-consuming and relatively costly. Therefore a cost-effective on-site tool that can quickly and accurately identify different types of algae and bacteria in a water sample is highly desired. By using the SAMSON system for data collection and a deep residual convolutional neural network, we were able to achieve an accuracy of 96% when classifying six different types of algae, either from the blue-green phylum or the green algae phylum. This end-to-end approach allows a multispectral image to be input to the deep learning model and the corresponding type of algae is identified. Furthermore, the main advantage of this method is that the neural network learns the optimal combination of spectral and spatial features. These initial results show that using a combination of fluorescence and absorption spectral data, along with the morphological data is a potentially effective method for on-site identification and monitoring of algae in a water body.

Contributions

JLD, CJ, and AW conceived and designed the SAMSON system. JLD collected the data, wrote the code and ran the experiments. JLD and AW designed the deep convolutional neural network for classification. JLD, CJ, and AW conducted the analysis of the experiments. All authors contributed to the writing of the manuscript.

Acknowledgements. The authors would like to thank the Canadian Phycological Culture Centre (CPCC) for preparing the algae samples, and Velocity Science for providing tools and resources for proper data collection. This research was funded by the Natural Sciences and Engineering Research Council of Canada (NSERC) and Canada Research Chairs program.

References

1. Toxic algae bloom in Lake Erie. NASA, October 2011. https://earthobservatory.nasa.gov/IOTD/view.php?id=76127
2. Barsanti, L., Gualtieri, P.: Algae: Anatomy, Biochemistry, and Biotechnology. CRC Press, Boca Raton (2014)
3. Canada, H.: Canadian Drinking Water Guidelines. Cyanobacterial Toxins - Microcystin-LR, July 2002
4. Coltelli, P., Barsanti, L., Evangelista, V., Frassanito, A.M., Gualtieri, P.: Water monitoring: automated and real time identification and classification of algae using digital microscopy. Environ. Sci. Process. Impacts **16**(11), 2656–2665 (2014)
5. Deglint, J.L., Tang, L., Wang, Y., Jin, C., Wong, A.: SAMSON: spectral absorption-fluorescence microscopy system for ON-site-imaging of algae. J. Comput. Vis. Imaging Syst. (2018)
6. Falconer, I.R.: Potential impact on human health of toxic cyanobacteria. Phycologia **35**(6S), 6–11 (1996)
7. He, K., Zhang, X., Ren, S., Sun, J.: Deep residual learning for image recognition. In: Proceedings of the IEEE Conference on Computer Vision and Pattern Recognition, pp. 770–778 (2016)
8. Minister of Health: Guidelines for Canadian Recreational Water Quality, 3rd edn. Health Canada, Ottawa (2012)
9. Huisman, J., Codd, G.A., Paerl, H.W., Ibelings, B.W., Verspagen, J.M., Visser, P.M.: Cyanobacterial blooms. Nat. Rev. Microbiol. **16**(8), 471 (2018)
10. Michalak, A.M., et al.: Record-setting algal bloom in lake erie caused by agricultural and meteorological trends consistent with expected future conditions. Proc. Natl. Acad. Sci. **110**(16), 6448–6452 (2013)
11. Murphy, D.B.: Fundamentals of Light Microscopy and Electronic Imaging. Wiley, New Jersey (2002)
12. Organization, W.H., et al.: Cyanobacterial Toxins: Microcystin-LR. Guidelines for Drinking Water Quality **2** (1998)
13. Otsu, N.: A threshold selection method from gray-level histograms. Automatica **11**(285–296), 23–27 (1975)
14. Poryvkina, L., Babichenko, S., Leeben, A.: Analysis of phytoplankton pigments by excitation spectra of fluorescence. In: EARSeL-SIG-Workshop LIDAR. Institute of Ecology/LDI, Tallinn, Estonia, pp. 224–232 (2000)

15. Sayers, M.J., et al.: Satellite monitoring of harmful algal blooms in the western basin of Lake Erie: a 20-year time-series. J. Great Lakes Res. **45**, 508–521 (2019)
16. Wynne, T., Stumpf, R.: Spatial and temporal patterns in the seasonal distribution of toxic cyanobacteria in western lake erie from 2002–2014. Toxins **7**(5), 1649–1663 (2015)

Medical Imaging and Analysis Using Deep Learning and Machine Intelligence

A Random Field Computational Adaptive Optics Framework for Optical Coherence Microscopy

Ameneh Boroomand[1], Bingyao Tan[1], Mohammad Javad Shafiee[1,2], Kostadinka Bizheva[1], and Alexander Wong[1,2(✉)]

[1] University of Waterloo, Waterloo, ON, Canada
a28wong@uwaterloo.ca

[2] Waterloo Artificial Intelligence Institute, Waterloo, ON, Canada

Abstract. A novel random field computational adaptive optics (R-CAO) framework is proposed to jointly correct for optical aberrations and speckle noise issues in optical coherence microscopy (OCM) and thus overcome the depth-of-field limitation in OCM imaging. The performance of the R-CAO approach is validated using OCM tomograms acquired from a standard USAF target and a phantom comprised of 1 µm diameter microspheres embedded in agar gel. The R-CAO reconstructed OCM tomograms show reduced optical aberrations and speckle noise over the entire depth of imaging compared to the existing state-of-the-art computational adaptive optics algorithms such as the regularized maximum likelihood computational adaptive optics (RML-CAO) method. The reconstructed images using the proposed R-CAO framework show the usefulness of this method for the quality enhancement of OCM imaging over different imaging depths.

Keywords: Computational adaptive optics · Optical coherence microscopy · Random field

1 Introduction

In optical coherence microscopy (OCM) [3], a recognized issue is the presence of optical aberrations, which lead to overall image quality degradations, particularly in out-of-focus regions. Different types of optical aberrations can be generated by both the optical design of the OCM system and the structure of the imaged object [1].

Overall, optical aberrations degrade the OCM image contrast and resolution and the effect is more pronounced with distance away from the focal plane. Speckle noise is another issue that causes degradation of the overall image quality

The authors would like to thank Natural Science and Engineering Research Counsel of Canada, Canadian Institutes of Health Research, and the Canada Research Chairs program.

F. Karray et al. (Eds.): ICIAR 2019, LNCS 11663, pp. 283–294, 2019.
https://doi.org/10.1007/978-3-030-27272-2_24

in OCM tomograms and therefore hinders the correct visualization and proper identification of micro-structures in the imaged sample.

The technology of adaptive optics (AO) has emerged as a successful approach for the aim of aberration compensation in optical imaging systems including the OCM imaging [9,16,22]. Combining OCM with AO technology for optical aberration correction leads to the improved lateral resolution, smaller speckle size and higher SNR in OCM images [1,10].

However, combining OCM with AO increases the complexity of the optical design and hardware, the physical size, as well as the overall cost of the AO-OCM system and in most cases limits the transmitted spectral bandwidth, which degrades the OCM system's axial resolution. It also limits the OCM scanning speed in case of on-line aberration correction optimization during the OCM imaging. Computational adaptive optics (CAO) is a relatively new approach for correction of optical aberrations that takes advantage of computational methods to compensate for the optical aberrations in OCM images. Since CAO is independent on the OCM hardware, it can be integrated in to any type of OCM imaging system. Furthermore, the CAO approach provides a number of advantages, such as significantly lower cost and compact design of the imaging system and possibly faster correction of the optical aberrations compared to the conventional adaptive optics technology. The integration of CAO with OCM can solve the depth-of-field limitation issue in OCM imaging using numerical methods.

Most of the previously published CAO methods are based on estimation of a phase correction term through either solving of an optimization problem [1,8,21] or by using various sub-aperture correlation approaches [4]. Therefore, the performance of those approaches is highly dependent on the correct estimation of the phase term that is sensitive to the sample motion as well as OCM system fluctuations [15]. In addition, most of the previously proposed CAO methods only account for the isotropic optical aberrations in OCM systems that have low NA [4] and therefore the optical aberrations over all imaging depths can be corrected using a spatially invariant phase correction term. A recent publication expanded upon the sub-aperture based CAO to correct for the out-of-focus anisotropic optical aberrations in an OCM imaging with high NA [5]. Deconvolution based CAO methods were also utilized to compensate for the system-related aberrations in OCM imaging by characterizing the aberration function of the OCM system [2,7,13,19]. Interferometric synthetic aperture microscopy (ISAM) [11,12] was recently proposed as a technique that takes advantage of inverse scattering modeling to reconstruct OCM images with less out-of-focus blurring caused by optical aberrations, and provides the same lateral resolution throughout the whole scanning range. A combination of ISAM and CAO was recently proposed for high-speed OCM imaging with sub-cellular resolution [8].

In this paper, we introduce a novel random field CAO (R-CAO) framework for OCM imaging to simultaneously correct for optical aberrations and reduce speckle noise using a unified computational framework. Two different experiments using a standard USAF resolution target and a phantom comprised of 1 μm diameter microspheres embedded in agar gel were performed to show the ability of proposed R-CAO framework in reconstructing OCM images with reduced optical aberrations and speckle noise. The paper is organized as follows. Section 2 provides a detailed description of the proposed R-CAO framework. Section 2.2 presents the experimental setup and provides a discussion on the experimental results for the two experiments performed. Section 3 presents the conclusions and a description of future work.

2 Methodology

2.1 Random Field Computational Adaptive Optics Framework

As a typical framework for the OCM imaging, the construction of an OCM image can be formulated using a forward problem,

$$A = D(V, H) \times \mathbb{N}, \tag{1}$$

where $A = \mathcal{F}[M_k]$, with $\mathcal{F}$ denoting the Fourier transform and M_k denoting the OCM acquisition in k-space domain. In this formulation, $D(.)$ models the overall OCM imaging degradation where it is a function of OCM optical aberration, H, as well as the aberration-corrected, noise-compensated OCM tomogram, V. In this work, the optical aberrations H are initially modeled using a general Gaussian function. In the formulation of Eq. (1), $\mathbb{N}$ denotes the multiplicative speckle noise that inherently exist in all types of OCM imaging.

Based on the forward model of Eq. (1), the aberration-corrected, noise-compensated OCM tomogram, V, can be calculated through solving an inverse problem,

$$\hat{V} = D^{-1}(A, H). \tag{2}$$

Here, the proposed R-CAO framework employs a maximum a posteriori (MAP) strategy to solve the inverse problem of Eq. (2) and find a true estimation of aberration-corrected, noise-compensated OCM tomogram V,

$$\hat{V} = \underset{V'}{argmax} P(V|A), \tag{3}$$

where, $P(V|A)$ is a posterior probability that defines the probability of aberration-corrected, noise-compensated OCM tomogram, V, given an OCM acquisition, A. The proposed R-CAO framework takes advantage of the graphical theory concept [18] such that it assumes a graphical model for both the aberration-corrected, noise-compensated OCM tomogram, V, as well as the OCM acquisition, A, and with the graph nodes defining the different locations of the OCM tomograms. Using such a graphical modeling, the posterior probability, $P(V|A)$, can be represented as,

$$P(V|A) = \frac{1}{Z(A)} \exp(-E(V, A)), \tag{4}$$

where, Z is a normalization term, referred to as a partition function in the CRF literature [6] and $E(.)$ represents an energy function of the following form,

$$E(V, A) = \sum_{i=1}^{n} \psi_u(v_i, A) + \sum_{l \in L} \psi_p(v_l, A), \tag{5}$$

which is defined over the random fields for the aberration-corrected, noise-compensated OCM tomogram, V, as well as OCM acquisition, A, and with, i, referring to each location in the assumed graph. In the proposed R-CAO framework, the energy function, $E(.)$, encodes the direct relationships that exist between the OCM acquisition, a_i, and aberration-corrected, noise-compensated OCM tomogram, v_i, at each location i in the graph and using a distance based unary potential function $\psi_u(.)$,

$$\psi_u(v_i, A) = \frac{1}{\sigma\sqrt{2\pi}} exp\left(\frac{(log(a_i) - \sum log(D(v_i, H))^2}{2\varphi^2}\right). \tag{6}$$

According to the formulation of Eq. 6, the designed unary potential function aims to enforce the data fidelity by obtaining the best estimate of aberration-corrected, noise-compensated OCM tomogram, v_i, at each single node, i, and with respect to the whole OCM acquisition, A. In the formulation of Eq. 6, φ is a control parameter which controls the effect the designed distance based weighting function in the unary term. Here, the logarithmic domain is used to transform the multiplicative speckle noise to an additive noise term that is common in forward modeling formulation. Furthermore, the energy function, $E(.)$, also models the interaction relationships between each pair of nodes v_i and v_j regarding to the OCM acquisition, A, using a pairwise potential function $\psi_p(.)$ defined over a specific clique structure L,

$$\psi_p(v_{l \in L}, A) = \exp\left(\frac{\|N_i - N_j\|^2}{\sigma_{cl}}\right)(v_i - v_j);\ L = \{i, j\}, \tag{7}$$

where, N_i and N_j respectively denote to specified neighborhood coordinates centered around the ith and j^{th} locations of the defined graphs for the OCM tomograms and they are utilized to compute a weighting exponential function for assessing the similarity of two nodes v_i and v_j in a defined neighborhood. Here, σ_{cl} is the standard deviation that controls the effect of pairwise potential function, $\psi_p(.)$, for a specific clique structure L.

The particular features of the incorporated pairwise potential function of Eq. (7) that results in a strong performance of the proposed R-CAO framework in terms of jointly compensating for the optical aberrations and speckle noise issues is mentioned here. First, the designed pairwise potential function, $\psi_p(.)$ utilizes a set of nodes to assess the nodes similarity which leads to the better robustness of the proposed R-CAO framework in the presence of speckle noise and artifacts. Second, the designed pairwise potential of Eq. (7) takes advantage of a recently proposed stochastic clique structure within a fully-connected random field modeling (SF-CRF) [14]. Using the SF-CRF modeling enforces higher probability to the pairs of nodes that are closer in the defined random field than pairs of nodes that are farther apart and therefore it helps in better preservation of image boundaries and edges in the final estimate of aberration-corrected, noise-compensated OCM tomogram, V.

To calculate the best estimate of aberration-corrected, noise-compensated OCM tomogram, V, the proposed R-CAO framework takes advantage of an approximation of graph cuts optimization method [20] to iteratively solve the MAP problem of Eq. (3) with the optimal solution obtained by minimizing the energy function $E(.)$ in Eq. (5),

$$V^{t+1} = V^t - \rho \frac{\nabla E(V, A)}{\nabla V}, \tag{8}$$

where, V^{t+1} and V^t are the solutions at iterations $t+1$ and t, $\frac{\nabla E(V,A)}{\nabla V}$ is the energy gradient, and ρ is the learning rate.

2.2 Experimental Setup

All OCM images were acquired with a high-speed, ultrahigh resolution spectral domain OCM system. The system has a compact fiber optic design and is powered by a supercontinuum laser (SUPER K, NKT Photonics) with a spectrum centered at $\lambda_c = 780$ nm, and spectral bandwidth of $\Delta\lambda = 250$ nm. The detection end of the OCM system consists of a high resolution commercial spectrometer (Wasatch Photonics) interfaced with a CCD camera (Piranha HS8K, Teledyne DALSA) with 8192 pixels to acquire interference fringes at 34 kHz data acquisition rate. The imaging probe of the system is comprised of an achromat collimator lens ($f = 10$ mm), a pair of galvanometric scanners (Cambridge Technologies), a beam expander (2 ahromat doublets with $f = 40$ mm and $f = 80$ mm) and a microscope objective (Nikon NIR APO 40X/0.8).

Using such an optical design, the ultrahigh resolution spectral domain OCM system provides 1.3 µm axial resolution in free space. Because the entrance aperture of the microscope objective is partially under-filled, the measured lateral resolution in free space is ~1 µm, which is larger than the theoretical resolution of the objective. All test samples were imaged with 750 µW optical power incident on the sample's surface. The system's SNR is 98 dB near the zero delay with roll-off of 12 dB over a scanning range of 1.2 mm.

To apply the proposed R-CAO framework, the aberration function H of the OCM imaging system needs to be characterized. In the proposed R-CAO framework, the aberration function H is modeled using a generalized Gaussian function where its standard deviation is characterized using imaging of a standard USAF resolution target and with the same OCM system. A chosen zoomed-in region of the OCM image of the USAF resolution target that includes three horizontal bars of group 6, element 2 is shown in Fig. 1(A).

3 Experimental Results

The performance of proposed R-CAO framework was tested using two different experiments that take advantage of (1) a standard USAF resolution target, and (2) a phantom comprised of 1 μm diameter microspheres embedded in agar gel. For all experiments, the results were compared to the extended version of the state of the art maximum likelihood approach [2], called regularized maximum likelihood computational adaptive optics (RML-CAO) method which takes advantage of Tikhonov regularization [17] to control the effect of speckle noise in reconstruction of RML-CAO OCM tomogram. All methods were implemented in embedded C++ code in MATLAB (The MathWorks, Inc.) and tested on an AMD Athlon II X3 3.10 GHz machine with 12 GB of RAM.

3.1 Experiment 1: Standard USAF Resolution Target

To test the performance of the proposed R-CAO using the standard USAF resolution target, the optical aberration function, H, was characterized using the USAF resolution target of Fig. 1(A) and incorporated to the modeling of R-CAO framework. The reconstructed aberration-corrected, noise-compensated resolution target image using the R-CAO framework is shown in Fig. 1(C). The proposed R-CAO framework was tested using different number of iterations where the optimal result was achieved using 30 iterations. For comparison, the state of the art RML-CAO was also applied to the same USAF resolution target image of Fig. 1(A) and the reconstructed image is shown in Fig. 1(B). To have a fair comparison between the results, the number of iterations was set the same for both the RML-CAO method and the proposed R-CAO framework.

Results in Fig. 1 show that the optical aberrations were successfully compensated in the R-CAO tomogram (Fig. 1(C)) such that the width of all horizontal bars are the same and they are within the same distance from each other compared to the original OCM image in Fig. 1(A). Furthermore, the reconstructed resolution target images using both RML-CAO method as shown in Fig. 1(B) as well as proposed R-CAO framework as shown in Fig. 1(C) show that the speckle noise was greatly reduced compared to the original OCM image in Fig. 1(A).

An intensity plot measured across the bars of the USAF resolution target at a location marked with the white lines in Figs. 1(A–C) is presented in Fig. 1(D). The intensity plots show smoother as well as more narrow width curves with using of both RML-CAO method and the R-CAO framework as can been seen by comparing of the red intensity plot with the blue and black plots in Fig. 1(D). However, the intensity plot related to the proposed R-CAO (black intensity plot) is much narrower compared to the original intensity plot (red intensity plot) that shows superior performance of the proposed R-CAO in optical aberrations compensation compared to the tested RML-CAO method.

For quantitative comparison of the 2 approaches, SNR values were calculated for all images in Figs. 1(A–C). The image SNR for the original OCM-USAF image was measured to be 14.7 dB, while the SNR for the RML-CAO and

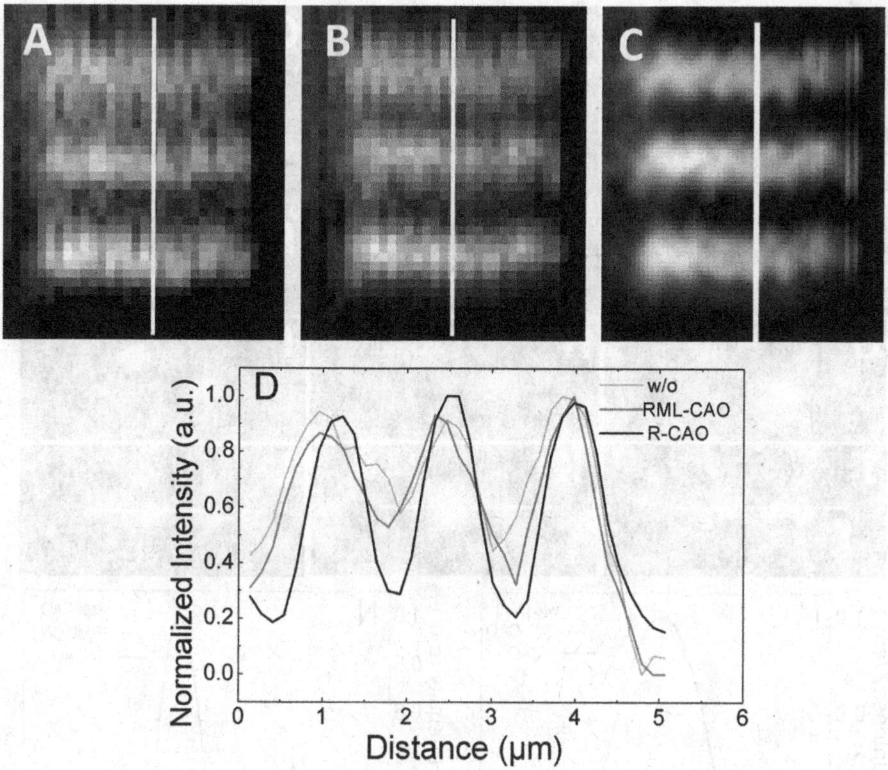

Fig. 1. (A) Out-of-focus, enface OCM image of USAF resolution target, group 6, element 2. (B) Same image processed with RML-CAO and (c) with R-CAO. (D) Intensity plots obtained from the images at the locations marked with the white lines.

R-CAO images was 15.3 dB and 18.6 dB respectively as shows the significant SNR improvement using the proposed R-CAO framework.

3.2 Experiment 2: Microspheres

To demonstrate the efficacy of the proposed R-CAO for producing nearly aberration-free OCM images, a phantom composed of 1 μm diameter polystyrene microspheres embedded in agar gel was imaged using the ultrahigh resolution spectral domain OCM system. A volumetric (512 × 512) OCM image was acquired from the microspheres phantom and the dispersion in the OCM images was compensated numerically up to the 9th order. The proposed R-CAO framework was used to calculate the final estimate of R-CAO phantom tomogram and with incorporation of the optimized aberration function H in to the framework of R-CAO. The proposed R-CAO framework was tested using a different number of iterations and optimal results were achieved using 25 iterations. The results were compared to the reconstructed image using the tested RML-CAO method where the same number of iterations was used to ensure a fair comparison between the results.

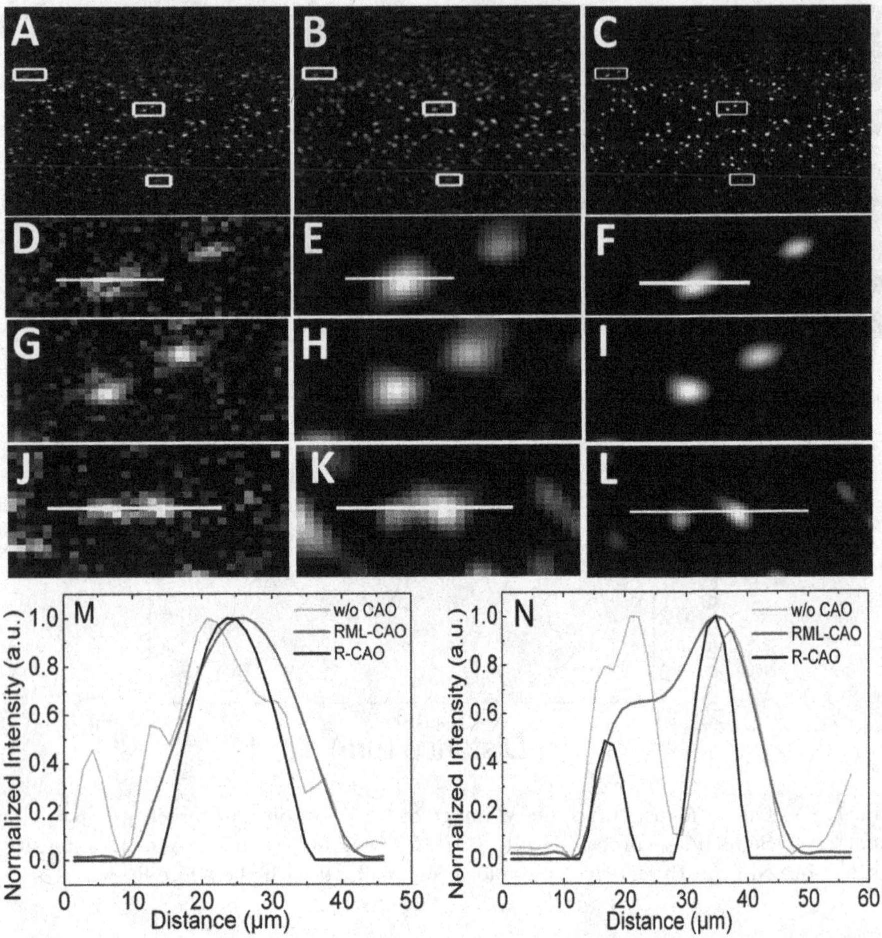

Fig. 2. (A) Cross-sectional OCM image of a gel phantom with embedded 1 µm polystyrene microspheres. (B) Same image produced with the RML-CAO and (C) R-CAO. White rectangles mark regions of interest (ROI above, at and below the focal plane). (D, G, J) Magnified copies of the marked ROIs in the original image, (E, H, K) RML-CAO image and (F, I, L) R-CAO image. (M) Intensity profiles measured along the white lines in images D, E and F, acquired from a location above the focal plane. (N) Intensity profiles measured along the white lines in images J, K and L, acquired from a location below the focal plane. (Color figure online)

Figure 2 shows a cross-sectional OCM image of the microspheres phantom (A) and the same image produced with RML-CAO (B) and the proposed R-CAO (C). Regions of interest (ROI) containing a few microspheres were selected for locations 110 µm above, approximately at and 120 µm below the focal plane in each image and marked with the white line rectangles. Magnified copies of the ROIs are presented in Fig. 2 for locations above (D–F), approximately at (G–I) and below the focal plane (J–L).

Overall, the reconstructed cross-sectional phantom images using both RML-CAO method and proposed R-CAO framework significantly compensate for the speckle noise. Images of the individual microspheres from ROIs above and below the focal plane appear blurred in the original OCM image, while the microspheres appear of smaller size, with sharp boundaries, almost round shape and of significantly higher contrast in the ROIs produced with using of the proposed R-CAO framework as shown in Figs. 2(F, L) as compared to the RML-CAO images in Figs. 2(E, K). While RML-CAO corrects for the optical aberrations to a certain degree, as observed by the shape of the microspheres in the resulting image, the microspheres still appeared blurred compared to the sharp, aberration corrected microspheres in the images produced using the proposed R-CAO framework. Furthermore, the RML-CAO method introduced significant undesired pixelation effect that can be observed around the microspheres compared to the proposed R-CAO framework.

The improvement of the lateral OCM resolution is demonstrated in Fig. 2(M) and Fig. 2(N), where intensity profiles are presented for locations across a chosen microsphere, shown by white horizontal lines in images of Figs. 2(D–F) and (J–L) from original (red color intensity plots) and the OCM images produced using RML-CAO (blue color intensity plots) and proposed R-CAO (black color intensity plots). The intensity profiles in Fig. 2(M) and Fig. 2(N) clearly show the better compensation of out-of-focus aberrations using the proposed R-CAO framework such that for example, the two microspheres in Fig. 2(J) can be easily distinguished form each other in the result of Fig. 2(L) after optical aberrations compensation using the R-CAO while this separation is impossible using the result of RML-CAO as shown in Fig. 2(K). The black color plot in Fig. 2(N) which is related to the result of R-CAO framework confirms this interpretation as the black color intensity plot shows the existence of two microspheres by showing an intensity plot with two distinguished peaks.

To better demonstrate the performance of proposed R-CAO framework in using of microsphere phantom imaging, the enface images acquired from the microspheres phantom are also shown in Fig. 3(A) at the focal plane and in Fig. 3(G) at 300 μm below the focal plane. The reconstructed enface phantom images with RML-CAO and R-CAO are respectively shown in Figs. 3(B, C) at focal plane and Figs. 3(H, I) at 300 μm below the focal plane.

ROIs containing a few microspheres were selected from those images (locations marked with the white line rectangles). Magnified versions of the ROIs are presented in Figs. 3(D–F) (focal plane) and Figs. 3(J–L) (at 300 μm below the focal plane). The original OCM tomogram acquired at 300 μm below the focal plane in Fig. 3(J) shows low reflective spots of larger size compared to the physical size of the microspheres, while the OCM image acquired close to the focal plane as shown in Fig. 3(D) shows high reflective spots of smaller size corresponding to the microspheres. The images in Figs. 3(F, L) produced with

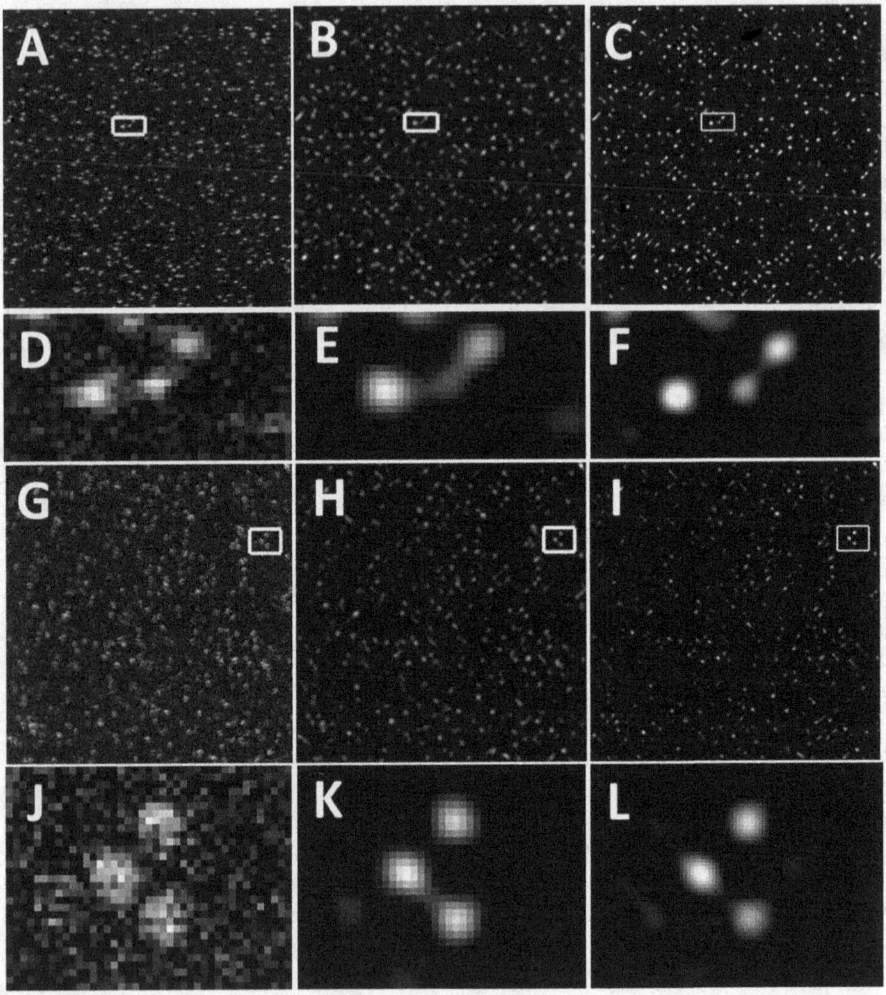

Fig. 3. Enface OCM image of polystyrene microspheres acquired at (A) the focal plane. Same region produced with the (B) RML-CAO method and (C) R-CAO framework with white rectangles marking ROIs. Enface OCM image of microspheres (G) acquired ~300 µ below the focal plane. Same region produced with the (H) RML-CAO method and (I) R-CAO framework. (D–F) Magnified images of the ROIs at the focal plane and (J–L) at ~300 µ below the focal plane.

R-CAO show better improvement in the shape and contrast for the microsphere images acquired at both near the focal plane and also at a depth of 300 µm below the focal plane and compared to the images in Figs. 3(E, K) produced with tested RML-CAO. Again, both of the RML-CAO method and R-CAO framework could reduce the speckle noise compared to the original images in Figs. 3(D, J), while the optical aberrations is better compensated using the proposed R-CAO framework and compared to the tested RML-CAO method while the RML-CAO method also results in some undesired pixelation artifact in reconstructed images of Figs. 3(E, K).

For all of the above experiments, a computation time analysis was performed to assess the computational efficiency of the proposed R-CAO method compared to the tested RML-CAO method, when the acquired time shows that the tested RML-CAO is in average 1.2 times faster than the proposed R-CAO method.

4 Conclusion

In conclusion, we proposed a novel random field computational adaptive optics framework (R-CAO) for the compensation of out-of-focus aberrations in OCM imaging. Our results showed that the R-CAO framework outperforms current state-of-the-art methods such as the regularized maximum likelihood computational adaptive optics (RML-CAO), as it results in higher image SNR and more image contrast. Our proposed R-CAO framework also has the advantage of reducing speckle noise simultaneously with the aberration correction. The proposed joint compensation framework has also the potential of compensating for the other OCM imaging issues such as motion artifact that can be incorporated in to the designed compensation algorithm and possibly improve the quality of *in-vivo* OCM imaging. Testing and evaluation of other methods for estimating of the overall OCM aberration function and motion correction is left for the future work.

References

1. Adie, S.G., Graf, B.W., Ahmad, A., Carney, P.S., Boppart, S.A.: Computational adaptive optics for broadband optical interferometric tomography of biological tissue. Proc. Nat. Acad. Sci. **109**(19), 7175–7180 (2012)
2. Hojjatoleslami, S., Avanaki, M., Podoleanu, A.G.: Image quality improvement in optical coherence tomography using lucy-richardson deconvolution algorithm. Appl. Opt. **52**(23), 5663–5670 (2013)
3. Izatt, J.A., Hee, M.R., Owen, G.M., Swanson, E.A., Fujimoto, J.G.: Optical coherence microscopy in scattering media. Opt. Lett. **19**(8), 590–592 (1994)
4. Kumar, A., Drexler, W., Leitgeb, R.A.: Subaperture correlation based digital adaptive optics for full field optical coherence tomography. Opt. Express **21**(9), 10850–10866 (2013)
5. Kumar, A., Kamali, T., Platzer, R., Unterhuber, A., Drexler, W., Leitgeb, R.A.: Anisotropic aberration correction using region of interest based digital adaptive optics in fourier domain OCT. Biomed. Opt. express **6**(4), 1124–1134 (2015)
6. Lafferty, J., McCallum, A., Pereira, F.: Conditional random fields: probabilistic models for segmenting and labeling sequence data. In: Proceedings of the Eighteenth International Conference on Machine Learning, ICML, vol. 1, pp. 282–289 (2001)
7. Liu, Y., Liang, Y., Mu, G., Zhu, X.: Deconvolution methods for image deblurring in optical coherence tomography. JOSA A **26**(1), 72–77 (2009)

8. Liu, Y.Z., et al.: Computed optical interferometric tomography for high-speed volumetric cellular imaging. Biomed. Opt. Express **5**(9), 2988–3000 (2014)
9. Merino, D., Dainty, C., Bradu, A., Podoleanu, A.G.: Adaptive optics enhanced simultaneous en-face optical coherence tomography and scanning laser ophthalmoscopy. Opt. Express **14**(8), 3345–3353 (2006)
10. Miller, D., Kocaoglu, O., Wang, Q., Lee, S.: Adaptive optics and the eye (super resolution OCT). Eye **25**(3), 321–330 (2011)
11. Ralston, T.S., Adie, S.G., Marks, D.L., Boppart, S.A., Carney, P.S.: Cross-validation of interferometric synthetic aperture microscopy and optical coherence tomography. Opt. Lett. **35**(10), 1683–1685 (2010)
12. Ralston, T.S., Marks, D.L., Carney, P.S., Boppart, S.A.: Interferometric synthetic aperture microscopy. Nat. Phys. **3**(2), 129–134 (2007)
13. Ralston, T.S., Marks, D.L., Kamalabadi, F., Boppart, S.A.: Deconvolution methods for mitigation of transverse blurring in optical coherence tomography. IEEE Trans. Image Process. **14**(9), 1254–1264 (2005)
14. Shafiee, M., Wong, A., Siva, P., Fieguth, P.: Efficient bayesian inference using fully connected conditional random fields with stochastic cliques. In: 2014 IEEE International Conference on Image Processing (ICIP), pp. 4289–4293. IEEE (2014)
15. Shemonski, N.D., Adie, S.G., Liu, Y.Z., South, F.A., Carney, P.S., Boppart, S.A.: Stability in computed optical interferometric tomography (part i): stability requirements. Opt. Express **22**(16), 19183–19197 (2014)
16. Shi, G., Dai, Y., Wang, L., Ding, Z., Rao, X., Zhang, Y.: Adaptive optics optical coherence tomography for retina imaging. Chin. Opt. Lett. **6**(6), 424–425 (2008)
17. Tikhonov, A.N., Arsenin, V.Y.: Solutions of Ill-Posed Problems (1977)
18. Wainwright, M.J., Jordan, M.I.: Graphical Models, Exponential Families, and Variational Inference. Foundations and Trends® in Machine Learning, vol. 1, no. 1–2, pp. 1–305 (2008)
19. Woolliams, P.D., Ferguson, R.A., Hart, C., Grimwood, A., Tomlins, P.H.: Spatially deconvolved optical coherence tomography. Appl. Opt. **49**(11), 2014–2021 (2010)
20. Yildiz, A., Akgul, Y.S.: A gradient descent approximation for graph cuts. In: Denzler, J., Notni, G., Süße, H. (eds.) DAGM 2009. LNCS, vol. 5748, pp. 312–321. Springer, Heidelberg (2009). https://doi.org/10.1007/978-3-642-03798-6_32
21. Yu, L., et al.: Improved lateral resolution in optical coherence tomography by digital focusing using two-dimensional numerical diffraction method. Opt. Express **15**(12), 7634–7641 (2007)
22. Zawadzki, R.J., et al.: Integrated adaptive optics optical coherence tomography and adaptive optics scanning laser ophthalmoscope system for simultaneous cellular resolution in vivo retinal imaging. Biomed. Opt. Express **2**(6), 1674–1686 (2011)

Deep Learning Approaches for Gynaecological Ultrasound Image Segmentation: A Radio-Frequency *vs* B-mode Comparison

Catarina Carvalho[1(✉)], Sónia Marques[2], Carla Peixoto[3,4], Duarte Pignatelli[3,4], Jorge Beires[3], Jorge Silva[1,2], and Aurélio Campilho[1,2]

[1] INESC TEC, Porto, Portugal
catarina.b.carvalho@inesctec.pt
[2] Faculdade de Engenharia da Universidade do Porto, Porto, Portugal
[3] Centro Hospitalar de São João, Porto, Portugal
[4] Faculdade de Medicina da Universidade do Porto, Porto, Portugal

Abstract. Ovarian cancer is one of the pathologies with the worst prognostic in adult women and it has a very difficult early diagnosis. Clinical evaluation of gynaecological ultrasound images is performed visually, and it is dependent on the experience of the medical doctor. Besides the dependency on the specialists, the malignancy of specific types of ovarian tumors cannot be asserted until their surgical removal. This work explores the use of ultrasound data for the segmentation of the ovary and the ovarian follicles, using two different convolutional neural networks, a fully connected residual network and a U-Net, with a binary and multi-class approach. Five different types of ultrasound data (from beam-formed radio-frequency to brightness mode) were used as input. The best performance was obtained using B-mode, for both ovary and follicles segmentation. No significant differences were found between the two convolutional neural networks. The use of the multi-class approach was beneficial as it provided the model information on the spatial relation between follicles and the ovary. This study demonstrates the suitability of combining convolutional neural networks with beam-formed radio-frequency data and with brightness mode data for segmentation of ovarian structures. Future steps involve the processing of pathological data and investigation of biomarkers of pathological ovaries.

Keywords: B-mode ultrasound data · Beam-formed ultrasound data · Image segmentation · Neuronal networks · Ovarian cancer

1 Introduction

Ovarian cancer (OC) is one of the pathologies with the worst prognostic in adult women. This is a silent and fast progressing disease and in more than a half of the patients, the disease is only found in advanced stages. The majority of ovarian

F. Karray et al. (Eds.): ICIAR 2019, LNCS 11663, pp. 295–306, 2019.
https://doi.org/10.1007/978-3-030-27272-2_25

cancers grows as cystic masses. Once these cysts rupture or leak, cancer cells can easily spread into the pelvic cavity affecting healthy tissues. Ovarian cysts and follicles are encapsulated collections of fluid and tissue, differing from each other because follicles contain a microscopic oocyte, while cysts may contain tissue not relevant for reproduction purposes or cancerous tissue [8].

Currently, the clinical evaluation of gynaecological ultrasound (US) images is performed visually, on brightness mode (B-mode) images, and it is dependent on the experience of the physician. In this type of US images, follicles are represented as smooth, hypoechogenic oval-shapped structures. Ovaries, on the other hand, present higher echogenicity which translates into an increased texture content. According to Rauh-Hain *et al.* [17], most ovarian masses detected by B-mode US screening are benign, corresponding to false-positives. Moreover, it is also known that, independently on the expertise of the specialists, there are specific type of ovarian masses that cannot be diagnosed with certainty until surgery is performed.

False-positives and uncertainty of diagnosis can then lead to unnecessary oophorectomys which have long term impact on both women's fertility and hormonal balance. Thus, research for computer-aided methods that can provide a second opinion to gynaecologists is recommended.

State-of-the-art methods within the field of gynaecologial US, are typically applied for large follicle detection and make use of classical image processing analysis. Potocnik *et al.* [16] reported, in 2012, a survey on follicle detection methods on ovarian US images and most of the approaches are based on texture analysis, thresholding, region growing and knowledge-based methods [4,10,19]. There were also some initial tests using cellular neural networks and support vector machines [13]. Major limitations of all these methods lay on the dependency on the feature's selection process, these only detect large and single follicles, do not consider the stroma for assessment and are dependent on the signal-to-noise ratio.

More recently, in 2017, Isah *et al.* [11] presented a work based on the extraction of geometric and texture features. The features that are best suited to the problem were selected by a Particle Swarm Optimization algorithm and were fed into a Multilayer Perceptron Artificial Neural Network, achieving an accuracy of 98.3% for follicle detection. Despite the good accuracy, the result is for follicle-wise detection, meaning that these consider the number and not the area of the follicles present in the ovary. Lastly, a 3D method based on wavelet transforms, adaptive multiscale search, and recursive convexity-based region splitting has been investigated for follicle selection [4]. Reported results are qualitative and applied to a limited dataset (30 images).

As for deep-learning approaches, to the best knowledge of the authors, there has been only one publication for follicle segmentation in US images. Wanderley *et al.* [7] showed the ability of a fully convolutional neural network to learn features to distinguish ovarian structures, achieving a mean DICE score of 0.677 for the segmentation of the stroma and of 0.784 for the follicles.

Regarding the type of images used in the state-of-the-art, only B-mode has been investigated for segmentation of the ovarian structures. However, the type of information that can be extracted from B-mode data is limited due the extensive post-processing it suffers. Alternatively, beam-formed radio-frequency (BRF) is a raw type of data from which both structural (lower-frequency) and textural (higher-frequency) information can be extracted from. The higher-frequency content of US images has been reported to be important for texture characterization problems [1,3,5,15].

The main contribution of this paper is to investigate the influence of using different types of US data, ranging from raw BRF data to B-mode images, in the performance of two convolutional neural networks (CNN) for the segmentation of follicles and ovary.

For this evaluation, two different CNNs, a U-Net and a fully connected residual network (FCRN), were implemented. These networks were trained using both a binary and a multi-class approach. The performance of both CNNs for the different combination of types of data and number of classes was evaluated and compared.

2 Methods

In this section, the dataset used in this work, which is based on the BRF data, is detailed, as well as the ground-truth (GT) for the binary and multi-class approaches. The two CNNs used (U-Net and FCRN) are presented, plus the loss function used for the networks' training.

2.1 Dataset

The dataset used in this work was based on the 107 original BRF transvaginal US images of the ovary. These images were acquired at Centro Hospitalar de São João, with consent of the patients, while these attended first time appointment for reproductive treatment planning. Each image contains one ovary with single or multiple follicles. The original BRF data was directly acquired using an Ultrasonix SonixTouch Q+, equipped with an EC9-5/10 endovaginal microconvex transducer (frequency range 9–5 MHz). The lateral and axial image resolution of these BRF images was of 0.046 mm and [0.0097, 0.017] mm, respectively, its original image dimensions are 192 × [2000, 6200] px. The axial dimension of these images is variable due to the different scanning depths selected.

Five different types of images were extracted from the original BRF data, namely, rawBRF, rawIQ, filteredIQ, B-mode and B-mode&BRF. RawBRF was obtained by computing the absolute value of the original BRF data and normalizing the obtained intensity to a range of [0, 255]. RawIQ data was attained by storing the magnitude and phase information obtained after quadrature signal demodulation, as a 3D array with two channels. FilteredIQ data was obtained after filtering both magnitude and phase channels of rawIQ with a Hamming window. Also in this case, a 3D array with two channels, was created using the filtered magnitude and filtered phase data. B-mode data was obtained after applying envelope detection and log compression to the filteredIQ data [2]. The parameters used during image acquisition were used during the data conversion processes. B-mode&BRF data was obtained by resizing the B-mode and the rawBRF images into the same spatial dimensions and concatenating the two, in a 3D array, with two channels.

The five different types of images were all resized to 512 $\times$ 512, to normalize the resolution of the CNNs input data. Moreover, resizing of the BRF data, along the depth direction, is a decimation step, used in the conversion of BRF to B-mode.

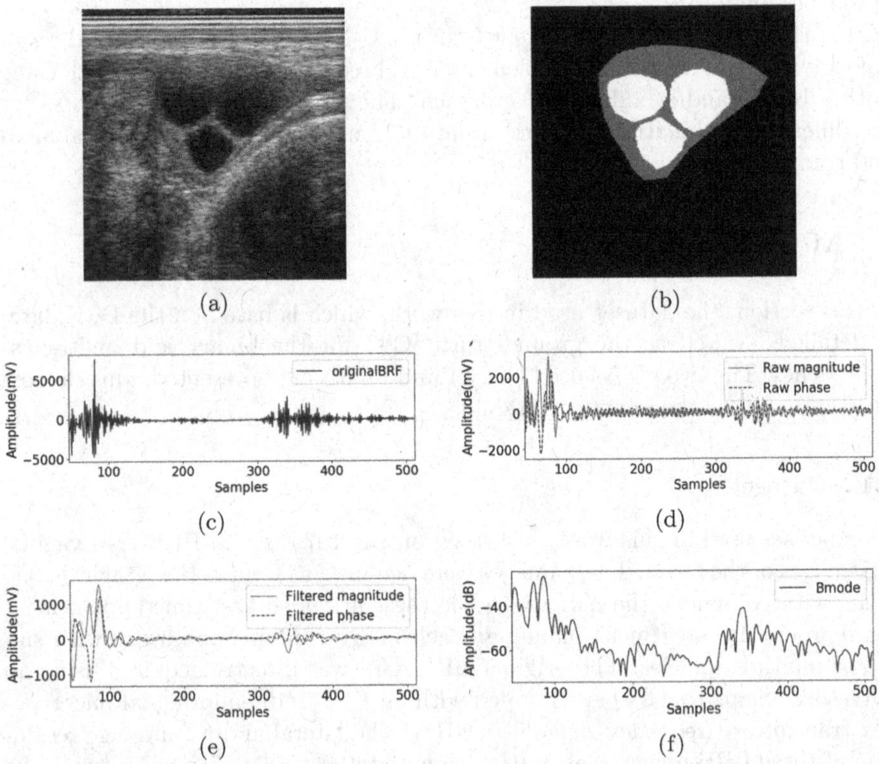

Fig. 1. Example of (a) B-mode; (b) ground-truth of (a) with follicles represented in white and stroma in grey; (c–f) intensity profiles along the central line of the: (c) original BRF; (d) rawIQ (magnitude and phase); (e) filteredIQ (magnitude and phase) and (f) B-mode images.

Figure 1a represents a linear B-mode image (reconstructed from the original BRF data) and Fig. 1b represents the corresponding GT image. GT contours of ovaries and follicles were drawn by a medical expert on the scan-converted B-mode images and mapped afterwards to the linear space, as represented in

Fig. 1b. Each pixel of the image is categorized as follicle, stroma and surrounding tissue, which was used for the multi-class approach. GT for binary ovary approach was produced with the union of the area of the follicles and stroma.

Five different datasets were constructed with the different types of data. For each, dataset division was as follows: 92 images were used for 5-fold cross-validation and 15 for test. Due to the uneven division of the number of images for 5-fold cross-validation, three of the folds were composed by 74 images for training and 18 for validation and the other two folds were composed by 73 images for training and 19 for validation.

2.2 Convolutional Neural Networks

In this section, the two CNNs, namely the U-Net [18] and a FCRN, used for the segmentation of follicles and ovary are presented. Figure 2 illustrates both architectures. U-Net was used due to its known good performance networks for segmentation of biomedical images [18], while FCRN was used for comparison purposes. The use of FCRN allows also to assess the variability of results produced when increasing the depth of the network and when including the residual learning scheme.

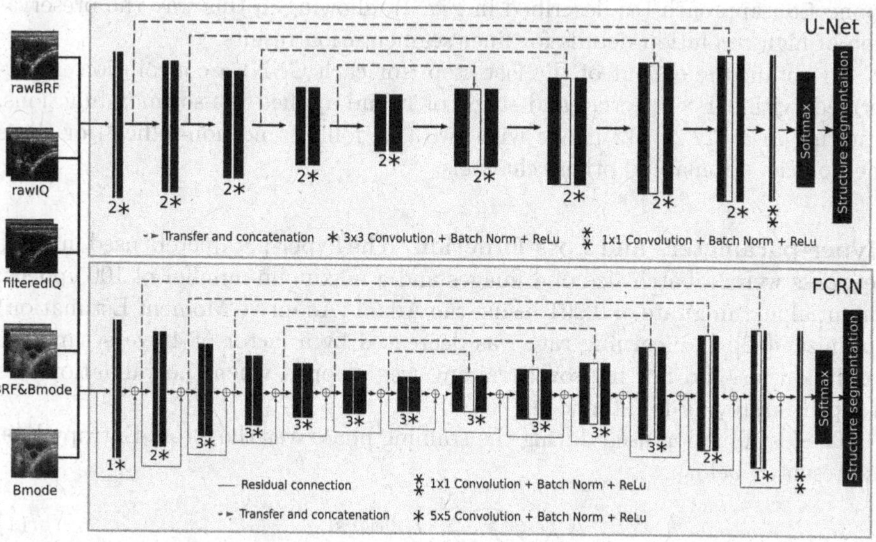

Fig. 2. Graphical representation of U-Net and FCRN network.

U-Net. The U-Net [18] has a contracting path, composed by five steps, whose output is then passed to an expanding path, composed by four steps. At each downsample (d)/upsample (u) step (s), the computed feature map is $y_s = f_{d|u,s}(x_s)$, where x_s is initial map of the step, and f represents two sequences of convolution, batch normalization and rectified linear unit (ReLU). In d and u occurs, respectively, the augmentation and reduction of the number of features. Between the steps of the contracting path it is applied max-pooling with a 2×2 kernel and stride of 2, while between the steps of the expanding path takes place a 2D transposed convolution with a scale factor of 2.

FCRN. The FCRN is an 2D adaptation of the V-Net [14] and re-uses the residual learning scheme of ResNet [9], since this learning scheme has been reported to address the gradient degradation problem [20] and has been proven to fasten the convergence [9].

At each downsample (d)/upsample (u) step (s), the computed feature map is $y_s = x_s + f_{d|u,s}(x_s)$, where x_s is the initial map of the step (*i.e.*, $x_s = y_{s-1}$) and f are sequences of convolution, batch normalization and ReLU.

The depth of the network (6 levels) was selected to allow for efficient representation of the segmentation problem through construction of hierarchical rules.

The convolutions performed in both CNNs use optimal zero-padding to preserve the image spatial size. The features obtained in each contracting step are concatenated with the features obtained after each expanding step via a skip-connection approach (as described in Fig. 2), allowing in this way the preservation of high resolution details for finer segmentation results.

To obtain the output of the last step (for each CNN) a convolution is performed, with a 1×1 kernel and stride of 1, and applied the softmax functions, resulting in a 512×512 image with two (i.e. follicle and non-follicle) or three (i.e. follicle, stroma and other) channels.

Hyper-parameters and Loss Function. The hyper-parameters used in these networks were: a batch size of 4 images and a maximum number of 100 epochs; an initial learning rate of 0.001, using the Adam (Adaptive Moment Estimation) optimizer [12]; the learning rate was decreased by a factor of 4 every time the validation loss did not improve; training was stopped when the validation loss stopped improving for 20 epochs.

The loss function used during the training phase was the Cross-Entropy loss, as presented below:

$$\mathrm{CE} = \sum_{i} \sum_{j=1}^{\mathrm{C}} t_{ij} \log(s_{ij}) \tag{1}$$

where i corresponds to an image pixel, C is the number of classes of the output, t_{ij} is the pixel's ground-truth value for that class and s_{ij} is the pixel's output probability score for that class.

U-Net and FCRN were trained using a binary and a multi-class approach. In the binary approach, the GT was binarized to represent the structure of interest (e.g. follicle) versus the other structures (e.g. stroma and surrounding tissue). In the multi-class approach, the model was optimized for the three classes simultaneously (as in Fig. 1b).

This code was implemented in Python 3.6.6 using Pytorch 0.4.1.

3 Results

This section presents experiments for the segmentation of follicles and ovary using the two different CNNs, FCRN and U-Net, and the different types of data (rawBRF, rawIQ, filteredIQ, B-mode and B-mode&BRF).

During test, a binary prediction, for follicles and ovary structures, was obtained by applying a threshold of 0.5 to the final pixel-wise probability maps. In the multi-class approach, ovary segmentation prediction was obtained by adding the probability maps of the follicle and of the stroma classes and thresholded afterwards.

For the evaluation of the performance of the trained models, test results were compared against the GT using the DICE score [6]. Models' performance analysis was performed considering the mean DICE scores of the images in the test-set, across the 5 folds of cross-validation.

A paired two tailed t-test analysis was used for comparing the performance of the different models, being the null hypothesis that the mean performance of the compared models was equal. The alpha level for all tests was set at 0.05.

Figure 3 illustrates the best and worse DICE performance for follicle and ovary segmentation, using the binary and the multi-class approach. The best and worst results here presented were obtained after performing the median DICE score per test image of the 5 cross-validation folds. The prediction image presented is the one that corresponds to the median.

The best performance is obtained for models that included B-mode images as input, while the worst performance is produced by models that use non-filtered versions of the data (rawBRF or rawIQ). The follicle segmentation with higher DICE scores were both obtained using the FCRN, while the ovary segmentation with higher DICE scores were obtained using the U-Net. The worst performance cases, for ovary and follicle segmentation, were all obtained with the U-Net.

Figure 4 presents the bar plots with the mean DICE scores of the images in the test-set, across the 5 cross-validation folds.

Statistical differences obtained for the binary segmentation of the follicles are presented in Table 1. Significant differences were found when comparing filtered data (B-mode, B-mode&BRF and filteredIQ) with rawBRF and rawIQ data. Similar results are found when comparing performance of multi-class follicle segmentation models, as shown in Table 2.

Table 3 shows that significant differences were found, for ovarian binary segmentation, when comparing the performance of the B-mode&BRF model, using the U-Net and models that use the U-Net as segmentation model but do not use B-mode as input data (i.e. rawBRF, rawIQ and filteredIQ). Significant differences are also found when comparing the performance of the U-Net method using B-mode versus B-mode&BRF data. As for the comparison between multi-class models that segment the ovary, no significant difference were found.

Table 1. p-value found for comparison between binary follicle segmentation models (alpha level was set at 0.05). Bold identifies the rejected null hypothesis cases.

		BRF		rawIQ		filteredIQ		B-mode& BRF		B-mode	
		FCRN	UNet	FCRN	UNet	FCRN	UNet	FCRN	UNet	FCRN	UNet
BRF	FCRN	-	0.963	0.423	0.321	0.052	**0.02**	**0.002**	**0.013**	**0.001**	**0.02**
	UNet		-	0.492	0.157	**0.015**	**0.002**	0	**0.002**	**0.001**	**0.003**
rawIQ	FCRN			-	0.142	**0.046**	**0.03**	**0.01**	**0.02**	**0.007**	**0.031**
	UNet				-	0.149	0.055	**0.005**	**0.034**	**0.006**	**0.048**
filteredIQ	FCRN					-	0.639	0.193	0.491	0.08	0.597
	UNet						-	0.315	0.706	0.06	0.907
B-mode&BRF	FCRN							-	0.491	0.216	0.309
	UNet								-	0.166	0.697
B-mode	FCRN									-	0.051
	UNet										-

Table 2. p-value found for comparison between multi-class follicle segmentation models (alpha level was set at 0.05). Bold identifies the rejected null hypothesis cases.

		BRF		rawIQ		filteredIQ		B-mode& BRF		B-mode	
		FCRN	UNet	FCRN	UNet	FCRN	UNet	FCRN	UNet	FCRN	UNet
BRF	FCRN	-	0.22	0.966	0.467	**0.001**	**0.007**	**0.001**	**0.004**	**0.001**	**0.003**
	UNet		-	0.242	0.84	**0**	**0.004**	**0.001**	**0.002**	**0.004**	**0.004**
rawIQ	FCRN			-	0.258	**0.001**	**0.005**	**0.001**	**0.004**	**0.001**	**0.003**
	UNet				-	**0.01**	**0.007**	**0.012**	**0.012**	**0.011**	**0.01**
filteredIQ	FCRN					-	0.903	0.968	0.681	0.492	0.254
	UNet						-	0.9	0.568	0.627	0.172
B-mode&BRF	FCRN							-	0.667	0.573	0.269
	UNet								-	0.908	0.169
B-mode	FCRN									-	0.421
	UNet										-

Table 3. p-value found for comparison between binary ovary segmentation models (alpha level was set at 0.05). Bold identifies the rejected null hypothesis cases.

		BRF		rawIQ		filteredIQ		B-mode& BRF		B-mode	
		FCRN	UNet	FCRN	UNet	FCRN	UNet	FCRN	UNet	FCRN	UNet
BRF	FCRN	-	0.33	0.38	0.299	0.647	0.363	0.547	0.213	0.185	0.806
	UNet		-	0.596	0.952	0.206	0.68	0.237	**0.026**	0.124	0.305
rawIQ	FCRN			-	0.581	0.425	0.682	0.331	0.209	0.198	0.887
	UNet				-	0.182	0.67	0.202	**0.008**	0.107	0.237
filteredIQ	FCRN					-	0.174	0.965	0.147	0.209	0.582
	UNet						-	0.235	**0.004**	0.056	0.135
B-mode&BRF	FCRN							-	0.274	0.276	0.652
	UNet								-	0.448	**0.002**
B-mode	FCRN									-	0.297
	UNet										-

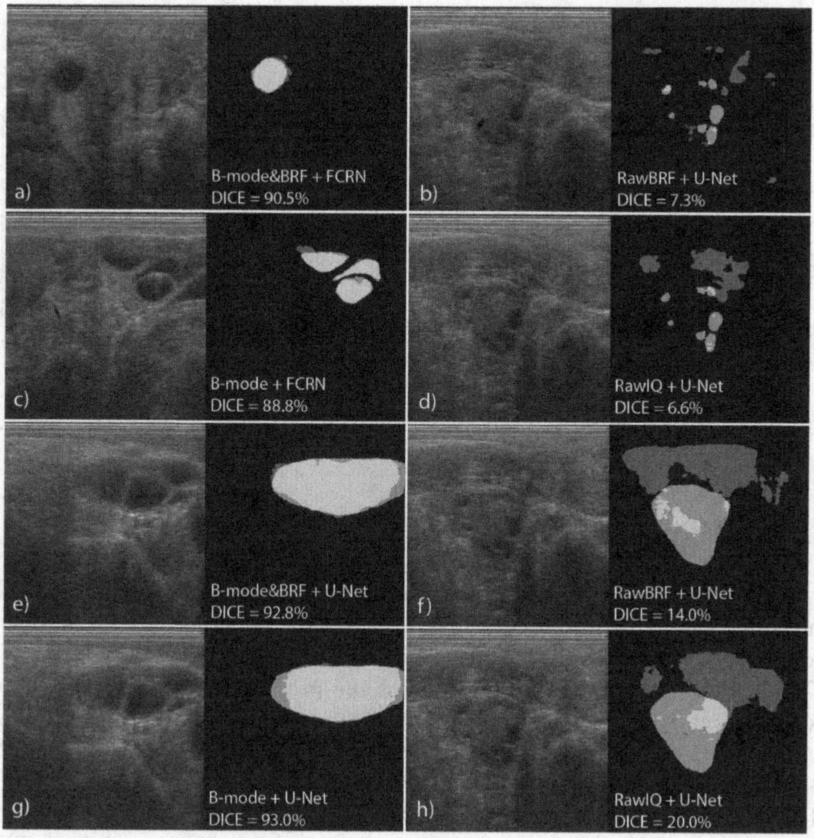

Fig. 3. DICE score for comparison between GT and segmentation results (true positives, false positives and false negatives are represented in yellow, red and green, respectively). Left column represents the four best DICE performance and the right column represents the four worst DICE performance; (a, b, e, f) represent results obtained using the binary approach while (c, d, g, h) represent results obtained using the multi-class approach. (a, b, c, d) correspond to follicle segmentation and (e, f, g, h) correspond to ovary segmentation. (Color figure online)

Also, no statistical differences were found when comparing the two CNNs independently on the type of input data. On the other hand, significant differences were found when comparing the performance of binary versus multi-class models for the ovary segmentation, when using the U-Net models trained on rawBRF, filteredIQ and B-mode data. For the follicle segmentation, a significant difference was obtained when comparing binary and multi-class models for B-mode data.

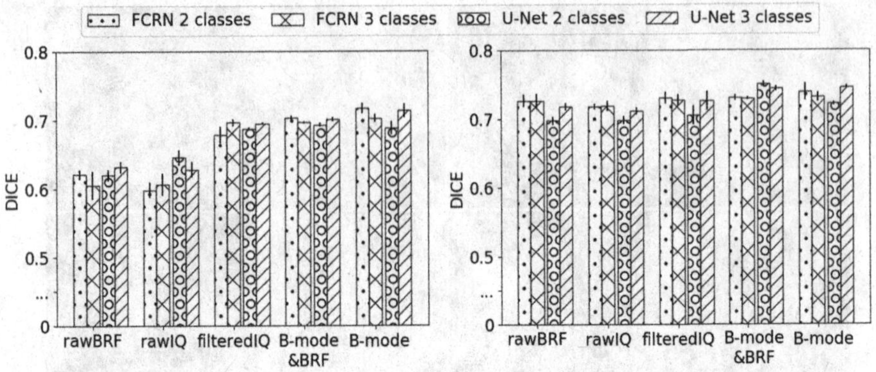

Fig. 4. Mean DICE scores of follicle (left) and ovary (right) segmentation results for each model on the test set.

4 Discussion

This work shows an extensive performance comparison of two different CNNs, trained and tested on different types of US data (ranging from rawBRF to B-mode data), for binary and multi-class problems.

One of the major research questions of the proposed paper regards the use of five different types of images extracted from the original BRF data. Due to such specifications, no other dataset containing these type of data was publicly available, limiting the evaluation of the developed methods on different data.

The qualitative results, shown in Fig. 3, demonstrate that the models trained with rawBRF or rawIQ data are not robust to noise in the unfiltered data. These results also indicate that B-mode and B-mode&BRF data are better for both follicle and ovary segmentation.

Significant differences found between follicle segmentation models that use B-mode data against the models that use unfiltered data (rawBRF and rawIQ) demonstrate that unfiltered data is not adequate for follicle segmentation. Lower performance of these models can be justified by the lower signal-to-noise ratio in follicles and by the reduced texture information, when compared to the stroma tissue. Unlike for follicle segmentation, no significant difference was found for ovary segmentation indicating that, in this case, the high-frequency content of unfiltered data helps the model to better characterize the ovarian structure.

Significant differences found for the different binary U-Net approaches, indicate that unless using B-mode&BRF data, it is challenging for the network to identify the spatial context of the ovarian region. This is likely to occur due to the small kernel sizes or the reduced depth of the U-Net.

The significant differences found when comparing binary against multi-class U-Net based models, for both ovary and of follicle segmentation, show that the optimization of the loss function, when following a multi-class approach, allow the U-Net model to better understand the spatial correlation between follicle and ovary.

These results show also that, despite the two different architectures used, no significant differences were found between these. Such results indicate that higher complexity of FCRN is an expensive solution that does entails improved performance.

5 Conclusion

The presented work extensively analyses the use of different types of ultrasound data (from beam-formed radio-frequency to B-mode data) as the input of distinct neural networks to solve the segmentation of follicles and ovary.

Results show that the best type of images for the segmentation of follicles is filtered ultrasound data, namely filtered IQ, B-mode and B-mode combined with beam-formed radio-frequency data.

As for ovary segmentation, all the different types of data used in this work produce similar results, indicating that noise reduction filters do not lead to an improvement of performance.

This work shows also that, when using U-Net, it may be beneficial to optimize the model with a multi-class ground-truth. Depth, along with kernel size, may also play an important role in ensuring the spatial context that the model can learn.

Despite, segmentation results obtained using beam-formed radio-frequency data also produce relatively accurate segmentation of the follicles and ovary. These results consolidate the assumption that beam-formed radio-frequency data contains detailed textural and structural information, and its high-frequency and fine-resolution information can be explored for segmentation and classification problems. To further benefit from the original beam-formed radio-frequency data, methods tailored for signal processing should be considered.

Future steps include the increasing of the dataset size, access to pathological data (benign and malignant ovarian cysts) and exploitation of the potential of ultrasound data for image classification regarding their malignancy.

Acknowledgments. This work is financed by National Funds through the Portuguese funding agency, FCT - Fundação para a Ciência e a Tecnologia as part of project "UID/EEA/50014/2019".

References

1. Al-Kadi, O.S., Chung, D.Y., Carlisle, R.C., Coussios, C.C., Noble, J.A.: Quantification of ultrasonic texture intra-heterogeneity via volumetric stochastic modeling for tissue characterization. Med. Image Anal. **21**(1), 59–71 (2015)
2. Ali, M., Magee, D., Dasgupta, U.: Signal processing overview of ultrasound systems for medical imaging. In: SPRAB12, Texas, pp. 1–27 (2008)
3. Brand, S., Weiss, E.C., Lemor, R.M., Kolios, M.C.: High frequency ultrasound tissue characterization and acoustic microscopy of intracellular changes. Ultrasound Med. Biol. **34**(9), 1396–1407 (2008)

4. Cigale, B., Zazula, D.: Directional 3D wavelet transform based on gaussian mixtures for the analysis of 3D ultrasound ovarian volumes. IEEE Trans. Pattern Anal. Mach. Intell. **41**(1), 64–77 (2019)
5. Dhanya, S., Kumari Roshni, V.S.: Comparison of various texture classification methods using multiresolution analysis and linear regression modeling. SpringerPlus **5**(1), 54 (2016)
6. Dice, L.R.: Measures of the amount of ecologic association between species. Ecology **26**(3), 297–302 (1945)
7. Wanderley, D.S., et al.: End-to-end ovarian structures segmentation. In: Vera-Rodriguez, R., Fierrez, J., Morales, A. (eds.) CIARP 2018. LNCS, vol. 11401, pp. 681–689. Springer, Cham (2019). https://doi.org/10.1007/978-3-030-13469-3_79
8. Furuya, M.: Ovarian cancer stroma: pathophysiology and the roles in cancer development. Cancers **4**(3), 701–724 (2012)
9. He, K., Zhang, X., Ren, S., Sun, J.: Deep Residual Learning for Image Recognition. zrXiv (2015)
10. Hiremath, P.S., Tegnoor, J.R.: automatic detection of follicles in ultrasound images of ovaries by optimal threshoding method. Int. J. Comput. Sci. Inf. Technol. **3**(2), 217-2 (2010)
11. Isah, O.R., Usman, A.D., Tekanyi, A.M.: A hybrid model of PSO algorithm and artificial neural network for automatic follicle classification. Int. J. Bioautomation **21**(1), 43–58 (2017)
12. Kingma, D., Ba, J.: Adam: a method for stochastic optimization. In: International Conference on Learning Representations (2014)
13. Lenic, M., Zazula, D., Cigale, B.: Segmentation of ovarian ultrasound images using single template cellular neural networks trained with support vector machines. In: Twentieth IEEE International Symposium on Computer-Based Medical Systems (CBMS 2007), pp. 205–212 (2007)
14. Milletari, F., Navan, N., Ahmadi, S.A.: V-Net: Fully Convolutional Neural Networks for Volumetric Medical Image Segmentation. arXiv (2016)
15. Olsen, L.O., Takiwaki, H., Serup, J.: High-frequency ultrasound characterization of normal skin. Skin thickness and echographic density of 22 anatomical sites. Skin Res. Technol. **1**(2), 74–80 (1995)
16. Potočnik, B., Cigale, B., Zazula, D.: Computerized detection and recognition of follicles in ovarian ultrasound images: a review. Med. Biol. Eng. Comput. **50**(12), 1201–1212 (2012)
17. Rauh-Hain, J.A., Krivak, T.C., Del Carmen, M.G., Olawaiye, A.B.: Ovarian cancer screening and early detection in the general population. Rev. Obstet. Gynecol. **4**(1), 15–21 (2011)
18. Ronneberger, O., Fischer, P., Brox, T.: U-net: convolutional networks for biomedical image segmentation. In: Navab, N., Hornegger, J., Wells, W.M., Frangi, A.F. (eds.) MICCAI 2015. LNCS, vol. 9351, pp. 234–241. Springer, Cham (2015). https://doi.org/10.1007/978-3-319-24574-4_28
19. Usman, A.D., Isah, O.R., Tekanyi, A.M.S.: Application of artificial neural network and texture features for follicle detection. Afr. J. Comput. ICT **8**(4), 2–9 (2015)
20. Veit, A., Wilber, M., Belongie, S.: Residual Networks Behave Like Ensembles of Relatively Shallow Networks, pp. 550–558 (2016)

Discovery Radiomics for Detection of Severely Atypical Melanocytic Lesions (SAML) from Skin Imaging via Deep Residual Group Convolutional Radiomic Sequencer

Helmut Neher[2(✉)], John Arlette[3], and Alexander Wong[1,2]

[1] Waterloo Artificial Intelligence Institute, University of Waterloo, Waterloo, ON, Canada

[2] Vision and Image Processing Research Group, University of Waterloo, Waterloo, ON, Canada

hneher@uwaterloo.ca

[3] Department of Surgery, Cumming School of Medicine, University of Calgary, Calgary, AB, Canada

Abstract. The incidence of severely atypical melanocytic lesions (SAML) has been increasing year after year. Early detection of SAML by skin surveillance followed by biopsy and treatment may improve survival and reduce the burden on health care systems. Discovery radiomics can be used to analyze a variety of quantitative features present in pigmented lesions that determine which lesions demonstrate enough atypical changes to pursue medical attention. This study utilizes a novel deep residual group convolutional radiomic sequencer to assess SAML. The discovery radiomic sequencer was evaluated against over 18,000 dermoscopic images of different atypical nevi to achieve a sensitivity of 90% and specificity of 83%. Furthermore, the radiomic sequences produced using the novel deep residual group convolutional radiomic sequencer are visualized and analyzed via t-SNE analysis.

Keywords: Radiomics · Melanoma · Deep residual group convolutional radiomic sequencers

1 Introduction

Over the past few decades the incidence of severely atypical melanocytic lesions (SAML) has increased, causing a significant burden on patients and financial costs to the healthcare system. Early recognition of abnormal lesions followed by appropriate investigation and treatment may improve patient progress and

The authors thank the Natural Sciences and Engineering Research Council of Canada, the Canada Research Chairs Program, and Elucid Labs.

F. Karray et al. (Eds.): ICIAR 2019, LNCS 11663, pp. 307–315, 2019.
https://doi.org/10.1007/978-3-030-27272-2_26

survival. Radiomics [3] can be used as screening of atypical pigmented lesions by analyzing quantitative features and characteristics seen in SAML and searching for those lesions identified as appearing abnormal.

Radiomics involves the high-throughput extraction and analysis of large amounts of quantitative features from medical imaging data to characterize tumor phenotype quantitatively. This framework is largely driven by quantitative imaging systems personalized for cancer decision support. By making personalized hand-held instruments and utilizing radiomics with proven efficacy, accuracy, and wide availability, individuals can be assessed and ranked by risk level. Traditional radiomics practice use quantitative features to identify the difference between healthy and abnormal malignant lesions. These can be limiting as they rely on traditional hand-engineered methods for characterizing texture and shape in skin lesions. The recent use of discovery radiomics in literature [1,2,4,6,7] ameliorates upon hand-engineered radiomic features by discovering a wider array of features directly from the wealth of collected skin lesion imaging data.

Discovery radiomics forgoes the notion of predefined feature models and discovers customized radiomics feature models learned from a corpus of available imaging data, thus, demonstrating an improved characterization of unique cancer phenotype for different forms of cancer. Highly unique characteristics are captured beyond what current predefined feature models are capable of.

The discovery framework consists of the following steps, as illustrated in Fig. 1. First, a wealth of standardized medical data from patients is first amassed and fed into the radiomics sequencer discovery engine where tailored radiomic sequencer is constructed based on the large amount of radiomic features discovered. These features capture unique characteristics and traits of tumors. Second, a new patient captures a medical image of the intended tumor and the discovery radiomics sequencer is then used to extract a wealth of rich imaging-based features from the medical imaging data of the new patient case for comprehensive, custom quantification of the tumor phenotype.

This study presents a novel deep residual group convolutional radiomic sequencer for the purpose of detecting SAML from skin imaging data. Traditional approaches which differ from the discovery radiomics approach involves hand-engineered features [12,13], skin lesion modelling [14], and computer-aided diagnosis using dermatology metrics which include asymmetry, border, color, and dermoscopic structure [15–17]. Although a recent study demonstrated an Inception-v3 deep convolutional neural network architecture achieving an accuracy of $72.1 \pm 0.9\%$ when discriminating between benign, malignant, and non-neoplastic lesions via dermatologist-labeled clinical images [8], the goal of this study is to detect severely atypical melanocytic lesions. This new deep residual group convolutional radiomic sequencer design leads to the creation of more discriminative, quantitative radiomic sequences, and can become a powerful tool to assist all medical professionals in improving atypical lesion identification and diagnosis.

The paper is organized as follows. First, Sect. 2 provides an overview of the general dermal discovery radiomics pipeline for SAML screening, as well and a detailed description of the design of the proposed deep residual group convolutional radiomic sequencer. Section 3 presents the experimental setup and experimental results using a large corpus of dermoscopic images are discussed. Finally, conclusions are presented in Sect. 4.

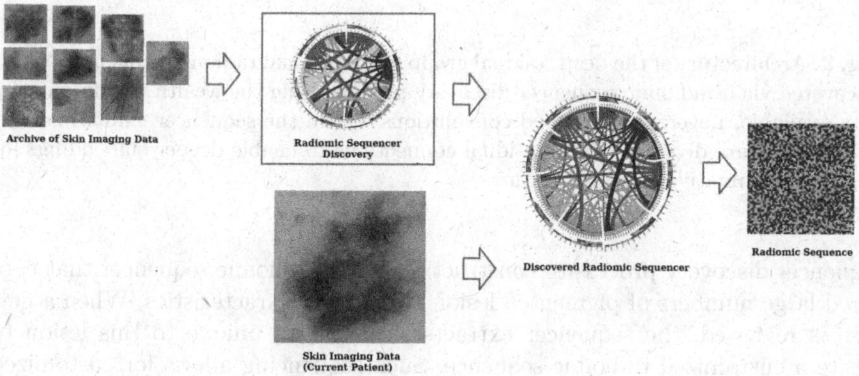

Fig. 1. The general dermal discovery radiomics pipeline for SAML screening. A radiomic sequencer (in this study, a deep residual group convolutional radiomic sequencer) is discovered via a radiomic sequencer discovery process using the wealth of skin imaging data available. The discovered radiomic sequencer can then be used to produce a radiomic sequence given an input skin image from a new patient.

2 Methodology

In this section, we will first discuss the general dermal discovery radiomics pipeline for SAML screening being presented in this study. Next, we will go into detail the design strategy for the proposed deep residual group convolutional radiomic sequencer.

2.1 Dermal Discovery Radiomics for SAML Screening

Unlike traditional approaches where predefined features are based on factors such as texture and color, dermal discovery radiomics directly obtains learned bio-marker features. The benefit of this approach is the gathering of intrinsic features that are not well-characterized by traditional approaches or not noticed by clinicians. The general pathway for atypical pigmented lesion evaluation by dermal discovery radiomics is shown in Fig. 1 which was inspired by the overall architectural layout of [18]. A comprehensive and quantitative characterization of skin phenotypes associated with SAML was built within a radiomic

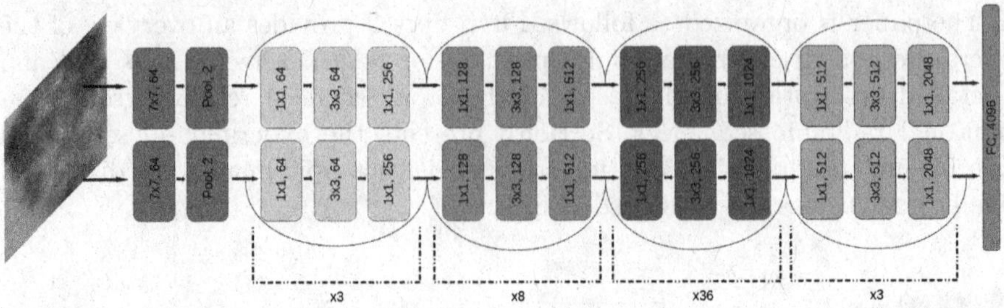

Fig. 2. Architecture of the deep residual group convolutional radiomic sequencer that is discovered via a radiomic sequencer discovery process using the wealth of skin imaging data available. Leveraging grouped convolutions within the sequencer enables greater radiomic feature diversity, while residual connections to enable deeper embeddings for highly discriminative radiomic features.

sequencer discovery process to construct a custom radiomic sequencer that captured large numbers of pigmented lesion traits and characteristics. When a new case is reviewed, the sequencer extracts the features unique to this lesion to create a customized radiomic sequence. Such sequencing allows for customized quantification of each lesion.

Table 1. Detailed configuration of the deep residual group convolutional radiomic sequencer.

Type	Output size	Configuration
gconv(2)	112×112	7×7, 64, stride 2
pool	56×56	3×3 maxpool, stride 2
gconv(2)	56×56	$[(1 \times 1, 64)\ (3 \times 3, 64)\ (1 \times 1, 256)] \times 3$
gconv(2)	28×28	$[(1 \times 1, 128)\ (3 \times 3, 128)\ (1 \times 1, 512)] \times 8$
gconv(2)	14×14	$[(1 \times 1, 256)\ (3 \times 3, 256)\ (1 \times 1, 1024)] \times 36$
gconv(2)	7×7	$[(1 \times 1, 512)\ (3 \times 3, 512)\ (1 \times 1, 2048)] \times 3$
FC		4096-d

2.2 Radiomic Sequencer Design

The radiomic sequencer introduced in this study is a custom deep residual group convolutional radiomic sequencer which sequences a total of 4096 quantitative radiomic features to characterize SAML. Figure 2 provides a graphical illustration of the overall radiomic sequencer design, with Table 1 outline the specific configuration of each component of the general architecture. The proposed deep residual group convolutional radiomic sequencer is characterized by two key traits: (i) grouped convolutions, and (ii) residual connections.

Grouped Convolutions. First, the proposed radiomic sequencer leverages the concept of grouped convolutions (as indicated by gconv(n) in Table 1, where n is the number of groups), where the components in the sequencer are divided into groups, with convolutions performed on the various channel groups separately. The use of grouped convolutions within the presented radiomic sequencer enables greater radiomic feature diversity and improved characterization performance. Such improvements are made while reducing the number of parameters needed to achieve the same level of accuracy in the case where grouped convolutions are not used. In addition, the use of two convolutional groups provide strong sensitivity and specificity measurements.

Residual Connections. Second, residual connections were leveraged in the proposed radiomic sequencer. For this study, residual connections were placed between each grouped convolution block after the pooling layer. The use of residual connections allows us to construct a deeper radiomic sequencer, and as such enables deeper feature embeddings to be discovered during the radiomic squencer discovery process. The ability to learn deeper feature embeddings results in the sequencer being able to produce highly discriminative radiomic features with strong tumor characterization capacity.

2.3 Radiomic Sequencer Discovery

The proposed deep residual group convolutional radiomic sequencer was discovered using a wealth of dermoscopic images via an iterative optimization strategy. More specifically, we leverage the Adam optimization strategy [10] to optimize a cross entropy loss function to discover the sequencer over 100 epochs, with batch size set as 6 and the adaptive learning rate decayed by 0.1 after every 25 epochs. Furthermore, we initialize the deep residual group convolutional radiomics sequencer using the Xavier weight initialization procedure [11] prior to the radiomic sequencer discovery process.

3 Results and Discussion

In this study, we evaluate the efficacy of the deep residual group convolutional radiomic sequencer for SAML detection from a large collection of dermoscopic images. First, we will discuss the data and evaluation setup, followed by a discussion of the experimental results both quantitatively and qualitatively.

3.1 Data

The efficacy of the presented deep residual group convolutional radiomic sequencer was evaluated against a collection set of 18,248 dermoscopic images of different atypical nevi. Figure 3 shows examples of dermoscopic images from the collected set spanning a spectrum of cases. Collected dermoscopic images

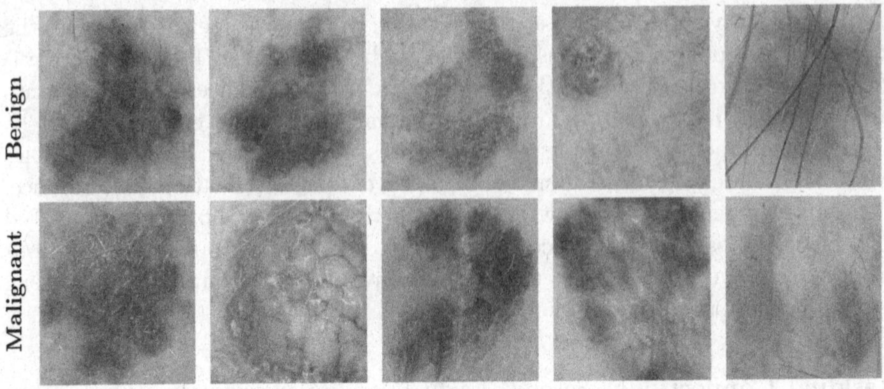

Fig. 3. Example dermoscopic images from the corpus of images used in this study.

like those shown in Figs. 1 and 3 were captured, after obtained written consent from patients referred for surgical management of SAML. The surgical procedure had been previously determined and discussed with the patient prior to being reviewed at a surgical center. The radiomic assessment on the dermoscopic images were done retrospectively and the results were benchmarked against clinical diagnosis and histopathology reports.

3.2 Evaluation Setup

The efficacy of the presented sequencer was evaluated by a random selection of 563 dermoscopic images for testing, comprised of 259 benign pigmented lesions and 264 malignant skin lesions. The radiomic sequencer produced was then fed into a fully-connected feed-forward neural network with three layers (200, 500 and 200 neurons, respectively) and an output layer with 2 neurons (for predicting malignant and benign). To quantitatively evaluate the performance of the presented sequencer, both sensitivity and specificity are computed across the entire collection of test dermoscopic images given that it is important to understand both the ability to correctly identify malignant lesions as well as avoid too many false positives.

Sensitivity is denoted by:

$$Sensitivity = \frac{TP}{TP + FN}$$

and specificity is denoted by:

$$Specificity = \frac{TN}{TN + FP}$$

where true positive (TP), false negative (FP), true negative (TN), and false positive (FP) correspond to the classification or misclassification of SAML.

3.3 Sensitivity and Specificity Analysis

The sensitivity and specificity results are shown in Table 2, alongside comparisons with previous studies by Shafiee et al. [7] and Wells et al. [5] showing quantitative evaluation of the efficacy of the proposed discovered radiomic sequencer. The sensitivity and specificity achieved with our deep residual group convolutional radiomic sequencer is 90% and 83%, respectively. In comparison, the study performed by Shafiee et al. [7] using a dataset of 9000 clinical images achieved a sensitivity and specificity of 90% and 73%. In the study by Wells et al. [5], it was found that dermatologists achieved a sensitivity and specificity of 80% and 43%, respectively, while MelaFind, a non-invasive high-based tool used for skin cancer screening, achieved a sensitivity of 96% and specificity of 8%. Although MelaFind achieved a higher sensitivity than the presented radiomic sequencer, MelaFind compromises specificity significantly. Furthermore, we are able to achieve a 10% increase in specificity when compared to the study by Shafiee et al. [7].

3.4 t-SNE Analysis

To visualize and analyze the efficacy of the radiomic sequencer, we project the 4096-dimensional radiomic sequences of each lesion in the test set generated by the presented radiomic sequencer into a two-dimensional feature space using t-Distributed Stochastic Neighbor Embedding (t-SNE) [9] analysis. T-SNE is a technique used for dimensionality reduction particularly for high-dimensional datasets. T-SNE captures local structure of high-dimensional data while also showing global structure in a single map by giving each data point a two dimensional map. Distances between each data point is proportional to the similarity of that lesion.

Table 2. Results of presented deep residual group convolutional (DRGC) radiomic sequencer in comparison to previous studies.

Study	Sensitivity	Specificity
DRGC sequencer	**90%**	**83%**
Shafiee et al. [7]	90%	73%
Dermatologist (Wells et al. [5])	80%	43%
MelaFind (Wells et al. [5])	96%	8%

In Fig. 4, we visualize the projected two-dimensional representations of the radiomic sequences in a two-dimensional feature space. Each lesion is symbolized as a point in representation space, with yellow indicating malignancy and purple indicating benign. It can be observed that the radiomic sequences generated using the proposed radiomic sequencer for malignant lesions are well-separated from the radiomic sequences for benign lesions. Some benign lesions were sequenced via the radiomic sequencer similarly to malignant lesions as some benign data points are interspersed within the malignant data point cluster of the t-SNE visualization. The interspersed benign data points within the t-SNE visualization supports the finding in Table 2 where the DRGC sequencer has a more challenging time identifying benign lesions as indicated with a specificity of 83% compared to the sensitivity of 90%.

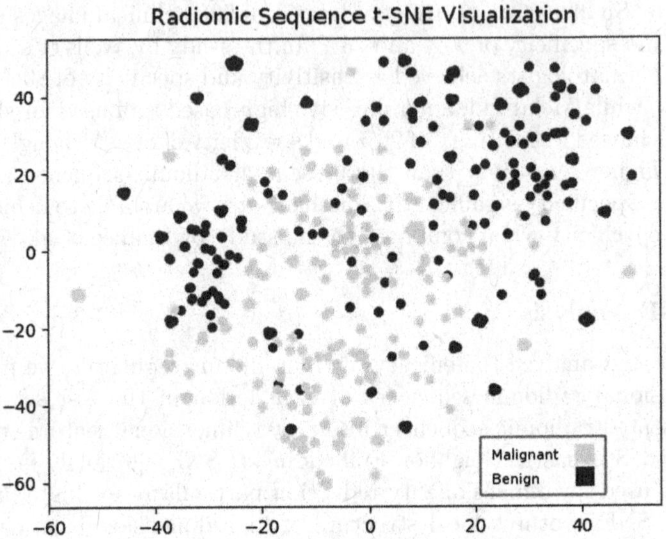

Fig. 4. A 2D visualization of the 4096 radiomic sequences extracted from the deep residual group convolutional radiomic sequencer using t-Distributed Stochastic Neighbor Embedding (t-SNE) [9]. Each point represents a lesion, where, yellow represents malignant and purple represents benign. The distance between each lesion is proportional to the similarity of that lesion. (Color figure online)

4 Conclusion

In this work we presented a discovery radiomics approach using a deep residual group convolutional radiomic sequencer for detecting atypical pigmented lesions for SAML. Given the above analysis using t-SNE as well as the aforementioned sensitivity and specificity results, it can be observed that the presented deep residual group convolutional radiomic sequencer can achieve superior performance when analyzing atypical pigmented lesions for SAML based on dermoscopic imaging data. The deep residual group convolutional radiomic sequencer presented demonstrates the efficacy of making this deep residual group convolutional radiomic sequencer a promising tool for early skin cancer screening.

References

1. Karimi, A.-H., et al.: Discovery radiomics via a mixture of deep convnet sequencers for multi-parametric MRI prostate cancer classification. In: Karray, F., Campilho, A., Cheriet, F. (eds.) ICIAR 2017. LNCS, vol. 10317, pp. 45–53. Springer, Cham (2017). https://doi.org/10.1007/978-3-319-59876-5_6
2. Kumar, D., Chung, A.G., Shaifee, M.J., Khalvati, F., Haider, M.A., Wong, A.: Discovery radiomics for pathologically-proven computed tomography lung cancer prediction. In: Karray, F., Campilho, A., Cheriet, F. (eds.) ICIAR 2017. LNCS, vol. 10317, pp. 54–62. Springer, Cham (2017). https://doi.org/10.1007/978-3-319-59876-5_7
3. Lambin, P., et al.: Radiomics: extracting more information from medical images using advanced feature analysis. Eur. J. Cancer **48**, 441–446 (2012)
4. Shafiee, M.J., Chung, A.G., Kumar, D., Khalvati, F., Haider, M., Wong, A.: Discovery radiomics via stochasticnet sequencers for cancer detection. In: NIPS Workshop on Machine Learning in Healthcare (2015)
5. Wells, R., Gutkowicz-Krusin, D., Veledar, E.A.E: Comparison of diagnostic and management sensitivity to melanoma between dermatologists and melafind: a pilot study. In: International Conference Image Analysis and Recognition (2012)
6. Wong, A., Chung, A.G., Kumar, D., Shafiee, M.J., Khalvati, F., Haider, M.: Discovery radiomics for imaging-driven quantitative personalized cancer decision support. J. Compt. Vis. Imaging Syst. (2015)
7. Shafiee, M.J., Wong, A.: Discovery radiomics via deep multi-column radiomic sequencers for skin cancer detection. J. Compt. Vis. Imaging Syst. **4**, 041305 (2017)
8. Esteva, A., et al.: Dermatologist-level classification of skin cancer with deep neural networks. Nature **542**, 115 (2017)
9. van der Maaten, L.J.P., Hinton, G.E.: Visualizing high-dimensional data using t-SNE. J. Mach. Learn. Res. **9**, 12 (2008)
10. Kingma, D., Ba, J.: Adam: a method for stochastic optimization. In: Proceedings of the 3rd International Conference on Learning Representations (2014)
11. Glorot, X., Bengio, J.: Understanding the difficulty of training deep feedforward neural networks (2010)
12. Amelard, R., Glaister, J., Wong, A., Clausi, D.A.: High-level intuitive features (HLIFs) for intuitive skin lesion description. IEEE Trans. Biomed. Eng. **62**, 820–831 (2015)
13. Cho, D., Clausi, D., Wong, A.: Dermal radiomics for melanoma screening. J. Comput. Vis. Imaging Syst. (2015)
14. Cho, D.S., Khalvati, F., Clausi, D.A., Wong, A.: A machine learning-driven approach to computational physiological modeling of skin cancer. In: Karray, F., Campilho, A., Cheriet, F. (eds.) ICIAR 2017. LNCS, vol. 10317, pp. 79–86. Springer, Cham (2017). https://doi.org/10.1007/978-3-319-59876-5_10
15. Barata, C., Celebi, M.E., Marques, J.S.: Development of a clinically oriented system for melanoma diagnosis. Pattern Recogn. **69**, 270–285 (2017)
16. Barata, C., Celebi, M.E., Marques, J.S., Rozeira, J.: Clinically inspired analysis of dermoscopy images using a generative model. Comput. Vis. Image Underst. **151**, 124–137 (2016)
17. Shimizu, K., Iyatomi, H., Celebi, M.E., Norton, K.A., Tanaka, M.: Four-class classification of skin lesions with task decomposition strategy. IEEE Trans. Biomed. Eng. **62**, 274–283 (2015)
18. He, K., Zhang, X., Ren, S., Sun, J.: Deep residual learning for image recognition. In: IEEE Conference on Computer Vision and Pattern Recognition (2016)

Identifying Diagnostically Complex Cases Through Ensemble Learning

Yan Yu(✉), Yiyang Wang(✉), Jacob Furst(✉), and Daniela Raicu(✉)

DePaul University, Chicago, IL 60601, USA
yyu45@mail.depaul.edu, {ywang192, jfurst}@depaul.edu, draicu@cdm.depaul.edu

Abstract. Computer-Aided Diagnosis systems have been used as second readers in the medical imaging diagnostic process. In this study, we aim to identify cases that are hard to diagnose and lead to interpretation variability among medical experts. We propose a combination of image features and advanced machine learning classifiers to predict the degree of malignancy and determine the level of diagnostic difficulty by looking where these classifiers collectively fail. Using the NIH/NCI Lung Image Database Consortium (LIDC) dataset and four ensemble learning algorithms (bagging, random forest, AdaBoost, and a heterogeneous ensemble with decision trees, support vector machines, and k-nearest neighbors), our results show that we can not only detect difficult cases, but we are also able to identify what imaging characteristics or features make these cases hard to diagnostically interpret.

Keywords: Ensemble learning · Computer-Aided Diagnosis · Diagnostic complexity

1 Introduction

In the radiology domain, Computer-Aided Diagnosis (CADx) systems have been proposed to assist radiologists in the diagnostic interpretation of different anatomical structures, such as lung [1], breast [2], and colon [3]. In general, there are two categories of approaches for developing CADx systems.

The traditional way involves extracting image features and then building classification models on image feature data. For example, by extracting mammogram features and implementing logistic regression as well as support vector machines (SVM) algorithms, Jing *et al.* [4] reported significant improvement in diagnosis accuracy. Kaya and Can [5] proposed a weighted-rule based method for malignancy prediction and achieved 82.52% classification accuracy. Goncalves *et al.* [6] used k-nearest neighbors (k-NN) and SVM to compute the malignancy likelihood of lung nodules with a performance of 0.96 for area under the receiver operator characteristic (AUC). Riely *et al.* [7] designed a selective iterative classification (SIC) approach for lung nodule classification.

The modern way employs deep learning approaches that diagnostically categorize the images without the need for using image features. Recently, Causey *et al.* [8]

F. Karray et al. (Eds.): ICIAR 2019, LNCS 11663, pp. 316–324, 2019.
https://doi.org/10.1007/978-3-030-27272-2_27

implemented deep learning convolutional neural networks (CNN) to predict lung nodule malignancy and achieved high accuracy for nodule malignancy classification with an AUC of 0.99. Liu *et al.* [9] proposed a multi-task deep learning framework with a novel margin ranking loss to investigate the relatedness between lung nodule classification and attribute score regression and achieved 93.9% classification accuracy. Hoo-Chang *et al.* [10] implemented deep convolutional neural networks to perform thoracic-abdominal lymph node detection and interstitial lung disease classification.

While all these studies focus on improving the prediction performance, only a few studies explored the factors (such as a case difficulty) affecting the performance of the classifiers for diagnostic interpretation. Analyzing the human observers, Lin *et al.* [11] proposed a content-boosted collaborative filtering (CBCF) to predict the difficulty level for each trainee in the radiology training system. Similarly, Wang *et al.* [12] developed a user model that predicted the likelihood of a trainee missing an abnormal location.

Rather than looking at the human observer level of expertise, other studies, including our previous work, focused on the use of image content to automatically detect when and why classifiers fail in predicting certain cases. Zamacona *et al.* [13] used decision tree to predict the malignancy ratings and differentiated easy and hard cases by applying a threshold value based on the distribution of the case error variance. Affenit *et al.* [14] proposed a new label set weighting approach to combine the experts' interpretations and their variability, as well as a SIC approach that was based on conformal prediction. Berglin *et al.* [15] defined the hardest cases by aggregating results from five different SIC techniques and identifying those that were above a threshold of difficulty.

Since our goal is not only to improve the malignancy prediction, but also to understand what makes a case difficult to interpret, we will focus on the first category of CADx systems. We introduce the concept of the "difficulty" of a case when collectively ensembles of classifiers fail to categorize the case based on its image content. Building upon our previous work [13], besides detecting the difficult cases, we propose to further determine the characteristics of the diagnostically difficult cases. We show our proof-of-concept in the context of the lung nodule diagnosis in Computed Tomography images, but the same approach can be applied to other anatomical structures and medical imaging modalities.

2 Methodology

2.1 The Lung Image Database Consortium (LIDC) Data and Low-Level Image Feature Extraction

The NIH/NCI Lung Image Database Consortium (LIDC) dataset [16] is a collection of Computed Tomography (CT) scans annotated by four different radiologists. Each radiologist provided nodule contours and ratings across nine semantic characteristics: calcification, internal structure, lobulation, malignancy, margin, sphericity, spiculation, subtlety, and texture. In this study, we focus on the prediction of the degree of malignancy ratings (1: highly unlikely; 2: moderately; 3: indeterminate; 4: moderately suspicious; 5: highly suspicious) and consider 829 nodules that have been annotated by all four radiologists.

From each image that contains a nodule, we extracted 64 low-level image features [17] shown in Table 1, that can be divided into four different categories: shape, size, intensity and texture. Figure 1 illustrates the feature extraction step and the rest of the CADx system as a way to identify hard cases.

Table 1. Image features, SD stands for standard deviation and BG for background

Shape Features	Size Features	Intensity
Circularity	Area	Min Intensity
Roughness	Convex Area	Max Intensity
Elongation	Perimeter	Mean Intensity
Compactness	Convex Perimeter	SD Intensity
Eccentricity	Equivalent Diameter	Min Intensity BG
Solidity	Major Axis Length	Max Intensity BG
Extent	Minor Axis Length	Mean Intensity BG
Radial Distance SD		SD Intensity BG
		Intensity Difference

Texture Features
11 Haralick features calculated from co-occurrence matrices (Contrast, Correlation, Entropy, Energy, Homogeneity, 3rd Order Moment, Inverse Variance, Sum Average, Variance, Cluster Tendency, Maximum Probability)
24 Gabor features are mean and standard deviation of 12 different Gabor images (orientation = 0°, 45°, 90°, 135° and frequency = 0.3, 0.4, 0.5)
5 Markov Random Fields (MRF) features are means of 4 different response images (orientation = 0°, 45°, 90°, 135°), along with the variance response image

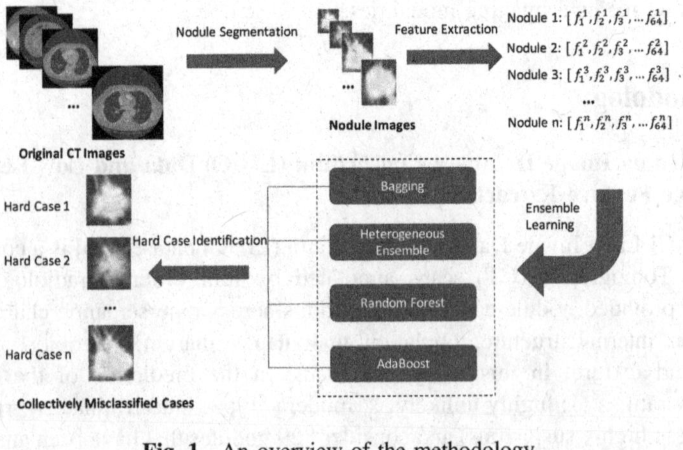

Fig. 1. An overview of the methodology

2.2 Data Preprocessing

Given the low number of cases for the second and fourth rating, we rescaled the malignancy by assigning ratings 1 and 2 to class 1 and ratings 4 and 5 to class 3, and rating 3 forming its own class 2. Furthermore, if the ratings for the same nodule varied among the radiologists, we considered the consensus label, the mode of four ratings, for the corresponding nodule when training and testing the CADx system.

We used 10-fold cross validation for testing and training. In this case, each instance is guaranteed one chance to be tested in a testing set.

2.3 Identifying Difficult Cases Through Ensemble Learning

Classification approaches range from single classifiers to ensemble of classifiers that are more robust, stable, and generalize well on complex data. Sometimes, no matter which type of algorithm is used, a case cannot be classified correctly based on its image content. For these situations, we introduce the concept of difficulty/complexity/hardness of a case to denote that a certain pattern cannot be learned from the image data even though the classification approach has been optimized with respect to the given data. In our current implementation, the classification approach is based on four ensembles of classifiers: bagging with decision trees (DT) [18], a heterogeneous ensemble based on a set of algorithms including decision trees, support vector machine (SVM) and k-nearest neighbors (k-NN), random forest [19], and AdaBoost with stump trees [20].

Bagging is a method for generating multiple versions of a prediction and using these to get an aggregated predictor. The multiple versions are formed by making bootstrapping of the training set and using these as new training sets to build different models. When predicting a class, the aggregated predictor does a plurality among the results of the models. Decision tree is our base classifier in Bagging. We implemented 10-fold cross validation method on the training sets and found the optimal number of trees that leads to the minimum cross validation error. The criteria of choosing the number of trees in Bagging is finding the knee point in the plot of relationship of number of trees to error. For the parameters in each decision tree, we let them grow fairly on each sampled data set, with no pruning. In our paper, the number of trees across ten training sets varies from eight to thirteen. The principle of Bagging algorithm is presented as follows:

$$N_j = \#\{k; \varphi(x, £_k) = j\}$$

$$\varphi_A(x) = argmax_j N_j \tag{1}$$

Where $£_k$ is a sequence of learning sets, φ is a single predictor, $\varphi(x, £_k)$ predicts a class $j \in \{1, \ldots, J\}$ and φ_A is a Bagging predictor.

The way heterogenous ensemble combines its base classifiers' result is the same as Bagging, a type of homogenous ensemble. We aggregated the results of base classifiers by voting. However, a heterogenous ensemble classifier is constructed by various algorithms as its base classifiers. In our paper, we used three base classifiers to build the heterogenous ensemble model: decision tree, SVM and k-NN.

Instead of using a single decision tree, the random forest algorithm creates a set of decision trees to improve the classification accuracy and assigns a prediction label by using a majority vote. There are two parameters in Random Forest Algorithm: the number of trees and the number of features per split. We chose the optimal parameter combination that leads to the minimum out of bag (OOB) error on the training sets.

The AdaBoost algorithm of Freund and Schapire was the first practical boosting algorithm. Adaboost, short for Adaptive Boosting, uses the conjunction of the weak learning algorithms to create a strong classifier. The output of the weak learners is combined into a weighted sum that represents the final output of the boosted classifier. An AdaBoost model can be formulated as follows:

$$H(x) = \sum\nolimits_{t=1}^{T} \alpha_t h_t(x) \tag{2}$$

Where $H(x)$ represents the final ensemble model, and $h_t(x)$ represents the hypothesis generated by the tth base classifier. α_t is the weight assigned to the tth base classifier. In order to find the number of iterations in Adaboost, we further separate a validation set from each training set. We chose the number of iterations that has the minimum difference between training accuracy and validation accuracy. In our paper, the number of iterations is 200.

A case is considered difficult if it is collectively misclassified by all ensembles as part of the testing set.

3 Results

3.1 Classification Accuracy and Distribution of Easy Versus Hard Cases

Tables 2 and 3 compared the mean values of 15 features that are significantly different between the easy cases and hard cases by performing the Welch's t-test, an unpaired t-test typically applied when two populations have unequal variances or sample sizes.

Table 2. Significant texture features

Features: mean values	Hard cases	Easy cases	P-value
Gabor Mean 1_1	62.93	67.07	0.05
Gabor Mean 2_1	48.45	53.46	0.03
Gabor SD 2_1	50.27	52.63	0.02
Gabor Mean 3_1	76.97	82.58	0.00
Contrast	64390.11	117896.03	0.00
Energy	0.00	0.00	0.00
Homogeneity	0.04	0.04	0.02
3rd Order Moment	3079755	10715780	0.00
Sum Average	488.41	553.33	0.00
Variance	105622.20	171999.10	0.00
Cluster Tendency	360990.20	575137.90	0.00

Table 3. Significant intensity features

Features: mean values	Hard cases	Easy cases	P-value
Max Intensity	1016.87	1269.09	0.00
Mean Intensity	561.65	652.63	0.01
SD Intensity	289.55	355.60	0.00
Intensity Difference	350.45	395.68	0.01

Table 4 shows the classification accuracy using 95% confidence interval (CI) given the 10 testing sets from the 10-fold cross-validation. Figure 2 shows the class distribution of identified difficult cases. If we only use one classifier, the random forest algorithm gives the least number of misclassified cases (288); while when we use two classifiers, the combination of random forest and bagging gives the least number of overlapped misclassified cases (156). For three classifiers, the combination of AdaBoost, random forest and bagging produces the least number of overlapped misclassified cases (119); when all four ensembles are used, the approach results in having 92 hard cases and 737 easy cases. Furthermore, we can see from Fig. 2 that class 2 ("indeterminate") is the majority class for difficult cases.

Table 4. Classification results on testing sets

Methods (Classifiers)	Accuracy (95% CI)
Random forest	64.65% ± 2.6%
Heterogeneous ensemble (DT, SVM & k-NN)	62.60% ± 3.0%
AdaBoost (Stump Trees)	62.31% ± 2.9%
Bagging (Decision Trees)	60.03% ± 3.5%

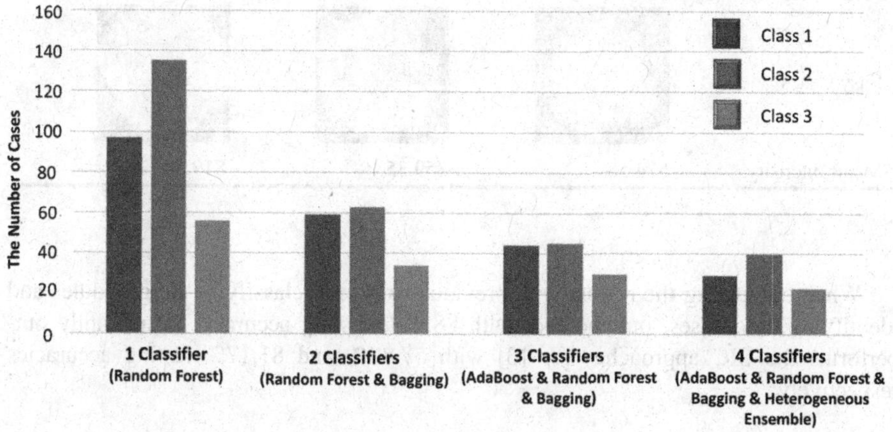

Fig. 2. Class distribution of identified difficult cases using different number of classifiers

3.2 Significant Features for Difficulty Identification

Using the Welch's t-test, we found that 15 out of the 64 features had significant mean differences between easy cases and hard cases at a 0.05 significance level. From Tables 2 and 3, we can see that difficult cases have significantly smaller mean intensity feature values and, with the exception of homogeneity, lower mean texture feature values. The features in Table 3 represent the maximum, mean and standard deviation of intensity values for those pixels within the boundary of the nodule. Intensity difference is the value of difference between the highest intensity pixel value and the lowest intensity pixel value. In Table 2, Gabor features were represented as 'Gabor Mean/SD x_y' format, where x represents four orientations (0°, 45°, 90°, and 135°) and y represents three frequencies (0.3, 0.4 and 0.5). Gabor mean 1_1, Garbor mean 2_1, Garbor mean 3_1 and Garbor SD 2_1 have the orientation and the frequency combination (45° and 0.4), (90° and 0.4), (135° and 0.4) and (90° and 0.4) respectively.

Smaller mean intensity feature values indicate the need to preprocess the images before their annotation and image feature extraction. In particular, contrast enhancement can improve the visual quality of the image and therefore, reduce the potential noise in the labeling of the image data as well as bringing the image data within the same intensity window. To illustrate the intensity differences between easy and hard cases, we present several examples of easy cases and hard cases in Table 5.

Table 5. Examples of hard vs. easy cases

Hard Cases	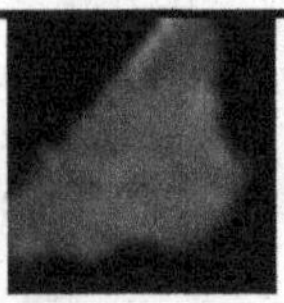	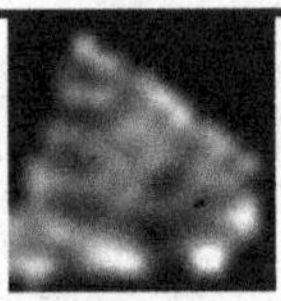	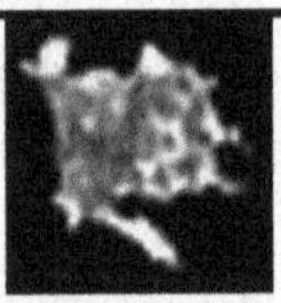
Mean Intensity	461.09	591.88	535.43
Easy Cases	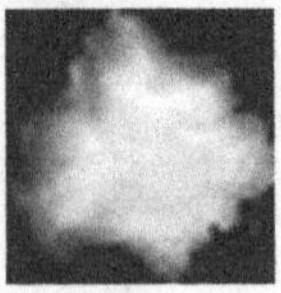	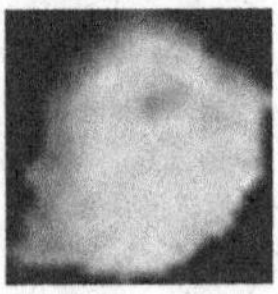	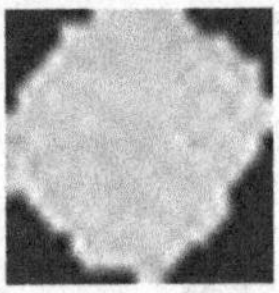
Mean Intensity	674.58	859.35	819.38

When comparing the results with previous works for classifying lung nodules and identifying hard cases, our method, with 88.90% testing accuracy, significantly outperforms the SIC approaches [7, 13] with 57.40% and 81.17% testing accuracies respectively.

4 Conclusions

In this study, we proposed ensemble learning algorithms to automatically identify difficult cases when predicting degree of malignancy based on image data. Our results show that not only we can detect these difficult cases, but also, we can differentiate the image characteristics between the difficult and easy cases.

The results of this work can help with the resource allocation problem by assigning more experts to a case only if it is a hard case to diagnose. Our findings also emphasize the need for contrast enhancement and data normalization when building CADx systems.

One limitation of this study is the lack of ground truth for validating the easy/hard classification. Future work will investigate measure of radiologist variation as a means of distinguishing easy/hard and compare to our predicted results.

References

1. Gong, J., Liu, J.-Y., Sun, X.-W., Zheng, B., Nie, S.-D.: Computer-aided diagnosis of lung cancer: the effect of training data sets on classification accuracy of lung nodules. Phys. Med. Biol. **63**(3), 035036 (2018)
2. Jalalian, A., Mashohor, S., Mahmud, R., Karasfi, B., Saripan, M.I.B., Ramli, A.R.B.: Foundation and methodologies in computer-aided diagnosis systems for breast cancer detection. EXCLI J. **16**, 113 (2017)
3. Tamai, N., et al.: Effectiveness of computer-aided diagnosis of colorectal lesions using novel software for magnifying narrow-band imaging: a pilot study. Endosc. Int. Open **5**(8), E690 (2017). Learning for Clinical Decision Support, pp. 74–82. Springer (2018)
4. Jing, H., Yang, Y.: Image retrieval for computer-aided diagnosis of breast cancer. In: 2010 IEEE Southwest Symposium on Image Analysis & Interpretation (SSIAI), pp. 9–12. IEEE (2010)
5. Kaya, A., Can, A.B.: A weighted rule based method for predicting malignancy of pulmonary nodules by nodule characteristics. J. Biomed. Inform. **56**, 69–79 (2015)
6. Goncalves, L., Novo, J., Cunha, A., Campilho, A.: Learning lung nodule malignancy likelihood from radiologist annotations or diagnosis data. J. Med. Biol. Eng. **38**(3), 424–442 (2017)
7. Riely, A., Sablan, K., Xiaotao, T., Furst, J., Raicu, D.: Reducing annotation cost and uncertainty in computer-aided diagnosis through selective iterative classification. In: Medical Imaging 2015: Computer-Aided Diagnosis, vol. 9414, p. 94141 K. International Society for Optics and Photonics (2015)
8. Causey, J.L., et al.: Highly accurate model for prediction of lung nodule malignancy with CT scans. Sci. Rep. **8**(1), 9286 (2018)
9. Liu, L., Dou, Q., Chen, H., Olatunji, I.E., Qin, J., Heng, P.-A.: MTMR-net: multi-task deep learning with margin ranking loss for lung nodule analysis. In: Stoyanov, D., et al. (eds.) DLMIA/ML-CDS -2018. LNCS, vol. 11045, pp. 74–82. Springer, Cham (2018). https://doi.org/10.1007/978-3-030-00889-5_9
10. Hoo-Chang, S., et al.: Deep convolutional neural networks for computer-aided detection: CNN architectures, dataset characteristics and transfer learning. IEEE Trans. Med. Imaging **35**(5), 1285 (2016)

11. Lin, H., Yang, X., Wang, W.: A content-boosted collaborative filtering algorithm for personalized training in interpretation of radiological imaging. J. Digital Imaging **27**(4), 449–456 (2014)
12. Wang, M., et al.: Predicting false negative errors in digital breast tomosynthesis among radiology trainees using a computer vision-based approach. Expert Syst. Appl. **56**, 1–8 (2016)
13. Zamacona, J.R., Niehaus, R., Rasin, A., Furst, J.D., Raicu, D.S.: Assessing diagnostic complexity: an image feature-based strategy to reduce annotation costs. Comput. Biol. Med. **62**, 294–305 (2015)
14. Affenit, R.N., Barns, E.R., Furst, J.D., Rasin, A., Raicu, D.S.: Building confidence and credibility into cad with belief decision trees. In: Medical Imaging 2017: Computer-Aided Diagnosis, vol. 10134, p. 101343Z. International Society for Optics and Photonics (2017)
15. Berglin, S., Shin, E., Furst, J., Raicu, D.: Efficient learning in computer-aided diagnosis through label propagation. In: 2019 Society of Photographic Instrumentation Engineers (SPIE) Medical Imaging (2019)
16. Armato III, S.G., et al.: The lung image database consortium (LIDC) and image database resource initiative (IDRI): a completed reference database of lung nodules on CT scans. Med. Phys. **38**(2), 915–931 (2011)
17. Zinovev, D., Raicu, D., Furst, J., Armato III, S.G.: Predicting radiological panel opinions using a panel of machine learning classifiers. Algorithms **2**(4), 1473–1502 (2009)
18. Breiman, L.: Bagging predictors. Mach. Learn. **24**(2), 123–140 (1996)
19. Breiman, L.: Random forests. Mach. Learn. **45**(1), 5–32 (2001)
20. Freund, Y., Schapire, R.E.: A decision-theoretic generalization of on-line learning and an application to boosting. J. Comput. Syst. Sci. **55**(1), 119–139 (1997)

tCheXNet: Detecting Pneumothorax on Chest X-Ray Images Using Deep Transfer Learning

Antonio Sze-To[1,2](✉) and Zihe Wang[3]

[1] Centre for Pattern Analysis and Machine Intelligence, University of Waterloo, Waterloo, ON N2L 3G1, Canada
hy2szeto@uwaterloo.ca

[2] Department of Systems Design Engineering, University of Waterloo, Waterloo, ON N2L 3G1, Canada

[3] Department of Mathematics, University of Waterloo, Waterloo, ON N2L 3G1, Canada
z622wang@edu.uwaterloo.ca

Abstract. Pneumothorax (collapsed lung or dropped lung) is an urgent situation and can be life-threatening. It is mostly diagnosed by chest X-ray images. Detecting Pneumothorax on chest X-ray images is challenging, as it requires the expertise of radiologists. Such expertise is time-consuming and expensive to obtain. The recent release of big medical image datasets with labels enabled the Deep Neural Network to be trained to detect diseases autonomously. As the trend moves on, it is expected to foresee more and more medical image big dataset will appear. However, the major limitation is that these datasets have different labels and settings. The know-how to transfer the knowledge learnt from one Deep Neural Network to another, i.e. Deep Transfer Learning, is becoming more and more important. In this study, we explored the use of Deep Transfer Learning to detect Pneumothorax from chest X-ray images. We proposed a model architecture tCheXNet, a Deep Neural Network with 122 layers. Other than training from scratch, we used a training strategy to transfer knowledge learnt in CheXNet to tCheXNet. In our experiments, tCheXNet achieved 10% better in ROC comparing to CheXNet on a testing set which is verified by three board-certified radiologists, in which the training time was only 10 epochs. The source code is available in https://github.com/antoniosehk/tCheXNet.

Keywords: Deep Learning · Transfer Learning · Medical Images · Chest X-rays · Pneumothorax

1 Introduction

Pneumothorax (collapsed lung or dropped lung) [1,2] refers to the entry of air into the pleural space, i.e. the space between the lungs and chest wall [2]. It is

F. Karray et al. (Eds.): ICIAR 2019, LNCS 11663, pp. 325–332, 2019.
https://doi.org/10.1007/978-3-030-27272-2_28

an urgent situation [1] and can be life-threatening emergency [2]. Pneumothorax is mostly diagnosed by chest X-ray images [2]. Figure 1 provides a graphical illustration of Pneumothorax, where (a) refers to a patient with no finding and (b) refers to a patient with Pneumothorax. Detecting Pneumothorax on chest X-ray images is challenging, as expertise of radiologists is required [3]. It is time-consuming and expensive to train a qualified radiologist. As a delayed diagnosis can cause harm to patients [3], it is important for the development of computer-aided detection approaches.

Recently, increasing studies [3] reported that researchers use Deep Learning [4] to detect diseases on chest X-ray images, and one [5] reported to achieve radiologist-level detection of pneumonia in chest X-ray image. In essence, Deep Learning refers to the use of Deep Neural Networks (DNN), defined as artificial neuron networks with at least 3 hidden layers [6]). Its success is built upon the advent of fast graphics processing units (GPU), and the availability of large amount of labeled data [4].

The driving force behind the emergence of these medical image Deep Neural Network can be attributed to the recent release of several big medical image datasets [7–9] with labels. For example, CheXpert [8] is a dataset that is recently released, containing 224,316 chest radiographs of 65,240 patients. There are 14 categories (observations) labeled with each of the chest radiographs, where one chest radiograph can be associated with multiple observations. As the trend moves on, there will be more and more big medical image datasets. However, the major limitation is that these datasets have different labels and settings. The know-how to transfer the knowledge learnt from one Deep Neural Network to another, i.e. Deep Transfer Learning [10,11], is becoming more and more important.

In this study, we explored the use of Deep Transfer Learning [10,11] to detect Pneumothorax [1,2] from chest X-ray images. We proposed a model architecture tCheXNet, a Deep Neural Network with 122 layers. Other than training from scratch, we used a training strategy to transfer knowledge learnt in CheXNet [5] to tCheXNet. Experimental results demonstrated that tCheXNet achieved 10% better in ROC comparing to CheXNet on a testing set verified by three board-certified radiologists using only a training time of 10 epochs. To our knowledge, it is the first systematic study to detect Pneumothorax on chest X-ray images using Deep Transfer Learning.

2 Methodology

2.1 Problem Definition

The detection task of Pneumothorax [1,2] from a frontal-view chest radiograph (or chest X-ray) image is defined as follows. Given a frontal-view chest X-ray image x_i, the output is a binary variable $y_i \in \{0, 1\}$, where 0 and 1 represents the absence and presence of Pneumothorax [1,2] in the X-ray image x_i respectively. From the point of view in machine learning, 0 represents the negative (−ve) classes, i.e. the chest X-ray images with the absence of Pneumothorax [1,2],

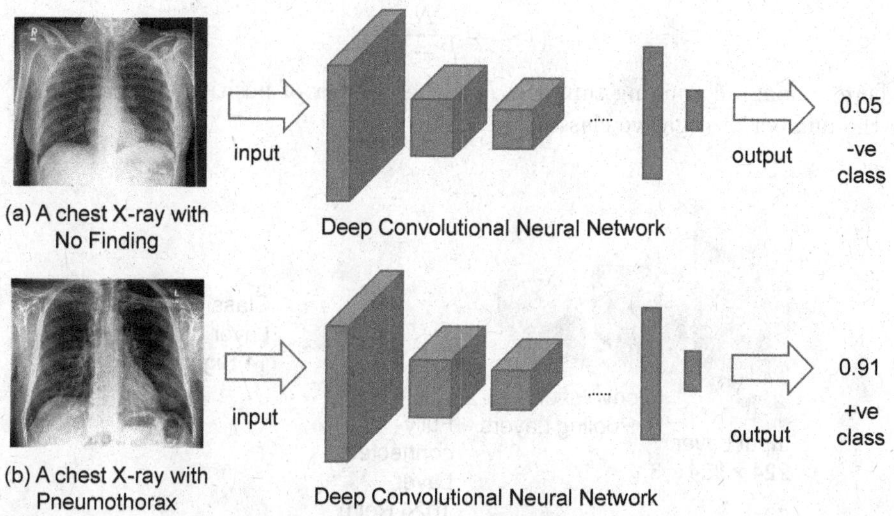

Fig. 1. An overview of the detection of Pneumothorax [1,2] on chest X-Ray images. Given a chest X-ray image, it is then inputted to a deep convolutional neural network. A real value between 0 and 1 inclusively is outputted. A threshold, such as 0.5, can be applied to assign a class label to the real-valued output to determine if there is Pneumothorax on the chest X-ray image. Absence of Pneumothorax is represented by negative (−ve) class, and presence of Pneumothorax is represented by positive (+ve) class. For illustration, two chest X-ray images were extracted from the validation set in CheXpert [8]. (a) is from the study 1 of patient64544, with the filename as view1_frontal.jpg. No finding was observed. (b) is from the study 1 of patient64547, with the filename as view1_frontal.jpg. Pneumothorax was observed. The observations were verified by three board-certified radiologists [8].

and 1 represents the positive (+ve) classes, i.e. the chest X-ray images with the absence of Pneumothorax [1,2]. Figure 1 provides a graphical illustration.

Let $S_{train} = \{(x_i, y_i)\}_{i=1}^{N}$ be a set of N training samples. Given S_{train}, the learning task is to learn a function $f : X \rightarrow Y$, such that

$$E_{(x,y)\sim D}[L(f(x); y)] \tag{1}$$

is minimized, where D is the data distribution over $X \times Y$, $x \in X$, $y \in Y$ and $L(z; y)$ is a loss function that measures the loss if we predict y as z. Equation 1 represents the generalization error of a learnt function.

As it is a binary classification problem, the binary entropy function was adopted as the loss function. Following [5], class weights were considered.

$$L(f(x_i); y_i) = -[w^+ y_i log_2(f(x_i)) + w^-(1 - y_i) log_2(1 - f(x_i))] \tag{2}$$

where w^+ is the ratio of positive classes among all training samples, and w^- is the ratio of negative classes among all training samples.

$$w^+ = \frac{P}{P + N} \tag{3}$$

$$w^- = \frac{N}{P+N} \quad (4)$$

where, among all training samples, P is the number of positive classes, and N is the number of negative classes.

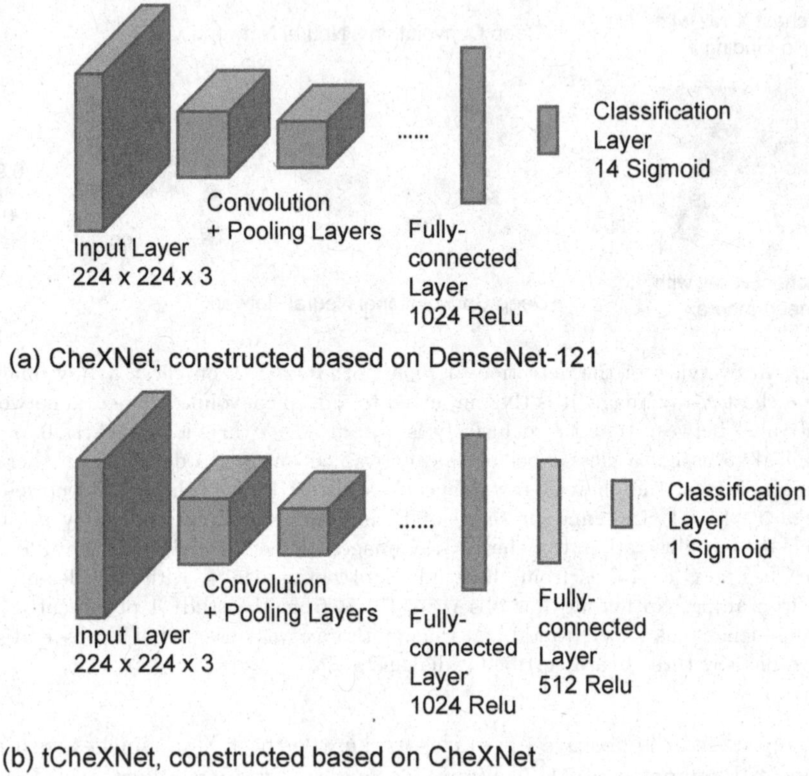

Fig. 2. An overview of the deep convolutional neural network models investigated in this study. (a) CheXNet [5] is a 121-layer convolutional neural network, constructed based on DenseNet-121 [12], that inputs a chest X-ray image and outputs the probability of pneumonia along with 13 other thoracic diseases including Pneumothorax. (b) tCheXNet, a model proposed by us, is a 122-layer convolutional neural network, constructed based on CheXNet [5], that inputs a chest X-ray image and outputs the probability of Pneumothorax.

2.2 Model Architecture

Two deep convolutional neural network models are investigated in this study. Figure 2 provides a graphical illustration. The first model, as shown in Fig. 2(a), is denoted as CheXNet [5]. it is a 121-layer convolutional neural network, constructed based on DenseNet-121 [12], that inputs a chest X-ray image and outputs the probability of pneumonia along with 13 other thoracic diseases including Pneumothorax. CheXNet [5] achieved radiologist-level disease detection particularly in the detection of pneumonia. It is thus the state-of-the-art model architecture.

The second model, as shown in Fig. 2(b), is denoted as tCheXNet, a model proposed by us. It is a 122-layer convolutional neural network, constructed based on CheXNet [5], that inputs a chest X-ray image and outputs the probability of Pneumothorax. Its first 120 layers are identical to those of CheXNet [5]. Two layers are then added on top, a fully-connected layer with 512 ReLu units, followed by a classification layer with 1 sigmoid unit. Hence, there are in total 122 layers in tCheXNet.

2.3 Training Strategy - Deep Transfer Learning

In order not to train tCheXNet, with 122 layers, from scratch, we developed a training strategy based on transfer learning. First. the model parameters of CheXNet [5] is used in the initialization of tCheXNet. Second, these model parameters are then locked in the training stage by setting the corresponding layers as non-trainable. Only the newly added layers are allowed to be trained. In other words, tCheXNet is pre-trained with the model parameters from CheXNet and those model parameters will remain in the training stage. The training strategy is summarized in Algorithm 1.

Algorithm 1. train-tCheXNet

Input: a set of training samples S_{train}, initialized model parameter $\theta_{CheXNet}$, epochs
Output: a model parameter $\theta_{tCheXNet}$
configure a model m as CheXNet
initialize m with $\theta_{CheXNet}$
set layers in m as non-trainable
remove the last layer from m
configure the model m as tCheXNet by adding two new layers
set the two new layers as trainable
set θ_m as the model parameters of m
for 1 to epochs **do**
  backprop-optimize(S_{train}, m, θ_m)
end for
$\theta_{tCheXNet} = \theta_m$
return $\theta_{tCheXNet}$

3 Experiments and Results

3.1 Dataset Preparation

In this study, we prepared training dataset, validation dataset and testing dataset to conduct experiments. A summary is provided in Table 1.

Training. The training set contains a total of 94,482 chest X-ray images, where 13,911 of them belong to the +ve class, and 80,571 of them belong to the −ve class. These chest X-ray images were obtained from the training set of CheXpert [8], selecting only the frontal chest X-ray.

Validation. The validation set contains a total of 23,620 chest X-ray images, where 2,869 of them belong to the +ve class, and 20,751 of them belong to the −ve class. These chest X-ray images were obtained from the training set of CheXpert [8], selecting only the frontal chest X-ray.

Testing. The testing set contains a total of 202 chest X-ray images, where 7 of them belong to the +ve class, and 195 of them belong to the −ve class. These chest X-ray images were obtained from the validation set of CheXpert [8], selecting only the frontal chest X-ray. It should be noted that the validation set of CheXpert [8] was verified by three board-certified radiologists.

Table 1. A summary of the datasets used in this study. The chest X-ray images were obtained and preprocessed from CheXpert [8]. The dataset has two classes: Negative (−ve) class and Positive (+ve) class, where the +ve class represents a presence of the Pneumothorax, and the −ve class represents an absence of the Pneumothorax.

	Positive (+ve)	Negative (−ve)	Total
Training	13,911	80,571	94,482
Validation	2,869	20,751	23,620
Testing	7	195	202

3.2 Data Preprocessing

While the testing set is validated by three board-certified radiologists, there are uncertainty entries (zeros and blanks), in addition to certain entries (positive ones and negative ones) in the training set and validation set. We followed the preprocessing procedure mentioned in [8] so that the entries with negative ones and zeros were considered to be negative (−ve) classes. The blank entries were also considered to be negative (−ve) classes. Only the entries with positive ones were consider to be (+ve) classes. All images were also preprocessed using the procedure mentioned in [12].

3.3 Experiments

tCheXNet was trained on the training set. Model selection was done using the validation set. The model with the lowest validation loss were selected. They were then evaluated on the testing set. Following [5,8], the performance of the models was evaluated by the area under the receiver operating characteristic curve (ROC) to enable the comparison over a range of prediction thresholds. CheXNet [5] was also evaluated on the same testing set.

3.4 Implementation and Parameter Setting

To build tCheXNet and re-implement CheXNet [5], the latest version (v2.2.4) of the deep learning library Keras (http://keras.io/) with Tensorflow backend [13] was adopted. The model weights of CheXNet was obtained from the link (https://github.com/brucechou1983/CheXNet-Keras). The number of training epochs and batch size were 10 and 16 respectively. Adam optimizer [14] was used in training. All parameters were set default unless further specified. Also, ROC was computed using the latest version (v0.20.3) of the machine learning library scikit-learn [15] with default parameter setting. All experiments were run on a computer with 8.0 GB DDR4 RAM, a Celeron G3900-2.80 GHz CPU (2 Cores) and two GTX 1070 Ti Graphics card. These settings were used in all experiments unless further specified. The source code is available in https://github.com/antoniosehk/tCheXNet.

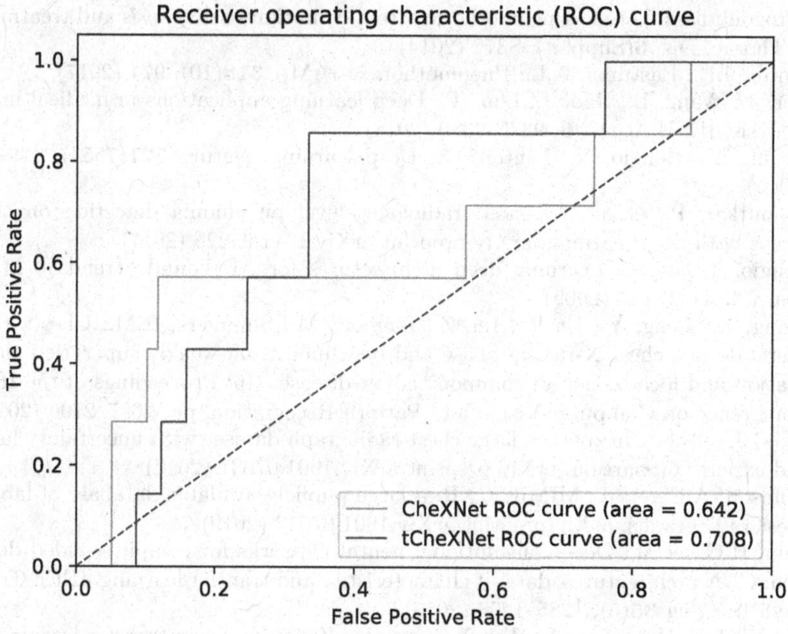

Fig. 3. A comparison of the prediction performance between CheXNet [5] and tCheXNet in terms of the area under the receiver operating characteristic (ROC) curve.

3.5 Results

Figure 3 shows the comparative results on the area under the ROC curve in the testing set. We observe that tChexNet obtained a higher ROC score (10% better) comparing to that obatained by CheXNet [5] in the testing set.

4 Conclusion

In this study, we proposed tCheXNet, a model architecture with 122 layers based on CheXNet [5], to detect Pneumothorax from chest X-ray images. We used a training strategy based on Deep Transfer Learning such that these 122 layers need not be trained from scratch by reusing and locking the model parameters from CheXNet [5]. Experimental resutls have demonstrated tChexNet, trained by our proposed strategy, obtained a 10% higher ROC on the detection of Pneumothorax from chest X-ray images, comparing to that obtained by CheXNet [5]. This study is made possible by a recent release of a large amount of labeled chest X-ray images in CheXpert [8]. Future extension of this work includes investigating if the training strategies work for observations in chest X-ray images in addition to Pneumothorax.

References

1. Zarogoulidis, P., et al.: Pneumothorax: from definition to diagnosis and treatment. J. Thorac. Dis. **6**(Suppl 4), S372 (2014)
2. Imran, J.B., Eastman, A.L.: Pneumothorax. JAMA **318**(10), 974 (2017)
3. Ker, J., Wang, L., Rao, J., Lim, T.: Deep learning applications in medical image analysis. IEEE Access **6**, 9375–9389 (2018)
4. LeCun, Y., Bengio, Y., Hinton, G.: Deep learning. Nature **521**(7553), 436–444 (2015)
5. Rajpurkar, P., et al.: Chexnet: radiologist-level pneumonia detection on chest x-rays with deep learning. arXiv preprint arXiv:1711.05225 (2017)
6. Bengio, Y., et al.: Learning deep architectures for AI. Found. Trends® Mach. Learn. **2**(1), 1–127 (2009)
7. Wang, X., Peng, Y., Lu, L., Lu, Z., Bagheri, M., Summers, R.M.: Chestx-ray8: hospital-scale chest X-ray database and benchmarks on weakly-supervised classification and localization of common thorax diseases. In: Proceedings of the IEEE Conference on Computer Vision and Pattern Recognition, pp. 2097–2106 (2017)
8. Irvin, J., et al.: Chexpert: a large chest radiograph dataset with uncertainty labels and expert comparison. arXiv preprint arXiv:1901.07031 (2019)
9. Johnson, A.E., et al.: MIMIC-CXR: a large publicly available database of labeled chest radiographs. arXiv preprint arXiv:1901.07042 (2019)
10. Shin, H.C., et al.: Deep convolutional neural networks for computer-aided detection: CNN architectures, dataset characteristics and transfer learning. IEEE Trans. Med. Imaging **35**(5), 1285–1298 (2016)
11. Yu, Y., Lin, H., Meng, J., Wei, X., Guo, H., Zhao, Z.: Deep transfer learning for modality classification of medical images. Information **8**(3), 91 (2017)
12. Huang, G., Liu, Z., Van Der Maaten, L., Weinberger, K.Q.: Densely connected convolutional networks. In: Proceedings of the IEEE Conference on Computer Vision and Pattern Recognition, pp. 4700–4708 (2017)
13. Abadi, M., et al.: Tensorflow: a system for large-scale machine learning. In: 12th {USENIX} Symposium on Operating Systems Design and Implementation ({OSDI} 2016), pp. 265–283 (2016)
14. Kingma, D.P., Ba, J.: Adam: a method for stochastic optimization. arXiv preprint arXiv:1412.6980 (2014)
15. Pedregosa, F., et al.: Scikit-learn: machine learning in Python. J. Mach. Learn. Res. **12**, 2825–2830 (2011)

Improving Lesion Segmentation for Diabetic Retinopathy Using Adversarial Learning

Qiqi Xiao[1], Jiaxu Zou[1], Muqiao Yang[1], Alex Gaudio[1], Kris Kitani[1], Asim Smailagic[1](✉), Pedro Costa[2], and Min Xu[1]

[1] Carnegie Mellon University, Pittsburgh, PA 15213, USA
{qiqix,jiaxuz,agaudio}@andrew.cmu.edu
{muqiaoy,kkitani,asim,mxu1}@cs.cmu.edu
[2] INESC TEC, Porto, Portugal
pedro.vendascosta@gmail.com

Abstract. Diabetic Retinopathy (DR) is a leading cause of blindness in working age adults. DR lesions can be challenging to identify in fundus images, and automatic DR detection systems can offer strong clinical value. Of the publicly available labeled datasets for DR, the Indian Diabetic Retinopathy Image Dataset (IDRiD) presents retinal fundus images with pixel-level annotations of four distinct lesions: microaneurysms, hemorrhages, soft exudates and hard exudates. We utilize the HEDNet edge detector to solve a semantic segmentation task on this dataset, and then propose an end-to-end system for pixel-level segmentation of DR lesions by incorporating HEDNet into a Conditional Generative Adversarial Network (cGAN). We design a loss function that adds adversarial loss to segmentation loss. Our experiments show that the addition of the adversarial loss improves the lesion segmentation performance over the baseline.

Keywords: Conditional generative adversarial networks · Deep learning · Segmentation · Medical image analysis

1 Introduction

Diabetic Retinopathy (DR) is an eye disease caused by damage to the retinal blood vessels of diabetic patients. Since the disease is relatively asymptomatic until the patient experiences loss of vision, physicians recommend regular screenings for diabetic patients. Analysis of high resolution fundus images obtained during the screening requires considerable time and effort by trained clinicians, as lesions can be hard to detect.

While the diagnosis of the disease ultimately requires a physician, automated detection of DR lesions can improve patient outcomes. Recent developments in

F. Karray et al. (Eds.): ICIAR 2019, LNCS 11663, pp. 333–344, 2019.
https://doi.org/10.1007/978-3-030-27272-2_29

machine learning and computer vision that enable accurate classification and localization are well suited to the DR detection task. Of particular interest are pixel level annotations of DR lesions that suggest to physicians where in the image the lesions should be. Automated detection methods save time and can reduce uncertainty in DR diagnosis.

The datasets available for DR strongly influence development of automated detection algorithms. Publicly available datasets for DR, such as Messidor [1], DRIVE [2], STARE [3] and DIARETDB [4], contain annotations of the whole image or of sub-regions of the image. Unfortunately, detection algorithms built from these datasets tend to make image level or patch level predictions, which by design has limited utility to a clinician who needs to explain the underlying factors leading to the diagnosis. A system capable of accurate pixel-level segmentation is more explainable and provides better value to clinicians.

In this work, we use the Indian Diabetic Retinopathy Image Dataset (IDRiD) [5]. To the best of our knowledge, IDRiD is the first public database for DR containing pixel level annotations of four typical DR lesions: microaneurysms (MA), hemorrhages (HE), hard exudates (EX), and soft exudates (SE). Physicians assess combinations of these lesions to diagnose various grades of DR (Fig. 1).

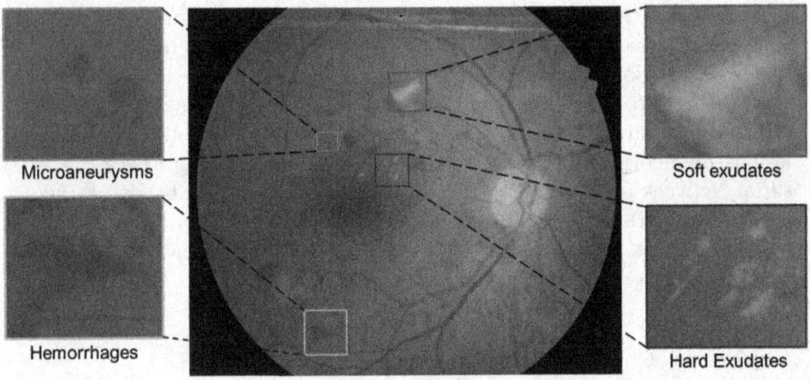

Fig. 1. Color fundus photograph containing different retinal lesions associated with diabetic retinopathy. Enlarged parts illustrating presence of Microaneurysms, Soft Exudates, Hemorrhages and Hard Exudates.

Our method uses the Holistically-Nested Edge Detection (HEDNet) network [7] to compute a segmentation map from a fundus image. To enhance HEDNet segmentation performance, we incorporate this model into a conditional Generative Adversarial Network (GAN) with a standard PatchGAN discriminator. Our method is end-to-end, and we show that the addition of adversarial loss can improve the lesion segmentation performance of diabetic retinopathy images.

2 Related Work

2.1 HEDNet in Semantic Segmentation

Semantic Segmentation is an image-to-image translation method that aims to identify regions and structures in an input image. These methods solve pixel-level classification problems, where the classes are pre-defined. For example, semantic segmentation of street view images produces classes like person, vehicle, building, etc. The result of such segmentation is fine-grained and thus contains more information about the scene than both simple classification and bounding box detection. In the context of the IDRiD dataset for DR, each pixel can be annotated as one of four lesion types or healthy.

Holistically-Nested Edge Detection (HEDNet) [7] is a state-of-art algorithm proposed to solve image-to-image problems with a deep convolutional neural network. Unlike traditional edge detectors, HEDNet can generate semantically meaningful edge maps that identify object contours. Experiments on Berkeley Segmentation Dataset show that HEDNet performs much better than traditional edge detection algorithms like Canny edge detection, and it also outperforms patch-based edge detection algorithms in terms of speed and accuracy [7]. Although it is originally proposed to solve edge detection for natural images, we show that HEDNet is capable of solving the segmentation problem as well.

Considering the effectiveness of HEDNet for edge detection and semantically meaningful contour maps, we choose to base our work on top of this architecture. We show that HEDNet is capable of solving the segmentation problem on the IDRiD dataset.

2.2 GAN in Semantic Segmentation

Classification algorithms, such as those for semantic segmentation, perform well when the task has a clearly defined objective. In practice, however, the objective function used often incorporates hidden assumptions that can be overly simplistic. For instance, the classification setting might assume that each pixel belongs to precisely one class, but in reality, a pixel could represent presence of both soft exudates (which occur in the Nerve Fiber Layer of the Retina) and hard exudates (which occur deeper in the retina). When we think about labeling these pixels, the multi-class setting breaks down. Therefore, in semantic segmentation tasks, the objective can be challenging to define because we need to consider all possible assumptions and we may not know in advance what they are.

Semantic segmentation tasks have been framed as adversarial generative modeling problems [15,16], where the generative model's objective function is learned. For instance, in the area of medical image processing, Splenomegaly Segmentation Network (SSNet) [22] utilizes conditional generative adversarial networks (cGAN) [23] to solve the spleen volume estimation problem, and the work shows significant improvement over the baseline on a medical dataset containing 60 MRI images.

While we use HEDNet to solve a straight-forward classification problem with the pixel-wise ground truth labels from IDRiD, we can also evaluate how realistic the HEDNet annotations are. Therefore, we present semantic segmentation on IDRiD as a generative modeling task, and we train HEDNet to both classify pixels correctly and generate realistic segmentation maps of typical DR lesions.

3 Methodology

In this section we start by showing how we preprocess the retinal images, then we explain how we use an image-to-image network to segment DR lesions and how we combine the GAN loss to further refine the segmentation results. An overview of our model structure is shown in Fig. 2.

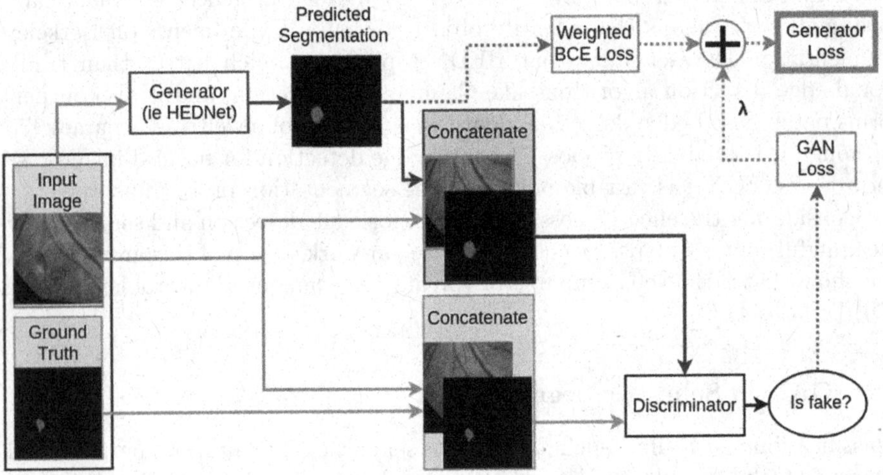

Fig. 2. Main framework of conditional generative adversarial network

3.1 Preprocessing Steps

Before we feed the raw images into our network, we consider using illumination correction and contrast enhancement techniques on the retinal images for better image enhancement.

Brightness Balance. Since the dataset is sampled from different lesions and tissues, there might exist some inconsistency in the brightness of the whole dataset. To avoid the imbalance of brightness among different images, we force each training and test image to have an average pixel intensity equal to the average pixel intensity of the training set.

Contrast Enhancement. Contrast enhancement ensures the pixel intensities cover a wide range of values, which can make details more readily apparent. We applied CLAHE (Contrast Limited Adaptive Histogram Equalization) for contrast enhancement. CLAHE affects small regions of the image instead of the entire image [24], and it can have significantly better performance than the regular histogram equalization.

Denoising. In practical situations, intrinsic and extrinsic conditions related to capture of the image result in different kinds of noise, and denoising is a fundamental challenge in image processing. Here we assume that the images contain Gaussian white noise, and apply the Non-local Means Denoising algorithm [25]. Additionally, we apply a bilateral filter the the image, which replaces the intensity of each pixel with a weighted average of intensity values from nearby pixels, thus preserving edge information while the noise is minimized.

3.2 Image to Image Network

The image to image network for segmentation we use is HEDNet [7]. HEDNet builds on VGGNet [19] by adding side outputs to the last convolutional layer in each stage and by removing the last stage and all fully connected layers. The VGGNet structure is initialized with weights pre-trained on ImageNet and then fine tuned. The side outputs are fused together via a trainable weighted-fusion layer; since each output corresponds to a different stage of VGGNet, the fusion enables a multi-scale representation of the output. This fully convolutional architecture allows HEDNet to maintain both high level information and low level details.

All side outputs from HEDNet are concatenated, and therefore each stage of the network contributes to the final pixel-wise binary cross-entropy (BCE) loss. This is known as deep supervision in the sense that each stage can be interpreted as an individual network output solving the learning task at a specific scales. Experiments have shown that with only the fusion layer loss, a large amount of edge information is lost on high level side outputs.

Diabetic Retinopathy lesions typically make up a very small proportion of a diseased fundus image and do not exist for images of healthy eyes. As a result, the ground truth is highly imbalanced. We use a class-balancing weight β, which differentiates cross-entropy loss for positive and negative samples:

$$Loss_{weight\_BCE} = -(\beta \cdot y \text{logp} + (1 - y)\text{log}(1 - p)) \tag{1}$$

where y is the binary indicator 0 or 1 and p is the predicted probability of observation of the positive class.

3.3 GAN Loss

Inspired by Splennomegaly Segmentation Network (SSNet) [22], we find that the variations in both size and shape of the lesions from the Diabetic Retinopathy can introduce a large number of false positive and false negative labelings, and conditional GAN [23] is an effective approach to improve generalization ability. The generator of SSNet is a Global Convolutional Network (GCN), which is inherently an image-to-image fully convolutional network with a large receptive field. Since we want to output an image of the same size with the input image, here we need an equivalent kernel size, therefore we propose to use HEDNet to replace the GCN for diabetic retinopathy.

Furthermore, a conditional GAN is used to discriminate the output, whose architecture is the same as infoGAN [26]. The discriminator utilizes the framework of PatchGAN [27], where the input image is split into smaller patches, and each small image patch is applied with a cross entropy loss to decide whether that patch is fake or real. The input to the discriminator is the concatenation of the original image patch and the corresponding segmentation output from the generator, which is a 4-channel tensor. Therefore, we can see that the discriminator learns the joint distribution of the input and the segmentation map conditioned on the input.

3.4 Loss Function

The final generator loss term is a weighted average of binary cross-entropy loss and GAN loss:

$$Loss_{generator} = Loss_{weighted\_BCE} + \lambda \cdot Loss_{GAN} \tag{2}$$

thus the goal of the network is to produce good segmentation with respect to ground truth as well as to make segmentation consistent such that the segmentation result seems real to the discriminator. Therefore, it is used to further refine the segmentation results.

4 Experiments

4.1 Datasets

We use the dataset from IDRiD challenge [5]. This sub-challenge can be divided in four different tasks, which are lesion segmentation of Microaneurysms (MA), Soft Exudates (SE), Hard Exudates (EX) and Hemorrhages (HE). Of the 54 training set images and 27 test set images, not all images contain all four lesion types. Table 1 shows the percent of images in the train and test sets respectively assigned to each of the four classes. We randomly divided the training set into training set with 80% images and validation set with 20% images. Each image has resolution of 4288 × 2848.

Table 1. Structure of IDRiD dataset. Percentages show amount of images containing the given lesion type.

Type	Dataset		
	Training set images	Testing set images	Total pathological images
Microaneurysms (MA)	54 (100%)	27 (100%)	81 (100%)
Soft exudates (SE)	26 (48%)	14 (52%)	40 (49%)
Hard exudates (EX)	54 (100%)	27 (100%)	81 (100%)
Hemorrhages (HE)	53 (98%)	27 (100%)	80 (99%)

4.2 Implementation Details

Hyperparameters. We use a pixel value in [0, 1] for each lesion image and ground truth segmentation. We use a patch size of 128 for the SE, EX and HE models and patch size of 64 for the MA model. We set the weight β in BCE loss to 10 to balance the positive and negative labels. We set the weight of the GAN loss $\lambda = 0.01$, as in SSNet. We use SGD as our optimizer for both HEDNet and the discriminator with an initial learning rate of 0.001 in both cases. For HEDNet, we decay the learning rate by 10% every 200 epochs. For the discriminator model, we decay the learning rate by 10% every 100 epochs. The momentum factor of the optimizer is 0.9. In addition, we apply L-2 weight decay with a rate of 0.0005. The training and validation batch size is 4 and the testing batch size is 1. For all experiments, the model is trained for 5000 epochs.

Preprocessing. For contrast enhancement, we apply the CLAHE technique with tiles of 8×8 pixels and a default contrast limit of 40. For denoising, we apply the Non-local Means Denoising algorithm with a filter strength of 10. We also normalize each channel of the lesion image to a mean of 0.485, 0.456, 0.406 and standard deviation of 0.229, 0.224, 0.225.

Data Augmentation. During training, we randomly crop each image to 512×512 pixels, and randomly rotate each image using a maximum angle of 20°.

4.3 Performance Evaluation Metrics

We use several performance metrics for evaluation, including Average Precision Score (AP), F-1 score and Precision-Recall Curve (PRC). All the 3 metrics reflect the precision and recall performance of the model on binary segmentation tasks from different perspectives. We compute the score of AP and F-1, and plot the PRC for each model on all the entire testing set. The evaluation is implemented using scikit-learn functions.

Table 2. Average precision on the test dataset on four lesions

Model	AP		
	UNET	HEDNet	HEDNet + cGAN
Microaneurysms (MA)	41.84%	**44.03%**	43.92%
Soft exudates (SE)	42.22%	43.07%	**48.39%**
Hard exudates (EX)	79.05%	83.98%	**84.05%**
Hemorrhages (HE)	41.93%	45.69%	**48.12%**

Table 3. F-1 score on the test dataset on four lesions

F-1 score	Model		
	UNET	HEDNet	HEDNet + cGAN
Microaneurysms (MA)	41.76%	39.81%	**42.98%**
Soft exudates (SE)	27.88%	40.12%	**43.98%**
Hard exudates (EX)	**69.90%**	68.94%	69.08%
Hemorrhages (HE)	44.97%	45.00%	**45.76%**

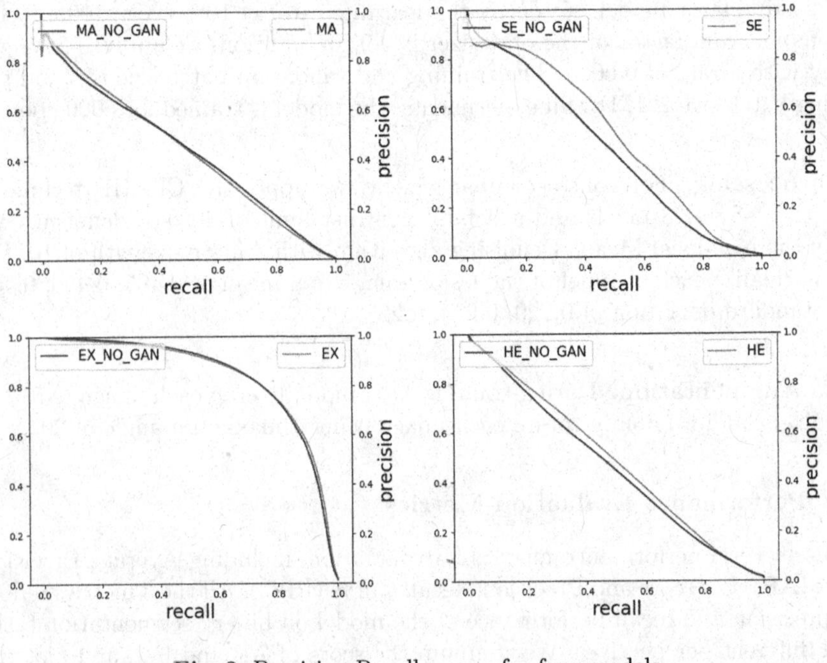

Fig. 3. Precision-Recall curves for four models

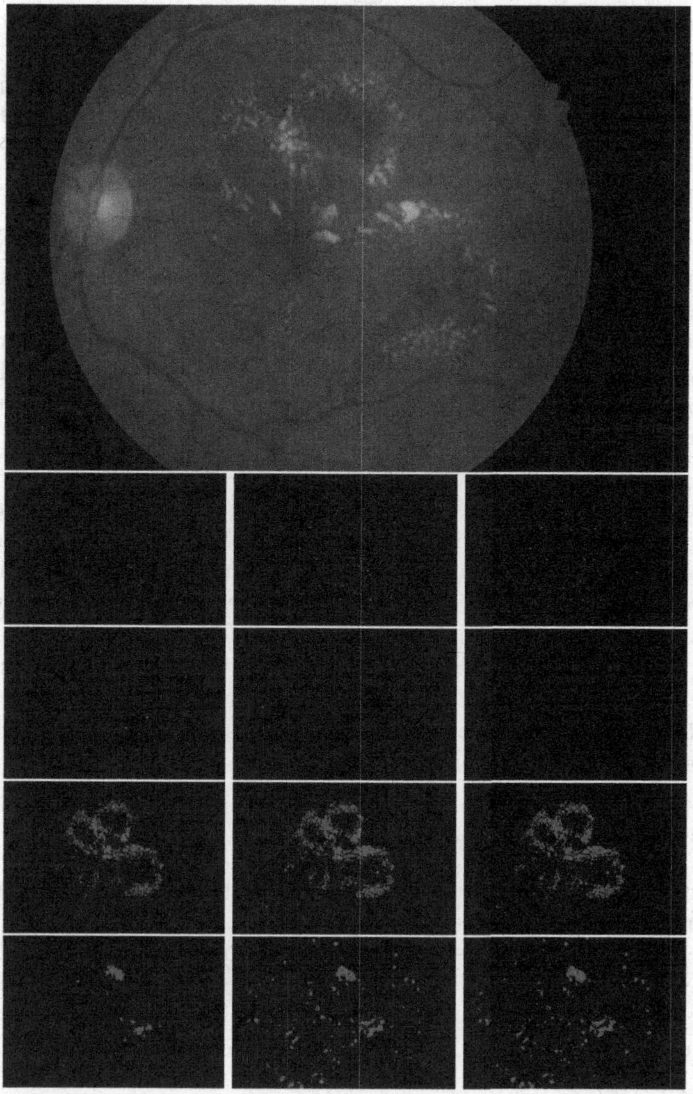

Fig. 4. Top: an example test set image presenting all four lesion types. Bottom: segmentation maps. Each row, from top to bottom, shows lesion types: MA, SE, EX and HE. Each column, from left to right, contains segmentation maps of ground truth, HEDNet output, and HEDNet + cGAN output, respectively.

4.4 Experimental Results

Quantitative Results. We compare three models: UNET, HEDNet and HEDNet with cGAN. UNET, which was originally proposed for biomedical image segmentation [8], is a standard and widely used model [9–11]. Results show that our HEDNet+cGAN model improves over both HEDNet and UNET. HED-

Net+CGAN improves average precision of SE, HE and EX segmentations, and it improves the F1 score for MA, SE and HE. The average precision and F-1 scores are shown in Tables 2 and 3 respectively. The results show that the model performs best on hard exudates, where it achieves the highest scores for both AP and F-1 score. This can be explained by the pathological features of EX lesions. Hard Exudates are small shiny white or yellowish white deposits deep to the retinal vessels with sharp margins, which leads to high contrast in the images. We do not see an obvious improvement on MA segmentation from the experimental results, which is also related to pathological features of MA. Compared to other 3 types of lesions, microaneurysms are very small, lower contrast and share higher similarity to blood vessels, which can confuse the model to certain extent. The nearly consistent improvements of the HEDNet+cGAN model over the HEDNet model on all 4 lesion types for both evaluation metrics demonstrates the model strength under the cGAN framework.

Qualitative Results. Figure 3 presents the qualitative results of a comparison between 2 frameworks by plotting the Precision-Recall curves. The ground truth segmentation is in the second column, and the segmentation results of HEDNet and cGAN are in the last two columns. From the results, EX shows the best performance. The other 3 lesion types do not have as good results as EX, but the segmentation result of cGAN framework is much closer to the ground truth than HEDNet only, which is consistent with the quantitative results. Figure 4 shows an example of the original lesion image from the test set and three segmentation maps for each of the four lesion types.

5 Conclusion

In this paper we have presented a method to improve the lesion segmentation performance on retinal images. We propose to use HEDNet to segment lesions in retinal images and, then, retinal image and segmentation pairs are fed to a PatchGAN discriminator that is trained to distinguish between ground truth pairs and predicted ones. The HEDNet segmentation model is then trained to both minimize a segmentation loss and to maximize the discriminator classification loss.

By using this approach, we show that it is possible to improve average precision on all lesion segmentation tasks. In particular, the AP of SE and HE segmentation improves by 5.3 and 3.1% points when using conditional GANs over using HEDNet alone. In the future we want to evaluate if this framework is able to improve the performance in combination with other segmentation models.

References

1. Decenciére, E., et al.: Feedback on a publicly distributed image database: the messidor database. Image Anal. Stereol. **33**(3), 231–234 (2004). https://doi.org/10.5566/ias.1155

2. Niemeijer, M., Staal, J.J., van Ginneken, B., Loog, M., Abramoff, M.D.: Comparative study of retinal vessel segmentation methods on a new publicly available database. In: Michael Fitzpatrick, J., Sonka, M. (eds.) SPIE Medical Imaging. SPIE, vol. 5370, pp. 648–656 (2004)
3. Hoover, A., Goldbaum, M.: Locating the optic nerve in a retinal image using the fuzzy convergence of the blood vessels. IEEE Trans. Med. Imaging **22**(8), 951–958 (2003)
4. Kauppi, T., et al.: DIARETDB1 diabetic retinopathy database and evaluation protocol. In: Proceedings of the 11th Conference on Medical Image Understanding and Analysis (2007)
5. Indian Diabetic Retinopathy Image Dataset. https://doi.org/10.21227/H25W98. Accessed 14 Mar 2019
6. Quellec, G., Charriére, K., Boudi, Y., Cochener, B., Lamard, M.: Deep image mining for diabetic retinopathy screening. Med. Image Anal. **39**, 178–193 (2017)
7. Xie, S., Tu, Z.: Holistically-nested edge detection. In: Proceedings of the IEEE International Conference on Computer Vision, pp. 1395–1403 (2015)
8. Ronneberger, O., Fischer, P., Brox, T.: U-net: convolutional networks for biomedical image segmentation. arXiv:1505.04597 (2015)
9. Zhou, Z., Rahman Siddiquee, M.M., Tajbakhsh, N., Liang, J.: UNet++: a nested U-net architecture for medical image segmentation. In: Stoyanov, D., et al. (eds.) DLMIA/ML-CDS -2018. LNCS, vol. 11045, pp. 3–11. Springer, Cham (2018). https://doi.org/10.1007/978-3-030-00889-5_1
10. Lachinov, D., Vasiliev, E., Turlapov, V.: Glioma segmentation with cascaded UNet. In: Crimi, A., Bakas, S., Kuijf, H., Keyvan, F., Reyes, M., van Walsum, T. (eds.) BrainLes 2018. LNCS, vol. 11384, pp. 189–198. Springer, Cham (2019). https://doi.org/10.1007/978-3-030-11726-9_17
11. Li, X., Chen, H., Qi, X., Dou, Q., Fu, C., Heng, P.: H-DenseUNet: hybrid densely connected unet for liver and tumor segmentation from CT volumes. IEEE Trans. Med. Imaging **37**, 2663–2674 (2018)
12. Gulshan, V., et al.: Development and validation of a deep learning algorithm for detection of diabetic retinopathy in retinal fundus photographs. Jama **316**(22), 2402–2410 (2016)
13. Payer, C., Štern, D., Bischof, H., Urschler, M.: Regressing heatmaps for multiple landmark localization using CNNs. In: Ourselin, S., Joskowicz, L., Sabuncu, M.R., Unal, G., Wells, W. (eds.) MICCAI 2016. LNCS, vol. 9901, pp. 230–238. Springer, Cham (2016). https://doi.org/10.1007/978-3-319-46723-8_27
14. Ronneberger, O., Fischer, P., Brox, T.: U-net: convolutional networks for biomedical image segmentation. In: Navab, N., Hornegger, J., Wells, W.M., Frangi, A.F. (eds.) MICCAI 2015. LNCS, vol. 9351, pp. 234–241. Springer, Cham (2015). https://doi.org/10.1007/978-3-319-24574-4_28
15. Luc, P., Couprie, C., Chintala, S., Verbeek, J.: Semantic segmentation using adversarial networks. arXiv:1611.08408 (2016)
16. Hung, W.C., Tsai, Y.H., Liou, Y.T., Lin, Y.Y., Yang, M.H.: Adversarial learning for semi-supervised semantic segmentation. arXiv preprint arXiv:1802.07934 (2018)
17. Ghafoorian, M., et al.: Location sensitive deep convolutional neural networks for segmentation of white matter hyperintensities. Sci. Rep. **7**(1), 5110 (2017)
18. Setio, A., et al.: Pulmonary nodule detection in ct images: false positive reduction using multi-view convolutional networks. IEEE Trans. Med. Imaging **35**(5), 1160–1169 (2016)
19. Simonyan, K., Zisserman, A.: Very deep convolutional networks for large-scale image recognition. arXiv preprint arXiv:1409.1556 (2014)

20. He, K., Zhang, X., Ren, S., Sun, J.: Deep residual learning for image recognition. In: Proceedings of the IEEE Conference on Computer Vision and Pattern Recognition, pp. 770–778 (2016)
21. Costa, P., et al.: Eyewes: weakly supervised pre-trained convolutional neural networks for diabetic retinopathy detection (2018)
22. Huo, Y., et al.: Splenomegaly segmentation using global convolutional kernels and conditional generative adversarial networks. In: Medical Imaging 2018: Image Processing, vol. 10574. International Society for Optics and Photonics (2018)
23. Mirza, M., Osindero, S.: Conditional generative adversarial nets. arXiv preprint arXiv:1411.1784 (2014)
24. Reza, A.: Realization of the contrast limited adaptive histogram equalization (CLAHE) for real-time image enhancement. J. VLSI Signal Process. Syst. Signal Image Video Technol. **38**(1), 35–44 (2004)
25. Buades, A., Coll, B., Morel, J.: Non-local means denoising. Image Process. Line **1**, 208–212 (2011)
26. Chen, X., Duan, Y., Houthooft, R., Schulman, J., Sutskever, I., Abbeel, P.: InfoGAN: interpretable representation learning by information maximizing generative adversarial nets. In: Advances in Neural Information Processing Systems, pp. 2172–2180 (2016)
27. Isola, P., Zhu, J., Zhou, T., Efros, A.: Image-to-image translation with conditional adversarial networks. In: Proceedings of the IEEE Conference on Computer Vision and Pattern Recognition, pp. 1125–1134 (2017)

Context Aware Lung Cancer Annotation in Whole Slide Images Using Fully Convolutional Neural Networks

Vahid Khanagha[1(✉)] and Sanaz Aliari Kardehdeh[2]

[1] Motorola Solutions Inc., Plantation, FL, USA
vahidkh62@gmail.com
[2] University of Maryland, College Park, MD, USA

Abstract. We propose a novel machine learning based methodology for detection and annotation of areas in Whole Slide lung Images (WSI) that are affected by lung cancer. Contrary to the trend of processing WSIs in small overlapping patches to generate a heat-map, we use a much larger patch with no overlap, aiming at capturing more of the context in each patch. As these larger patches are less likely to completely fall into one of the cancer/co-cancer classes, we use a pixel-level image segmentation approach consisting of a custom Fully Convolutional Neural Networks (FCNN). As opposed to the trend of using very deep neural networks, we carefully design a small FCNN, while avoiding the trainable upsampling layers, in order to cope with small training data and inaccurate region-based labeling of WSIs. We show that such an efficient architecture achieves better accuracy compared to the heat-map based approach. Apart from the descent results of our small network, this study shows that FCNNs are capable of learning region-based human labeling of biomedical images that sometimes does not correspond to a texture or a bounded object as a whole, but is more like drawing a line around a region containing a scattered number of small malignant tissues.

Keywords: Biomedical image analysis · Lung cancer detection · Deep neural networks · Fully Convolutional Neural Networks

1 Introduction

Lung cancer is the cancer with the highest rate of fatalities for both men and women. In 2017, more than 160000 Americans died of the lung cancer [2] and as such, the development of tools and approaches for accurate diagnosis of the patients could save lives of many. One of the essential steps in early diagnosis and treatment of Lung cancer is expert evaluation of microscopic histopathology slides, to determine the types and sub-types of lung cancer, which in turn defines the type of treatment. Histopathology imaging can also provide insights about the probability of the survival of the patient [13]. However, the evaluation of biopsy tissues by experts is a time-consuming process. This motivates

F. Karray et al. (Eds.): ICIAR 2019, LNCS 11663, pp. 345–352, 2019.
https://doi.org/10.1007/978-3-030-27272-2_30

the integration of computer aided approaches in the workflow of pathologists, to expedite the diagnosis process of lung cancer [4]. This is made possible by the advent of digital Whole Slide Imaging (WSI), which involves scanning of the glass histology slides of biopsy tissues to capture a gigapixel digital image. Figure 1 shows a sample segment of a WSI containing cancer tissues. Once appropriate tools and algorithms are created for systematic analyzing such gigantic sized images, automated analysis of WSIs provides more efficiency and accuracy to the workflow of an expert pathologists.

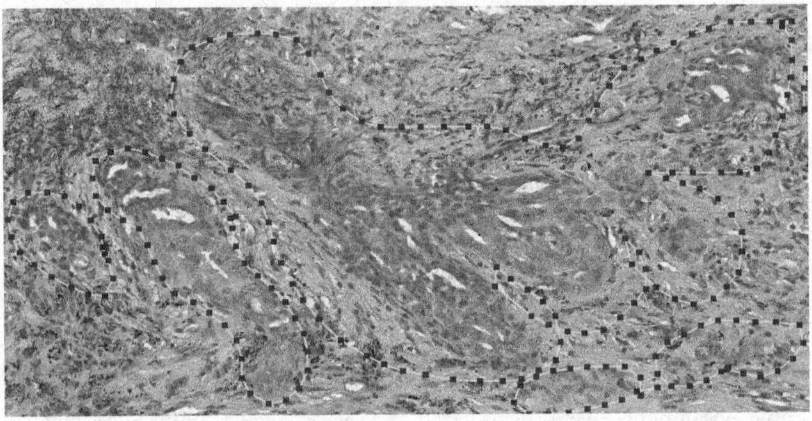

Fig. 1. A segment of a lung WSI with polygons annotating regions containing lung cancer tissues (175 um). Note that the annotations are a little loose in the sense that some of the areas containing normal tissues are also included in the polygon.

In this paper, we explore the use of a powerful neural network architecture for detection of areas in WSIs that contain cancer tissues. This task is a challenging one, because of small amount of available training data, the huge size of WSIs (millions of pixels) and inaccuracies in labeling of the training data. More specifically the architecture we use is a light Fully convolutional Neural Network that is designed with special care to deal with these challenges.

1.1 Related Work

Conventional approaches for detection of malignant tissues in histopathology images includes the use of hand-crafted features such as histogram, grey-level co-occurrence matrix and grey-level run-length matrix along with conventional classifiers such as Support Vector Machines that are applied for automatic detection of breast and oral cancers [10]. In recent years, with the advent of efficient training techniques for deep neural networks, a number of end-to-end learning methodologies are introduced for analysis (feature extraction and classification) of biomedical image. The majority of these approaches employ a particular deep

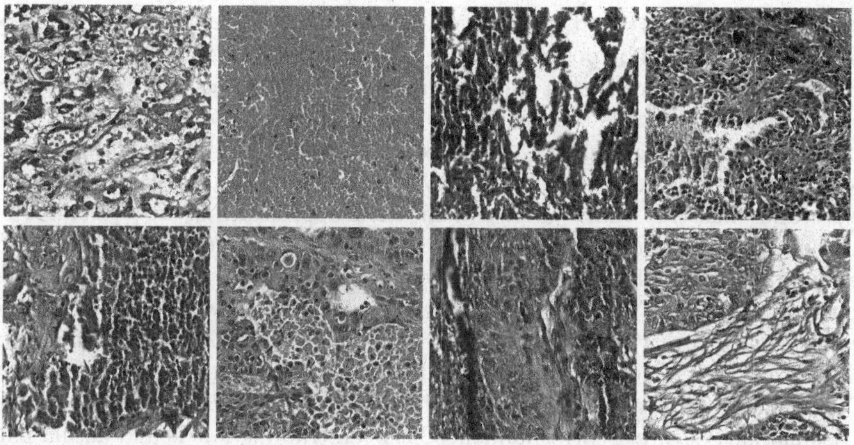

Fig. 2. Few examples of 1024 × 1024 pixel patches from Lung WSIs. First row shows examples of patches that are annotated as normal tissues by the expert pathologist and the second row shows examples of patches that are marked as containing cancer.

learning architecture called Convolutional Neural Networks (CNN) [6]. when enough training material is available, CNNs are shown to be powerful in creating rich features for all kinds of computer vision problems. Usually, multiple layers of CNNs are stacked together and followed by a fully connected neural network whose role is to perform the final classification using CNN features.

In [7], a method is proposed to apply a very powerful CNN based classifier (Inception [12]) to aid breast cancer metastasis detection in whole slide images. The approach is based on classifying small overlapping 100 × 100 pixel patches of WSI using the CNN network to generate a heatmap from which final classification is made by application of a global threshold. The authors show that their method yields state-of-the-art sensitivity in detecting small patches of tumor, while reducing the false negative rate to a quarter of a pathologist and less than half of the previous best result. This heatmap based approach is applied in [5] for the case of Lung cancer annotation. The authors performed a comprehensive evaluation of application of several well-known CNN based classifier in classifying small 256 × 256 patches of WSIs and shown the potential of CNNs for detecting cancer regions. In [3], to localize and classify sub-types of lung cancer (small-cell, non-small lung squamous cell and non-small cell lung adenocarcinoma).

1.2 Contributions

In this paper we conduct an exploratory research aiming at improving the performance of Lung cancer annotation in WSI images using an architecture that is usually used for pixel-level classification (semantic segmentation) of images (rather than the whole patch classification used in [7]). The reason we opted for this approach is that as opposed to the heatmap based approaches [7] that use patches as small as 100 × 100 pixels, we wanted to use a larger patch-size (1024 × 1024) so that it would be possible to take larger contexts into account. One intuition behind this choice is that even for human eye, detecting an object is easier when the whole object is seen in a wider view, compared to a zoomed-in view that captures only parts of a bigger object. However, when using a larger patch size, the corresponding annotations may now include both normal and cancer tissues and thus the whole-patch classification approaches as in [7] cannot be used anymore and thus the pixel-level semantic segmentation would be a more appropriate choice. The architecture we employ is a custom Fully Convolutional Neural Network (FCNN) [8]. FCNNs are shown to be powerful in end-to-end classification of every pixel of an image into one of the target object classes (when provided with enough training data with accurate pixel-level labels).

The challenge in application of FCNNs in annotation of Lung WSIs is the occasional lack of direct correspondence between training labels and actual patterns in WSIs. On one hand, the manual labels drawn around cancer regions are not precise at pixel level (Fig. 1) in the way a FCNN requires. This is a big challenge by itself and is studied to some extent in other domains, using semi-supervised training approaches [9]. On the other hand, sometimes it is hard to find pixel level evidence of cancer in all the pixels annotated as cancer regions. These regions usually do not correspond to an actual object with clear boundaries, as it is usual in photographic images. For instance, a car has clear boundaries and a distinct color in an image; but it is hard to draw a hard boundary around a region containing cancer tissues. Sometimes, a whole region is labeled as cancer tissues because a number of malignant cells are observed in that region, while the surrounding patterns look similar to the patterns seen in other regions annotated as non-cancer. This can be seen in the bottom row of Fig. 2 that contains few patches from regions entirely marked as cancer tissue. As such, the application of FCNN for finding the areas in WSI that are labeled as cancer regions, is more like aiming at learning the way of thinking of the expert pathologist rather than detection of objects with clear boundaries and specific textures, as is usual in semantic image segmentation tasks.

Aiming at dealing with these challenges, we design a custom FCNN network, by dropping the trainable upsampling convolutional filters and generating a coarse 32 × 32 pixels classification map using only convolutional and pooling layers. We avoid the use of very deep architectures to avoid over-fitting to the small training set we have and also to have shorter training time. The resulting network is almost 10 times smaller than the famous very deep networks that are usually employed (using transfer learning) and achieves better classification accuracy than the baseline heatmap based approach that makes use of the very deep inception v3 [7]. This shows the power of our small coarse pixel-level FCNNs in learning to annotate, even when the labels do not have a clear correspondence with the textures and boundaries in the images.

2 Context Aware Fully Convolutional Neural Network

The architecture we use to annotate cancer regions in Lung WSIs is inspired by the FCNN architecture introduced in [8] for pixel level semantic segmentation of images. The FCNN in [8] extends on some of the well-known network architectures like VGG network [11] that use a very deep Convolutional Neural Network (CNN) for feature extraction, followed by a fully connected neural network that performs image level classification. In the FCNN, the fully connected layer of the classifier is dropped and replaced by few more layers of CNNs to achieve coarse pixel level classification map. Subsequently, several deconvolution layers (upsampling and convolutional filters) are used to attain pixel level classification. The training is performed end-to-end, at pixel level to assign each pixel in the image to one of the available classes.

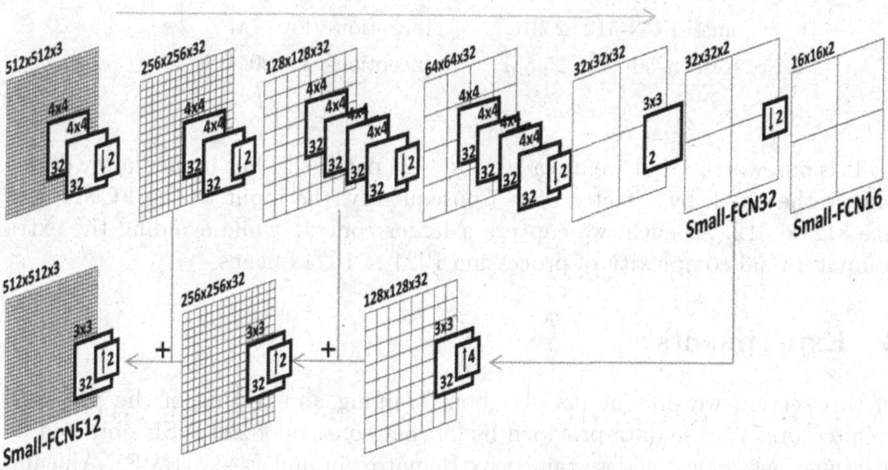

Fig. 3. The three FCNN architectures we use for annotation of lung cancer: small-FCN32, small-FCN16 and small-FCN512.

For the task of Lung Cancer annotation in WSI, we design a significantly smaller network shown in Fig. 3. The choice of smaller network is because of the nature of problem we are dealing with (Sect. 1.2) and also the much smaller training data we have (to lower the risk of over-fitting to the small training dataset). We have used 4 × 4 convolutional filters to increase the receptive field at different level, because we are aiming at labeling *regions* of WSIs rather than finding of the exact boundaries of objects.

We evaluate 3 alternatives shown in Fig. 3 by taking final output at different points in the network: *Small-FCN-32* does not even use the upsampling deconvolution filters and generates the final 1024 × 1024 mask by simple repetition of values at each pixel. *Small-FCN-16* goes even at a coarser level with an additional pooling layer, aiming at achieving region based labeling of human eyes.

Finally, in order to compare the ability of the trainable upsample in region-based labeling, we use *small-FCN-512*, which uses trainable deconvolution layers to get the mask at 512 × 512 resolution. Table 1 shows that all the networks we use are at least 30 times smaller than the well-known DNN architectures that are considered the state-of-the-art and are used in most of the current biomedical imaging DNN based approaches [6]. For training of these three architectures we use the spatial loss function defined as sum of cross-entropy loss function at each pixel.

Table 1. Number of parameters in different DNN architectures.

Architecture	Parameters	Architecture	Parameters
small-FCN-16	182K	VGG	138M
small-FCN-32	182K	AlexNet	61M
small-FCN-512	253K	Inception-v1	7M
ResNet-50	25.5M	Inception-v3	20M

It is noteworthy that we use a 1024 × 1024 patch-size but immediately downsample the patch by a factor of 2. Consequently, the input to the FCNN is of size 512 × 512. As such, we capture a larger context while avoiding the extra computational complexity of processing 1024 × 1024 images.

3 Experiments

In this section we present details about training and testing of the proposed architecture. We use data provided by [5] that consists of 200 WSIs obtained by scanning histological slides stained by Hematoxyin and Eosin (H&E). All samples were digitized using the same Olympus VS120 scanner with 20x objective magnification. Experienced pathologists have manually annotated the cancer regions on tissue level for each WSI.

For training of our network, we sample 1024 × 1024 patches from 150 of these WSIs, and use Adam optimizer [1] with a decaying learning rate that starts with 1e-4, to optimize the weights of these networks. We use a batch size equal to 10 for training on an NVIDIA Pascal GPU and the network starts to converge after about 2 hours of training. Figure 4, shows an example annotation generated by small-FCN-32. It can be seen that this small network is capable of predicting regions in WSI annotated as cancer regions by expert pathologists. There are also small regions in bottom left corner of the segment, where the generated annotation does not match the ground truth.

For a formal evaluation of the resulting annotations we use the remaining 50 WSIs as our test set and use Dice coefficient as the performance metric:

$$\frac{2TP}{2TP + FN + FP} \tag{1}$$

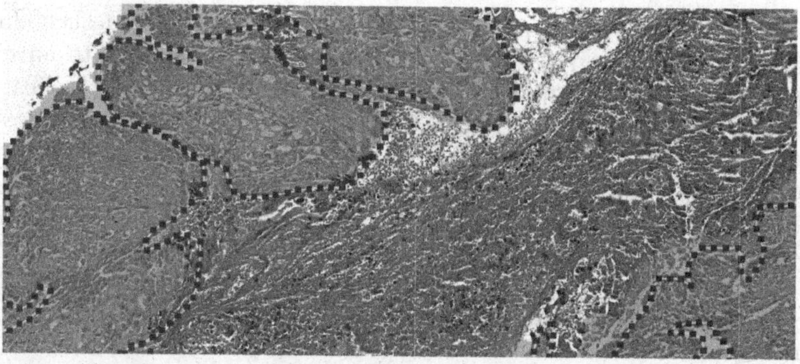

Fig. 4. A large segment of a Lung WSI in which cancer regions are marked by polygons around them. The prediction of our smallFCN-32 architecture is shown as green highlights overlaid on the original WSI. (Color figure online)

where TP indicates number of True Positives pixels, FP is the number of False Positives and FN is the number of False negatives. We compare our results to those of the heatmap based approach that was introduced in [7] for detection and localization of breast cancer metastases and was applied in [5] to the case of Lung cancer. For the baseline heatmap based approach we use Inception v3 [12] architecture on 256 × 256 pixels patches to generate the heatmap and apply a threshold of 0.5, with an overlap of 128 pixels between adjacent patches. The results are presented in Table 2. It can be seen that our small-FCN-32 achieves better results compared to the heatmap based approach [5].

Table 2. Test set performance for different approaches.

Approach	Patch size	Overlap	Average dice coef.
small-FCN-16	1024 × 1024	-	69.95
small-FCN-32	1024 × 1024	-	71.24
small-FCN-512	1024 × 1024	-	69.88
ImagenetFCN	1024 × 1024	-	73.54
Heatmap based [5]	256 × 256	128	67.45

4 Conclusions

In this research we introduced a new approach for annotation of cancer regions in Lung WSIs that rather than classifying small patches from the WSI as a whole, aims at classifying each pixel in larger patches using image segmentation methods. We introduced three custom FCNNs that are at least 30 times smaller than the well-known deep learning architectures. We showed that such efficient architecture is indeed capable of annotating Lung WSIs similar to an expert pathologist annotates cancer regions. Moreover, it outperformed the heat-map based approach that relies on a very deep neural network with much more computations. In this paper we focused on exploring the use of small FCNN architectures for lung cancer annotation and these results were achieved without any pre-processing and standardization of WSIs, that are shown helpful in improving the performance of machine learning based histopathology image analysis.

Acknowledgement. This research was sponsored under NVIDIA developer grant program.

References

1. Adam: a method for stochastic optimization. CoRR abs/1412.6980 (2014). http://arxiv.org/abs/1412.6980
2. American Cancer Society: Surveillance research, cancer facts & figures (2017.) https://www.cancer.org/research/cancer-facts-statistics/all-cancer-facts-figures/cancer-facts-figures-2017.html. Accessed March 2019
3. Graham, S., Shaban, M., Qaiser, T., Koohbanani, N.A., Khurram, S.A., Rajpoot, N.: Classification of lung cancer histology images using patch-level summary statistics (2018). https://doi.org/10.1117/12.2293855
4. Hipp, J., et al.: Computer aided diagnostic tools aim to empower rather than replace pathologists: lessons learned from computational chess. J. Pathol. Inform. **2**(1), 25 (2011)
5. Li, Z., et al.: Computer-aided diagnosis of lung carcinoma using deep learning - a pilot study. Computer Vision and Pattern Recognition arXiv:1803.05471
6. Litjens, G.J.S., et al.: A survey on deep learning in medical image analysis. CoRR abs/1702.05747 (2017). http://arxiv.org/abs/1702.05747
7. Liu, Y., et al.: Detecting cancer metastases on gigapixel pathology images. CoRR abs/1703.02442 (2017). http://arxiv.org/abs/1703.02442
8. Long, J., Shelhamer, E., Darrell, T.: Fully convolutional networks for semantic segmentation. In: The IEEE Conference on Computer Vision and Pattern Recognition (CVPR), June 2015
9. Papandreou, G., Chen, L.C., Murphy, K.P., Yuille, A.L.: Weakly- and semi-supervised learning of a deep convolutional network for semantic image segmentation
10. Rahman, T., Mahanta, L., Chakraborty, D.A.K., Sarma, J.D.: Textural pattern classification for oral squamous cell carcinoma. J. Microsc. **269**, 85–93 (2017)
11. Simonyan, K., Zisserman, A.: Very deep convolutional networks for large-scale image recognition. CoRR abs/1409.1556 (2014). http://arxiv.org/abs/1409.1556
12. Szegedy, C., Vanhoucke, V., Ioffe, S., Shlens, J., Wojna, Z.: Rethinking the inception architecture for computer vision. In: Proceedings of IEEE Conference on Computer Vision and Pattern Recognition (2016). http://arxiv.org/abs/1512.00567
13. Yu, K.H., et al.: Predicting non-small cell lung cancer prognosis by fully automated microscopic pathology image features. Nat. Commun. **7**, 12474 (2016)

Optimized Deep Learning Architecture for the Diagnosis of Pneumonia Through Chest X-Rays

Gabriel Garcez Barros Sousa(✉), Vandécia Rejane Monteiro Fernandes(✉), and Anselmo Cardoso de Paiva(✉)

Universidade Federal do Maranhão, São Luis, MA, Brazil
gabrielgarcezbsousa@hotmail.com, vandecia@ecp.ufma.br, paiva@nca.ufma.br

Abstract. One of the most common exams done in hospitals is the chest radiograph. From results of this exam, many illnesses can be diagnosed such as Pneumonia, which is deadliest illness for children. The main objective of this work is to propose a convolutional neural network model that performs the diagnosis of pneumonia through chest radiographs. The model's proposed architecture is automatically generated through optimization of hyperparameters. Generated models were trained and validated with an image base of chest radiographs presenting cases of viral and bacterial pneumonia. The best architecture found resulted in an accuracy of 95.3% and an AUC of 94% for diagnosing pneumonia, while the best architecture for the classification of type of pneumonia attained an accuracy of 83.1% and AUC of 80%.

Keywords: Pneumonia · Chest radiography · Deep neural network · Diagnosis

1 Introduction

About 450 million people are affected by pneumonia every year, resulting in approximately 4 million deaths [1]. In 2015, pneumonia accounted for 15% of the deaths of children under the age of 5, which made it the most deadly infectious disease in children [2]. In addition, pneumonia is estimated to cause over 11 million deaths by 2030 [3].

The most common types of pneumonia are those caused by bacteria or viruses. This disease can be treated more effectively if its method of transmission is quickly and correctly determined. To assist in the diagnosis of pneumonia, patients undergo an imaging exam called the chest radiograph, also known as chest X-ray (CXR). The product of this exam is a visual representation of the internal state of the patient's chest.

The chest X-ray is the most common type of radiological examination, which results in a high amount of images being generated each day. With an automatic method of detecting pneumonia, radiologists can be offered an objective second

F. Karray et al. (Eds.): ICIAR 2019, LNCS 11663, pp. 353–361, 2019.
https://doi.org/10.1007/978-3-030-27272-2_31

opinion to accelerate the diagnosis process. Since CXRs are images, this renders the process suitable for automation through the use of Deep Learning, which is an area of machine learning that is based on abstracting complex information through deep processing layers.

A model that makes use of Deep Learning has the ability to automatically distinguish features and classify images. This technique is already widely studied for use in the medical field for the diagnosis of diseases that can be diagnosed by the use of visual information such as images or volumes. As an example, Deep Learning has been applied in the detection of glaucoma [4], brain tumors [5] and skin cancer [6].

The main issue with using Deep Learning models is finding a suitable architecture for the problem being tackled. Complex architectures are robust and can be used for many problems but require long hours of training and significant computing power to be employed, while simple architectures might not possess the robustness needed to give accurate results. This problem can be explored through the use of hyper-parameter optimization [11].

Therefore, this work aims to present an automatic method to detect pneumonia through chest radiography by means of automatically generated deep convolutional networks (CNNs). In addition, the technique will also be applied in order to try to differentiate whether the patient is afflicted by bacterial or viral pneumonia. Several other authors have tackled this problem with varying degrees of success. Oliveira et al. [7] made use of different combinations of wavelets and achieved an AUC of 97% on a small base of 20 test images. More recently, Rajpurker et al. [8] and Kermany et al. [9] both used different CNN architectures to automatically extract features and classify images. They achieved AUCs of 76.8% and 96.8% respectively on different image bases.

This paper is organized as followed: Sect. 1 presents the proposed methodology use in detail. Experimental results along with tables and graphs are presented in Sect. 2.4. Section 3.2 concludes this paper with final considerations and future work.

2 Proposed Methodology

Two different convolutional neural network models will be generated by following the flowchart in Fig. 1. The first model will be able to diagnose pneumonia from a chest X-ray scan while the second will be able to differentiate whether the type of pneumonia is bacterial or viral through the same scan.

2.1 Dataset

The dataset used to measure the performance of the proposed methodology was initially collected and labeled by [9]. It presents 5,232 chest X-rays from routine exams done on children, where 3,883 (2,538 bacterial and 1,345 viral) were labeled as presenting pneumonia and 1,349 as normal. A patient may possess more than image in the dataset and the X-rays are stored in JPEG format with varying resolutions.

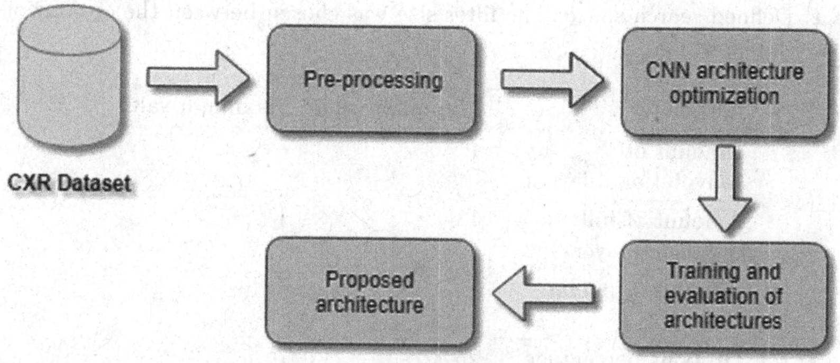

Fig. 1. Diagnosis and classification methodology flowchart.

To avoid biased and therefore invalid classifications, the author separated 624 images with no patients in common with the training set as the testing set. From these images, 234 of them are classified as normal and 390 as afflicted with pneumonia (242 bacterial and 148 viral). This is also the testing set used in this work.

2.2 Pre-processing

As mentioned, the images in the dataset come in varying resolutions and were even saved in a three-dimensional color scheme, despite the content of the image being in grayscale. To correct this, all of the images were redimensioned to a 300 × 300 pixel resolution and saved in a one-dimensional format to reduce the computational effort required for convolutional neural network training.

2.3 CNN Architecture Optimization

To solve the problem of finding an efficient architecture, a search space was defined. Each element in this space corresponds to a CNN architecture, which includes continuous parameters (number of neurons in each layer) and discrete ones (filter size, dropout rate, optimizer function and amount of each type of layer). A model's accuracy achieved with the testing set is the value to be optimized to as close to 100% as possible.

The optimization function used for this search was the Tree-structured Parzen Estimator (TPE), which is the algorithm that presented the best results in the study of hyper-optimization algorithms performed in a study by Bergstra et al. [11].

This search space is delimited in such a way that the encountered architectures require a lower need of computational processing. This was done in order to search for highly specialized models for each problem that can be easily used in computers or mobile devices with reduced computational power. The search space can be seen in Table 1.

Table 1. Defined search space. The filter size was chosen between the options of 3 × 3 and 5 × 5 pixels

Parameter	Minimum value	Maximum value
Amount of convolutional layers	1	7
Amount of fully connected layers	1	4
Amount of pooling layers	1	7
Dropout percentage	25%	75%
Amount of neurons in FC layer 1	512	2048
Amount of neurons in FC layer 2–4	64	512
Amount of neurons in convolutional layers 1–4	16	64
Amount of neurons in convolutional layers 5–7	32	128

2.4 Training and Evaluation of Architectures

Training sessions were performed by evaluating at least 50 different CNN architectures in each session. The sessions were divided into two classes: One to find models that could detect pneumonia between healthy or normal radiographs; and the other to find models that classified pathological radiographs between bacterial and viral pneumonia.

The training set was divided into training and validation sets, where the validation set was passed through the model at the end of each epoch. The training and validation bases were also completely identical throughout a specific session, this fact allows for a fair comparison between the results of the architectures in a given session.

Each architecture was trained for 100 epochs, where an epoch was defined as the application of all images in the training set on the model. After the 100 epochs, the model then receives the testing set where its accuracy is calculated and fed into the TPE algorithm to perform the search through the search space. A training session lasted for about 40 h in total for pneumonia diagnosis models and about 30 h for pneumonia classification models.

3 Experimental Results

3.1 Evaluation Metrics

All of the evaluation metrics for this work are derived from True Positive (TP), True Negative (TN), False Positive (FP) and False Negative (FN) values. These metrics are Sensitivity (SN), Specificity (SP), Accuracy (ACC) and the Area Under Curve (AUC). SN is the rate of which a model detects a disease while it is present, while SP is the rate of which a model estimates the non-presence of a disease where it isn't present.

A Receiver Operating Characteristic (ROC) curve is a visual representation of the relationship between the True Positive Rate and False Positive Rate. From this curve, the aforementioned AUC value can be derived. This value represents how well a model is distinguishing between different classes, where a value closer to 1 suggests more accurate classifications while a value closer to 0.5 the opposite.

3.2 Results

For the diagnosis of pneumonia, the best performing model achieved an AUC of 95.3% while for the classification of type of pneumonia, the best model attained a much lower 83.1% on each respective testing set. Table 2 shows the values of the other evaluation metrics.

The accuracy and sensitivity values for the diagnosis model were very high, while the specificity rate was moderate. These values show that the model is better at detecting pneumonia than detecting normal radiographies. Meanwhile, the values achieved by the classification model were relatively low, showing that it presented difficulties in identifying the differences between bacterial and viral pneumonia. This is due to how subtle the differences of these diseases are on a CXR scan.

Table 2. Results from the best generated models

Problem type	ACC	AUC	SN	SP
Diagnosis of pneumonia	95.3%	94%	99.7%	88%
Classification of pneumonia type	83.1%	80%	91.3%	69.6%

Figure 2 shows the how the best diagnosis model found behaved during its training. As it can be seen, the model quickly stabilizes at around 20 epochs of training aside from a spike at the 80 epoch mark. This spike is most likely caused by untrained neurons in the dropout layer and would stabilize with further training.

For the classification of pneumonia type model, Fig. 3 demonstrates how it performed during its training session. It is noticeable that the model started to quickly overfit due to how training and validation values constantly distanced itself. This shows that the model is completely unsuitable to handle this type of problem so further hyperparamenter search sessions should be explored.

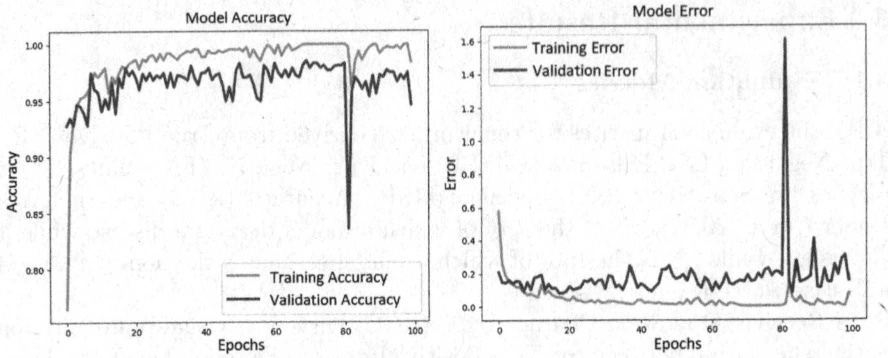

Fig. 2. Accuracy and error by epoch curves for the best model found for the diagnosis of pneumonia.

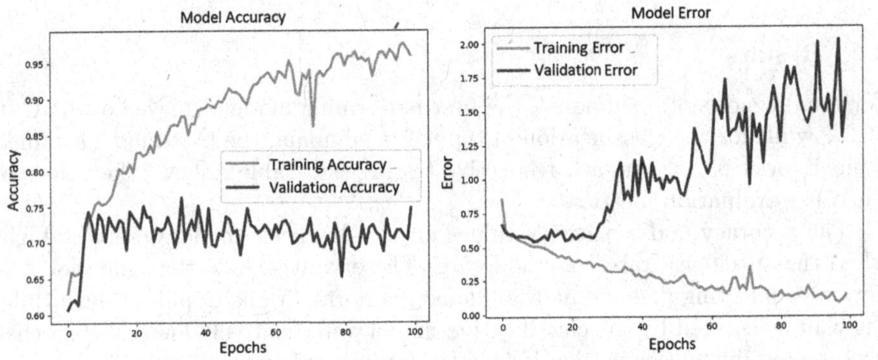

Fig. 3. Accuracy and error by epoch curves for the best model found for the classification of bacterial or viral pneumonia.

Tables 3 and 4 show the architectures and amount of trainable parameters of the best models found for each problem studied in this work.

Table 5 shows a comparison between similar works with the previously mentioned evaluation metric and the amount of hyperparameters the particular model used. Kermany et al. [9] was the creator of the dataset used for this work while Rajpurkar et al. [8] used the ChestX-ray14 [10] dataset for the training and evaluation of their model. This dataset contains 112,120 X-ray images with only 1,353 of them being labeled as presenting pneumonia. The labels of this dataset were automatically generated through natural language processing with an accuracy of 88.9% for the pneumonia label. This uncertainty in the labeling of radiographs can result in very inaccurate classifications and may be one of the reasons behind the author's low AUC.

For diagnosis, our model exceeded results obtained by Kermany et al. in terms of ACC and SN, and achieved only slightly lower values for the other metrics except for the amount of hyperparameters used. Our model necessitates

Table 3. Architecture of the best model found for diagnosis

Layer type	Input	Filter size	Activation function	Output	Amount of parameters
Convolutional 1	300 × 300 × 1	3 × 3	ReLU	150 × 150 × 16	160
Pooling 1	150 × 150 × 16	3 × 3		74 × 74 × 16	0
Pooling 2	74 × 74 × 16	3 × 3	ReLU	37 × 37 × 32	4640
Pooling 2	37 × 37 × 32	3 × 3		18 × 18 × 32	0
Convolutional 3	18 × 18 × 32	3 × 3	ReLU	9 × 9 × 16	4624
Pooling 3	9 × 9 × 16	3 × 3		4 × 4 × 16	0
Convolutional 4	4 × 4 × 16	3 × 3	ReLU	2 × 2 × 128	18560
Fully connected 1	512		ReLU	512	262656
Fully connected 2	512		ReLU	512	262656
Fully connected 3	512		ReLU	256	131328
Fully connected 4	256		ReLU	128	32896
Fully connected 5	128		Sigmoid	2	258

Table 4. Architecture of the best model found for classification

Layer type	Input	Filter size	Activation function	Output	Amount of parameters
Convolutional 1	300 × 300 × 1	5 × 5	ReLU	150 × 150 × 16	160
Pooling 1	150 × 150× 16	3 × 3		74 × 74 × 16	0
Convolutional 2	74 × 74 × 16	3 × 3	ReLU	37 × 37 × × 64	9280
Convolutional 3	37 × 37 × 64	3 × 3	ReLU	19 × 19 × 32	18464
Pooling 2	19 × 19 × 32	3 × 3		9 × 9 × 32	0
Convolutional 4	9 × 9 × 32	3 × 3	ReLU	5 × 5 × 128	36992
Pooling 3	5 × 5 × 128	3 × 3		2 × 2 × 128	0
Fully connected 1	512		ReLU	1024	525312
Fully connected 2	1024		ReLU	64	65600
Fully connected 3	64		ReLU	512	33280
Fully connected 4	512		ReLU	512	262656
Fully connected 5	512		Sigmoid	2	1026

a drastically lower amount of hyperparameters compared to the dataset's creator. This fact shows that the creation of simpler, highly specialized models for specific problems is feasible and increases the amount of computing devices that can make use of such models.

4 Conclusion and Future Works

Diagnosing diseases through chest X-rays is a common practice in hospitals. This work presented techniques to accelerate diagnosis for pneumonia. The technique used in this work was deep learning, which is a technique frequently used for image classification and recognition in the literature. One of the main problems of using this is finding a suitable classification architecture, thus this work

Table 5. Comparison of results

Problem type	Author	Amount of X-rays with pneumonia	ACC	AUC	SN	SP	Amount of hyperparameters
Diagnosis	Kermany et al. [9]	3,883	92.8%	96.8%	93.2%	90.1%	23 million
	Rajpurkar et al. [8]	1,353	-	76.8%	-	-	0.8 million
	Proposed methodology	3,883	95.3%	94%	99.7%	88%	0.77 million
Classification	Kermany et al. [9]	3,883	90.7%	94%	88.6%	90.9%	23 million
	Proposed methodology	3,883	83.1%	80%	91.3%	69.6%	0.52 million

presented a method to automatically generate and test different convolutional neural network models.

The results were very satisfactory for the diagnosis of the disease, surpassing the accuracy and sensitivity of the dataset's creator while presenting a comparably lower necessity of computational power. This last fact renders the model more applicable in suboptimal situations. For the classification of whether the pathology was caused by bacteria or virus, the simple models failed to present acceptable levels of classification due to their differences being considerably more subtle in chest radiographs.

For future works, exploring the usage of segmentated lungs from X-rays to accelerate and ease the feature extraction process should be done while also expanding the repertoire of possible generated model architectures, including more complex techniques such as transition layers. Different search space optimization algorithms similar to TPE should also be studied and applied in order to determine if there are better options in literature.

References

1. Lodha, R., Kabra, S.K., Pandey, R.M.: Antibiotics for community-acquired pneumonia in children. Cochrane Database Syst. Rev. (6). Article No. CD004874 (2013). https://doi.org/10.1002/14651858.CD004874
2. World Health Organization. http://www.who.int/news-room/fact-sheets/detail/pneumonia. Accessed 15 Feb 2019
3. Save the Children Organization. https://reliefweb.int/report/world/pneumonia-kill-nearly-11-million-children-2030. Accessed 12 Feb 2019
4. Cerentini, A., et al.: Automatic identification of glaucoma using deep learning methods. In: Studies in Health Technology and Informatics, PubMed (2017)
5. Havaei, M., et al.: Brain tumor segmentation with deep neural networks. Med. Image Anal. **35**, 18–31 (2017)
6. Esteva, A., et al.: Dermatologist-level classification of skin cancer with deep neural networks. Nature **524**, 115–118 (2014). https://doi.org/10.1038/nature21056
7. Oliveira, L.L.G., et al.: Computer-aided diagnosis in chest radiography for detection of childhood pneumonia. Int. J. Med. Inform. **77**(8), 555–564 (2008). https://doi.org/10.1016/j.ijmedinf.2007.10.010
8. Rajpurkar, P., et al.: CheXNet: radiologist-level pneumonia detection on chest X-rays with deep learning. In: Computing Research Repository, eprint 1711.05225, arXiv (2017)

9. Kermany, D., et al.: Identifying medical diagnoses and treatable diseases by image-based deep learning. Cell **172**(5), 1122–1131 (2018). https://doi.org/10.1016/j.cell.2018.02.010
10. Wang, X., et al.: ChestX-ray8: hospital-scale chest x-ray database and benchmarks on weakly-supervised classification and localization of common thorax diseases. In: Computing Research Repository, eprint 1705.02315, arXiv (2018)
11. Bergstra, J, et al.: Algorithms for hyper-parameter optimization. In: Proceedings of the 24th International Conference on Neural Information Processing Systems, pp. 2546–2554. Curran Associates Inc., Granada (2011)

Learned Pre-processing for Automatic Diabetic Retinopathy Detection on Eye Fundus Images

Asim Smailagic[1], Anupma Sharan[1], Pedro Costa[2](✉), Adrian Galdran[3], Alex Gaudio[1], and Aurélio Campilho[2,4]

[1] Carnegie Mellon University, Pittsburgh, USA
[2] INESC TEC, Porto, Portugal
ei10011@fe.up.pt
[3] École de Tecnologie Superieure, Montreal, Canada
[4] Faculty of Engineering, University of Porto, Porto, Portugal

Abstract. Diabetic Retinopathy is the leading cause of blindness in the working-age population of the world. The main aim of this paper is to improve the accuracy of Diabetic Retinopathy detection by implementing a shadow removal and color correction step as a preprocessing stage from eye fundus images. For this, we rely on recent findings indicating that application of image dehazing on the inverted intensity domain amounts to illumination compensation. Inspired by this work, we propose a Shadow Removal Layer that allows us to learn the pre-processing function for a particular task. We show that learning the pre-processing function improves the performance of the network on the Diabetic Retinopathy detection task.

Keywords: Retinal image preprocessing · Diabetic retinopathy detection · Color balancing

1 Introduction

Diabetic Retinopathy (DR) is an eye disease that affects more than 25% of the estimated 425 worldwide diabetic patients [1]. Consequently, DR is a leading cause of blindness in the working-age population of the world and, therefore, screening all diabetic patients is of paramount importance. With the growth in the prevalence of diabetes, the burden on ophthalmologists to screen the entire diabetic population also grows. For these reasons, a system capable of detecting DR is becoming increasingly important.

Screening for DR in the US and UK relies mainly on the right interpretation of a digital retinal image to recognize pathological features. Prompt acknowledgement and treatment of this pathology can save sight, and for this reason much research has been devoted in recent years to the design of machine learning pipelines that can help in its correct diagnosis. Unfortunately, lesions that

F. Karray et al. (Eds.): ICIAR 2019, LNCS 11663, pp. 362–368, 2019.
https://doi.org/10.1007/978-3-030-27272-2_32

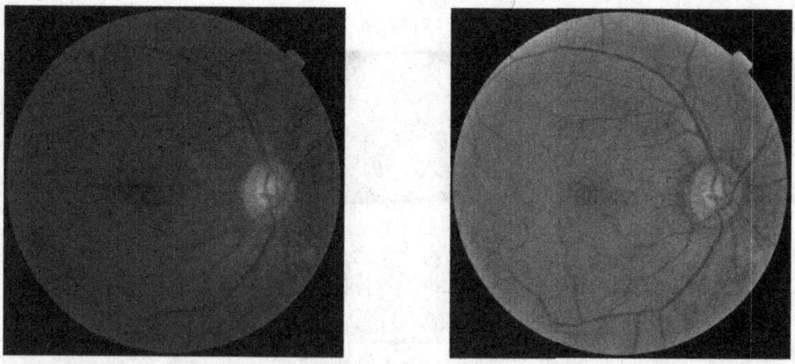

Fig. 1. Example of an eye fundus image. Left: unprocessed retinal image. Right: illumination-compensation by shadow removal.

characterize early stages of this disease are subtle, and when improperly illuminated by a fundus camera in acquisition time they can be confounded with other non-harmful signs of similar appearance.

A reasonable approach to deal with this problem is to improve the quality of the image by obtaining a shadow free version of the image. Although this step can be performed in a manual way [2–4], it may be preferable to learn the preprocessing function with minimal intervention, directly from the data. We propose to do so by implementing a U-net architecture [5], which is the convolutional neural network architecture of choice for biomedical image segmentation.

2 Related Work

The pre-processing of retinal images has been proposed in several papers before. One of the first proposed techniques for improving the visual appearance of this kind of data was introduced in [2]. The authors estimated an illumination field by first removing foreground pixels and then fitting a Gaussian model to the background. Similarly, the technique proposed in [6] relies on Laplace interpolation and a multiplicative model of illumination to remove its impact. In [7], an image formation model involving scattering and background illumination was proposed and inverted to retrieve well-illuminated images. A different model, based on cataracts formation, was used in [8] to reduce blurriness and improve contrast. Also recently, the authors of [4] introduce a luminosity correction technique with a focus on avoiding the creation of visual artifacts on regions of the image that were initially well-illuminated. It is important to stress that all these methods are designed and applied on retinal images in a static manner. This means that any subsequent automatic image understanding task for diagnostic purposes remains isolated from the pre-processing stage.

In this paper, we follow previous observations from [3,9] that fog/haze removal can be interpreted as illumination compensation when applied to inverted intensities on retinal images, as shown in Fig. 1. The standard model used to describe hazy images is given by the haze imaging equation [10–13]:

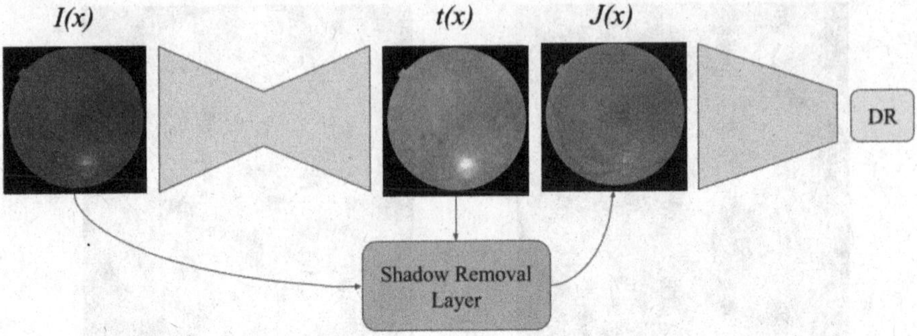

Fig. 2. Pipeline of the proposed method. A segmentation CNN is used to estimate the transmission map $t(x)$. Then, the input image $I(x)$ and $t(x)$ are provided to a Shadow Removal Layer that outputs the normalized image $J(x)$. Finally, $J(x)$ is given as input to a classifier CNN that outputs if the image has Diabetic Retinopathy or not. Both CNNs can be trained to minimize the classification error.

$$I(x) = J(x)t(x) + A(1 - t(x)). \tag{1}$$

Therefore, haze removal involves estimating the transmission map t (depth map), soft matting for its refinement, estimating the atmospheric light A and recovering the scene radiance J. While we also aim to apply the above model, in contrast with previous techniques our goal in this paper is to automatically learn to estimate these unknowns in such a way that they are optimal for the downstream task of diabetic retinopathy detection, which will be simultaneously solved.

3 Method

Pre-processing the images to have more consistent illumination and colors across the dataset can help improve the performance of DR detection. In this paper, we aim to remove shadows from eye fundus images by dehazing the inverted image [3]. Dehazing methods require the estimation of the transmission map t using heuristics that may not be optimal. To overcome this issue, we pose the problem of transmission map estimation as an optimization problem, and propose to learn the function that maps an eye fundus image to a transmission map $t(x)$ by minimizing a classification error. This allows us to optimize the transmission map estimation for a particular classification task.

3.1 Shadow Removal Layer

In order to accomplish this, we develop a Shadow Removal Layer. This layer uses an estimated transmission map $t(x)$ and an input image $I(x)$ and outputs a pre-processed image $J(x)$, with shadows removed. This layer applies the following equation:

$$J(x) = 1 - (\frac{(1 - I(x)) - A}{t(x)} + A). \tag{2}$$

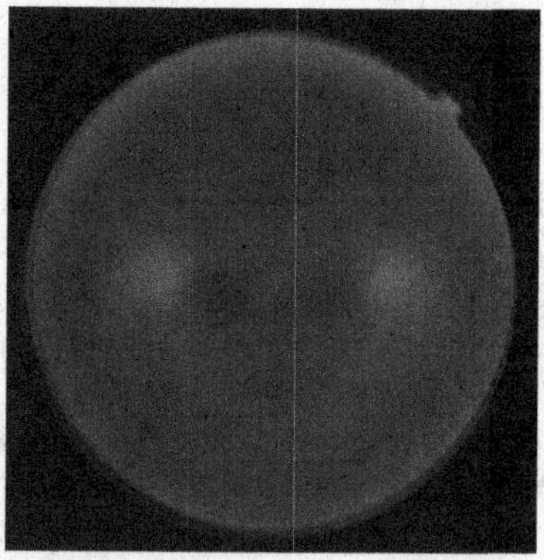

Fig. 3. Average depth map computed manually from the entire dataset of eye fundus images, used as additional supervision to the transmission map.

We can assume that $A = 1$ if we white balance the images before applying the illumination estimation function as shown in [3]. The equation then reduces to $I(x)/t(x)$ *i.e.* simply dividing the input image intensities with the transmission map. In this work, we use a Segmentation Convolutional Neural Network (CNN) to learn the function $t(x)$.

The problem is that we do not have the ground-truth data to train the segmentation model $t(x)$. To solve this issue, we derive the training signal from a classification CNN that learns to detect DR from $J(x)$. Therefore, the segmentation CNN learns to output the transmission map that minimizes the classification CNN error. This is possible as Eq. 2 is differentiable, and the training signal can flow to the segmentation CNN's parameters. The entire architecture is shown in Fig. 2.

3.2 Transmission Map Supervision

For the transmission map estimation model to be able to learn something close to the depth map of the image, we add a term to the loss. On top of the classification loss we minimize the mean squared error between $t(x)$ and a reference transmission map M. This reference transmission map is obtained by computing the depth maps for each image in the dataset manually as per the Dark Channel Prior theory [14] and taking an average over all the depth maps, as shown in Fig. 3. The objective of the network is hence modified to decrease the difference between the manually computed reference depth map and the learned depth map. The new loss function is:

$$J(x, \theta_c, \theta_s) = \mathcal{L}(x, \theta_c, \theta_s) + MSE(x, \theta_s), \quad (3)$$

where $\mathcal{L}$ is the classification loss, θ_c are the classification network's parameters and θ_s are the segmentation network's parameters. In this paper we used Binary Cross-Entropy as the classification loss $\mathcal{L}$.

4 Experiments

4.1 Implementation Details

We used a network inspired by U-Net as the segmentation CNN that estimates the transmission map $t(x)$ and a pre-trained Inception v3 network as the classification network. The eye fundus images are resized to 512×512 and provided to the U-Net. The pre-processed images that are given to the Inception v3 network are also 512×512. To accomodate for the larger input image size, we remove the last layer of the Inception v3 network and add a global average pooling layer followed by a Fully-Connected layer with a single output.

The two models are trained using the Adam optimizer with a learning rate of 2×10^{-4}. The training process consists of 2 phases:

1. Fitting: Here, the parameters of the Inception network are frozen and the U-net alone is trained;
2. Fine-tuning: Here, the layers of the Inception network are made trainable and thus fine tuned along with the U-net parameters

Both fitting and fine-tuning are performed for 100 epochs each with a batch-size of 4.

4.2 Dataset

The Messidor dataset [15] is a collection of eye fundus images of healthy and unhealthy patients. It consists of 1200 eye fundus color numerical images acquired by 3 ophthalmologic departments. The image sizes are 1440×960, 2240×1488 or 2304×1536 pixels. The retinopathy grade has been provided by medical experts, where a grade of 0 corresponds to healthy and grades 1,2 and 3 correspond to unhealthy.

The training data consists of 949 images, 441 healthy and 508 unhealthy, and the test data consists of 238 images, 106 healthy and 132 unhealthy. The images in both training an test set are distributed equally among the 3 opthalmologic departments.

The images are center cropped and resized. Each image corresponds to 4 images, the original image, a randomly rotated image by an angle in the range of 230°, and the horizontally flipped version of both.

Table 1. Our shadow removal layer improves the classification accuracy over the baseline.

Results	Test accuracy
Inception V3	89.50%
U-Net+Shadow Removal+Inception v3	90.34%

4.3 Results

We trained the classifier on the original dataset for the task of DR detection and obtained 89.50% accuracy. Our pre-processing method achieves a test accuracy of 90.34% after fine-tuning, as shown in Table 1, giving an improvement 0.84% in the test set over the baseline. Our model converges better than the baseline and also improves the detection.

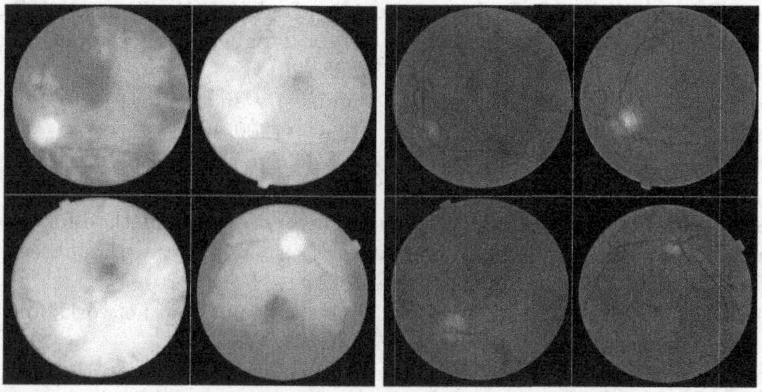

Fig. 4. Transmission map learned by the U-Net and corresponding output of the Shadow Removal Layer.

Furthermore, we can visually inspect the estimated transmission maps $t(x)$. As shown in Fig. 4, we can verify that the U-Net was able to output valid transmission maps, different from the mean transmission map M. Moreover, the images produced by the Shadow Removal Layer have similar illumination, indicating that the learned pre-processing step is effectively removing shadows from the eye fundus images.

5 Conclusion and Future Work

In this paper we proposed a method to learn how to pre-process eye fundus images for the task of DR detection. We draw inspiration from haze/shadow removal methods and devise a methodology to train a segmentation CNN to estimate the transmission map of the input eye fundus image. Then, we apply a Shadow Removal Layer to pre-process the input image and then provide that image to a classifier. The entire system can be trained to minimize the classification error.

We show that, by learning to pre-process eye fundus images to a particular task, the performance of DR detection is improved. As future work, we plan to verify if the learned pre-processing function is useful for other retinal tasks, such as vessel segmentation.

Acknowledgments. This work is financed by the ERDF - European Regional Development Fund through the Operational Programme for Competitiveness and Internationalisation - COMPETE 2020 Programme, by National Funds through the FCT - Fundação para a Ciência e a Tecnologia (Portuguese Foundation for Science and Technology) within project CMUP-ERI/TIC/0028/2014.

References

1. Ruta, L.M., Magliano, D.J., Lemesurier, R., Taylor, H.R., Zimmet, P.Z., Shaw, J.E.: Prevalence of diabetic retinopathy in type 2 diabetes in developing and developed countries. Diabet. Med. **30**(4), 387–398 (2013)
2. Foracchia, M., Grisan, E., Ruggeri, A.: Luminosity and contrast normalization in retinal images. Med. Image Anal. **9**(3), 179–190 (2005)
3. Savelli, B., et al.: Illumination correction by dehazing for retinal vessel segmentation, pp. 219–224, June 2017
4. Saha, S., Fletcher, A., Xiao, D., Kanagasingam, Y.: A novel method for automated correction of non-uniform/poor illumination of retinal images without creating false artifacts. J. Vis. Commun. Image Represent. **51**, 95–103 (2018)
5. Ronneberger, O., Fischer, P., Brox, T.: U-net: convolutional networks for biomedical image segmentation. CoRR, abs/1505.04597 (2015)
6. Leahy, C., O'Brien, A., Dainty, C.: Illumination correction of retinal images using Laplace interpolation. Appl. Opt. **51**(35), 8383–8389 (2012)
7. Xiong, L., Li, H., Xu, L.: An enhancement method for color retinal images based on image formation model. Comput. Methods Program. Biomed. **143**, 137–150 (2017)
8. Mitra, A., Roy, S., Roy, S., Setua, S.K.: Enhancement and restoration of non-uniform illuminated fundus image of retina obtained through thin layer of cataract. Comput. Methods Program. Biomed. **156**, 169–178 (2018)
9. Galdran, A., Bria, A., Alvarez-Gila, A., Vazquez-Corral, J., Bertalmío, M.: On the duality between retinex and image dehazing. In: 2018 IEEE/CVF Conference on Computer Vision and Pattern Recognition, pp. 8212–8221, June 2018
10. Narasimhan, S.G., Nayar, S.K.: Vision and the atmosphere. Int. J. Comput. Vis. **48**(3), 233–254 (2002)
11. Narasimhan, S.G., Nayar, S.K.: Chromatic framework for vision in bad weather. In: Proceedings of the IEEE Conference on Computer Vision and Pattern Recognition (2000)
12. Fattal, R.: Single image dehazing. ACM Trans. Graph. **27**(3), 72:1–72:9 (2008)
13. Tan, R.: Visibility in bad weather from a single image, June 2008
14. He, K., Sun, J., Tang, X.: Single image haze removal using dark channel prior. IEEE Trans. Pattern Anal. Mach. Intell. **33**(12), 2341–2353 (2011)
15. Decencière, E., et al.: Feedback on a publicly distributed database: the messidor database. Image Anal. Stereol. **33**(3), 231–234 (2014)

TriResNet: A Deep Triple-Stream Residual Network for Histopathology Grading

Rene Bidart[1,2] and Alexander Wong[1,2](✉)

[1] Waterloo Artificial Intelligence Institute, University of Waterloo, Waterloo, ON, Canada
[2] Vision and Image Processing Research Group, University of Waterloo, Waterloo, ON, Canada
a28wong@uwaterloo.ca

Abstract. While microscopic analysis of histopathological slides is generally considered as the gold standard method for performing cancer diagnosis and grading, the current method for analysis is extremely time consuming and labour intensive as it requires pathologists to visually inspect tissue samples in a detailed fashion for the presence of cancer. As such, there has been significant recent interest in computer aided diagnosis systems for analysing histopathological slides for cancer grading to aid pathologists to perform cancer diagnosis and grading in a more efficient, accurate, and consistent manner. In this work, we investigate and explore a deep triple-stream residual network (**TriResNet**) architecture for the purpose of tile-level histopathology grading, which is the critical first step to computer-aided whole-slide histopathology grading. In particular, the design mentality behind the proposed TriResNet network architecture is to facilitate for the learning of a more diverse set of quantitative features to better characterize the complex tissue characteristics found in histopathology samples. Experimental results on two widely-used computer-aided histopathology benchmark datasets (CAMELYON16 dataset and Invasive Ductal Carcinoma (IDC) dataset) demonstrated that the proposed TriResNet network architecture was able to achieve noticeably improved accuracies when compared with two other state-of-the-art deep convolutional neural network architectures for histopathology grading. Based on these promising results, the hope is that the proposed TriResNet network architecture could become a useful tool to aiding pathologists increase the consistency, speed, and accuracy of the histopathology grading process.

Keywords: Deep neural network · Histopathology grading · Residual learning

The authors thank the Natural Sciences and Engineering Research Council of Canada, the Canada Research Chairs Program, and the Queen Elizabeth II Graduate Scholarship in Science & Technology for partially supporting this research. Furthermore, the authors thank Nvidia for the GPUs used in this study that were provided as part of a hardware grant.

F. Karray et al. (Eds.): ICIAR 2019, LNCS 11663, pp. 369–382, 2019.
https://doi.org/10.1007/978-3-030-27272-2_33

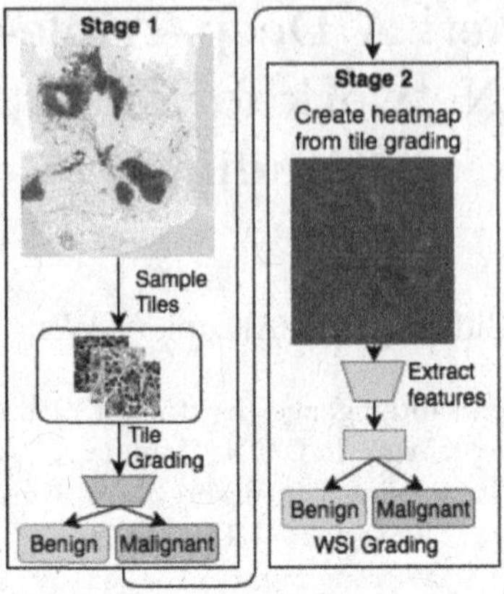

Fig. 1. An overview of the deep learning-driven computer-aided whole slide image (WSI) histopathology grading pipeline. In the first stage, tiles from the WSI are extracted and tile-level histopathology grading is performed using a deep convolutional neural network (CNN). In the second stage, the histopathology gradings for all tiles in the WSI are combined to create a malignancy probability heatmap. Features are then extracted from this heatmap, and are used to generate a final WSI-level grading. In this paper, we focus on improving tile-level histopathology grading using the proposed TriResNet network architecture.

1 Introduction

The microscopic analysis of hematoxylin and eosin (H&E) stained histopathological slides is generally considered as the gold standard method for diagnosing and grading cancers [10,18]. However, the current method for performing such an analysis requires the manual visual inspection of human pathologists, and as such can be limiting in several aspects. First of all, histopathological diagnosis and grading via manual visual inspection relies on the qualitative analysis of images from a microscope by a human pathologist, and as such can suffer from high inter-observer and intra-observer variability, particularly with the lack of standardization in the diagnosis and grading process. Second, the visual inspection of histopathological slides is an extremely time-consuming and labor intensive process, especially considering the large volume of slides that a typical pathologist must analyze, with each slide containing millions of cells [2,9,27]. These issues associated with the current method for performing histopathological diagnosis and grading are problematic in developed countries, but are far greater in developing countries where there is a severe lack of trained pathologists [5]. As such, there has been significant recent interest in computer aided diagnosis systems for analysing histopathological slides for cancer grading to aid pathologists to perform cancer diagnosis and grading in a more efficient, accurate, and consistent manner.

Amongst the different strategies proposed for the purpose of computer aided histopathology grading, one of the most promising recent developments has been the leveraging of machine learning for building computational predictive models learnt directly from the wealth of histopathological slides. Earlier methods that leveraged machine learning for computer aided histopathology grading utilized human-engineered quantitative features extracted from a histopathological image, followed by the application of a machine learning-driven classification model on these extracted features [3,4,8,13,23,26]. For example, [26] utilized tissue texture features by performing cell segmentation and calculating nuclei density and position as extracted features to be fed into a quadratic classifier. Other approaches have utilized a heterogeneous mix of human-engineered features ranging from simple features such as hue, saturation, and intensity to more complex features such as texture-based features (e.g., Haralick features and Gabor features) as well as graph-based features, followed by the application of support vector machines on these extracted features [8]. However, such earlier methods that leverage human-engineered features have been limited in their performance due to the significant difficulties for human experts to manually design a comprehensive set of features that can comprehensively capture the complex tissue characteristics exhibited in histopathological slides. Therefore, methods that can learn a comprehensive set of important quantitative features for discriminating between benign and cancerous tissue directly from histopathological slides themselves is highly desired.

In recent years, the concept of deep learning [19] has revolutionized the area of computer-aided histopathology diagnosis and grading by automatically learning discriminative quantitative features from the wealth of available histopathological images in a direct manner, rather than being constrained by the limitations of human-engineered features. In particular, a type of deep neural network known as deep convolutional neural networks (CNN), which demonstrated state-of-the-art performance on visual perception compared to other machine learning algorithms [17], has been leveraged for computer-aided histopathology grading to great success [20–22,28,31]. These deep learning-driven computer-aided whole slide image (WSI) histopathology grading approaches tend to share the same general pipeline. More specifically, the vast size of whole slide image make them computational intractable to be processed by a deep convolutional neural network in a single inference pass, as is commonly performed in general image classification where the images are significantly smaller in size.

To handle this size and complexity issue, these approaches breaks the task of WSI histopathology grading into two main stages (an overview of this two-stage approach is illustrated in Fig. 1). In the first stage, tissue image tiles are extracted from the WSI after preprocessing is used to reduce the irrelevant white space in the slide. A CNN trained to perform tile-level tissue grading is then used to grade each of the individual tiles extracted over the entire WSI. In the second stage, the histopathology gradings for all tiles in the WSI are then combined together to create a malignancy probability heatmap, and from this heatmap a number of WSI-level geometrical and morphological features are then extracted.

These extracted WSI-level features are then used by a machine learning classification model to generate the final WSI-level histopathology grading. As such, improvements to either of these two stages would yield benefits for the overall WSI histopathology grading processing. In this paper, we place our focus on improving the first stage of the computer-aided WSI histopathology grading pipeline by improving the performance of the tile-level tissue grading process through the introduction of an improved CNN network architecture.

The key contribution of this paper is the introduction of a novel deep triple-stream residual network (TriResNet) architecture for the purpose of improved tile-level histopathology grading. The proposed TriResNet architecture incorporates three different streams comprised of a deep stack of residual blocks, with the underlying motivation that, through careful training, each residual stream will learn a different set of quantitative features for better characterizing different aspects of the complex tissue characteristics captured in histopathology images than what can be achieved by a single-stream network. A multi-stage targeted training procedure is also introduced to overcome the difficulty of training such a large network architecture as well as better encouraging feature diversity within the network.

2 Deep Triple-Stream Residual Network

The proposed deep triple-stream residual network (TriResNet) architecture is designed based on the idea of extracting a more diverse set of discriminative quantitative features for better characterizing the diverse and complex tissue characteristics exhibited in histopathological images. A more detailed description of the proposed network architecture as well as the multi-stage targeted training policy used to train this network is provided below.

2.1 Network Architecture

The underlying goal behind the design of the proposed TriResNet network architecture is to better learn a larger, more diverse set of quantitative features for characterizing complex and varied tissue characteristics exhibited in histopathology images. To achieve this goal, we leverage the notion of residual learning first proposed in [12], which has not only demonstrated state-of-the-art performance for a wide variety of applications such as general image recognition [12], but has been recognized in research literature for its terrific ability to perform well both for feature extraction and fine-tuning [16].

The strategy we leverage in the proposed TriResNet network to encourage greater feature diversity is to incorporate multiple streams of residual blocks, with the underlying premise being that each of these independent streams, when trained appropriately, will be able to capture different nuances within the tissue characteristics in histopathology images. More specifically, as shown in Fig. 2, the proposed TriResNet architecture comprises of three separate residual streams consisting of deep stacks of residual blocks for a total of 34 layers in

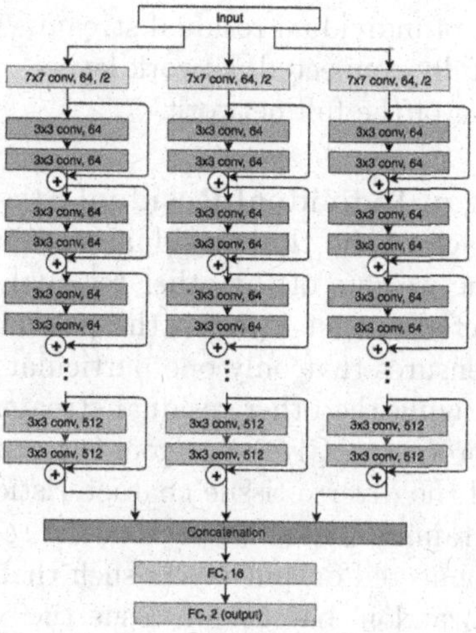

Fig. 2. Deep triple-stream residual network (TriResNet) architecture. An input layer feeds three separate residual streams, which each residual stream composed of a deep stack of residual blocks with a total of 34 layers. Each of these residual streams extract different sets of quantitative features, which are then fed into a concatenation layer, followed by two fully connected layers that result in a final grading prediction of the input histopathological image tile as being either malignant or benign tissue.

each stream, with each stream made up of a different set of learned weights to capture diverse feature sets. To explicitly encourage feature diversity of individual residual streams and learn to capture different tissue nuances amongst the streams, each residual stream undergoes pre-training exposure to different data collections, which will be described in detail in Sect. 2.2 where the multi-stage targeted training policy is outlined.

The features of the last residual blocks in each of the three residual streams within the proposed TriResNet architecture are combined in a concatenation layer, which is then fed into a 16-neuron fully connected layer, followed by a ReLU layer, which then feeds into a final fully connected layer where the number of neurons is equal to the number tissue grades to provide the final prediction output.

2.2 Multi-stage Targeted Training Policy

One of the challenges with leveraging the proposed TriResNet architecture for tile-level histopathology grading is that training such a complex network is extremely difficult because of the large number of parameters within this network (which makes converging to an appropriate solution quite challenging given this large parameter size) as well as the dangers of over-fitting. In order to tackle the aforementioned problem, we leverage a multi-stage targeted training policy consisting of the following three main stages:

1. Targeted pre-training of individual residual streams.
2. Targeted training of fully connected network layers.
3. End-to-end fine-tuning of the full network.

Targeted Pre-training of Individual Residual Streams. As the first stage of the training policy, each of the three residual streams are pre-trained independently by freezing the weights of the other residual streams, and augmenting a proxy fully connected output layer to the particular residual stream we wish to pre-train. This ensures that only one particular residual stream will be pre-trained at a time, leaving the other residual streams unaffected during the individual pre-training processes. Given our goal is to encourage diverse feature learning to better model the diverse tissue characteristics in histopathology, we utilize a stochastic pre-training policy for each of the residual streams via their individual proxy fully connected output layers such that the individual streams are exposed to different random batches of tissue tiles during the pre-training process. This ensures that each residual stream will converge to a different set of weights, and thus will be capable of capturing a diverse set of quantitative features compared to the other residual streams during inference. To speed up the pre-training process, each residual stream was initialized with pre-trained weights based on the ImageNet Challenge Dataset [7]. This pre-training process is repeated for each of the residual streams, and the proxy layers are removed at the end of the pre-training processes.

Targeted Training of Fully Connected Network Layers. After the targeted training of individual residual streams, we now focus on the targeted training of the fully connected network layers. The rationale behind this is that, because the random initialization of these layers, there is strong potential for convergence issues if the entire network architecture is trained end-to-end at this point. By freezing the weights of the individual residual streams while the fully connected layers begin to learn, we allow the fully connected layers to converge to a good set of weights without the convergence issues associated with training the entire network at this point. Furthermore, because backpropagation is performed only on the fully connected layers, the time to convergence is greatly accelerated.

End-to-End Fine-Tuning of the Full Network. After the fully-connected layers in the network have been trained using the targeted training process, the entire network undergoes an end-to-end fine-tuning process to further improve the performance of the full network architecture. In this part of the training process, we backpropogate the gradient though the entire network, including each of the three residual streams and the fully connected layers as a whole, thus optimizing the weights of the entire network. This is done at a lower learning rate that is a factor of 10 times lower than the initial learning rate. This end-to-end fine-tuning phase also encourages the individual residual streams to work cohesively together as a complete network architecture.

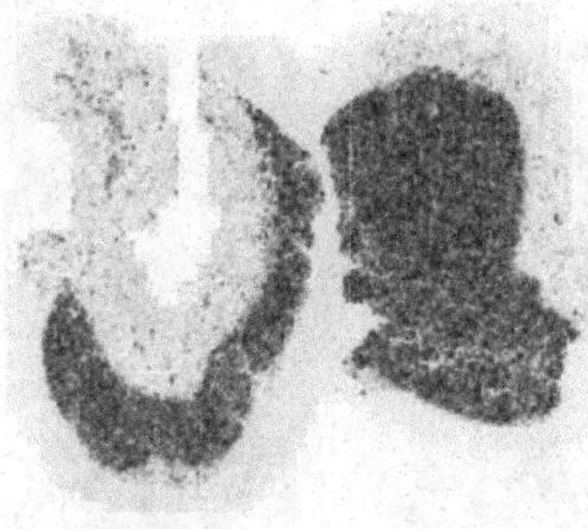

Fig. 3. An example of a whole slide image from the CAMELYON16 dataset, showing the large amount of irrelevant background in white.

3 Experiments

To study the efficacy of the proposed TriResNet network for the purpose of tile-level histopathology grading, we performed a series of experiments using two widely-used histopathological image benchmark datasets. The details of these datasets as well as the experimental setup are presented below.

3.1 Data

We investigate two publicly-available histopathological image benchmark datasets: (i) CAMELYON16 [1] dataset, and (ii) Invasive Ductal Carcinoma (IDC) [6,14] dataset.

CAMELYON16 Dataset. The CAMELYON16 dataset contains lymph node tissues of breast cancer patients, with the goal being to find metastasis of breast cancer. CAMELYON16 consists of 400 whole slide images (WSI) divided into 270 for training and 160 for testing. Ground truth is provided by a mask corresponding to each slide, which is an image with pixel level annotation indicating the cancerous regions. Both the mask and the WSI are very high resolution (100,000 × 200,000 pixels), with a single file being about 5 gigabytes. These are stored in a multi-resolution format, meaning that each file contains the high resolution image, as well as down sampled versions to a minimum size of about 512 × 1024. An example WSI from the CAMELYON16 dataset is shown in Fig. 3.

Due to the large size of the high resolution WSI slides making it difficult to handle and even perform simple operations on the slides in a direct manner, OpenSlide [11] is used to read in subsections of the WSI at a lower resolution.

Preprocessing. Because of the large size of the WSIs, the background is segmented from the actual tissue to greatly reduce the computational requirements in dealing with the histopathological images. This is accomplished in this paper using the preprocessing approach described in [31]:

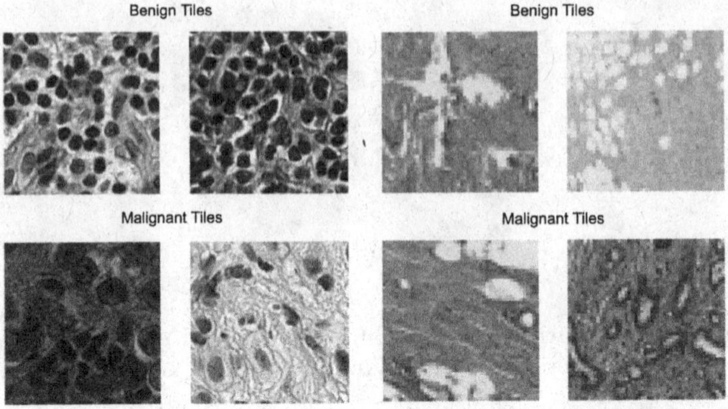

Fig. 4. Examples of tissue image tiles from the CAMELYON16 (left) and IDC (right) datasets showing benign and malignant tissues. These tissue image tiles are extracted at the highest magnification (40x), with a size of 224×224 pixels.

1. Read in WSI at resolution about 3072 × 7168 pixels, and convert from RGB to HSV.
2. Use Otsu's algorithm [24] to separate the background from foreground, then take the union of the result with the H and S channels to generate a tissue mask.

Dataset Generation. In many circumstances, 270 images would be considered too few data points to train a CNN. However, due to the fact that we have pixel-level annotations and very high resolution images, a much larger training dataset can be generated from subsections of the original WSI slides and the labels from the pixel-level annotations, using a similar approach as in previous research literature [30,31]. More specifically, we create a dataset of 224 × 224 sized tissue image tiles at the highest magnification available, as past research literature has shown that it is most useful to look at the WSIs at the highest magnification [22, 31]. Example tissue image tiles obtained from the CAMELYON16 dataset are shown in Fig. 4(left).

Class Imbalance. Given that the WSIs contain far more benign than malignant tissue, this can lead to a significant data imbalance problem when training CNNs. Therefore, we oversample the malignant class to create a balanced dataset of half malignant and half benign tiles.

To generate the dataset, we alternate sampling between malignant and benign tissue. In the case of malignant tissue, we select a malignant slide and sample from the region indicated by the malignancy mask. In the case of benign tissue, because malignant slides also contain benign tissue, we select any slide, and make sure that the area we sample in is inside the tissue mask and but not in the malignancy mask.

In both cases the malignancy mask is down-sampled to be the same magnification as the tissue mask, and sampling is done at this magnification. These points are then converted to the highest magnification, and we read in the tile at this level. No color normalization is used because it proved to be ineffective in other research [22].

Invasive Ductal Carcinoma (IDC) Dataset. The Invasive Ductal Carcinoma (IDC) dataset [6,14] is generated from 162 whole slide images of breast cancer, scanned at 40x magnification. From these slides, 198,738 images were sampled of size 50 × 50 pixels, with 78,786 of these images containing IDC. Because of the small size of these images, they were resized to the minimum acceptable size for the network during training (197 × 197), as is done in previous literature. The dataset is already in the format of a standard image classification dataset, so no special preprocessing is needed. Example tissue image tiles from the IDC dataset are shown in Fig. 4(right).

3.2 Experimental Setup

In this paper, we compare the proposed TriResNet network to two state-of-the-art deep convolutional neural networks in order to gauge its performance for the purpose of tile-level histopathology grading. Details of these experiments are shown below.

Test-Train-Validation Split

The CAMELYON16 dataset was split between by WSI into 80% for training and 20% for validation, and the independent test set given by the CAMELYON16 competition was used for testing and evaluation. For each of the WSIs we extracted malignant and benign tiles, balancing the number of benign and malignant samples, as described above. For the IDC dataset, a split of 70% training, 15% for validation, and 15% for test set was used.

Tested Deep Convolutional Neural Networks

To evaluate and compare the performance of the proposed TriResNet, we compare it to two state-of-the-art deep convolutional neural networks: (i) Liu et al. [22], and (ii) Li et al. [21]. We optimized the performance for the two tested networks to the best of our abilities for high histopathology grading performance on the two datasets.

- **Liu et al.** [22]: This state-of-the-art network architecture based on Inception-v3 [29] was shown to achieve state-of-the-art performance on the CAMELYON16 histopathology competition [22]. Because of this network's demonstrated impressive performance in computer-aided histopathology diagnosis, this network is a good choice for comparing the overall performance of the proposed TriResNet network to.
- **Li et al.** [21]: This state-of-the-art network architecture based on ResNet-34 [12] is compared with the proposed TriResNet as it was shown to provide state-of-the-art performance on histopathology grading [21,28]. Furthermore,

it was compared with the proposed TriResNet also to get a clearer idea of the benefits of a triple-stream network architecture in capture more diverse features for improved performance when compared to a single-stream network architecture. The network has the same number of residual blocks and layers as a single residual stream of TriResNet, thus making the comparison more direct in terms of potential benefits.

All tested networks are implemented using PyTorch [25], and were initialized with pre-trained weights on the ImageNet Challenge Dataset [7] to improve the speed of convergence. The Adam optimizer [15] was used for training. Data augmentation was relatively standard, with random flips, rotations, and brightness transformations.

Performance Metrics

For both the CAMELYON16 and IDC datasets, we evaluated the performance of each tested network on their ability to grade tissue image tiles as either malignant or benign. For each network and dataset we evaluated the following three performance metrics on the test set:

1. $sensitivity = TP/(TP + FN)$
2. $specificity = TN/(TN + FP)$
3. $accuracy = (TP + TN)/(TP + TN + FP + FN)$.

4 Results and Discussion

Tables 1 and 2 show the grading performance (in terms of accuracy, sensitivity, and specificity) of the tested networks for the test sets of the CAMELYON16 dataset and the IDC dataset, respectively. A number of interesting observations can be made from the quantitative results. First of all, it can be clearly seen that for both benchmark datasets, the proposed TriResNet network achieved improved overall accuracy compared to both the tested networks.

When compared to [22], the proposed TriResNet achieves higher overall accuracy on both datasets, with an increase of 1.8% and 1.7% for the CAMELYON16 dataset and the IDC dataset, respectively. Since this network has been demonstrated to provide strong performance in histopathology image grading [22] as well as general image classification problems [29], this demonstrates that the proposed TriResNet can be a very effective network for histopathology grading.

The comparison with [21] demonstrates that a multi-stream network architecture clearly has merits compared to a single-stream network architecture for histopathology grading in terms of capturing a more diverse and discriminative set of quantitative features for characterizing tissue complexities in histopathology images, with the accuracy of the proposed TriResNet being higher by 3.6% and 1.2% on the CAMELYON16 and IDC datasets, respectively.

It can also be observed that the proposed TriResNet achieved higher sensitivity and specificity compared to the other tested networks for the IDC dataset, which illustrates the efficacy of the proposed network. Furthermore, what is particularly interesting to note is, while achieving lower specificity compared to the other tested networks, the increase in sensitivity achieved by the proposed TriResNet is quite pronounced for the CAMELYON16 dataset, where the sensitivity achieved by the proposed TriResNet network is 6.3% and 9.1% compared to [22] and [21], respectively. The higher sensitivity achieved by the proposed TriResNet network is particularly important for the case of histopathology grading, as it is more important to identify all instances of malignancy than to have a very low number of false positives, because of the risks associated with missed malignant tissues leading to patients not being treated for malignant cancer.

Rather than simply discuss the strengths of the proposed TriResNet network for the purpose of tile-level histopathology grading, we also study the limitations of its abilities by looking at some example tissue image tiles that are incorrectly graded by the proposed TriResNet, as shown in Fig. 5. It can be observed that both the proposed TriResNet as well as [21] have some systematic difficulties grading in certain circumstances. For example, one repeated issue experienced by both TriResNet and [21] was the difficulty associated with grading when there was a large amount of adipose tissue. In addition to this, the networks experienced difficulties when the color of the tissue is different from what is considered the norm; for example, as more malignant tissues tend to look more purple, the networks falsely used this as an indication of malignancy in some benign tissues. Greater diversity of tissues and stains used during training of the networks should alleviate these issues. Finally, it is important to note that while the proposed TriResNet network achieves very strong performance compared to the other tested networks, it is also noticeably larger in terms of network size compared to the other networks, although for clinical purposes accuracy is in general more important than inference speed.

Table 1. Comparison of tested networks on tile-level grading for the test set of the CAMELYON16 dataset. Numbers shown indicate test set performance, and best performance for each category is highlighted in **bold**

Network	Accuracy	Sensitivity	Specificity
[22]	85.3%	75.9%	95.9%
[21]	83.5%	73.1%	**96.5%**
TriResNet	**87.1%**	**82.2%**	91.2%

Table 2. Comparison of tested networks on tile-level grading for the test set of the IDC dataset. Numbers shown indicate test set performance, and best performance for each category is highlighted in **bold**

Network	Accuracy	Sensitivity	Specificity
[22]	89.2%	91.4%	83.1%
[21]	89.7%	92.3%	82.9%
TriResNet	**90.9%**	**93.1%**	**85.1%**

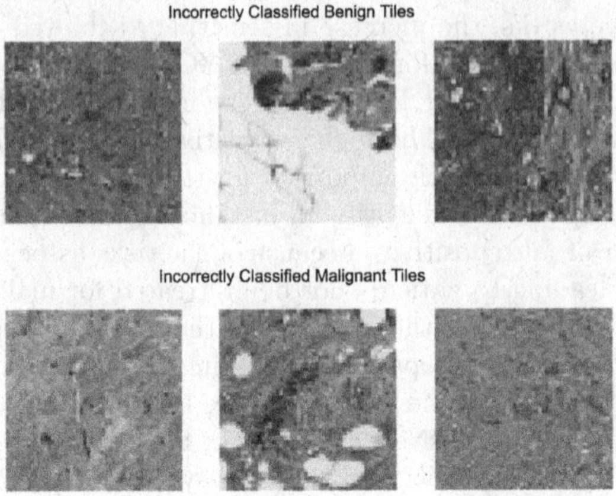

Fig. 5. Examples of tissue image tiles that were misclassified by both TriResNet and [21]. The top row shows examples that are actually benign tissue, but were falsely considered malignant, and the bottom set shows malignant tissue that was considered benign.

5 Conclusion and Future Work

In this paper, we introduced a deep triple-stream residual network (TriResNet) architecture designed to better learn more diverse and discriminative features for characterizing complex tissue characteristics, and thus provide improved tile-level histopathology grading. Experimental results across two widely-used benchmark datasets demonstrated the efficacy of the proposed TriResNet in achieving increased accuracy when compared to two state-of-the-art networks. The promising results achieved using the proposed TriResNet network indicate that such a network could be a useful tool to aid pathologists in improving the consistency, accuracy, and speed of analyzing large volumes of whole histopathology slides containing millions of cells. In the future, we hope to leverage improved data augmentation strategies to handle some issues experienced by the proposed TriResNet network associated with staining diversity, as well as more comprehensive testing and evaluation with a larger variety of histopathology image data. Furthermore, a more comprehensive and fundamental trade-off analysis between the number of streams within the network and the level of performance achieved would be quite useful to better understand network design.

References

1. Camelyon (2016). https://camelyon16.grand-challenge.org/. Accessed: 2018–02-01
2. Allende, D., et al.: Inter-observer and intra-observer variability in the diagnosis of dysplasia in patients with inflammatory bowel disease: correlation of pathological and endoscopic findings. Colorectal Dis. **16**(9), 710–718 (2014)

3. Altunbay, D., Cigir, C., Sokmensuer, C., Gunduz-Demir, C.: Color graphs for automated cancer diagnosis and grading. IEEE Trans. Biomed. Eng. **57**(3), 665–674 (2010)
4. Basavanhally, A., et al.: Multi-field-of-view framework for distinguishing tumor grade in ER+ breast cancer from entire histopathology slides. IEEE Trans. Biomed. Eng. **60**(8), 2089–2099 (2013)
5. Benediktsson, H., Whitelaw, J., Roy, I.: Pathology services in developing countries: a challenge. Arch. Pathol. Lab. Med. **131**(11), 1636–1639 (2007)
6. Cruz-Roa, A., et al.: Automatic detection of invasive ductal carcinoma in whole slide images with convolutional neural networks. In: Medical Imaging 2014: Digital Pathology, vol. 9041, p. 904103. International Society for Optics and Photonics (2014)
7. Deng, J., Dong, W., Socher, R., Li, L.J., Li, K., Fei-Fei, L.: ImageNet: a large-scale hierarchical image database. In: CVPR (2009)
8. Doyle, S., Agner, S., Madabhushi, A., Feldman, M., Tomaszewski, J.: Automated grading of breast cancer histopathology using spectral clustering with textural and architectural image features. In: 5th IEEE International Symposium on Biomedical Imaging: From Nano to Macro, ISBI 2008, pp. 496–499. IEEE (2008)
9. Elmore, J.G., et al.: Diagnostic concordance among pathologists interpreting breast biopsy specimens. Jama **313**(11), 1122–1132 (2015)
10. Fischer, A.H., Jacobson, K.A., Rose, J., Zeller, R.: Hematoxylin and eosin staining of tissue and cell sections. Cold Spring Harb. Protoc. **2008**(5), pdb-prot4986 (2008)
11. Goode, A., Gilbert, B., Harkes, J., Jukic, D., Satyanarayanan, M.: OpenSlide: a vendor-neutral software foundation for digital pathology (2013). https://doi.org/10.4103/2153-3539.119005. http://www.jpathinformatics.org/article.asp?issn=2153-3539;year=2013;volume=4;issue=1;spage=27;epage=27;aulast=Goode;t=6
12. He, K., Zhang, X., Ren, S., Sun, J.: Deep residual learning for image recognition. In: Proceedings of the IEEE Conference on Computer Vision and Pattern Recognition, pp. 770–778 (2016)
13. He, L., Long, L.R., Antani, S., Thoma, G.R.: Histology image analysis for carcinoma detection and grading. Comput. Methods Program. Biomed. **107**(3), 538–556 (2012)
14. Janowczyk, A., Madabhushi, A.: Deep learning for digital pathology image analysis: a comprehensive tutorial with selected use cases. J. Pathol. Inform. **7** (2016)
15. Kingma, D.P., Ba, J.: Adam: a method for stochastic optimization. arXiv preprint arXiv:1412.6980 (2014)
16. Kornblith, S., Shlens, J., Le, Q.V.: Do better ImageNet models transfer better? arXiv preprint arXiv:1805.08974 (2018)
17. Krizhevsky, A., Sutskever, I., Hinton, G.E.: ImageNet classification with deep convolutional neural networks. In: Pereira, F., Burges, C.J.C., Bottou, L., Weinberger, K.Q. (eds.) Advances in Neural Information Processing Systems, vol. 25, pp. 1097–1105. Curran Associates, Inc., New York (2012). http://papers.nips.cc/paper/4824-imagenet-classification-with-deep-convolutional-neural-networks.pdf
18. Kumar, V., Abbas, A.K., Fausto, N., Aster, J.C.: Robbins and Cotran Pathologic Basis of Disease. Elsevier Health Sciences, Amsterdam (2014). Professional Edition e-book
19. LeCun, Y., Bengio, Y., Hinton, G.: Deep learning. Nature **521**(7553), 436 (2015)
20. Lee, B., Paeng, K.: Breast cancer stage classification in histopathology images (2017)

21. Li, Y., Ping, W.: Cancer metastasis detection with neural conditional random field. In: International conference on Medical Imaging with Deep Learning (2018)
22. Liu, Y., et al.: Detecting cancer metastases on gigapixel pathology images. arXiv preprint arXiv:1703.02442 (2017)
23. Monaco, J.P., et al.: High-throughput detection of prostate cancer in histological sections using probabilistic pairwise Markov models. Med. Image Anal. **14**(4), 617–629 (2010)
24. Otsu, N.: A threshold selection method from gray-level histograms. IEEE Trans. Syst. Man Cybern. **9**(1), 62–66 (1979). https://doi.org/10.1109/TSMC.1979.4310076
25. Paszke, A., et al.: Automatic differentiation in PyTorch (2017)
26. Petushi, S., Garcia, F.U., Haber, M.M., Katsinis, C., Tozeren, A.: Large-scale computations on histology images reveal grade-differentiating parameters for breast cancer. BMC Med. Imaging **6**(1), 14 (2006)
27. Raab, S.S., et al.: Clinical impact and frequency of anatomic pathology errors in cancer diagnoses. Cancer **104**(10), 2205–2213 (2005)
28. Shah, M., Wang, D., Rubadue, C., Suster, D., Beck, A.H.: Deep learning assessment of tumor proliferation in breast cancer histological images (2017)
29. Szegedy, C., Vanhoucke, V., Ioffe, S., Shlens, J., Wojna, Z.: Rethinking the inception architecture for computer vision. In: Proceedings of the IEEE Conference on Computer Vision and Pattern Recognition, pp. 2818–2826 (2016)
30. Vang, Y.S., Chen, Z., Xie, X.: Deep learning framework for multi-class breast cancer histology image classification. CoRR abs/1802.00931 (2018). http://arxiv.org/abs/1802.00931
31. Wang, D., Khosla, A., Gargeya, R., Irshad, H., Beck, A.H.: Deep learning for identifying metastatic breast cancer. arXiv preprint arXiv:1606.05718 (2016)

BEM-RCNN Segmentation Based on the Inadequately Labeled Moving Mesenchymal Stem Cells

Jingxiong Li[1], Yaqi Wang[2], and Qianni Zhang[1](✉)

[1] Queen Mary University of London, London E1 4NS, UK
jingxiong.li@se18.qmul.ac.uk, qianni.zhang@qmul.ac.uk
[2] Hangzhou Dianzi University, Hangzhou 310018, China
wangyaqi@hdu.edu.cn

Abstract. This paper addresses the challenging task of moving mesenchymal stem cell segmentation in digital time-lapse microscopy sequences. A convolutional neural network (CNN) based pipeline is developed to segment cells automatically. To accommodate the data in its unique nature, an efficient binarization enhancement policy is proposed to increase the tracing performance. Furthermore, to work with datasets with inadequate and inaccurate ground truth, a compensation algorithm is developed to enrich the annotation automatically, and thus ensure the training quality of the model. Experiments show that our model surpassed the state-of-the-art. Result of our model measured by SEG score is 0.818.

Keywords: Cell segmentation · Binarization · Compensation · Inadequate label · CNN

1 Introduction

Mesenchymal stem cells (MSCs) is a heterogeneous subset of stromal stem cells that distributed in adult tissues [4]. MSCs can differentiate into mesodermal lineage cells (e.g. bone, fat cells) and has differentiate potential for endodermic and neuroectodermic cells (e.g. neuron, lung cells). MSCs participate in many elemental biological processes, including immune response and disease spreading [19], where cell categorization, division and tracking is the key to achieve reliable and quantitative analysis [18]. Usually, meaningful messages can only be extracted from large amount of monitor data due to the high complexity of biological processes [21]. Traditionally, it requires time consuming human labor to examine the captured image, posing problems in generating quantitative and reproducible result. Hence it is urgent to develop accurate automated cell tracking systems that can automatically detect cell boundaries and track cell movements over time, providing information about their velocities and trajectories, and detecting cell-lineage changes as a result of cell division or cell death. Several methods have been proposed in the literature achieving decent results [12],

F. Karray et al. (Eds.): ICIAR 2019, LNCS 11663, pp. 383–391, 2019.
https://doi.org/10.1007/978-3-030-27272-2_34

but all have to rely on good-sized training sets. When only a small amount of training data is available, such as the dataset considered in this paper [3], the problem becomes more difficult to solve since inadequate training of the model may easily lead to overfitting [7].

Recognizing MSCs out of detected image is a challenging task. Usually, MSCs are high fluence and deformable cells with weak features. It requires a sensitive model for detecting each target cell, and at the same time, maintaining high accuracy under a high noise condition [2]. To balance between sensitivity and accuracy, we design a specialized model based on convolutional neural networks (CNN) and special processing techniques.

It is well known that CNNs have rapidly improved the accuracy and semantic segmentation quality by sensitively analyzing features extracted from input images. Some works has shown their potential in medical image analysis such as classifying breast cancer [20] and segmenting lungs for chest X-Rays [13].

The advances in CNN encouraged researchers to develop more powerful networks, such as R-CNN [6] in 2014, Fast/Faster R-CNN [5,15], Fully Convolutional Network (FCN) [10] in 2015. These models provided concepts and solutions for semantic segmentation, image recognition, and object localization. In 2015, based on FCN, U-Net has been specially designed for medical images and used for producing state-of-the-art result for ISBI cell tracking challenge [16]. Extended and optimized from Faster R-CNN, Mask R-CNN was proposed in 2017 and outperformed other models in object detection and semantic segmentation [8].

In this paper, the task of cell segmentation is tackled, with potential application in cell tracking, following the experiment requirements set out by ISBI cell tracking competition. From the point of view of machine learning, the challenges this task are:

(1) Small dataset size: the MSCs dataset only contains 96 annotated images for both training and testing;
(2) Ground truth (GT) annotations are inadequate and inaccurate;
(3) The images are noisy and low-contrast, with vague object (cell) boundaries.

To deal with these problems, we design a cell segmentation model including the following key components:

(1) Binarization enhanced pre-processing method.
(2) Ground truth compensation algorithm for improving inaccurate annotations.
(3) BEM-RCNN to segment high-fluid deformable targets.

2 Methods

2.1 Binarization Enhancement and Image Pre-processing

The dataset we focus on is split into two subsets for training and testing purposes, each contains 48 manually annotated images. Each annotation stands for a MSC. Figure 1 shows some instances from this dataset. As described above, there are several intrinsic difficulties in training a model based on this dataset, because the frames are low in signal to noise ratio, low in contrast between cells and background and including high fluid deformable cells. What is more, the size of the dataset is far from enough for training of a reasonable deep CNN model such as Inception or ResNet [17].

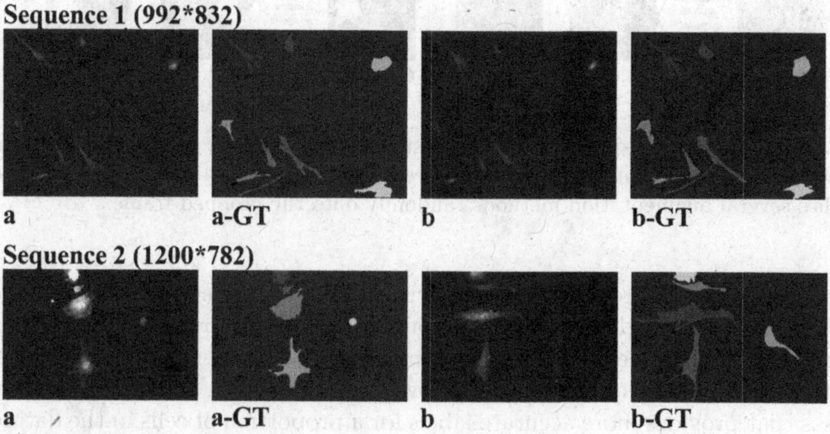

Fig. 1. Image and ground truth masks from the first sequence (a) and the second sequence (b) of Fluo-C2DH-MSC. The resolution is 992 × 832 pixels for of sequence 1 and 1200 × 782 pixels for sequence 2.

To obtain sufficient data for training a robust model, we use a binarization enhancement (BE) method to augment the training set. All the instances are pre-processed by different thresholds based on the normalised images. A pixel's value V is set to 1 when it is larger than the threshold, otherwise it is set to 0 as:

$$V = \begin{cases} 1, & \text{if } V \geq \text{ threshold} \\ 0, & \text{otherwise} \end{cases} \tag{1}$$

For each image, the applied thresholds are 0.155, 0.175, 0.195 and 0.210. The binarized images are saved as additional training samples and fed into the model together with the original training data, using the same annotation. Thus, the binarization process increases the amount of data by 400%.

Moreover, we randomly crop the images to 512 × 512 pixels before each training epoch, along with some common augmentation methods including rotation, translation, scaling, flipping, shearing and blurring. Note that the ground truth are converted into the corresponding shape for augmented training data. The pre-processing pipeline is shown in Fig. 2.

2.2 Ground Truth Compensation

In this dataset, some ground truth masks do not cover all targets in the scope. When training on a large scale dataset, few inaccurate labels may not severely

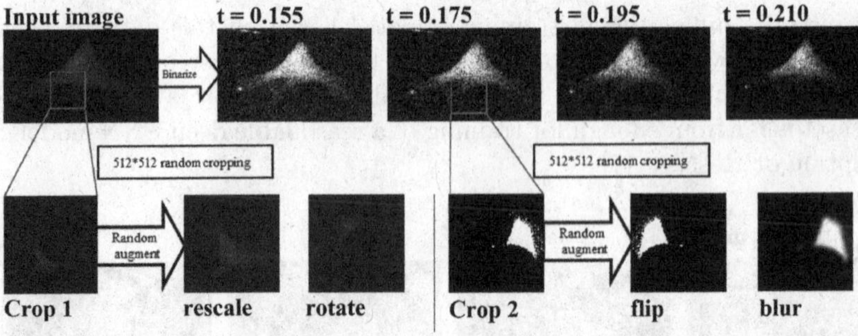

Fig. 2. Pipeline of pre-processing. The first row shows a part of real dataset frame provided, using different threshold to generate four sets of data files. The second row applies several augmentation methods randomly onto the cropped frame.

affect the detection result. However, with a small training set, the detection quality of the trained model may be largely influenced by inaccurate ground truth. The dataset includes 2 sets of annotation masks, a set of tracking masks that includes all cells in a relatively low accuracy, and a set of segmentation masks that provides more accurate labels for a proportion of cells in the dataset. Taking the advantage of this dual annotation, a ground truth compensation method is proposed here to sidestep the issue of inaccurate annotation.

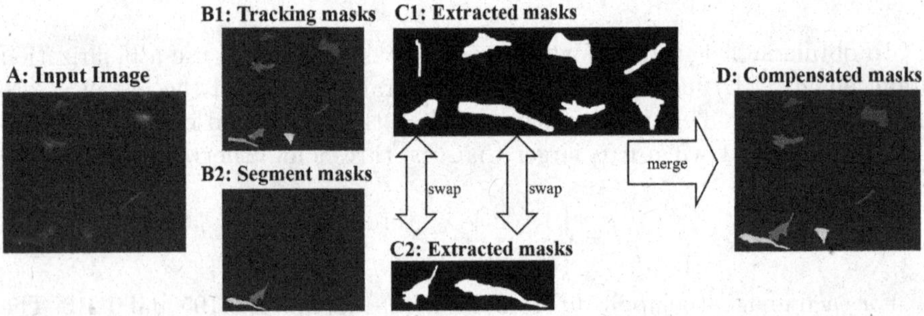

Fig. 3. Less-labeled ground truth compensation pipeline. The input image (A) is has a fully annotated inaccurate tracking masks (B1) and accurately but partially annotated segment masks (B2). Our algorithm extracted masks from both sets (C1 and C2), taking all segment masks and compensate the targets without a mask with tracking masks. The compensated masks include information from both tracking masks and segment masks (D).

As shown in Fig. 3, each training example has 2 set of labels. When the segmentation masks are inadequate, tracking masks will replenish the missing annotations. When masks are available for a cell in both tracking and segmentation ground truth, the segmentation mask will be used. All the chosen annotation are merged to one file for training. In such a way, it is guaranteed that each cell has a annotation mask, and if both annotations are available, the one with the best quality is used. The resulting annotation masks are referred to as compensated annotation.

2.3 Cell Identification Network

We propose a automatic cell identification and segmentation method that employs deep neuron network, namely BEM-RCNN. The architecture of the network is illustrated in Fig. 4, which is adapted the Mask R-CNN. A CNN (e.g. ResNet), pre-trained on MS-COCO data, is used to extract feature map for input images. Then, pre-set candidate bounding boxes, i.e. candidate Region of Interest (RoI), are distributed for each anchor point in the map, called a Region Proposal Network (RPN). Then the candidate RoIs are distinguished into foreground and background, to screen out some false RoIs. In the next stage, features are refined by RoIAlign [8], corresponding to the feature map and the RoIs. Finally, fixed size feature maps are put into the mask head to classify RoIs, perform bounding box regression and generate mask inside each RoI in parallel. To draw a mask for a RoI with semantic sense, the mask branch employs a Feature Pyramid Network (FPN) [9] as its backbone. RoI classification and bounding box regression are performed by a full connected network.

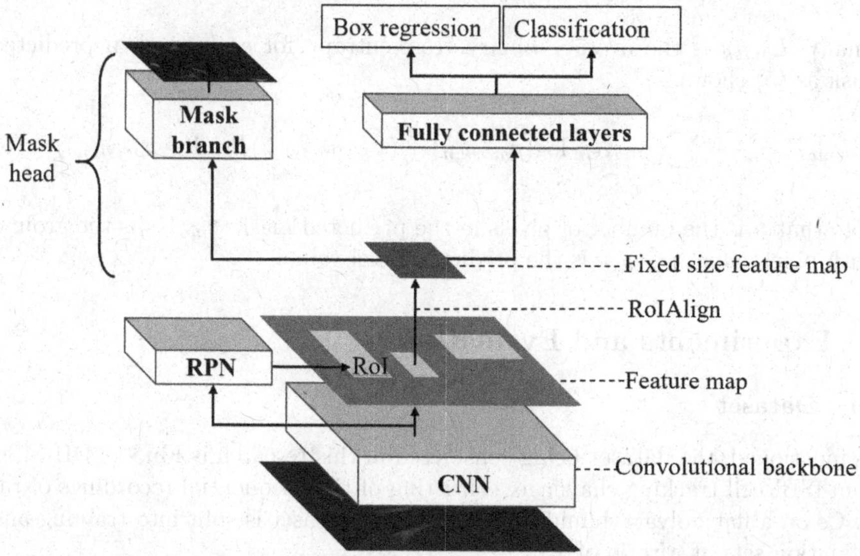

Fig. 4. The architecture of cell identification network. The input image is mapped into a feature map by CNN. The Region of Interest (RoI) is generated by Region Proposal Network (RPN). On the RoIs, box regression, classification and mask generation are operated for final results.

Formally, the multi-task loss L has been defined as (2)

$$L = L_{cls} + L_{box} + L_{mask} \tag{2}$$

In which L_{cls} can be divided into L_{rpn_cls} for RPN classify loss and L_{mask_cls} for mask classify loss. As it shows in (3), L_{rpn_cls} stands for classification loss between GT and predicted bounding box generated by RPN network. L_{mask_cls} is loss for GT and predicted masks. both loss are calculated by cross-entropy.M and N are the quantity of classes, y_{rpn_cls}, y_{mask_cls} are GT class for RPN and masks.p_{rpn_cls}, p_{mask_cls} are logits predicted by RPN and mask head.

$$\begin{aligned} L_{cls} &= L_{rpn\_cls} + L_{mask\_cls} \\ &= -\sum_{a=1}^{M} y_{rpn\_cls,a} \log(p_{rpn\_cls,a}) - \sum_{b=1}^{N} y_{mask\_cls,b} \log(p_{mask\_cls,b}) \end{aligned} \tag{3}$$

Similarly, L_{box} consists L_{rpn_box} and L_{mask_box}. Both represents the loss for bounding boxes generted by RPN and mask head. it is calculated by smooth l1 loss [15]. Calculation of L_{rpn_box} is shown in (4), where y_{rpn_box} is GT bounding box, p_{rpn_box} is predicted box.

$$L_{rpn\_box} = \begin{cases} 0.5 \times (y_{rpn\_box} - p_{rpn\_box})^2, & \text{if} |y_{rpn\_box} - p_{rpn\_box}| < 1 \\ |y_{rpn\_box} - p_{rpn\_box}| - 0.5, & \text{otherwise} \end{cases} \tag{4}$$

Finally, L_{mask} is the average binary cross-entropy for each pixel in predicted mask as (5) shows.

$$L_{mask} = -\frac{1}{n} \sum_{n} (y_{mask,n} \log(p_{mask,n}) + (1 - y_{mask,n}) \log(1 - p_{mask,n})) \tag{5}$$

Note that n is the number of pixels in the predicted mask, $y_{mask,n}$is the ground truth pixel value, $p_{mask,n}$ is the predicted pixel value.

3 Experiments and Evaluation

3.1 Dataset

As mentioned, the dataset being considered in this research is Fluo-C2DH-MSC from ISBI cell tracking challenge, consisting of time sequential recordings of rat MSCs on a flat polyacrylamide substrate. The dataset is split into training and validation sets at a ratio of 4:1.

3.2 Network Training

All the images are randomly cropped to the same size of 512 × 512 before each epoch of training. For each image, there are 512 RoIs [9], and the ratio between positive and negative RoIs is 1:3. A positive RoI must have a Intersection over Union (IoU) value for at least 0.5. Otherwise, the RoI will be considered as negative. Masks are defined on positive RoIs only. The model is trained on a Nvdia RTX 2070 GPU. The learning rate is 0.001, with a weight decay of 0.0001 and the momentum is 0.9. The network converges after 200 epochs of training.

3.3 Results

Figure 5 shows an example image with its groundtruth, masks generated by our BEM-RCNN model and masks generated without binarize enhancement and GT compensation steps. As it can be observed, the proposed method (BEM-RCNN) can detect and draw masks accurately for each target. We evaluate the segmentation result by SEG benchmark, which based on the Jaccard similarity index [14]. Table 1 shows our BEM-RCNN yeilds superior performance to other methods proposed on ISBI cell tracking challenge [11].

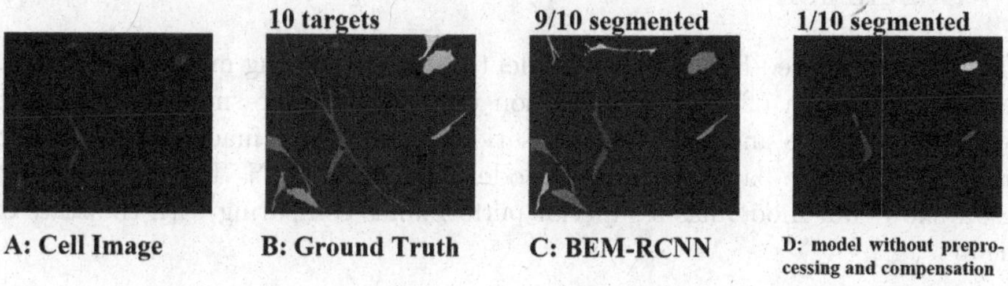

Fig. 5. A cell image from validation set (A); the ground truth from the dataset (B); our proposed BEM-RCNN model (C); model without binarize enhancement and GT. compensation (D).

Table 1. SEG performance of models.

Models	SEG score
Model without enhancement and compensation	0.075
KTH-SE	0.590
FR-Fa-GE	0.617
BGU-IL	0.645
BEM-RCNN (ours)	**0.818**

GT compensation also shows a positive effect on increasing robustness of the model. The number of successfully segmented cell is shown in Table 2. The proposed model tracked 98.1% of target cells, comparing with 79.9% of targets detected by model trained without GT compensation.

Table 2. Model comparison on valid segmented cells.

	Ground truth	BEM-RCNN (ours)	Model without compensation
Cell count	517	**507 (98.1%)**	413 (79.9%)

3.4 Discussions

In semantic segmentation computer vision tasks Mask R-CNN has achieved state-of-the-art [8]. In this paper, we presented our BE-MRCNN trained on a very small dataset, targets on detecting high fluid stem cells from low quality images. The model proposed includes better data augmentation method, and GT compensating algorithm, which has been proved to boost the performance of our model. In the future, we will specific the model more carefully and expand it to more datasets then compare with the result of other models.

4 Conclusion

This paper proposed BEM-RCNN model to segment moving mesenchymal stem cells, including an effective binarization enhancement for small dataset with low quality iamges and a GT compensation algorithm for inadequately labeled ground truth. The backbone of our model is Mask R-CNN. The segmentation result shows our model has a superior performance comparing with the state of the art.

Acknowledgements. The authors thank the IEEE International Symposium on Biomedical Imaging 2019 (ISBI19) cell tracking challenge [1] for providing the datasets aiding the development of this work.

References

1. Cell tracking challenge. http://celltrackingchallenge.net/
2. Akram, S.U., Kannala, J., Eklund, L., Heikkilä, J.: Cell tracking via proposal generation and selection. arXiv preprint arXiv:1705.03386 (2017)
3. Amat, F., et al.: Fast, accurate reconstruction of cell lineages from large-scale fluorescence microscopy data. Nat. Methods **11**(9), 951 (2014)
4. Caplan, A.I.: Mesenchymal stem cells. J. Orthop. Res. **9**(5), 641–650 (1991)
5. Girshick, R.B.: Fast R-CNN. In: 2015 IEEE International Conference on Computer Vision (ICCV), pp. 1440–1448 (2015)
6. Girshick, R.B., Donahue, J., Darrell, T., Malik, J.: Rich feature hierarchies for accurate object detection and semantic segmentation. In: Proceedings of the 2014 IEEE Conference on Computer Vision and Pattern Recognition, CVPR 2014, pp. 580–587 (2014)
7. Hawkins, D.M.: The problem of overfitting. J. Chem. Inform. Comput. Sci. **44**(1), 1–12 (2004)
8. He, K., Gkioxari, G., Dollár, P., Girshick, R.B.: Mask R-CNN. In: 2017 IEEE International Conference on Computer Vision (ICCV), pp. 2980–2988 (2017)

9. Lin, T.Y., Dollár, P., Girshick, R.B., He, K., Hariharan, B., Belongie, S.J.: Feature pyramid networks for object detection. In: 2017 IEEE Conference on Computer Vision and Pattern Recognition (CVPR), pp. 936–944 (2017)
10. Long, J., Shelhamer, E., Darrell, T.: Fully convolutional networks for semantic segmentation. In: 2015 IEEE Conference on Computer Vision and Pattern Recognition (CVPR), pp. 3431–3440 (2015)
11. Maška, M., et al.: A benchmark for comparison of cell tracking algorithms. Bioinformatics **30**(11), 1609–1617 (2014)
12. Neumann, B., et al.: Phenotypic profiling of the human genome by time-lapse microscopy reveals cell division genes. Nature **464**(7289), 721 (2010)
13. Rashid, R., Akram, M.U., Hassan, T.: Fully convolutional neural network for lungs segmentation from chest X-rays. In: Campilho, A., Karray, F., ter Haar Romeny, B. (eds.) ICIAR 2018. LNCS, vol. 10882, pp. 71–80. Springer, Cham (2018). https://doi.org/10.1007/978-3-319-93000-8_9
14. Real, R., Vargas, J.M.: The probabilistic basis of Jaccard's index of similarity. Syst. Biol. **45**(3), 380–385 (1996)
15. Ren, S., He, K., Girshick, R.B., Sun, J.: Faster R-CNN: towards real-time object detection with region proposal networks. In: Proceedings of the 28th International Conference on Neural Information Processing Systems, NIPS 2015, vol. 1, pp. 91–99 (2015)
16. Ronneberger, O., Fischer, P., Brox, T.: U-Net: convolutional networks for biomedical image segmentation. In: Navab, N., Hornegger, J., Wells, W.M., Frangi, A.F. (eds.) MICCAI 2015. LNCS, vol. 9351, pp. 234–241. Springer, Cham (2015). https://doi.org/10.1007/978-3-319-24574-4_28
17. Szegedy, C., Ioffe, S., Vanhoucke, V., Alemi, A.A.: Inception-v4, inception-resnet and the impact of residual connections on learning. In: Thirty-First AAAI Conference on Artificial Intelligence (2017)
18. Trepat, X., Chen, Z., Jacobson, K.: Cell migration. Compr. Physiol. **2**(4), 2369 (2012)
19. Uccelli, A., Moretta, L., Pistoia, V.: Mesenchymal stem cells in health and disease. Nat. Rev. Immunol. **8**(9), 726 (2008)
20. Xie, X., Li, Y., Shen, L.: Active learning for breast cancer identification. arXiv preprint arXiv:1804.06670 (2018)
21. Zimmer, C., et al.: On the digital trail of mobile cells. IEEE Signal Process. Mag. **23**(3), 54–62 (2006)

Image Analysis and Recognition for Automotive Industry

Inceptive Event Time-Surfaces for Object Classification Using Neuromorphic Cameras

R. Wes Baldwin, Mohammed Almatrafi, Jason R. Kaufman, Vijayan Asari(✉), and Keigo Hirakawa

University of Dayton, Dayton, OH 45469, USA
{baldwinr2,almatrafim2,jkaufman1,vasari1,khirakawa1}@udayton.edu
https://www.udayton.edu/engineering/research/centers/vision_lab
http://issl.udayton.edu

Abstract. This paper presents a novel fusion of low-level approaches for dimensionality reduction into an effective approach for high-level objects in neuromorphic camera data called Inceptive Event Time-Surfaces (IETS). IETSs overcome several limitations of conventional time-surfaces by increasing robustness to noise, promoting spatial consistency, and improving the temporal localization of (moving) edges. Combining IETS with transfer learning improves state-of-the-art performance on the challenging problem of object classification utilizing event camera data.

Keywords: Object classification · Dynamic vision · Neuromorphic vision · Dimensionality reduction

1 Introduction

A standard image sensor is comprised of an array of Active Pixel Sensors (APS). Each APS circuit reports the pixel intensity of the image formed at the focal plane by cycling between a period of integration (wherein photons are collected and counted by each pixel detector) and a readout period (where digital counts are combined from all pixels to form a single frame). Motion detected and estimated across frames has useful applications in computer vision tasks. Unfortunately, detecting fast moving objects can be challenging due to the limitations of the integration and read out circuit. Object motion that is too fast relative to the integration period induces blurring and other artifacts. Additionally, since all pixels have a single exposure setting, parts of the scene may be underexposed while other parts are saturated. Both of these issues degrade the image quality of the captured video frames, reducing our ability to detect or recognize objects by their shapes or their motions. While high-speed cameras with very fast frame

This work is funded in part by Ford University Research Program.

F. Karray et al. (Eds.): ICIAR 2019, LNCS 11663, pp. 395–403, 2019.
https://doi.org/10.1007/978-3-030-27272-2_35

rates can resolve blur issues, they are expensive, consume lots of power, generate large amounts of data, and require adjusting exposure settings.

Event-based cameras were engineered to overcome these limitations of the APS circuitry found on conventional framing cameras. As described below, these neuromorphically inspired cameras can operate at extremely high temporal resolution (>800 kHz), low latency (20 ms), wide dynamic range (>120 dB), and low power (30 mW). They report only changes in the pixel intensity, requiring a new set of techniques to perform basic image processing and computer vision tasks—examples include optical flow [3,8], feature extraction [4,12,13], gesture recognition [2,11], and object recognition [5,14].

"Time-surface" is one such technique with proven usefulness in pattern recognition by encoding the event-time as an intensity [10]. However, time-surfaces are sensitive to noise and to multiple events corresponding to the same image edge with some latency when the intensity changes are large. Both have an effect on time-surfaces similar to the ways that blurring affects APS data. An improved time-surface technique called Filtered Surface of Active Events (FSAE) [1] was introduced in a corner detection and tracking algorithm. FSAE yields an improved time-surface by only utilizing the initial event of a series—effectively removing events corresponding to the same edge. Yet, while FSAE is shown to be very effective for representing simple features such as corners, object classification tasks deal with significantly more complex objects.

In this work, we propose IETS, aimed at extracting noise-robust, low-latency features that correspond to complex object edge contours over a temporal window. IETS extends FSAE to achieve higher object recognition accuracy while removing over 70% of FSAE events. We verify the effectiveness of our object classification framework on multiple datasets.

1.1 Event Cameras

Each event-based camera pixel operates asynchronously with no notion of frame rate across the focal plane. Instead of a fixed integration time, pixels generate events only when the rate of detected photons varies above or below a predefined threshold. A log-based threshold gives the event camera an extreme dynamic range. If the scene is changing slowly, the sensor naturally compresses the data since few events are generated. In contrast, fast moving objects trigger events almost instantaneously—allowing object tracking within microseconds. Example event generation for a single pixel is illustrated in Fig. 1(a).

In a Prophesee Asynchronous Time-based Image Sensor, used in N-CARS [17], each event comprises a row, column, time, and polarity. Row and column are the pixel coordinates. The time entry records when the change was detected in microseconds, and the polarity is a binary value indicating if the intensity increased or decreased.

Event camera data is often noisy and requires filtering for many applications. Previous algorithms rely on the assumption that when a pixel is triggered, neighboring pixels are also activated [7,15] and large intensity changes generate

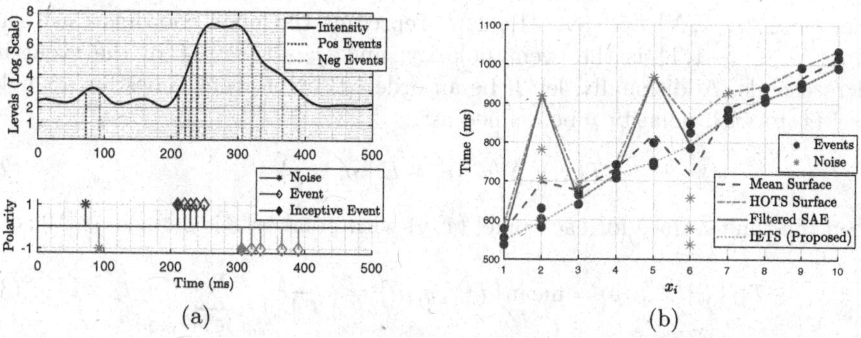

Fig. 1. Event generation. (a) On a per pixel level, intensity variations trigger events at each log-scaled level crossing. The first event in a series of consecutive events is called an inceptive event. (b) Time-Surface generation in the presence of noise.

multiple events at a single pixel. These assumptions motivate the use of spatial-temporal density as a way to isolate valid events from noise, but this approach fails when motion is slow (i.e. sparse valid events are removed as noise) and when noise is high (i.e. dense noise mislabeled as real events).

1.2 N-CARS Dataset

The N-CARS dataset is a large, real-world, event-based, public dataset for car classification. It is composed of 12,336 car samples and 11,693 non-cars samples (background). The camera was mounted behind the windshield of a car and gives a view similar to what the driver would see. Each sample contains exactly 100 milliseconds of data with 500 to 59,249 events per sample.

Figure 2 shows a sequence from N-CARS; each point in the three dimensional cube (2D space, 1D time) represents a reported event. Object velocity can be inferred when this cube is viewed from the time-space plane (Fig. 2(a)), while the object shape is better identifiable from the 2D space plane (Fig. 2(b)). Spiral patterns near the rear wheel of the car highlight high-speed rotational motion—a challenging set of relevant features to preserve during dimensionality reduction.

2 Related Works

Object classification from event data is an active area of research. There are a number of applications that require feature extraction from the raw event detection camera data in order to carry out classification tasks. Time-surface is a technique used as an intermediary step to feature extraction by reducing the spatial-temporal structure in Fig. 2 to a two dimensional image representation. More specifically, let E denote a set comprised of events generated by an event detection camera sensor of frame size $M \times N$:

$$E(x, y) = \{(t_i, p_i)\}_{i=1}^{I}, \tag{1}$$

where $x \in [1, ..., N]$ and $y \in [1, ..., M]$ represent the pixel coordinates in the frame; $p_i \in \{-1, 1\}$ is the event polarity; and t_i is the time of the event in microseconds. Additionally, let T be an ordered set of event times for a single pixel (x, y) with polarity p be defined as:

$$T(x, y, p) = \{e_i \in E \mid p_i = p\}. \tag{2}$$

Then the time-surface for each pixel (x, y) with polarity p is defined as [10]:

$$\mathcal{TS}\{T\}(x, y, p) = \text{mean}\{T(x, y, p)\} = \frac{1}{|T|} \sum_{(t_i, p_i) \in T(x,y,p)} t_i. \tag{3}$$

Variations to time-surface can be implemented by replacing the "mean" operator in (3) with minimum, maximum, median, etc.

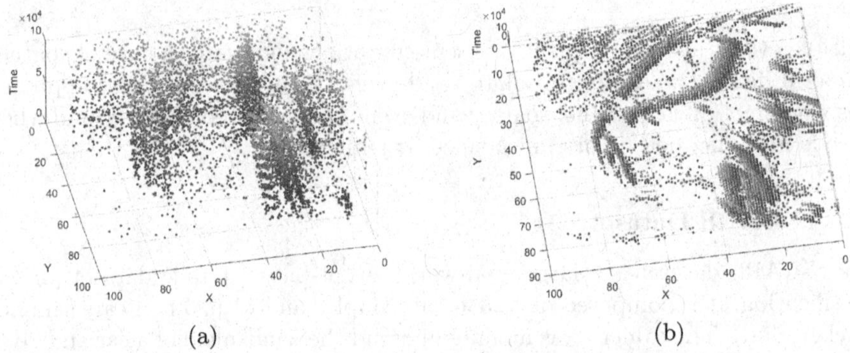

Fig. 2. N-CARS dataset example. (a) 3D plot of event data colored by time. (Blue/old to green/new). (b) Same data viewed under different orientation. (Color figure online)

Time-surface has been used successfully in object recognition tasks. For example, Hierarchy of Time-Surfaces (HOTS) [10] utilized straightforward time-surfaces for feature generation, but it did not attempt to limit the impact of noise directly, instead relying on clustering. While this method performed well on simple shapes like numbers and letters, it does not extend well to more complex-shaped objects with wider variations (like cars).

The Histograms of Averaged Time-Surfaces (HATS) algorithm [17] localizes the motion vector representation for a specific region of the sensor (cell) using a region-based time-surface. This improved robustness to noise by averaging across the reported times of the events within each cell. A major disadvantage to HATS is the loss of fine spatial features, which is exacerbated by the low sensor resolution of current event cameras.

FSAE is a method to directly improve time-surface by eliminating redundant events [1]. The FSAE filter is defined as:

$$\mathcal{FSAE}(x, y, p) = \{t_i \in T(x, y, p) \mid (t_i - t_{i-1}) > \tau^-\}, \tag{4}$$

where τ^- is a pre-defined threshold. Intuitively, events occurring in succession typically correspond to the same edge, and so redundant events can be eliminated by discarding events that are not temporally separated from prior events.

3 Proposed Method: Inceptive Event Time-Surfaces

To advance object classification using event data, we propose a novel concept called Inceptive Event Time-Surfaces (IETS). IETS is an extension of FSAE aimed at improving dimensionality reduction and noise robustness. IETS retains features critical to object classification (i.e. corners and edges) by fitting time-surfaces to a subset of events. Unlike previous approaches that focused on generating handcrafted features from noisy event data, IETS uses deep convolutional neural networks (CNNs) to learn features from time-surface images with less noise. As demonstrated by the experiments using the N-CARS, IETS combined with CNNs achieves a new state-of-the-art in classification performance.

We begin by the observation that a single log-intensity change often trigger multiple events in temporal sequence. As shown by Fig. 1(a), the first event indicates an "arrival" of an edge, which we refer to as an "inceptive event" (IE). Intuitively, IEs describe the shape of the moving object within the scene. On the other hand, the subsequent events correspond to the magnitude of the log-intensity change, which we refer to as "scaling events." As such, edge magnitude as indicated by successive scaling events do not necessarily describe the edge shape well. The comparison between inceptive and scaling events in Fig. 1(a) make this clear. While scaling events are more useful for intensity-based inferences, the effect the latency (relative to the edge arrival) has on the time-surface is similar to image blur. Furthermore, scaling events are subject to degradation by two hardware designs: a low-pass filter and a regulated "refractory period"—a period of time after an event trigger that a pixel must wait before triggering again (due to the limitations of read out and reset circuits).

Object detection tasks require a clear representation of the object boundaries that define the shape of the object-of-interest. Recall (2). To successfully filter events prior to time-surface generation, we propose the following:

$$\mathcal{IE}(x,y,p) = \{t_i \in T(x,y,p) | (t_i - t_{i-1}) > \tau^- \ \wedge \ (t_{i+1} - t_i) < \tau^+\}, \quad (5)$$

where τ^+ and τ^- are predefined threshold parameters. One may notice that by comparing (5) to (4) that $\mathcal{IE} \subset \mathcal{FSAE}$, meaning there are necessarily fewer IEs than FSAE events. The proposed $\mathcal{IETS}$ is then defined as a time surface constructed from $\mathcal{IE}$:

$$\mathcal{IETS}(x,y,p) = TS\{\mathcal{IE}\}(x,y,p). \quad (6)$$

We propose to carry out the object classification by training a CNN on IETS surfaces. There are three input image channels to the proposed CNN. First two input channels are IETS surfaces of both polarities: $\mathcal{IETS}(x,y,+1)$ and $\mathcal{IETS}(x,y,-1)$, which are mapped to images of 8-bit intensity values.

The third input channel is generated based on a simple count of unfiltered events (i.e. $E(x, y)$) at each pixel. This channel can improve machine learning by acting as a weight for the other channels. All channels are scaled from 0 to 1, and pixels with no events in the entire dataset are set to zero. With $\tau^- = \tau^+ = 12$ ms, IETS removes over 85% of events in N-CARS. Discriminating noise from real events can be challenging, degrading time-surfaces significantly. Figure 1(b) highlights the effectiveness of IETS in removing noise while accurately fitting the time-surface, compared to other methods.

Due to the extremely sparse number of events (<1 k) in some N-CARS datasets, likely captured during periods of little camera or target motion, IETS filtering occasionally makes object identification even more challenging. For that reason, if a pixel does not contain an IE, the mean time of all events for that pixel is used in its place. Although this reintroduces noise to each image, the overall classification accuracy on N-CARS improved by over 12% when mean event time for non-IE data was appended. Additional data, even if very noisy, is preferred when using deep neural networks. Figure 3 highlights how effectively IETS can reduce dimensionality while at the same time removing noisy events.

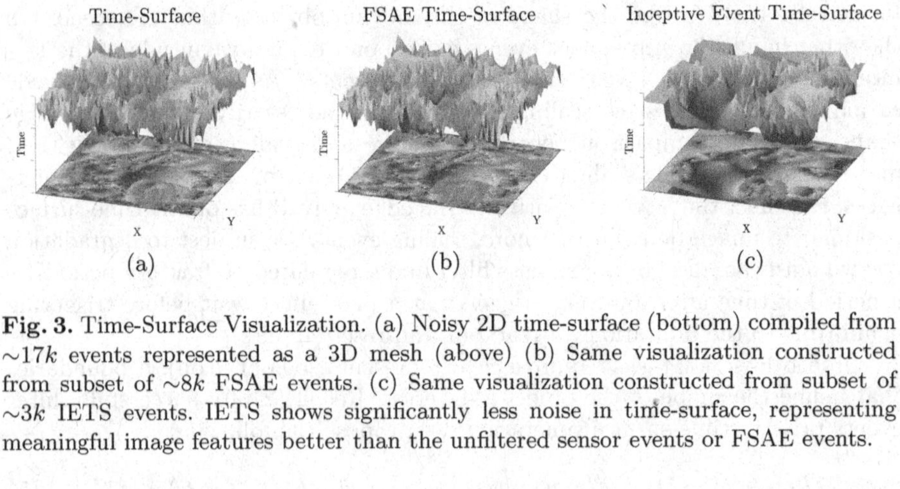

Fig. 3. Time-Surface Visualization. (a) Noisy 2D time-surface (bottom) compiled from ~17k events represented as a 3D mesh (above) (b) Same visualization constructed from subset of ~8k FSAE events. (c) Same visualization constructed from subset of ~3k IETS events. IETS shows significantly less noise in time-surface, representing meaningful image features better than the unfiltered sensor events or FSAE events.

Previous event-based features [6,10] are limited in the same way as many custom-designed descriptors. Leveraging CNNs to learn optimal features is typically a superior approach over custom-designed features. Of course, deep convolutional neural networks currently require millions of labeled images—something that does not yet exist for event cameras. Since no vast archive of labeled event camera data exist, IETS images are generated in a way that makes them optimal to utilize transfer feature learning from millions of real-world images via GoogLeNet [9,18]. IETS is highly parallelizable and quick to train since transfer learning converges rapidly. IETS generates images at the full resolution of the event camera. This means resolution, which is typically poor for event cameras, is not lost prior to classification as with algorithms employing cells.

IETS has excellent performance as all events in a given time window are processed simultaneously—removing the requirement to iterate over each event. Additionally, a non-optimal implementation of IETS processed over 100k events/sec, significantly faster than real-time requirements.

4 Experiments

Each N-CARS sample was processed into an image using IETS. Examples from IETS processing are shown in Fig. 4. Algorithm evaluation was accomplished via the standard metrics of accuracy rate and Area Under Curve (AUC).

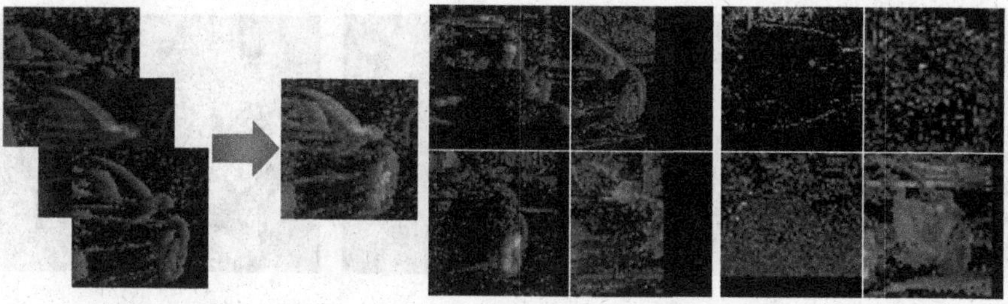

(a) (b) (c)

Fig. 4. (a) Example input to CNN is two IETSs (positive/negative polarity) and the event count per pixel (shown here as RGB). Examples from N-CARS dataset that were (b) correctly and (c) incorrectly labeled as 'cars'.

The maximum score was produced after augmenting the training data by using IETS images that had also been flipped. The maximum accuracy score obtained by IETS was 0.973. Comparison to other state-of-the-art algorithms is shown in Table 1, and is a considerable improvement over the HATS published score of 0.902. AUC also improved from 0.945 to 0.997. To ensure performance gains were not entirely from replacing the Support Vector Machine (SVM) with a CNN, HATS features were used to train the same GoogLeNet architecture. These results are also included Table 1 as HATS/CNN. Additionally, to show the improvement IETS offers in generating a time-surface, FSAE images were used to train the architecture and are also included for comparison.

Table 1. Classification results on N-CARS.

Algorithm	H-First	HOTS	Gabor	HATS	HATS	FSAE	IETS
Classifier	SNN	SVM	SNN	SVM	CNN	CNN	**CNN**
Accuracy	0.561	0.624	0.789	0.902	0.929	0.961	**0.976**
AUC	0.408	0.568	0.735	0.945	0.984	0.993	**0.997**

To further test the results from IETS, an IniVation Davis Dynamic Vision Sensor (DVS) 240C was used to collect cars driving near the University of Dayton. This dataset was significantly different in the fact targets were acquired using a camera from a different manufacturer, at a further range, images were uncropped, and the camera was stationary. The vehicles collected were side on as shown in Fig. 5. Seven datasets were recorded with durations ranging from 2.76 to 8.30 s—resulting in 5,236 samples. Using four datasets for training and three for testing resulted in a classification accuracy of 0.9951 and AUC score of 0.9999. Although the dataset proved less challenging, the results indicate that supplementing with additional variation in sensor models, viewing angles, and camera positions will allow the algorithm to extend to more general use cases.

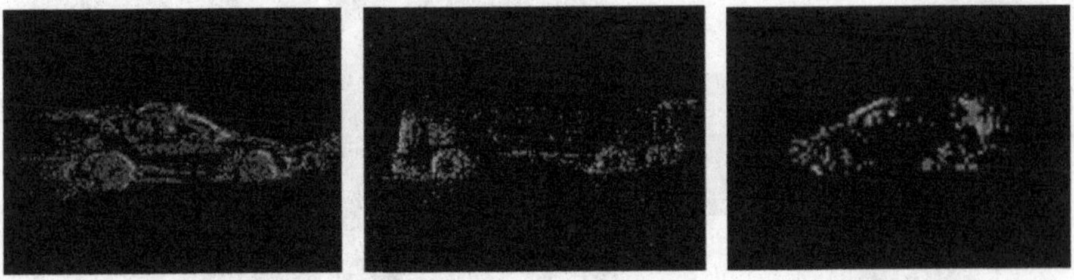

Fig. 5. Three IETS images generated from data collected near the University of Dayton used for additional testing. Data included multiple cars, buses, and trucks.

5 Conclusion and Future Work

Overall, there are a wide range of future applications for event-based sensors due to their speed, size, low memory requirements, and high dynamic range. This paper presents an algorithm that improves state-of-the-art performance for object classification of cars. As classification rates near 100% for the N-CARS, the lack of large labeled datasets will limit advancement in this area. Multiple simulators now exist for generating synthetic data [13,16], which have been used successfully in several papers for testing. Although these simulators may be useful in the short term, real-world data is always preferred as noise, calibration, and manufacturing defects are challenging to reliably simulate.

Two limitations of IETS should be addressed with future work. First, IETS relies on the fact that edges triggering events rarely generate large, overlapping time-surfaces within 100 ms. This may not be true for all scenarios. For example, a spinning fan, pulsing light, or very fast moving object would generate overlapping surfaces and likely limit the utility of IETS in these cases. The IETS algorithm currently averages overlapping surfaces, but this is not optimal as these unique signatures are undetectable to a standard camera. Second, after the time-surfaces are generated from IEs, no effort is made to recover data originally filtered as noise. A two-stage filter design will help recover events and allow for a broader application of the algorithm.

References

1. Alzugaray, I., Chli, M.: Asynchronous corner detection and tracking for event cameras in real time. IEEE Robot. Autom. Lett. **3**(4), 3177–3184 (2018)
2. Amir, A., et al.: A low power, fully event-based gesture recognition system. In: Proceedings of the IEEE Conference on Computer Vision and Pattern Recognition, pp. 7243–7252 (2017)
3. Bardow, P., Davison, A.J., Leutenegger, S.: Simultaneous optical flow and intensity estimation from an event camera. In: Proceedings of the IEEE Conference on Computer Vision and Pattern Recognition, pp. 884–892 (2016)
4. Barranco, F., Teo, C.L., Fermuller, C., Aloimonos, Y.: Contour detection and characterization for asynchronous event sensors. In: Proceedings of the IEEE International Conference on Computer Vision, pp. 486–494 (2015)
5. Barua, S., Miyatani, Y., Veeraraghavan, A.: Direct face detection and video reconstruction from event cameras. In: 2016 IEEE Winter Conference on Applications of Computer Vision (WACV), pp. 1–9. IEEE (2016)
6. Clady, X., Maro, J.M., Barré, S., Benosman, R.B.: A motion-based feature for event-based pattern recognition. Front. Neurosci. **10**, 594 (2017)
7. Czech, D., Orchard, G.: Evaluating noise filtering for event-based asynchronous change detection image sensors. In: 2016 6th IEEE International Conference on Biomedical Robotics and Biomechatronics (BioRob), pp. 19–24. IEEE (2016)
8. Haessig, G., Cassidy, A., Alvarez, R., Benosman, R., Orchard, G.: Spiking optical flow for event-based sensors using IBM's truenorth neurosynaptic system. IEEE Trans. Biomed. Circ. Syst. **12**(4), 860–870 (2018)
9. Krizhevsky, A., Sutskever, I., Hinton, G.E.: ImageNet classification with deep convolutional neural networks. In: Advances in Neural Information Processing Systems, pp. 1097–1105 (2012)
10. Lagorce, X., Orchard, G., Galluppi, F., Shi, B.E., Benosman, R.B.: HOTS: a hierarchy of event-based time-surfaces for pattern recognition. IEEE Trans. Pattern Anal. Mach. Intell. **39**(7), 1346–1359 (2017)
11. Lee, J.H., et al.: Real-time gesture interface based on event-driven processing from stereo silicon retinas. IEEE Trans. Neural Netw. Learn. Syst. **25**(12), 2250–2263 (2014)
12. Mitrokhin, A., Fermüller, C., Parameshwara, C., Aloimonos, Y.: Event-based moving object detection and tracking. In: 2018 IEEE/RSJ International Conference on Intelligent Robots and Systems (IROS), pp. 1–9. IEEE (2018)
13. Mueggler, E., Rebecq, H., Gallego, G., Delbruck, T., Scaramuzza, D.: The event-camera dataset and simulator: event-based data for pose estimation, visual odometry, and slam. Int. J. Robot. Res. **36**(2), 142–149 (2017)
14. Orchard, G., Meyer, C., Etienne-Cummings, R., Posch, C., Thakor, N., Benosman, R.: HFirst: a temporal approach to object recognition. IEEE Trans. Pattern Anal. Mach. Intell. **37**(10), 2028–2040 (2015)
15. Padala, V., Basu, A., Orchard, G.: A noise filtering algorithm for event-based asynchronous change detection image sensors on truenorth and its implementation on truenorth. Front. Neurosci. **12**, 118 (2018)
16. Rebecq, H., Gehrig, D., Scaramuzza, D.: ESIM: an open event camera simulator. In: Conference on Robot Learning, pp. 969–982 (2018)
17. Sironi, A., Brambilla, M., Bourdis, N., Lagorce, X., Benosman, R.: HATS: histograms of averaged time surfaces for robust event-based object classification. In: Proceedings of the IEEE Conference on Computer Vision and Pattern Recognition, pp. 1731–1740 (2018)
18. Szegedy, C., et al.: Going deeper with convolutions. In: Proceedings of the IEEE Conference on Computer Vision and Pattern Recognition, pp. 1–9 (2015)

An End-to-End Deep Learning Based Gesture Recognizer for Vehicle Self Parking System

Hassene Ben Amara(✉) and Fakhri Karray

Department of Electrical and Computer Engineering, Centre for Pattern Analysis and Machine Intelligence (CPAMI), University of Waterloo, Waterloo, ON, Canada
hassene.benamara@gmail.com

Abstract. Hand gesture recognition have become versatile in numerous applications. In particular, the automotive industry has benefited from their deployment, and human-machine interface designers are using them to improve driver safety and comfort. In this paper, we investigate expanding the product segment of one of America's top three automakers through deep learning to provide an increased driver convenience and comfort with the application of dynamic hand gesture recognition for vehicle self parking. We adapt the architecture of the end-to-end solution to expand the state of the art video classifier from a single image as input (fed by monocular camera) to a multiview 360 feed, offered by a six cameras module. Finally, we optimize the proposed solution to work on a limited resource embedded platform that is used by automakers for vehicle-based features, without sacrificing the accuracy robustness and real time functionality of the system.

Keywords: Gesture recognition · Car parking · Deep learning

1 Introduction

Automotive gesture recognition market size is estimated to reach USD 13.6 billion by 2024 according to a new research report by Global Market Insights, Inc [5]. The application of gesture recognition to advanced driver assistance systems can improve driving safety to some degree. The driver can use gestures to control various functions of the car or to modify various parameters of the car, hence pay more attention to reducing road accidents.

The automotive industry is now looking for the future of the driver-less parking systems. There are several device-based solutions for vehicle self-parking that are offered by automakers nowadays:

– Remote-controlled Solutions: A button on the vehicle display key activates the remote-controlled parking function from outside the car. This procedure is monitored by Park Distance Control (PDC), the Parking assistant and the Surround View sensors.

F. Karray et al. (Eds.): ICIAR 2019, LNCS 11663, pp. 404–416, 2019.
https://doi.org/10.1007/978-3-030-27272-2_36

- Smartphone Controlled Solutions: Using a mobile app, the driver can automatically park his vehicle in and out of a parking spot without being behind the wheel.
- Smartwatch Controlled Solutions: The parking operation is triggered by a configurable wave gesture that is recognized by the smart watch and transmitted to the vehicle over wireless connection. The transmitted hand gesture gives the vehicle the signal to initiate the parking operation.

Although the device-based solutions for vehicle driver-less parking systems stated above seem promising and are already available in the market for end users, these systems, whether the remote-based or smartwatch-controlled, represents the following disadvantages:

- Device dependant: the presented solutions require an additional hardware to be fully functional (*e.g.* smart key fob, smart watch). Therefore, any damage to the device (*e.g.* caused by water, low battery) or unfavorable conditions (*e.g.* rain or snowy weather) will render the feature unusable.
- User experience/convenience: Even though the above mentioned systems use a very common human-machine interaction medium (touch screen), it still presents an inconvenience to the user as it requires an intermediary medium between the user and the car.

2 Multiview Vision-Based Hand Gesture Recognition for Vehicle Self Parking

The proposed vision-based multiview gesture recognition for self parking system consists of two main modules: person detection and frames extraction module and gesture recognition module. The input stream is a multiview 360° feed, offered by a six cameras system. The person detection module performs the detection of all subjects present in the six frames video input. The resulted frames are then passed to a dynamic hand gesture classification module which

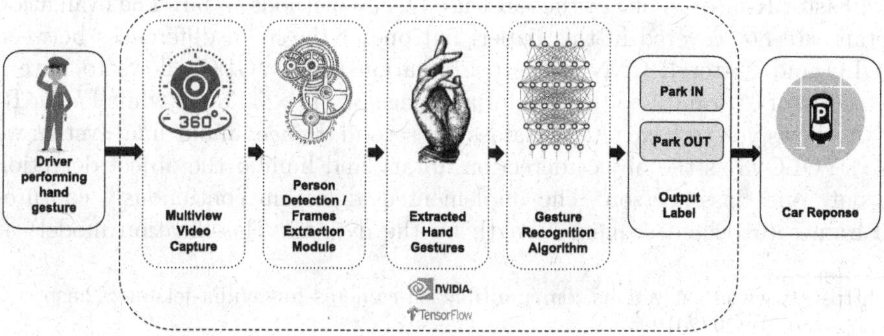

Fig. 1. Proposed multiview hand gesture recognition system overview

finally decides whether to initiate the parking operation or not. The overall architecture of the end-to-end system is shown in Fig. 1. For capturing 360° video frames, many hardware solutions exists on the market, and our choice was the HexCamera (e-CAM30_HEXCUTX2) from e-con systems[1] which consists of a multiple camera solution for NVIDIA Jeson TX1/TX2 developer kit. The setup consists of six cameras with 3.4MP each and an adaptor board to interface with the J22 connector on the Jetson. The camera can stream 720p (HD) and 1080p (Full HD) at 30 fps in uncompressed YUV422 Format.

2.1 Person Detection and Frames Extraction Module

This module is the first core component of our end-to-end system. As mentioned in the previous section, the output of the multiview camera is a six frames stream representing 360 degree view. One of the main challenges, is to adapt the output of the multiview camera to the hand gesture recognition module presented in Sect. 2.2. Our dynamic hand gesture classifier was trained on video frames of size 176×100 where every video consists of one single subject performing the hand gesture. Given that the multiview camera output may contain multiple subjects in crowded environments (e.g. parking lot), the first step the person detection and frames extraction module performs, is the detection of all subjects present in the six frames video input. This module detects all the persons present in the 360 camera view feed, calculates the bounding box coordinates and finally crops over every 30 frames (required input length for the gesture recognition module) and saves separate image files for every subject. Once this step is complete, the resulted frames are passed to the 3D-CNN network to perform the hand gesture recognition. It's important to note that the authentication of the car's owner is out of the scope of this work, which means any subject performing one of the two gestures (Swiping Hand Left and Swiping Hand Right) would trigger the parking operation.

The person detection module uses an underlying object detection library. We evaluated two object detection tools that were released recently using the convolutional neural networks: Faster R-CNN and YOLO. We chose these tools because YOLO allows to get the best results on VOC2007[2] data and VOC2012[3] and Faster R-CNN is one of the most used CNN methods so far. The evaluation details are not covered in this paper, but one of the main differences between YOLO and Faster R-CNN is the computation time, YOLO allows to have a detection of 37 frames per second for an image of $445 \times 445 \times 3$ while Faster R-CNN allows you to have only 5 frames per second. Hence, in our final system we used YOLOv3 as the object detection library and limited the object detection to only one class: Person. The implemented algorithm continuously captures 30 frames (expected sequence length by the dynamic classification model) at

[1] https://www.e-consystems.com/multiple-csi-cameras-for-nvidia-jetson-tx2.asp, accessed: 01/29/2019.

[2] http://host.robots.ox.ac.uk/pascal/VOC/voc2007/, last accessed: 02/20/2019.

[3] http://host.robots.ox.ac.uk/pascal/VOC/voc2012/, last accessed: 02/20/2019.

12 frames/s and passes them to the YOLO based person detector. The latter, only looks at the first frame of the 30 frames input and detects all the persons present, calculates the bounding boxes and finally crops all of the 30 frames based on the respective boxes coordinates. The cropped videos are then saved in memory to be passed one at a time to the gesture recognition module.

2.2 Dynamic Hand Gesture Recognition Module

The hand gesture recognition module represents the second core component of our end-to-end system after the person detection module. It encompasses mainly our dynamic hand gesture classifier which details will be presented in the next section. Once the persons detection and cropping step is complete and the output frames are extracted, we resize them to match the dimensions of the expected input video by the 3D-CNN classifier, in our case with height × width × frames equal to 176 × 100 × 30. Then, we pass every input (consisting of 30 frames with the format shown in Fig. 2) to the hand gesture recognition network for classification. The output of this module can be one of the three classes: Swiping Hand Left (Park IN), Swiping Hand Down (Park OUT) or Doing Other Things (ignored by the system). Once one of the relevant classes (Park IN or Park OUT) is detected, the algorithm drops the rest of the input cropped videos and trigger the corresponding parking action.

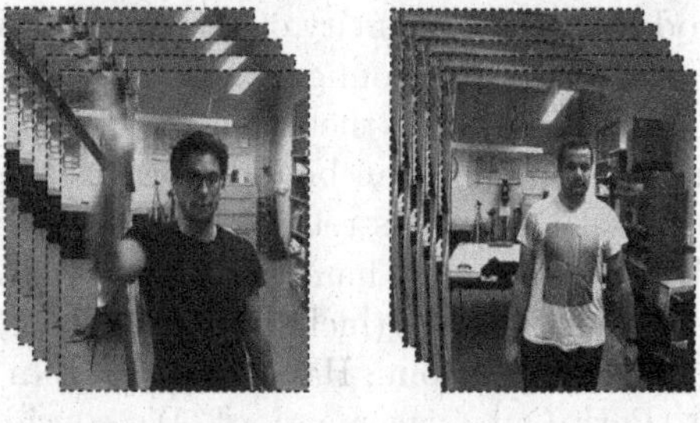

Fig. 2. Sample cropped persons images: Left image shows a detected person performing the "Swiping Hand Left" gesture (used as Park IN trigger). Right image shows a detected person not performing any hand gesture.

3 Proposed 3D-CNN Dynamic Hand Gesture Classifier

Hand gesture recognition can be treated as a multiclass classification problem that maps an input video sequence to one of the three classes our model has learned: C1 = Swiping Hand Left (Park In), C2 = Swiping Hand Down (Park Out) and C3 = Doing Other Things. The experimental results presented in Sect. 3.1 will serve to evaluate the performance of the proposed gesture model, and to compare it with the state of the art method applied to this paper's use case. In this section, we present the machine learning methodology we followed in order to build the dynamic hand gesture classifier. First, the deep neural network architecture and training process are presented. Then, the different experiments leading to the tuning of the hand-gesture classification network are described. Finally, the different test scenarios conducted while assessing the classifier as well as their corresponding results are reported.

3.1 Training Dataset

The 20BN-JESTER dataset consists of a large collection of densely-labeled video sequences taken by a static camera (webcam or laptop camera) that show humans performing pre-defined hand gestures. This dataset was collected thanks to a large number of crowd workers and made available by the German company TwentyBN [9] as free of charge for academic research. In this database, we find a total of 148092 video sequences. The data was provided as a big archive containing directories numbered from 1 to 148092. Each folder corresponds to one video clip (single gesture) and contains JPEG images that were extracted at 12 fps having a height of 100 px and variable widths. The length of sequences differs from one sequence to another. The dataset groups together 27 classes that represent the different hand gestures, namely: Swiping Hand Left, Swiping Hand Down, Rolling Hand Forward, Doing Other Things, No Gestures, etc. In each class, the hand gesture is performed by participants that represent a generalized distribution of different gender, age, skin color, and with different speeds. The latter, makes this dataset one of the largest data collections available to build a robust deep learning-based gesture classifiers. A study of our dataset revealed that the hand can produce a great diversity of gestures. However, it is extremely difficult to recognize all the possible configurations of the hand from its projection in an image. Indeed, according to the orientation of the hand in relation to the camera, some parts of the hand can be hidden. It is then necessary to consider an appropriate subset of gestures related to our application. In our work, the goal is to recognize three dynamic hand gestures for parking in and parking out actions as well as other gestures (including no gesture). The two gestures that we want to recognize are: Swiping Hand Left (Park In trigger action) and Swiping Hand Down (Park Out trigger action). We considered these two gestures because they are among the most used in human-human interaction and will be perfectly adapted to a natural man-car interaction. Furthermore, among other possible gestures available from 20BN-Jester dataset, the high neural discriminability (i.e. decodability) between the two chosen gestures contributed in giving us the best model performance during our experiments.

Due to the fact that video sequences from 20BN-JESTER dataset have different length (variable number of frames), the first step in our data preparation phase is to sub-sample every video down to 30 frames. So a 31-frames video and a 45-frames video will both be reduced to 30 frames, with the 45-frames video essentially being fast-forwarded. The decision to fix the sequence length to 30 was made after the inspection of the 20BN-JESTER dataset which is mostly composed of videos with a length that varies from 27 to 46 frames. Also, a data cleaning step was performed to limit samples to only videos having a duration greater than the sequence lengths, therefore discarding all shorter videos (*e.g.* 28 frames).

Data Splitting. For the context of our work, our model is trained to classify three gestures: Park In (Swiping Hand Left), Park Out (Swiping Hand Down) and Doing Other Things (which covers other possible gestures including no gesture). For that purpose, we used 20BN-JESTER dataset to extract a subset of data containing all videos for the aforementioned three classes. We divided our dataset into 3 subsets: training (D_{train}), validation (D_{valid}) and evaluation (D_{eval}), the latter two being generally smaller than the first. It is through the ratio (Training: 75%, Validation: 12.5%, Testing: 12.5%) that we can ensure the capacity of the model to generalize well and avoid overfitting. Our training data set consists of 2601 video sequences for the Park In gesture (Swiping Hand Left), 2641 videos for the Park Out gesture (Swiping Hand Down) and 8601 videos for "Doing Other Things". The latter class has more than 3 time the number of video sequence to represent real life scenarios, as most gestures do not belong to the first two classes.

There are many machine learning methods in the literature that work well on temporal classification tasks as encountered in our dynamic hand gestures classifier. After a review of many of these methods and reported results, we limited our experiments to the following learning algorithms: 3D Convolutional Neural Networks and Long-term Recurrent Convolutional Networks.

4 3D-CNN Dynamic Hand Gesture Classifier

A 2D CNN is composed of convolution layer(s), Pooling layer(s) and finally fully connected Layer(s). The fully connected layer(s) are often used as the network output. Usually, a convolution layer is followed by an activation function and then a pooling layer, this sequence can be repeated several times up to the fully connected layer to form a convolution network that is often denoted under the CONVNET notation. It is also common to use more than one fully connected layer before the output of the network. On the other hand, 3D-CNN applies a third dimensional filter to the dataset and the filter moves 3-directions (x, y, z) to learn the low-level feature representations. Their output shape is a 3-dimensional volume space such as cube.

Our model will therefore consists of 8 convolution layers, 5 layers of max-pooling, 2 fully connected layers and finally a softmax output layer. Figure 3 shows the final 3D-CNN architecture of our gesture model for classifying 3 different types of dynamic hand gestures.

To determine the optimal architecture and parameters of our gesture model (number of convolution layers, number of neurons per layer, number of max-pooling layers, etc.), many models with different configurations have been trained on the dataset presented in Sect. 3.1. The results obtained from those experiments have helped us determine the best model architecture that produced the highest performance for our use case. One of the drawbacks of DNN is the difficulty to select the network hyper-parameters which makes the network tuning one of the major phases in a connectionist modeling based machine learning application.

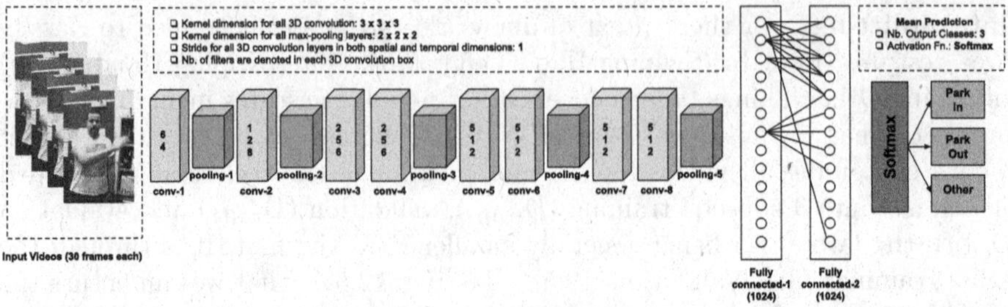

Fig. 3. Our final model architecture: 3D ConvNet network for dynamic hand gesture recognition

4.1 Network Training

The purpose of our classification is to decide whether a video contains one of the two relevant gestures for our use case: Swiping Hand Left (Parking in) or Swiping Hand Down (Parking out). To resolve this problem, training the classifier was performed using a subset of labeled RGB images from 20BN-Jester dataset as previously detailed in Sect. 3.1. For the implementation of the training algorithm, we used Keras, an open source neural network library written in Python and TensorFlow as backend, all running on a NVIDIA GPU with 16GB of RAM.

The input to the 3D-CNN network is 30 frames from the training dataset of a given dynamic hand gesture reshaped to (176 × 100 × 3) size. We used the back-propagation algorithm to adjust the networks weights and ReLu as the activation function, with a batch size of 6 (experimented with higher values of batch size to speedup training but rapidly hit the memory limit). Also, a dropout of 0.5 was used between the two fully connected layers which helped avoid overfitting. We compute the validation error (aka. loss) after each epoch with an early stopping patience value set to 5, to stop the training once the validation error stops decreasing for 5 consecutive epochs. Training our classifier took ~11 h and went through a total of 10 epochs. Figure 4 shows the loss and accuracy curves for validation and training when the network is being trained.

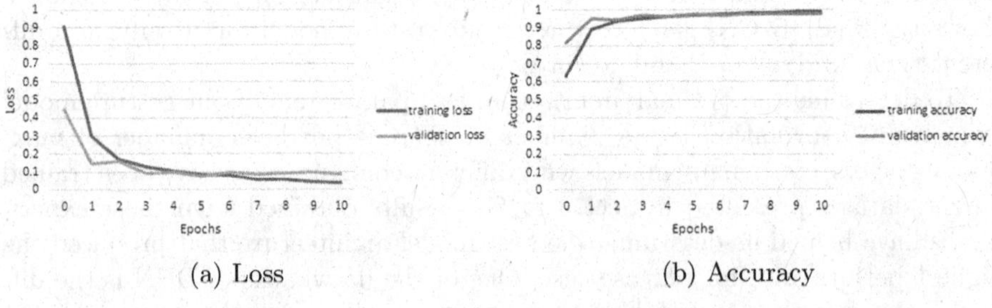

(a) Loss (b) Accuracy

Fig. 4. Training and validation curves v.s. training epochs (3D-CNN)

Our trained 3D-CNN gesture classifier is considered as a good fit model based on the obtained loss/accuracy curves. We can see that our model did not experience a blatant case of overfitting. Validation loss reached its lowest value of 0.074 at the fifth epoch where the validation accuracy was at 0.977. Whereas, training loss continued decreasing to reach a minimum of 0.039 at the tenth epoch with a training accuracy of 0.989.

5 LRCN Dynamic Hand Gesture Classifier

This model proposed by Jeff Donahue in 2016 represents a Long-term Recurrent Convolutional Network (LRCN) which combines a deep hierarchical visual feature extractor (such as a CNN) with an LSTM model that can learn to recognize and synthesize temporal dynamics for tasks involving sequential data, visual, linguistic, or otherwise [2]. The reported state-of-the art results in this paper on three vision problems (activity recognition, image description and video description) made Long-term Recurrent Convolutional Network one of the approaches we considered to solve our problem of dynamic hand gesture recognition. The steps of the LRCN model training are detailed in the following sections. CNNs have been proved powerful in image related tasks like computer vision, image classification, object detection etc. LSTMs are used in modelling tasks related to sequence-based predictions. LSTMs are widely used in NLP related tasks like machine translation, sentence classification and generation. LRCN, also known as CNN-LSTM model was specifically designed for sequence prediction problems with spatial inputs, like images or videos. We trained an LRCN network on the same gesture dataset used for training our 3D-CNN model by feeding 30 input frames representing one hand gesture to a feature extractor layer (CNN) and combine it with LSTMs to support the sequence prediction.

5.1 Network Training

The training of the LRCN classifier was performed using the same computer specifications (GPU, RAM, etc,) used for training the 3D-CNN classifier and on the same training/validation dataset. We used the Adam optimizer with a learning rate of 1e−5, decay of 1e−6 and applied a dropout of 0.5 before the LSTM layer for dimensionality reduction. The total duration of the training using a batch size of 6 was ∼36 h which is more than 3 times longer than the training duration of the 3D-CNN classifier due the much slower training speed of LSTMs [1]. It went through a total of 37 epochs before the model started to converge. We examined the training and validation curves, shown in Fig. 5, when the network is being trained and we observed that the validation loss stopped decreasing after the 23th epoch to reach a minimum of 0.248 at the 32th epoch and then started increasing again until the early stopping mechanism triggered to stop the training 5 epochs later. In comparison with the 3D-CNN classifier training, where a much lower validation loss of 0.074 was reached in much shorter amount of time. At the same time, validation accuracy reached a maximum of

0.927 at the 36th epoch compared to 0.977 for 3D-CNN. Based on the LRCN training data analysis, the obtained model can be considered as a good fit model since no remarkable overfitting symptoms are observed.

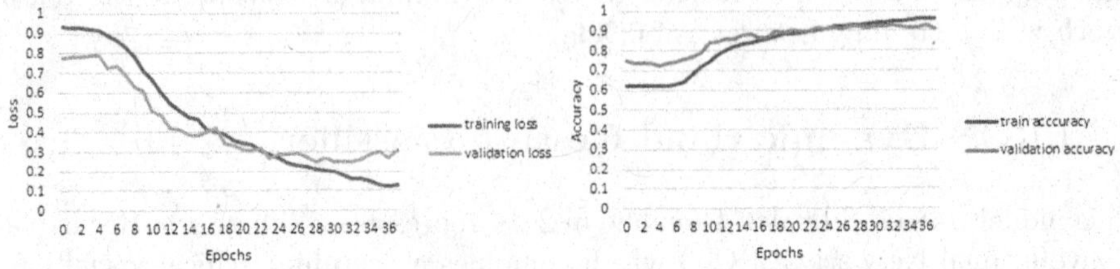

(a) Loss (b) Accuracy

Fig. 5. Training and validation curves v.s. training epochs (LRCN)

It's still difficult at this stage to draw conclusions about the model that allows the best performance on our task of dynamic hand gesture recognition. Therefore, in the following section, we will present our evaluation results of both models tested on our evaluation dataset.

6 Experimental Results and Discussion

This section is devoted to the presentation of the experimental results relating to the two models introduced in Sects. 3 and 5, namely the 3D-CNN model and the LRCN model. As mentioned earlier, one of the most important motivations behind the introduction of these two models is their generalisation capacity in comparison with other approaches in literature. The experiments therefore were carried out on dynamic hand gesture recognition task using our evaluation dataset presented in Table 1. In addition, the experimental results presented in this section will also serve to evaluate the performances of the two model, and to compare the proposed 3D-CNN model to the state of the art on the issue studied. Table 1 shows the performance of two different classifiers on each class. The results shows that the 3D-CNN classifier is dominating LRCN on the three classes (Swiping Hand Left, Swiping Hand Down and Doing Other Things). The performance of the two classifiers is similar on the average precision, especially for the Swiping Hand Left and Swiping Hand Down classes, than that on recall and F1-measure. Furthermore, the table also shows that while the LRCN classifier achieved a high precision for Swiping Hand Left and Swiping Hand Down classes that is comparable to that of the 3D-CNN, we notice on the other hand a relatively poor recall on the same two classes; which means the LRCN system classifies more samples into Doing Other Things, hence the high recall value for the latter class and poor precision. Now going back to our use case in this project: a gesture recognition self parking system, both metrics, precision and recall, are important; we would like to achieve a high precision on the Swiping Hand Left

(Park In) and Swiping Hand Down (Park Out) classes, but most importantly a high recall value to give a better user experience to the driver using the system while avoiding cases where the driver need to repeat the hand gesture many times to trigger the parking action. The confusion matrices on the validation set can be seen below in Fig. 6, the overall accuracy of the LRCN classifier is **0.8544** whereas that of our 3D-CNN classifier is at **0.9502**. The confusion matrix for LRCN shows clearly that many samples of Swiping Hand Left and Swiping Hand Down are classified as Doing Other Things, hence the poor recall noticed earlier. As expected, the LRCN model performed poorer that 3D-CNN. The proposed explanation is that he position of the hand in each of the 30 frames will differ from sample to sample, which leads to feeding the LSTM with different positions of the hand in the respective indexes of the 30 frames. This could confuse the LSTM which is reflected in the the number of false negatives.

Table 1. Per class performance comparison between LRCN and 3D-CNN

Class	LRCN			3D-CNN (ours)		
	Precision	Recall	F1-Measure	Precision	Recall	F1-Measure
Swiping Hand Left (Park In)	0.96	0.83	0.89	0.99	0.93	0.96
Swiping Hand Down (Park Out)	0.94	0.80	0.86	0.99	0.93	0.96
Doing Other Things	0.73	0.94	0.82	0.88	0.99	0.93
Average	**0.88**	**0.85**	**0.86**	**0.95**	**0.95**	**0.95**

7 Transfer Learning and Final Model Fine-Tuning

One of the big challenges in machine learning applications is that training data can be slightly different from the real-world data faced by the algorithm. Hence, the performance of the end-to-end system once faced with real data may not be at the desired level. We noticed that the trained 3D-CNN classifier did not perform well when tested live. Two main factors had a major impact on the performance of our system:

- Driver to Camera Distance: The closer the driver is to the multiview camera, the higher is the accuracy of the system. A camera distance within a range of [60 cm, 110 cm] produced the best performance. Whereas, in the real-world scenario, the car driver would have a distance of at least 2 m from the car to trigger the auto parking.
- Height of the Multiview Camera System: We noticed also during our end-to-end testing of the system that the camera system needs to be at a certain height (slightly lower than the user) in order to achieve the best system performance and accuracy. Once we place the multiview camera at the same level or slightly higher than the user, gesture detection accuracy starts to degrade.

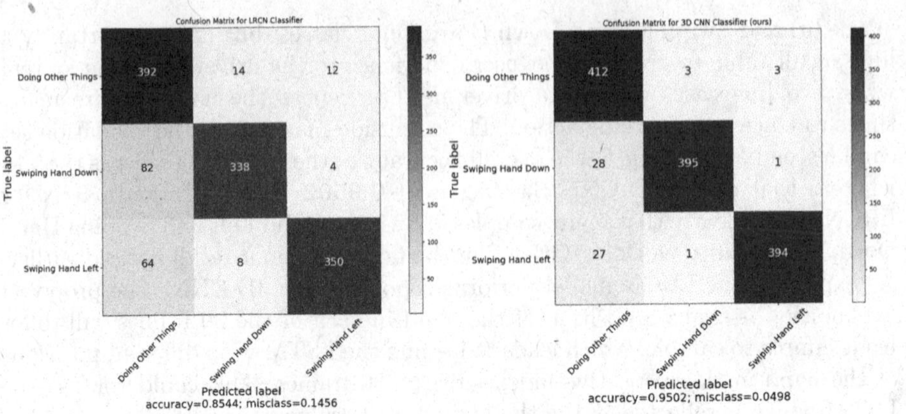

(a) LRCN gesture classifier (b) 3D CNN Gesture Classifier (ours)

Fig. 6. Confusion matrices for both LRCN and 3D CNN hand gesture classifiers

The previous observations can be explained by the nature of the 20BN-Jester dataset we used to train our gesture model. In fact, most of the video samples in 20BN-Jester dataset are taken using a laptop or desktop computer webcam placed at a relatively close distance (50 to 100 cm) and slightly lower level from the user. Hence, the sensitivity of our end model to those factors. In order to overcome these limitations, enhance the system performance and end user experience, we fine-tuned our model using transfer learning techniques. The following section would describe the contingency steps that were taken to overcome the aforementioned challenges.

7.1 Transfer Learning: Dataset Augmentation

A dataset containing generalized gesture videos that are relevant to our use case of autonomous parking was not available. Therefore, we collected a second dataset in our lab and used data augmentation techniques to generate more data samples. The created dataset consists of a reasonable amount of videos where many subjects performed the Swiping Hand Left and Swiping Hand Down gestures at variable distance from the camera system and at different setup heights. On the background of the user, we placed a green screen that enabled us to use the Chroma Keying technique (a.k.a. green screen keying, used for decades in film studios by placing human characters in otherworldly situations without them having to leave the studio) to create new videos using parking lot backgrounds, reflecting the real-world scenario of parking situations, and various other backgrounds for data augmentation purpose. Figure 7 shows the process we followed to generate the new dataset using Chroma Keying. The early layers of the 3D-CNN network already trained with the 20BN-Jester large dataset can extract generic features, so we used methods that further tunes a pre-trained model. Given the relatively small dataset (220 videos) compared

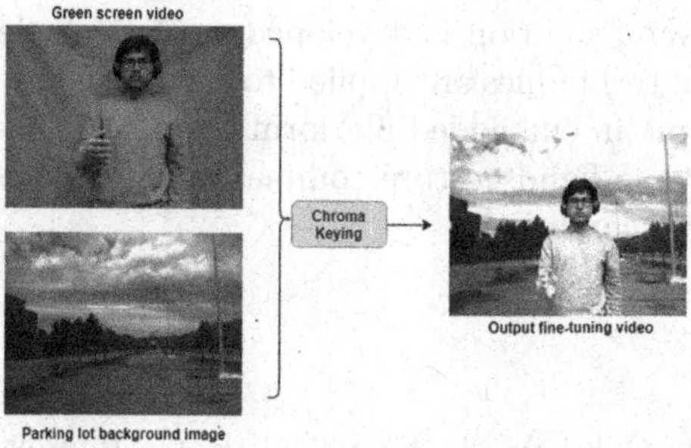

Fig. 7. Data generation using Chroma Keying

to the 20BN-Jester dataset, we did only fine-tune the last layer of our 3D-CNN which enhanced significantly the classification performance. The evaluation metric for live tests was empirical and based on the automaker satisfaction of the performance. After the dataset augmentation, the automaker reported a twice as good performance.

8 Conclusion

Our main motivation for this paper was to eliminate the intermediate medium between the car and the driver to offer a friendly user interface for the self-park feature. To achieve the aforementioned attribute, we solely rely on a vision-based gesture recognition solution. For simplicity, the developed feature has two commands, represented by two hand gestures "swiping hand left" and "swiping hand down". As a first step to recognize the hand gesture, the solution requires a person detection algorithm at the front of the pipeline. YOLO paired with a six-camera based sensor offers a pre-processing module that detects and identifies all instances of "persons" in the 360 view of the vehicle. Each of the identified objects (person present within the vehicle field of view), is then processed by a 3D-CNN classifier. The latter is a multi-class classification, which maps the first hand gesture (swiping hand left) to the park-in command and the second hand gesture (swiping hand down) to the park-out command. A third class (garbage model) is necessary to capture any gesture that doesn't fall in the aforementioned buckets. We achieve an accuracy of 95.02% with the selected 3D-CNN, while alternatives such as LRCN, performed at a maximum accuracy of 85.44%. The reported results were based on experiments ran in a lab environment. Once tested in a real world setting, we noticed a significant drop in accuracy, due to the varying distance and height of the user with respect to the camera. This is expected, as all of the training dataset consists of laptop/webcam collected videos which implies a limited range of distance and height of the person performing the gesture. To overcome this limitation of our training data, we decide to leverage transfer learning and collect custom made data that would generalize our model on different backgrounds, distances and heights of the classified subject. This end-to-end solution is developed as the vehicle for a host. Hence, multiple optimization techniques are applied to ensure the resulting model would operate in real-time on an embedded platform (NVIDIA Jetson TX2): less than 2 s of processing for one hand gesture command, which is considered as a successful real-time implementation.

References

1. Chen, X., Liu, X., Gales, M. J., Woodland, P. C.: Improving the training and evaluation efficiency of recurrent neural network language models. In: 2015 IEEE International Conference on Acoustics, Speech and Signal Processing (ICASSP), pp. 5401–5405. IEEE (2015)
2. Donahue, J., et al.: Long-term recurrent convolutional networks for visual recognition and description. In: Proceedings of the IEEE Conference on Computer Vision and Pattern Recognition, pp. 2625–2634 (2015)
3. Gupta, O., Raviv, D., Raskar,R.: Deep video gesture recognition using illumination invariants. arXiv preprint arXiv:1603.06531 (2016)
4. BMW Media Information. BMW at the consumer electronics show (ces) 2016 in las vegas. https://www.bimmerpost.com/goodiesforyou/autoshows/ces2016/bmw-ces-2016.pdf (2016)
5. Global Market Insights. Automotive gesture recognition market to exceed 13 billions by 2024. https://www.gminsights.com/pressrelease/automotive-gesture-recognition-market (2019)
6. Koesdwiady, A., Bedawi, S.M., Ou, C., Karray, F.: End-to-end deep learning for driver distraction recognition. In: Karray, F., Campilho, A., Cheriet, F. (eds.) ICIAR 2017. LNCS, vol. 10317, pp. 11–18. Springer, Cham (2017). https://doi.org/10.1007/978-3-319-59876-5_2
7. Ohn-Bar, E., Trivedi, M.M.: Hand gesture recognition in real time for automotive interfaces: a multimodal vision-based approach and evaluations. IEEE Trans. Intell. Transp. Syst. **15**(6), 2368–2377 (2014)
8. Strezoski, G., Stojanovski, D., Dimitrovski, I., Madjarov, G.: Hand gesture recognition using deep convolutional neural networks. In: Stojanov, G., Kulakov, A. (eds.) International Conference on ICT Innovations. Advances in Intelligent Systems and Computing, pp. 49–58. Springer, Cham (2016)
9. TwentyBN. The 20bn-jester dataset v1. https://20bn.com/datasets/jester (2018)
10. Di, W., et al.: Deep dynamic neural networks for multimodal gesture segmentation and recognition. IEEE Trans. Pattern Anal. Mach. Intell. **38**(8), 1583–1597 (2016)

Thermal Image SuperResolution Through Deep Convolutional Neural Network

Rafael E. Rivadeneira[1(✉)], Patricia L. Suárez[1], Angel D. Sappa[1,2], and Boris X. Vintimilla[1]

[1] Facultad de Ingeniería en Electricidad y Computación, CIDIS, ESPOL Polytechnic University, Escuela Superior Politécnica del Litoral, ESPOL, Campus Gustavo Galindo Km. 30.5 Vía Perimetral, P.O. Box 09-01-5863, Guayaquil, Ecuador
{rrivaden,plsuarez,asappa,boris.vintimilla}@espol.edu.ec

[2] Computer Vision Center, Edifici O, Campus UAB, 08193 Bellaterra, Barcelona, Spain

Abstract. Due to the lack of thermal image datasets, a new dataset has been acquired for proposed a super-resolution approach using a Deep Convolution Neural Network schema. In order to achieve this image enhancement process, a new thermal images dataset is used. Different experiments have been carried out, firstly, the proposed architecture has been trained using only images of the visible spectrum, and later it has been trained with images of the thermal spectrum, the results showed that with the network trained with thermal images, better results are obtained in the process of enhancing the images, maintaining the image details and perspective. The thermal dataset is available at http://www.cidis.espol.edu.ec/es/dataset.

Keywords: Thermal infrared images · Thermal cameras · Image enhancement · Convolutional neural networks

1 Introduction

The electromagnetic spectrum, as shown in Fig. 1, can be split up into several regions, such as the visible spectrum, ultraviolet, X-ray, infrared, radar, radio, among others. The infrared region can be additionally divided into the near (NIR: near-infrared), short (SWIR: short-wavelength infrared), middle (MWIR: mid-wavelength infrared), long (LWIR: long-wavelength infrared) and far (FIR: far-infrared) spectral bands, where the long-wavelength infrared is also known as thermal. All objects emit infrared radiation by themselves, independently of any external energy source, and depending on their temperature they emit a different wavelength in the long wavelength infrared spectrum (i.e., thermal). Thermal cameras capture information in this long wavelength spectral band; they are passive sensors that capture infrared radiation emitted by all objects with a temperature above absolute zero [8], thus it can provide valuable extra

F. Karray et al. (Eds.): ICIAR 2019, LNCS 11663, pp. 417–426, 2019.
https://doi.org/10.1007/978-3-030-27272-2_37

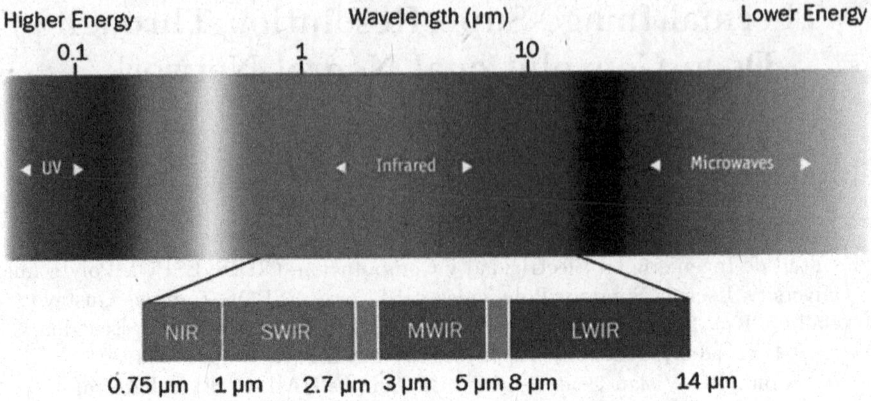

Fig. 1. Electromagnetic spectrum with sub-divided infrared spectrum

information to the visible one (e.g., RGB camera). In particularly, those applications that can be affected by poor lighting conditions, for instance in security and object recognition, where nothing can be captured in total darkness. Contrariwise, thermal cameras are not affected by this lack of illumination. As shown in Fig. 2 thermal images are represented as grayscale images, with dark pixels for cold spots and the whites one for hot spots.

In recent years, infrared imaging field has grown considerably; nowadays, there is a large set of infrared cameras available in the market (e.g, Flir[1], Axis[2], among others) with different technical specifications and costs. Innovative use of infrared imaging technology can therefore play an important role in many applications, such as medicine [16], military [9], objects or materials recognition [3], among others, as well as detection, tracking, and recognition of humans, or even applied for Vegetation Index Estimation [17].

Depending of the thermal camera's specifications, the cost can vary between \$ 200.00 and more than \$ 20000.00; the latter one has better resolution and higher frame rate. On the contrary, cheap existing thermal cameras have resolution smaller than commercial RGB cameras. This lack of resolution, at a moderate price, is a big limitation when thermal cameras need to be used for general purpose solutions. Hence, a possibility to overcome this limitation could be based on the development of new algorithms that allow to increase image resolution. This possibility has been largely exploited in the visible spectrum domain, where different super-resolution approaches have been proposed from a conventional interpolation (e.g., [7,10,18]). Recently, novel deep learning based approaches have been introduced with large improvements in performance (e.g., [5,11,15,19]). Hence, inspired on those approaches, some contributions have been proposed in the literature to tackle this challenging limitation of thermal imaging; most of these approaches are deep learning based (e.g., [4,13]).

[1] https://www.flir.com.
[2] https://www.axis.com.

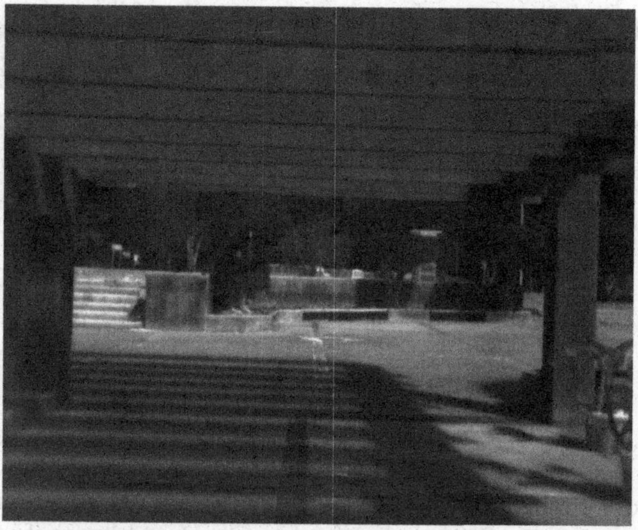

Fig. 2. Thermal image capture with a Tau2 Camera

One of the most relevant approaches for image enhancement has been presented in SRCNN [5]; the approach is based on a convolutional neural network (CNN), where the architecture is trained to learn how to get a high-resolution image from an image with a lower resolution. The authors explored the performance by using different color space representations. They conclude that the best option is obtained by using the Y-channel from the YCbCr color space. The main limitation of their contribution is related with the training time. The approach, named "Accelerating the Super-Resolution Convolutional Neural Network" [6], from the same authors of the previous work, proposes accelerating and compacting their SRCNN structure for faster and better super resolution (SR). The authors introduce a deconvolution layer at the end of the network and adopt smaller filter size but more mapping layers. Yamanaka et al. [19] propose a CNN based approach referred to as "Deep CNN with Residual Net, Skip Connection and Network in Network" (DCSCN) for visible spectrum image super-resolution. According to the authors, this approach has a computation complexity of at least 10 time smaller that state of the art (e.g. VDSR [11], RED [15] and DRCN [12]). Like in the SRCNN in DCSCN the given images are converted to the YCbCr color space and only the Y-channel is considered. All these approaches have been proposed for images enhancement from the visible spectrum.

A CNN based approach for enhancing thermal images has been introduced by Choi et al. in [4], inspired by the proposal in [5]. The authors in [4] compare the accuracy of a network trained in different image spectrum to find the best representation of thermal enhancement. They conclude that a grayscale trained network provided better enhancement than the MWIR-based network

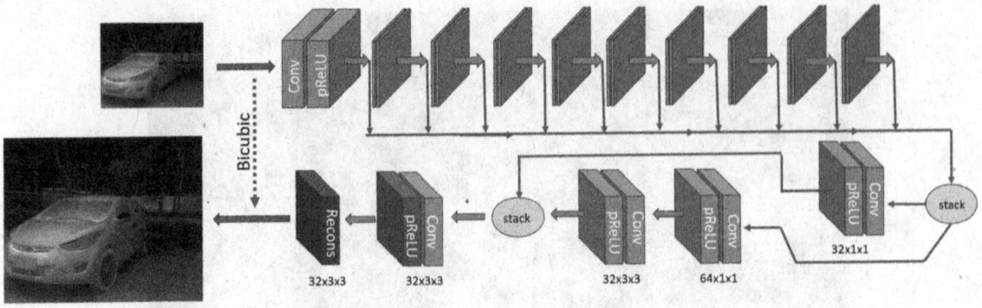

Fig. 3. Proposed convolutional neural network architecture

for thermal image enhancement. On the other hand, Lee et al. [13] also propose a convolutional neural network based on image enhancement for thermal images. The authors evaluate four RGB-based domains, namely, gray, lightness, intensity and V (from HSV color space) with a residual-learning technique. The approach improves the performance of enhancement and speed of convergence. The authors conclude that the V representation is the best one for enhancing thermal images. In [14] the authors proposed a parallelized 1×1 CNNs, named Network in Network to perform image enhancement with a low computational cost; also in [14], uses this technique for image reconstruction.

In most of the previous approaches thermal images have not been considered during the training stage, although intended for thermal image enhancement. They propose to train their CNN based approaches using images from the visible spectrum at different color space representations. On the contrary to all of them, in the current work thermal images are considered for training the proposed CNN architecture. The current work has two main contributions, the first one is the thermal image dataset acquisition used for training and validation. The second is proposed a CNN model designed for thermal spectrum images. The second one is to propose a CNN model designed for thermal spectrum images. Through this paper, terms "thermal images enhancement" and "images super resolution" will be indistinctly used.

The rest of the paper is organized as follows. Section 2 details the collected dataset and describe the approach proposed to enhance thermal images. Experimental results are presented in Sect. 3; and finally, Sect. 4 summarize main contributions of current work.

2 Proposed Approach

In the current work a deep CNN architecture with a residual net and dense connections are proposed. The network uses a thermal dataset to perform a super-resolution to maintain image details.

The architecture, presented in Fig. 3, has a part of the architecture dedicated to obtain the high level characteristics of the image, and another part, to perform the reconstitution of the image. All layers have dropouts and use parametric

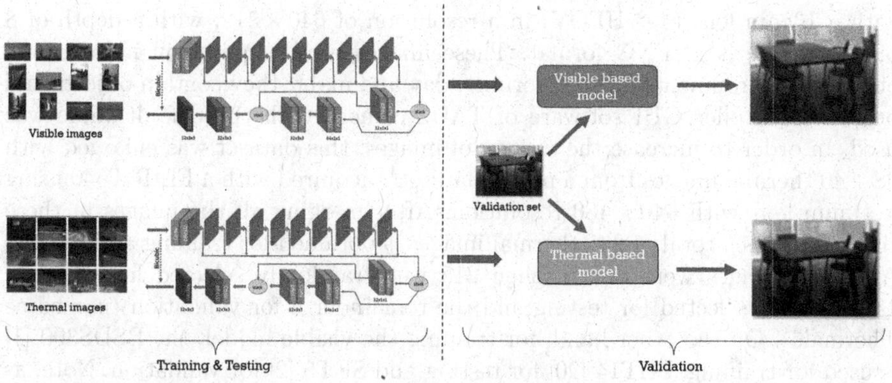

Fig. 4. Training process design of two datasets, using the proposal architecture, to generate two models for validation process.

ReLU as activator (preventing from learning a large negative bias term and getting better performance). Additionally, based on the work of [19], the image generated by bicubic interpolation has been used to enhance the output of the network.

This architecture is used for obtaining thermal image SR. On the contrary to the state-of-the-art approaches, where CNN based architectures are trained with visible spectrum images and used with thermal images. In this work the network is trained with thermal images in order to obtain better results. The latter hypothesis is validated by training the networks twice, one with visible images and one with thermal images. This training process results in two models (see Fig. 4), which are finally validated with thermal images. More details are given below.

3 Experiments Results

In this section, the dataset acquisition and preparation for training and testing are explained. Then the network setup information is provided, and finally the comparison of the two models are depicted.

3.1 Datasets for Training and Testing

As mention above the current work the architecture presented is trained twice, one with visible and other with thermal images. In this section the two datasets used for these training processes are detailed.

Due to the fact that there are not enough thermal image datasets, and the few ones available are in low resolution, a new dataset of 101 thermal images was generated (Fig. 5). This dataset was acquired using a TAU2[3] thermal camera

[3] https://www.flir.com/products/tau-2/.

with a 13 mm lens (45° HFOV) in a resolution of 640 × 512, with a depth of 8 bits and save it in PNG format. These images were acquired in indoors and outdoors environments, in the morning, day and night; they contain objects and people. Controller GUI software of TAU2 camera with the default value was used. In order to increase the variety of images, this dataset was enlarged with 98 + 40 thermal images from a public dataset[4], acquired with a FLIR T640 using a 41 mm lens with 640 × 480 resolution. After merging all the images in these three datasets a total of 231 thermal images is obtained for training and testing. All these images were mixed, then 215 were randomly selected for training, 18 randomly selected for testing and the remainder 6 for validation (named as Thermal6). On the other hand, for training the visible model, the BSDS300 [1] is used for training, SET14 [20] for testing and SET5 [2] for validation. Note, as shown in Fig. 4, that the thermal images validation set is used to evaluate both models.

In order to increase the number of training images, a *data augmentation* process is performed, rotating and flipping from top to bottom, from left to right all images. The quality and resolution of the images is maintained getting a total of 1720 and 2400 images for thermal and visible respectively.

3.2 Training

The proposed architecture, has been training using a dense network, also, uses the image generated by bicubic interpolation to improve image details, also the layers for feature extractor uses dropout and ReLU operations, also a learning rate of 0.002 is applied to the model, and uses MSE as a loss function to measure the difference between the ground truth and the output. The model uses Adam Optimizer, which is an adaptive learning rate method, which means, it computes individual learning rates for different parameters. Its name is derived from adaptive moment estimation, and the reason it's called that is because Adam uses estimations of first and second moments of gradient to adapt the learning rate for each weight of the neural network. Each epoch train with a batch of 100000 patches for a total of 63 epochs. Mean Squared Error (MSE) between the ground truth and output is used as a basic loss value.

As presented above, in order to evaluate the proposed approach, the same architecture was trained with the two different datasets, the 1720 thermal images were split up into 48 × 48 patches with 25 pixels overlapping of adjacent patches, having a total batch of 185760. The 2400 visible images also were split up into 48 × 48 patches with 25 pixels overlapping, having a batch of 108000 (note that although there are more visible than thermal images the number of thermal patches is larger since thermal images have larger resolution.

The patches obtained above are used as ground truth, while the input patches are obtained by resizing them to half their original resolution. In the current work there is not noise added to the input.

[4] https://sites.google.com/view/multispectral/dde.

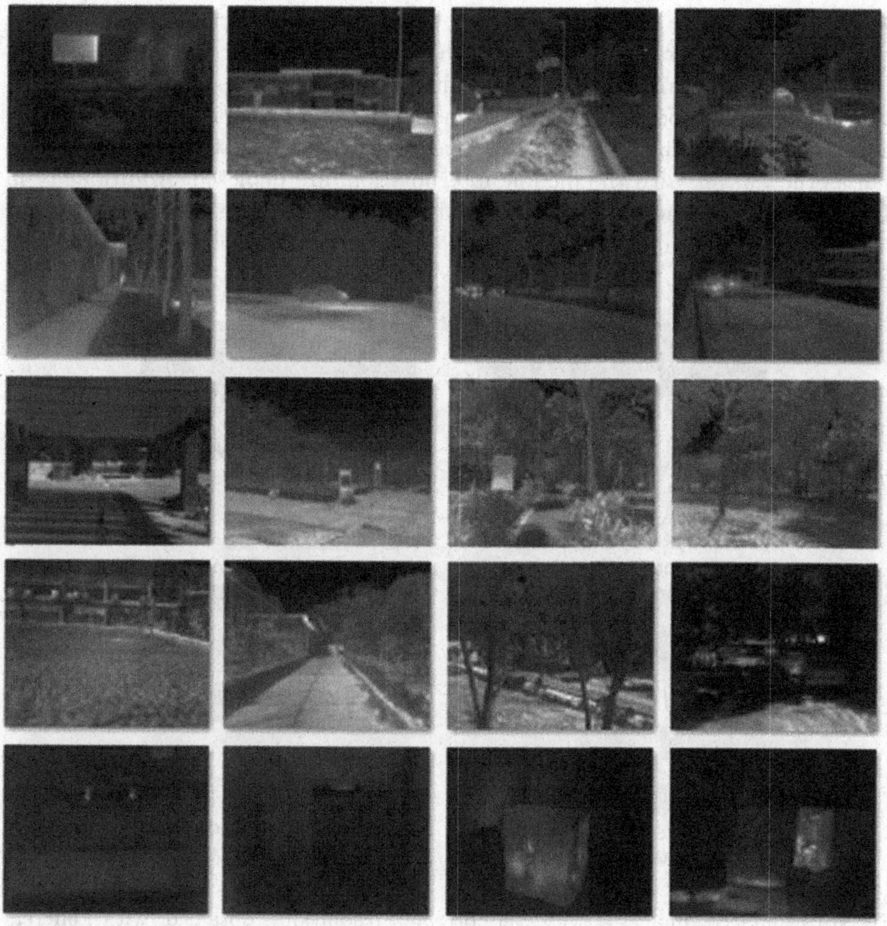

Fig. 5. Acquired thermal image dataset, with 640×512 resolution, using a Tau2 thermal camera.

The training is performed in Windows Server 2012, with a dual 2.50 GHz CPU E5-2640, using one GPU K20m of 4 GB. Each training consumes approximately 5 GB of RAM and takes approximately 25 h. This architecture is implemented using Tensorflow and Python.

3.3 Results

A fair comparison between the two models trained using the same infrastructure with the same number of batches per epochs and hyper parameters were used.

As show in Fig. 4, two models have been trained with the different dataset, each trained network was validated with a set of six thermal images (Thermal6) and five RGB images (SET5), obtaining a Visible Based Model and a Thermal

Based Model. Table 1 shows that with Thermal6, the thermal trained model shown a PSNR average value higher than the PSNR average value obtained with the Visible trained model. Also, it shows that SET5 got better PSNR values on visible model than thermal model. A qualitative comparison can be appreciated in Fig. 6, where the SR images obtained with the two models, as well as the images with the bicubic interpolation, are depicted. Additionally in this figure the ground truth is presented (values in brackets correspond to the average PSNR presented in Table 1).

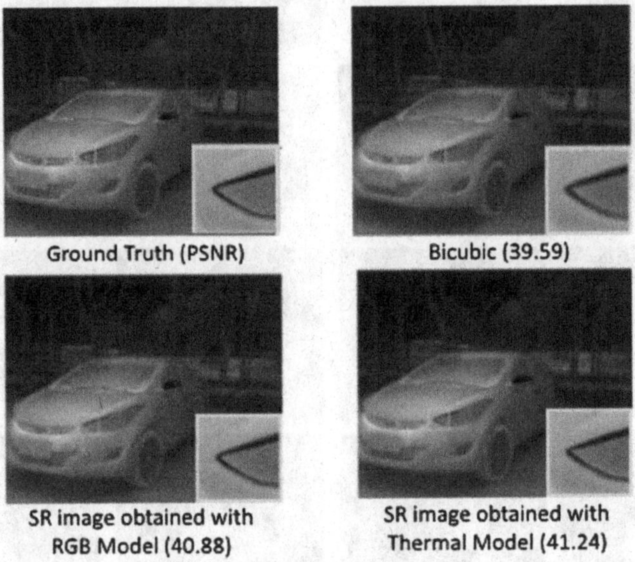

Fig. 6. Enhanced images (twice the original resolution) obtained with different approaches.

Table 1. Average result of PSNR with proposed architecture

Dataset	Scale	Bicubic based model	Visible based model	Thermal
Thermal6	×2	39.59	40.88	**41.24**
	×3	37.68	39.14	**39.62**
	×4	34.98	37.17	**37.85**
SET5	×2	33.64	**37.69**	37.46
	×3	30.37	**34.01**	33.74
	×4	28.41	**31.69**	31.25

4 Conclusions

In the current work, the usage of the proposal network has been considered to obtain thermal image SR. Two models have been obtained by training the same network with two different datasets in order to seek for the best options when thermal images are considered. The experimental results indicate that the network model trained with thermal image dataset is better than using visible image dataset. As an additional contribution a thermal image dataset has been acquired, which is publicly available. As a future work, new CNN architecture will be designed specifically intended for thermal images. Additionally, training the model using a dataset obtained from the combination of different domains (e.g., Y-channel, V-Brightness, Gray and Thermal) will be considered.

Acknowledgment. This work has been partially supported by: the ESPOL project PRAIM (FIEC-09-2015); the Spanish Government under Project TIN2017-89723-P; and the "CERCA Programme/Generalitat de Catalunya". The authors thanks CTI-ESPOL for sharing server infrastructure used for training and testing the proposed work. The authors gratefully acknowledge the support of the CYTED Network: "Ibero-American Thematic Network on ICT Applications for Smart Cities" (REF-518RT0559) and the NVIDIA Corporation for the donation of the Titan Xp GPU used for this research.

References

1. Arbelaez, P., Maire, M., Fowlkes, C., Malik, J.: Contour detection and hierarchical image segmentation. IEEE Trans. Pattern Anal. Mach. Intell. **33**(5), 898–916 (2011)
2. Bevilacqua, M., Roumy, A., Guillemot, C., Alberi-Morel, M.L.: Low-complexity single-image super-resolution based on nonnegative neighbor embedding. BMVA press (2012)
3. Cho, Y., Bianchi-Berthouze, N., Marquardt, N., Julier, S.J.: Deep thermal imaging: proximate material type recognition in the wild through deep learning of spatial surface temperature patterns. In: Proceedings of the 2018 CHI Conference on Human Factors in Computing Systems, p. 2. ACM (2018)
4. Choi, Y., Kim, N., Hwang, S., Kweon, I.S.: Thermal image enhancement using convolutional neural network. In: 2016 IEEE/RSJ International Conference on Intelligent Robots and Systems (IROS), pp. 223–230. IEEE (2016)
5. Dong, C., Loy, C.C., He, K., Tang, X.: Image super-resolution using deep convolutional networks. IEEE Trans. Pattern Anal. Mach. Intell. **38**(2), 295–307 (2016)
6. Dong, C., Loy, C.C., Tang, X.: Accelerating the super-resolution convolutional neural network. In: Leibe, B., Matas, J., Sebe, N., Welling, M. (eds.) ECCV 2016. LNCS, vol. 9906, pp. 391–407. Springer, Cham (2016). https://doi.org/10.1007/978-3-319-46475-6_25
7. Duchon, C.E.: Lanczos filtering in one and two dimensions. J. Appl. Meteorol. **18**(8), 1016–1022 (1979)
8. Gade, R., Moeslund, T.B.: Thermal cameras and applications: a survey. Mach. Vis. Appl. **81**, 89–96 (2014)

9. Goldberg, A.C., Fischer, T., Derzko, Z.I.: Application of dual-band infrared focal plane arrays to tactical and strategic military problems. In: Infrared Technology and Applications XXVIII, vol. 4820, pp. 500–515. International Society for Optics and Photonics (2003)
10. Keys, R.: Cubic convolution interpolation for digital image processing. IEEE Trans. Acoust. Speech Signal Process. **29**(6), 1153–1160 (1981)
11. Kim, J., Kwon Lee, J., Mu Lee, K.: Accurate image super-resolution using very deep convolutional networks. In: Proceedings of the IEEE Conference on Computer Vision and Pattern Recognition, pp. 1646–1654 (2016)
12. Kim, J., Kwon Lee, J., Mu Lee, K.: Deeply-recursive convolutional network for image super-resolution. In: Proceedings of the IEEE Conference on Computer Vision and Pattern Recognition, pp. 1637–1645 (2016)
13. Lee, K., Lee, J., Lee, J., Hwang, S., Lee, S.: Brightness-based convolutional neural network for thermal image enhancement. IEEE Access **5**, 26867–26879 (2017)
14. Lin, M. Chen, Q., Yan, S.: Network in network. In: International Conference on Learning Representations (ICLR) (2014)
15. Mao, X., Shen, C., Yang, Y.B.: Image restoration using very deep convolutional encoder-decoder networks with symmetric skip connections. In: Advances in Neural Information Processing Systems, pp. 2802–2810 (2016)
16. Ring, E.F.J., Ammer, K.: Infrared thermal imaging in medicine. Physiol. Meas. **33**(3), R33 (2012)
17. Suárez, P.L., Sappa, A.D., Vintimilla, B.X.: Vegetation index estimation from monospectral images. In: Campilho, A., Karray, F., ter Haar Romeny, B. (eds.) ICIAR 2018. LNCS, vol. 10882, pp. 353–362. Springer, Cham (2018). https://doi.org/10.1007/978-3-319-93000-8_40
18. Watson, D.F., Philip, G.M.: Neighborhood-based interpolation. Geobyte **2**(2), 12–16 (1987)
19. Yamanaka, J., Kuwashima, S., Kurita, T.: Fast and accurate image super resolution by deep CNN with skip connection and network in network. CoRR, abs/1707.05425 (2017)
20. Zeyde, R., Elad, M., Protter, M.: On single image scale-up using sparse-representations. In: Boissonnat, J.D., et al. (eds.) Curves and Surfaces 2010. LNCS, vol. 6920, pp. 711–730. Springer, Heidelberg (2012). https://doi.org/10.1007/978-3-642-27413-8_47

Adaptive Methods for Ultrasound Beamforming and Motion Estimation

Compensated Row-Column Ultrasound Imaging Systems with Data-Driven Point Spread Function Learning

Ibrahim Ben Daya[1,2](✉), John T. W. Yeow[3], and Alexander Wong[1,2]

[1] Vision and Image Processing Research Group, University of Waterloo, Waterloo, Canada
ibendaya@uwaterloo.ca

[2] Water Artificial Intelligence Institute, Waterloo, Canada

[3] Advanced Micro and Nano Devices Lab, Waterloo, Canada

Abstract. Ultrasound imaging systems are invaluable tools used in applications ranging from medical diagnostics to non-destructive testing. The concept of row-column imaging using row-column-addressed arrays has received a lot of attention recently for 3-D ultrasound imaging. However, it suffers from a few intrinsic limitations: data sparsity, speckle noise, and a spatially varying point spread function. These limitations cannot be addressed by transducer design alone. In this research, we propose PL-UIS, a compensated ultrasound imaging system that combines physical modeling with data-driven spatially varying point spread function learning within a random field framework to address the limitations of row-column ultrasound imaging. Experimental results using the proposed ultrasound imaging system show the effectiveness of our proposed PL-UIS system compared to state-of-the-art compensated ultrasound imaging systems.

Keywords: Ultrasound imaging · Non-stationary point spread function · Conditional random fields · Point spread function learning

1 Introduction

Ultrasound imaging is a valuable tool in many areas ranging from medical image diagnostics to non-destructive testing. Conventional 2-D ultrasound is widely used, but the lack of anatomy and orientation information makes viewing 3-D anatomic structures difficult as clinicians and technicians must mentally imagine the volume with planar 2-D images; capturing 3-D volumes circumvents this. 3-D volumes are also valuable to material scientists as they can more accurately infer material properties from volumetric data [1].

There are two main ways to acquire 3-D ultrasound images: mechanical movement of transducers, or using 2-D array transducers [2]. 2-D arrays are preferred

F. Karray et al. (Eds.): ICIAR 2019, LNCS 11663, pp. 429–441, 2019.
https://doi.org/10.1007/978-3-030-27272-2_38

since mechanically moving a transducer can introduce unwanted artifacts and increase image acquisition time. A fully addressed 2-D $N \times N$ array requires N^2 connections and poses a challenge in terms of addressing these connections and handling the large amount of data needed; so a few 2-D array simplification methods have been proposed. One method that received a lot of attention recently is row-column imaging using row-column-addressed arrays [3,5,7–11,23].

Originally proposed in [6], the row-column imaging method consists of two sets of orthogonally positioned 1-D array; one set responsible for transmit beamforming, the other for receive beamforming. This method reduces the required number of connections to $N + N$, making it much more practical. Despite its promise to enabling practical, operational 3-D ultrasound imaging, the row-column imaging method still suffers from a few intrinsic limitations: (i) data is inherently sparse, images suffer from speckle noise, and (ii) the point spread function (PSF) of the system - the response of the imaging system to a point source - is spatially varying to a great degree. There is a steadily growing body of research that is attempting to address some of the row-column limitations through transducer design [5,7,9,25], but improved transducer design alone cannot fully address these inherent limitations.

A complimentary approach for addressing the inherent limitations of row-column imaging is the notion of computationally compensated ultrasound imaging. Computationally compensated row-column systems were first proposed in [10], where leveraging physical models within a random field based framework was used to address the limitations of the row-column method. This work has been extended to higher order random fields to better preserve edges [11]. Both of these systems leveraged the commonly accepted Tuphlome-Stephanisshen model for spatial impulse response [24] to account for the spatially varying PSF. However, a closer study of the PSF done in [11] revealed notable differences between the PSF derived using a physical model such as the Tuphlome-Stephanisshen model and that of the PSF for a row-column ultrasound imaging system. Furthermore, different configurations of row-column ultrasound imaging systems can result in noticeably different spatially varying PSFs, making it difficult to leverage the same physical model across different imaging systems. This leads us to the motivation behind this work: instead of relying purely on a physical model, we propose a data-driven approach to learning the PSF within the framework of a computationally compensated row-column ultrasound imaging system. This is the basis of PL-UIS, the proposed compensated row-column ultrasound imaging system in this work.

The rest of the paper is organized as follows. Section 2 outlines the theory and methodology behind the proposed PL-UIS system. Section 3 describes experimental setup and presents the experimental results. Finally, conclusions are drawn in Sect. 4.

2 Methodology

The proposed compensated row-column ultrasound imaging system with data-driven point spread function learning (which we will refer to as PL-UIS) has two steps: (i) characterization, and (ii) compensation. The characterization step uses a set of models that describe the ultrasound imaging system. This includes an image formation model, a noise model, and a point spread function model (which in the proposed PL-UIS system is learned); all of which aim to address some of the limitations of the underlying ultrasound imaging system. The compensation step unifies these models in a random field framework that aims to reconstruct ultrasound images while compensating for the limitations of the system. We will look at both steps in more detail here.

2.1 Characterization

The characterization step uses three models to describe the ultrasound imaging system: an image formation model, a noise model, and a point spread function model. Respectively, each will address data sparsity, speckle noise, and the spatially varying point spread function of ultrasound imaging systems. In the proposed PL-UIS system, we introduce a novel spatially varying PSF learning approach to obtain an improved characterization than what can be achieved using existing physical models.

Image Formation Model. An observed ultrasound RF image g_r can be mathematically described as:

$$g_r(x, y, z) = M(x, y, z)[f(x, y, z) * h(x, y, z) + u(x, y, z)] \tag{1}$$

where $M(x, y, z)$ is the sampling function that determines where measurements take place, $f(x, y, z)$ is the tissue reflectivity function, $h(x, y, z)$ is the spatially dependant point spread function of the ultrasound imaging system, '$*$' is the convolution operator, $u(x, y, z)$ is the noise component taking into account measurement noise as well as physical phenomenon not accounted for by the convolution model [10], and x, y, z are the Cartesian coordinates of the imaged space.

Noise Model. Speckle noise affects all scans from coherent imaging modalities. It is a result of the interfering echoes of transmitted waveforms emanating from the heterogeneities of the studied object. Previous work in literature has shown that the Fisher-Tippett model [12] provides the best fit for speckle noise in envelope detected observed image. The Fisher Tippett distribution is given by:

$$p(I(x, y, z)) = 2\exp\left[(2I(x, y, z) - \ln 2\sigma^2) - \exp\left[2I(x, y, z) - \ln 2\sigma^2\right]\right], \tag{2}$$

where $I(x, y, z)$ is the pixel intensity and σ is the standard deviation.

Point Spread Function. For ultrasound imaging systems, the PSF is spatially variable. This is due to the nature of sound waves: sound pressure weakens as it moves, creating a varying beam profile [4]. Previous work characterized and accounted for this when compensating for the ultrasound imaging system using physical models. More specifically, past systems leveraged a PSF derived base on the Tuphlome-Stephanisshen model for spatial impulse response, which was further derived in [15] for the pulse-echo case. However, as stated earlier in the paper, this physical model has notable deviations from the PSF for row-column ultrasound imaging systems. It is also difficult to leverage this same physical model across different imaging systems with different setups. Driven to address these fundamental limitations of using purely a physical model for the PSF, we introduce a data-driven approach for PSF learning to obtain a more representative PSF for the underlying row-column ultrasound imaging system.

The proposed data-driven PSF learning method extends upon the approach introduced in Pan *et al.* [26] to enable the learning of spatially variable PSFs found in row-column imaging systems, and can be described as follows. To find the optimal spatially varying PSF based on the underlying acquisition at hand, the PSF learning method alternates between two processes: (i) estimating the latent tissue reflectivity function $f(x, y, z)$

$$\min_{f} ||f(x,y,z) * h(x,y,z) - g(x,y,z)||_2^2 + \lambda R(f(x,y,z)), \tag{3}$$

and (ii) estimating the spatially varying PSF $h(x, y, z)$,

$$\min_{h} ||f(x,y,z) * h(x,y,z) - g(x,y,z)||_2^2 + \gamma ||h(x,y,z)||_2^2, \tag{4}$$

where $R(f(x, y, z))$ is a regularized prior on tissue reflectivity magnitude and gradient, λ and γ are constraints for the PSF and latent tissue reflectivity function.

To minimize Eq. 3, an auxiliary variable $a(x, y, z)$ with respect to $f(x, y, z)$ is introduced as well as $v(x, y, z)$ corresponding to the tissue reflectivity gradient. With these two variables, the objective function is re-written as:

$$\begin{aligned}\min_{f,a,v} ||f(x,y,z) * h(x,y,z) - g(x,y,z)||_2^2 + \eta ||f(x,y,z) - a(x,y,z)||_2^2 \\ + \mu ||\nabla f(x,y,z) - v(x,y,z)||_2^2 + \lambda(\sigma ||a(x,y,z)||_0 + ||v(x,y,z)||_0),\end{aligned} \tag{5}$$

Here σ is a weight that balances the regularized priors, η and μ are penalty parameters. The values of $a(x, y, z)$ and $v(x, y, z)$ are first initialized to zeros, and in each iteration, the latent tissue reflectivity function is obtained by solving

$$\begin{aligned}\min_{f} ||f(x,y,z) * h(x,y,z) - g(x,y,z)||_2^2 + \eta ||f(x,y,z) - a(x,y,z)||_2^2 \\ + \mu ||\nabla f(x,y,z) - v(x,y,z)||_2^2,\end{aligned} \tag{6}$$

Given $f(x, y, z)$, $a(x, y, z)$ and $v(x, y, z)$ are then computed separately by

$$\min_{a} \eta ||f(x,y,z) - a(x,y,z)||_2^2 + \lambda\sigma ||a(x,y,z)||_0, \tag{7}$$

$$\min_{v} \mu ||\nabla f(x,y,z) - v(x,y,z)||_2^2 + \lambda ||v(x,y,z)||_0. \tag{8}$$

Algorithm 1. Solving (5)

Input: g and h
$f \leftarrow g$, $\eta \leftarrow 2\lambda\sigma$
repeat
  solve for a using (7)
  $\mu \leftarrow 2\lambda$
  repeat
    solve for v using (8)
    solve for f using (6)
    $\mu \leftarrow 2\mu$
  until $\mu > \mu_{max}$
  $\eta \leftarrow 2\eta$
until $\eta > \eta_{max}$
Output: Intermediate latent tissue reflectivity f

The main steps for solving for the latent tissue reflectivity function can be summarized through the following algorithm:

Given $f(x, y, z)$, (4) becomes a least squares minimization problem. The spatially varying PSF can be estimated by:

$$\min_h ||\nabla f(x, y, z) * h(x, y, z) - \nabla g(x, y, z)||_2^2 + \gamma ||h(x, y, z)||_2^2. \quad (9)$$

As such, the algorithm for learning the spatially varying PSF can be summarized as:

Algorithm 2. Spatially Varying PSF Learning

Input: g
initialize h using coarse-to-fine process
for $i = 1 \rightarrow 5$
  solve for f using Algorithm 1
  solve for h using (9)
  $\lambda \leftarrow \max\{\lambda/1.1, 1e^{-4}\}$
endfor
Output: PSF h and intermediate latent tissue reflectivity function f

Given the aforementioned spatially varying PSF learning approach, we now can address data sparsity through incorporating the image formation model, account for speckle noise through the noise model, and learn the spatially varying PSF using the proposed data-driven algorithm. All three models are used in a unified compensation framework that will be described in the next section.

2.2 Compensation

The compensation stage leverages the models defined in the characterization stage to find a solution for the inverse problem of Eq. 1. This is essentially an image reconstruction problem, where we are given a sampled observed noisy image and need to find an estimate of the ideal image. We formulate the image reconstruction problem as a Maximum a Posteriori (MAP) problem, where we wish to maximize the posterior distribution $P(F|G)$:

$$F^* = \underset{\bar{F}}{argmin}\{E(F, G, Cr)\}. \tag{10}$$

where F^* denotes the MAP solution, $\bar{F}$ denotes the possible result set, and G denotes the observation.

To model $P(F|G)$, we can leveraging the notion of conditional random fields (CRFs). This gives us the flexibility of modeling the conditional probability without specifying a prior model, but instead with a set of potential functions $\psi(\cdot)$ [14]. The general form for CRFs is:

$$P(F|G) = \frac{1}{Z(G)} \exp\left(- \psi(F, G)\right) \tag{11}$$

where Z is the partition function.

The potential function $\psi(\cdot)$ is a combination of unary and pairwise potential functions:

$$\psi(F, G) = \sum_{i=1}^{n} \psi_u(f_i, G) + \sum_{c \in C} \psi_p(f_c, G) \tag{12}$$

C here is a clique structure for each node. With this framework, neighbours in a clique structure are considered with the same degree of certainty, which isn't the case when dealing with incomplete or sparse data. This necessitates the addition of a layer that takes into account the degree of uncertainty, which is what multilayered conditional random fields (MCRF) accounts for. Equation 11 can be rewritten as:

$$P(F|Cr, G) = \frac{1}{Z(G)} \exp\left(- \psi(F|Cr, G)\right) \tag{13}$$

where C_r is the uncertainty layer, a zero-to-one plane that indicates where measurements exist, with $C_r = 0$ where readings are available.

The unary potential function ψ_u plays the role of the data driven function. It incorporates the observation into the random field model as well as taking into account the spatially varying PSF. Since we believe the ideal image is degraded according to the noise model shown in Eq. 2, the unary potential function is formulated after the Fisher Tippett distribution:

$$\psi_u(f_i, G, Cr_i) = \frac{1 - C_r}{\sigma} \exp\left(- \alpha \frac{\log G - \log H(f_i)}{\sigma}\right) . \exp\left(- \frac{\log G - \log H(f_i)}{\sigma}\right) \tag{14}$$

where *alpha* determines how much contribution the unary potential has, $H(.)$ is the function that takes into account factors pertaining to the imaging system like PSF and sensor noise.

The pairwise potential function ψ_p is a spatially driven function, incorporating spatial information within a local clique structure into the random field model. The potential function in the proposed system consists of two penalty terms: the first penalizes pixels that are farther away (since it's less likely they belong to the same label) referred to as spatial proximity penalty w_{sp}, the second penalizes pixels with different intensities (outlining tissue transitions more clearly) referred to as the first order variation penalty w_{fov}. ψ_p is formulated as:

$$\psi_p(f_c, G) = \exp(-\beta|f_i - f_j|w(g_i, g_j)), \tag{15}$$

where β determines how much contribution the pairwise potential has, w is the combined penalty function consisting of the spatial proximity penalty:

$$w_{sp}(i,j) = \exp\left(\frac{-d_E(i,j)}{2\sigma_{sp}^2}\right), \tag{16}$$

and the first order variation penalty:

$$w_{fov}(g_i, g_j) = \exp\left(-\frac{||g_i - g_j||}{2\sigma_{fov}^2}\right) \tag{17}$$

with σ_{sp} and σ_{fov} being control factors setting the strength of the corresponding penalty function, and $d_E(i,j)$ is the Euclidian distance between nodes i and j.

Now that the potential functions are defined, an energy function driving the MAP problem can be set up as:

$$E(F, G, Cr) = \sum_{i=1}^{n} \psi_u(f_i, G, Cr_i) + \sum_{c \in C} \psi_p(f_c, G). \tag{18}$$

With this energy function, the MAP problem in (10) can be rewritten as:

$$F^* = \underset{F}{argmin}\{E(F, G, Cr)\}. \tag{19}$$

To solve the MAP problem, gradient descent algorithm is used.

3 Results

To evaluate our proposed PL-UIS system, we compared the performance of our PL-UIS system with previously proposed row-column imaging systems in literature, including the original compensated row-column ultrasound imaging system CRC-UIS [10], the edge-guided compensated system EG-CRCUIS [11], a baseline row-column system [7], a system that uses integrated apodization to correct for some of the row-column limitation through transducer design [5], and a fully addressed 2-D array. In this section, we will outline the experimental setup, metrics used to evaluate the performance, visual evaluation, and quantitative evaluation.

3.1 Experimental Setup

In this work, Field II MATLAB Toolkit [15] was used for simulation of row-column ultrasound imaging systems. This includes phantom generation as well as ultrasound beamforming. More specifically, the ultrasound imaging systems were implemented with 32 × 32 2-D addressing. Center frequency was set at 6 MHz, F-number on receive was set at 4. Attenuation was not applied.

Two phantoms were tested in this work, shown in Fig. 1. The first phantom is a series of 4 cysts with decreasing diameter, each placed 10 mm apart. The bottom two cysts are placed at 5 mm and 10 mm off the center axis. The second phantom is an L shape made up of three 6 mm by 6 mm squares. To ensure fully developed speckle during the simulation, 500,000 scatterers were set in the scanning region.

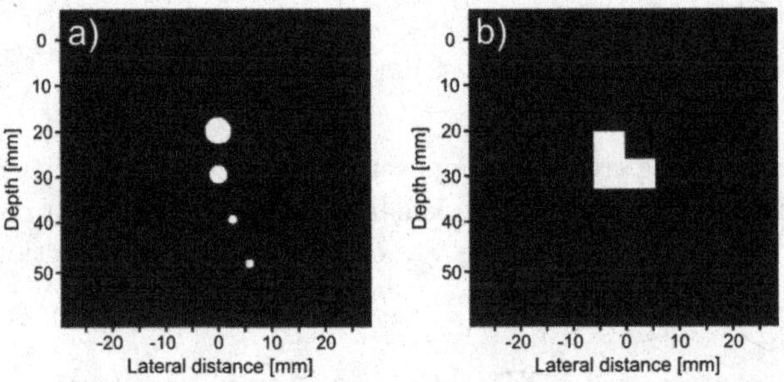

Fig. 1. Phantoms tested in this study. The phantom in (a) consists of four cysts of decreasing size, with the bottom two offset away from the middle axis. The phantom in (b) is a homogeneous 'L' shape.

3.2 Metrics for Comparison

For the purpose of our implementation, we use peak signal-to-noise ratio (PSNR) to provide a quality measure based on the power of the ideal and reconstructed image, expected number of looks (ENL) to provide a measure of speckle removal (as it give a measure of statistical fluctuations), and coefficient of correlation (CoC) to provide a measure of edge preservation. All metrics are used in accordance to recent literature definitions [10,11,16–22].

3.3 Quantitative Evaluation

Quantitative results for the first phantom are summarized in Table 1. The proposed PL-UIS outperforms all other methods in reconstructing the phantom across all metrics, achieving higher ENL and CoC and thus indicating better speckle removal and edge preservation. All compensated systems show higher performance in these metrics when compared against the baseline RC as well as the integrated apodization systems.

Table 1. Quantitative results for the first phantom

System	PSNR	ENL	CoC
PL-UIS (proposed)	**22.1649**	**3.5466**	**0.37784**
EG-CRCUIS [11]	20.2834	1.1456	0.30495
CRC-UIS [10]	20.2541	1.5587	0.34094
Baseline RC [7]	18.6101	2.2711	0.2234
Integrated apodization [23]	18.7266	0.49454	0.33837
Fully addressed 2-D array	16.8628	2.9858	0.21104

Quantitative results for the second phantom are summarized in Table 2. The proposed PL-UIS once again outperforms the other tested row-column imaging systems in terms of PSNR and CoC, indicating better reconstruction and edge preservation. CRC-UIS performs the highest in ENL indicating better speckle removal.

Table 2. Quantitative results for the second phantom

System	PSNR	ENL	CoC
PL-UIS (proposed)	**15.0724**	35.0585	**0.21247**
EG-CRCUIS [11]	14.3523	80.6775	0.19492
CRC-UIS [10]	12.4017	**89.5186**	0.17279
Baseline RC [7]	10.6971	1.473	0.13585
Integrated apodizzation [23]	11.1029	5.9159	0.16998
Fully addressed 2-D array	12.9316	5.9159	0.18795

3.4 Visual Evaluation

Reconstruction of the first phantom is shown in Fig. 2, with a closer look at the cysts in Fig. 3. The results of PL-UIS are remarkably close to the phantom, with sharp edges and homogeneous regions that reflect the underlying phantom. The top cysts loses some of its round shape when compared to other compensated systems, which may be due to the data-driven nature of the PSF estimation, the other cysts retain their shape better than other systems. The sizes of the cysts are most consistent in PL-UIS. This is particularly noticeable in all three compensated systems with the top and bottom cysts that are farthest from the line of focus, which is indicative of the value of variable PSF compensation.

Reconstruction of the second phantom is shown in Fig. 4. PL-UIS shows a significant improvement over its predecessors, particularly when compared with CRC-UIS. While visually it looks like a better reconstruction of the phantom when compared with the uncompensated row-column systems, the fully addressed array still retains the closest shape, particularly with the corners; though speckle is still an issue.

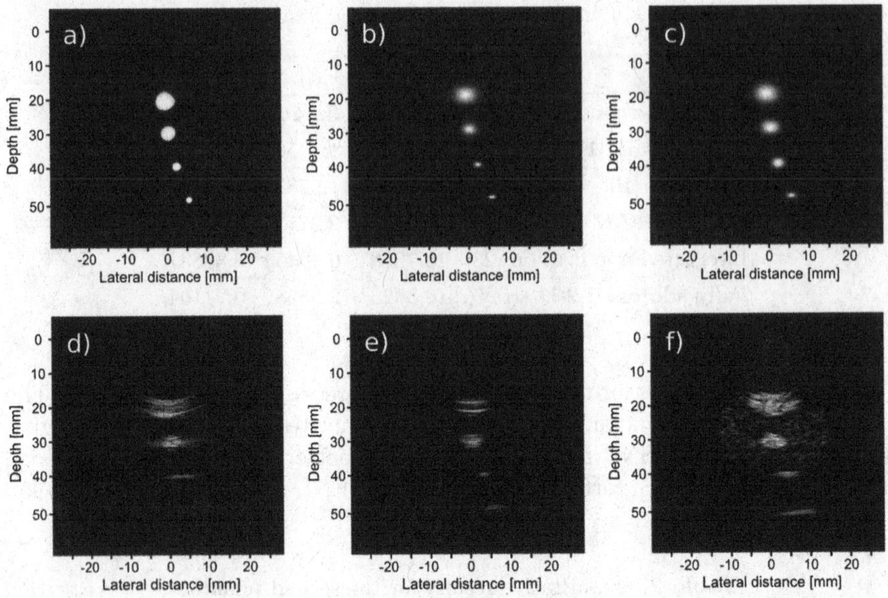

Fig. 2. First phantom visual assessment of the proposed PL-UIS system (top left) as opposed to other systems in literature. The PL-UIS reconstruction is shown in (a), the EG-CRCUIS reconstruction [11] is shown in (b), CRC-UIS [10] is shown in (c), baseline RC [7] is shown in (d), integrated apodization [5] system is shown in (e), and the fully addressed 2-D array is shown in (f). All scans are shown at a dynamic range of 40 dB.

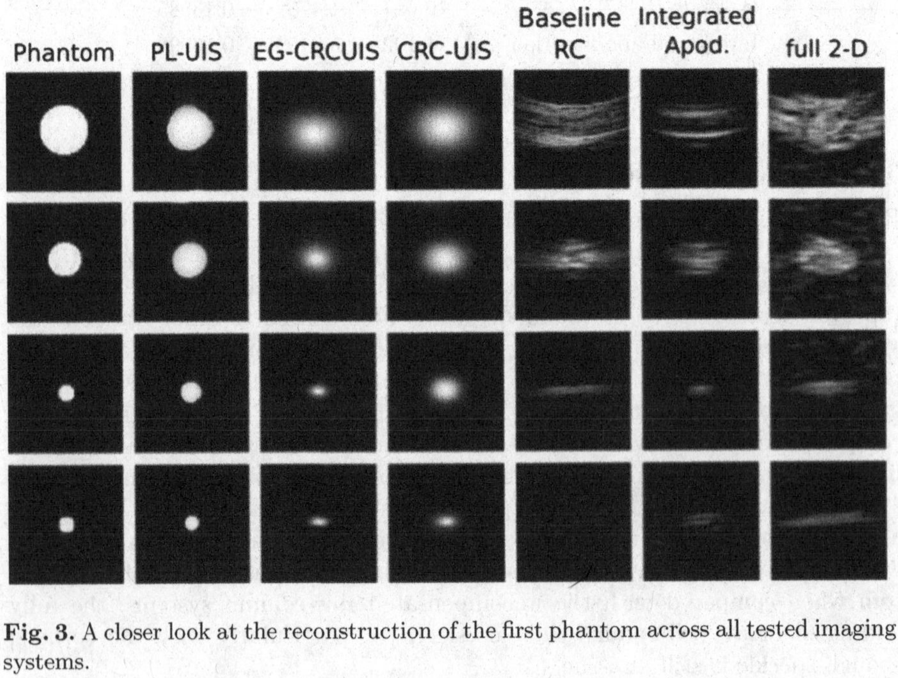

Fig. 3. A closer look at the reconstruction of the first phantom across all tested imaging systems.

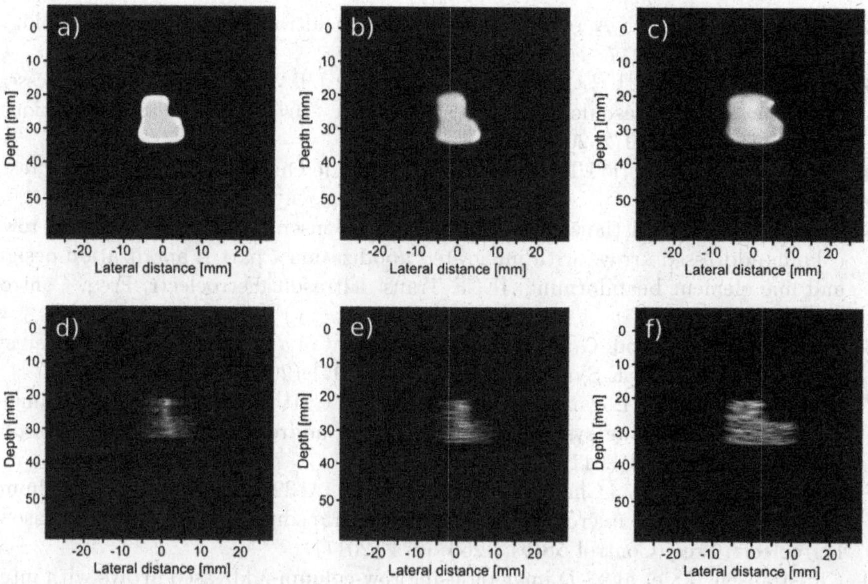

Fig. 4. Second phantom visual assessment of the PL-UIS (top left) as opposed to other systems in literature. The PL-UIS reconstruction is shown in (a), the EG-CRCUIS reconstruction [11] is shown in (b), CRC-UIS [10] is shown in (c), baseline RC [7] is shown in (d), integrated apodization [5] system is shown in (e), and the fully addressed 2-D array is shown in (f). All scans are shown at a dynamic range of 40 dB.

4 Conclusion

In this work, we proposed PL-UIS, a compensated row-column ultrasound imaging based on a unified multilayered random field framework that combines physical models as well as a data-driven approach for spatially varying point spread function learning. The proposed PL-UIS system was tested against other row-column imaging systems - both compensated and uncompensated - from literature, with promising results that demonstrate the value of introducing data-driven approaches to improve the characterization of row-column imaging systems to enhance compensation capabilities.

Future work includes incorporating higher order random fields, as the integration of additional energy potentials for improved image quality.

Acknowledgement. This work was supported by the Natural Sciences and Engineering Research Council of Canada's Collaborative Research and Training Experience (NSERC-CREATE) Program, and the Canada Research Chairs Program.

References

1. Smith, R.A., Nelson, L.J.: 2D transmission imaging with a crossed-array configuration for defect detection. Insight J. Br. Inst. NDT **51**, 82–87 (2009)

2. Huang, Q., Zeng, Z.: A review on real-time 3D ultrasound imaging technology. BioMed Res. Int. **2017**, 1–20 (2017)
3. Wong, L., Chen, A.I.H., Li, Z., Logan, A.S., Yeow, J.T.W.: A row-column addressed micromachined ultrasonic transducer array for surface scanning applications. Ultrasonics **54**(8), 2072–2080 (2014)
4. Szabo, T.L.: Diagnostic Ultrasound Imaging: Inside Out. Elsevier Academic Press, Amsterdam (2004)
5. Rasmussen, M., Christiansen, T., Thomsem, E., Jensen, J.: 3-D imaging using row-column-addressed arrays with integrated apodization - part I: apodization design and line element beamforming. IEEE Trans. Ultrason. Ferroelectr. Freq. Control **62**(5), 947–958 (2015)
6. Morton, C., Lockwood, G.: Theoretical assessment of a crossed electrode 2-D array for 3-D imaging. IEEE Symp. Ultrason. **1**, 968–971 (2003)
7. Chen, A., Wong, L., Logan, A., Yeow, J.T.W.: A CMUT-based real-time volumetric ultrasound imaging system with row-column addressing. IEEE Int. Ultrason. Symp. **1**, 1755–1758 (2011)
8. Logan, A., Wong, L., Chen, A., Yeow, J.T.W.: A 32 × 32 element row-column addressed capacitive micromachined ultrasonic transducer. IEEE Trans. Ultrason. Ferroelectr. Freq. Control **58**(6), 1266–1271 (2011)
9. Christiansen, T., et al.: 3-D imaging using row-column-addressed arrays with integrated apodization - part II: transducer fabrication and experimental results. IEEE Trans. Ultrason. Ferroelectr. Freq. Control **62**(5), 959–971 (2015)
10. Ben Daya, I., Chen, A.I.H., Shafiee, M.J., Wong, A., Yeow, J.T.W.: Compensated row-column ultrasound imaging system using fisher tippett multilayered conditional random field model. PLoS ONE **10**(12), e0142817 (2015)
11. Daya, I.B., Chen, A.I.H., Shafiee, M.J., Wong, A., Yeow, J.T.W.: Compensated row-column ultrasound imaging system using multilayered edge guided stochastically fully connected random fields. Sci. Rep. **7**, 10644 (2017)
12. Michailovich, O., Tannenbaum, A.: Despeckling of medical ultrasound images. IEEE Trans. Ultrason. Ferroelectr. Freq. Control **53**(1), 64–78 (2006)
13. Jensen, J.A., Svendsen, N.B.: Calculation of pressure fields from arbitrarily shaped, apodized, and excited ultrasound transducers. IEEE Trans. Ultrason. Ferroelectr. Freq. Control **39**(2), 262–267 (1992)
14. Lafferty, J.D., McCallum, A., Pereira, F.C.N.: Conditional random fields: probabilistic models for segmenting and labeling sequence data. In: Proceedings of the Eighteenth International Conference on Machine Learning, pp. 282–289 (2001)
15. Jensen, J.A.: Field: a program for simulating ultrasound systems. In: 10th Nordic-Baltic Conference on Biomedical Imaging Published in Medical Biological Engineering Computing, vol. 34, pp. 351–353 (1996)
16. Achim, A., Bezerianos, A., Tsakalides, P.: Novel Bayesian multiscale method for speckle removal in medical ultrasound images. IEEE Trans. Med. Imaging **20**(8), 772–783 (2001)
17. Shruthi, G., Usha, B.S., Sandya, S.: Article: a novel approach for speckle reduction and enhancement of ultrasound images. Int. J. Comput. Appl. **45**(20), 14–20 (2012)
18. Wu, S., Zhu, Q., Xie, Y.: Evaluation of various speckle reduction filters on medical ultrasound images. In: Engineering in Medicine and Biology Society, pp. 1148–1151, July 2013
19. Sivakumar, R., Gayathri, M.K., Nedumaran, D.: Speckle filtering of ultrasound b-scan images- a comparative study between spatial and diffusion filters. In: IEEE Conference on Open Systems, pp. 80–85, December 2010

20. Nageswari, C., Prabha, K.: Despeckle process in ultrasound fetal image using hybrid spatial filters. In: International Conference on Green Computing, Communication and Conservation of Energy, pp. 174–179, December 2013
21. Srivastava, R., Gupta, J., Parthasarthy, H.: Comparison of PDE based on other techniques for speckle reduction from digitally reconstructed holographic images. Opt. Laser. Eng. **48**(5), 626–635 (2010)
22. Michailovich, O., Tannenbaum, A.: Blind deconvolution of medical ultrasound images: a parametric inverse filtering approach. IEEE Trans. Image Process. **16**(12), 3005–3019 (2007)
23. Rasmussen, M., Jensen, J.: 3-D ultrasound imaging performance of a row-column addressed 2-D array transducer: a measurement study. In: IEEE International Ultrasonics Symposium, pp. 1460–1463, July 2013
24. Jensen, J.: A model for the propagation and scattering of ultrasound in tissue. J. Acoust. Soc. Am. **89**(1), 182–191 (1991)
25. Engholm, M., Havreland, A., Thomsen, E., Beers, C., Tomov, B., Jensen, J.: A row-column-addressed 2D probe with an integrated compound diverging lens. In: IEEE International Ultrasonics Symposium (IUS), pp. 1–4 (2018)
26. Pan, J., Hu, Z., Su, Z., Yang, M.: L_0-regularized intensity and gradient prior for debluring text images and beyond. IEEE Trans. Pattern Anal. Mach. Intell. **39**, 342–355 (2017)

Channel Count Reduction for Plane Wave Ultrasound Through Convolutional Neural Network Interpolation

Di Xiao(✉), Billy Y. S. Yiu, Adrian J. Y. Chee, and Alfred C. H. Yu

Research Institute for Aging and Department of Electrical and Computer Engineering, University of Waterloo, Waterloo, ON N2L 3G1, Canada
di.xiao@uwaterloo.ca

Abstract. Plane wave ultrasound imaging has helped to achieve high frame rate ultrasound, however the data required to achieve frames rates over 1000 fps remains challenging to handle, as the transfer of large amounts of data represents a bottleneck for image reconstruction. This paper presents a novel method of using a fully convolutional encoder-decoder deep neural network to interpolate pre-beamformed raw RF data from ultrasound transducer elements. The network is trained on *in vivo* human carotid data, then tested on both carotid data and a standard ultrasound phantom. The neural network outputs are compared to linear interpolation and the proposed method captures more meaningful patterns in the signal; the output channels are then combined with the non-interpolated channels and beamformed to form an image, showing not only significant improvement in mean-squared error compared to the alternatives, but also 10–15 dB reduction in grating lobe artifacts. The proposed method has implications for current ultrasound research directions, with applications to real-time high frame rate ultrasound and 3D ultrasound imaging.

Keywords: Convolutional neural network · Channel interpolation · Ultrasound · Plane wave imaging · Encoder-decoder

1 Introduction

Ultrasound is a conventional medical imaging modality that sees widespread popularity due to its ease-of-use, noninvasive nature, relative affordability and ability to image both tissue and blood flow. Traditionally, ultrasound imaging is performed in the brightness mode (B-mode) where ultrasonic waves are iteratively emitted from transducer elements focused in a beam or line, then the reflected signals are read back to form the image line by line. In recent years, new developments in the ultrasound transmit and receive framework have led to the emergence of plane wave imaging, where ultrasonic waves are transmitted through a broad planar wave front, as opposed to line by line. As the wave propagates, it insonifies the entire imaging view and the subsequent reflections, or echoes, are then detected and beamformed to reconstruct a complete image for each transmission event [1, 2]. Because of this ability to transmit

F. Karray et al. (Eds.): ICIAR 2019, LNCS 11663, pp. 442–451, 2019.
https://doi.org/10.1007/978-3-030-27272-2_39

and receive one plane wave instead of many lines, as few as one transmission is required for an image reconstruction and so it has become a strong enabler for high frame rate ultrasound (HiFRUS).

A frame rate increase for a real-time imaging modality such as ultrasound naturally comes with additional data transfer requirements and computation costs as there are many more frames to be processed and reconstructed independently - upwards of 10 GB/s of data is collected and processed for plane wave ultrasound at over 1000 frames per second [3]. While the computing challenges of plane wave ultrasound have been addressed in previous works such as [4], these methods are still bottlenecked by the amount of data transferrable per second for real-time imaging. Without addressing the amount of data transferred, the framerate of plane wave imaging on conventional hardware remains constricted – few works aim to reduce the amount of data gathered despite the restrictions posed by the data bottlenecking. Compressive sensing has been applied to tackle and reduce the samples collected, but it uses a slower, iterative approach unsuited for HiFRUS and required additional hardware implementation at the front-end [5]. Another work that attempts to use neural networks to address the data intake is [6]; however, their framework is limited to B-mode acquisitions through the construction of their neural network. Another earlier work that applies neural networks and tries to reduce channel count is [7], but their network is a post-processing technique without *in vivo* validation.

This paper aims to present a novel approach to reducing the data transfer requirements from the ultrasound probe by half through deep learning interpolation, with a the additional possibility of reducing the probe's physical channel count. By noting that there exist redundancies in the raw radiofrequency (RF) data from the transducer channels from the geometric properties of wave reflection, we hypothesize salient features form when the RF data is stacked channel-wise to form an image, even when some channels are taken away. Because of its effectiveness in similar interpolation tasks, we propose a convolutional encoder-decoder neural network model to be trained on *in vivo* data in order to first learn an encoded representation of the types of the features that exist across channels and then to interpolate missing channels. By splitting the interleaving channels of a 128-channel count probe into input and output pairs for neural network training, our goal is to examine the performance of such a neural network model for both accurate interpolation and image reconstruction.

2 Background Considerations

2.1 Transducer Channel Redundancy

The physical principles underlying pulse-echo ultrasound image formation lends credence to the idea that some of the information in each channel, acquired by a single transducer element on the probe, contain shared information between channels that can be leveraged. Figure 1 shows a model with three transducer elements receiving the reflected signal from a point source – after a plane wave is transmitted from the transducers, the lowermost transducer receives the reflected signal first as it is geometrically the closest to the point source and the uppermost transducer receives the reflected signal last. This is the fundamental principle behind delay-and-sum beamforming for image formation as the total receive and transmit delay is calculated and the channel data is summed. Because the lower, middle, and upper channels are all receiving information from the same source at different times, the information of the middle channel can be inferred from the information for the two neighboring channels.

By noting that there is a salient structure to the reflected echoes across channels, feature extraction type of techniques can potentially be applied through treating the signals from the channels as an $n \times m$ image, where n is the number of samples per channel and m is the number of channels. The expected types of features include lines or arcs appearing across several RF channels. The core idea is that if the middle channel were missing, the neighboring channels can potentially be used to interpolate or reconstruct the missing information through the detected features.

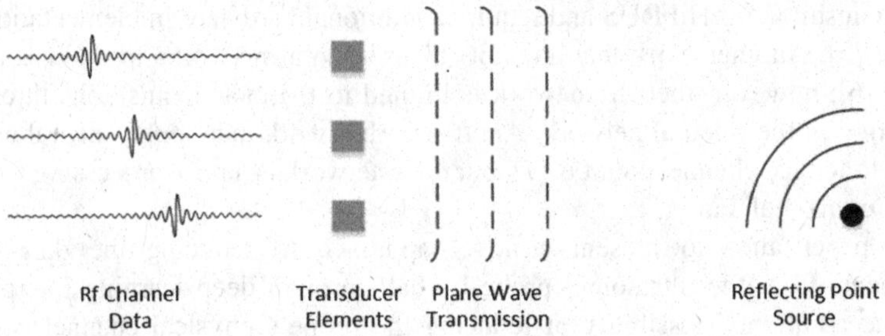

Fig. 1. A simple representation of the physical principles behind plane wave pulse-echo imaging. The transducer elements first emit a plane wave transmission which is reflected by the object of interest. The same transducers receive the reflected waves and convert the acoustic signal into an electrical signal.

2.2 Convolutional Neural Networks

The convolutional neural network (CNN) is a popular tool in the machine learning and pattern recognition fields that has seen much recent success for feature extraction and more [8, 9]. While classic neural networks learn dense connections between individual neurons, CNNs instead learn small convolutional kernels which are applied to images while still creating nonlinearity through the activation function. When trained on images, the kernels will often start learning edge detector types of patterns [9], and, when combined with pooling and upsampling layers, can be used sequentially to form an encoder-decoder architecture [10].

The encoder-decoder deep learning architecture has shown results in literature in other fields where the input and the output have similar spatial characteristics, such as image inpainting or denoising [11]. With a deep learning approach, the ideal is for the encoder to learn a representation of the source in terms of its trained features and the decoder to interpret the representation in a sensible fashion. This is the motivation for attempting this approach on ultrasound RF data stacked to form an image; the encoder learns the geometric features unique to the pulse-echo reflections across channels and the decoder learns to interpret the feature space representation to interpolate the channels that are removed.

3 Neural Network Model

3.1 Architecture

In determining the architecture for the neural network to be used for RF data interpolation, key design considerations included the number of channels that the convolutional kernels needed to capture and how each layer downsamples the representation. The chosen neural network structure used for this paper is depicted in Fig. 2. The first and last layers used a larger kernel size of (6, 6) to try to better encapsulate the expected, curved, geometrical features. While many convolutional encoder-decoder networks use max pooling layers after the convolutional layers, Springenberg et al. has shown in [12] that stride based encoder-decoder structures perform at a comparable level to pooling and upsampling layers without the need to discard information. The neural network structure includes the zero-padding and cropping layers at the start and end of the sequence of layers to transform the data to a clean multiple of 2 as each convolutional layer uses a stride length of 2 in the RF data direction. Additionally, the stride length in the channel direction is 1 – no reduction is performed in the channel-wise direction. Each convolutional layer uses a ReLU activation function to introduce nonlinearity, while the recombination layer required to regenerate the image uses a standard choice of hyperbolic tangent activation function. Because ultrasound is a real-time imaging modality, the total number of layers was limited to minimize the additional computational complexity required for an implementation.

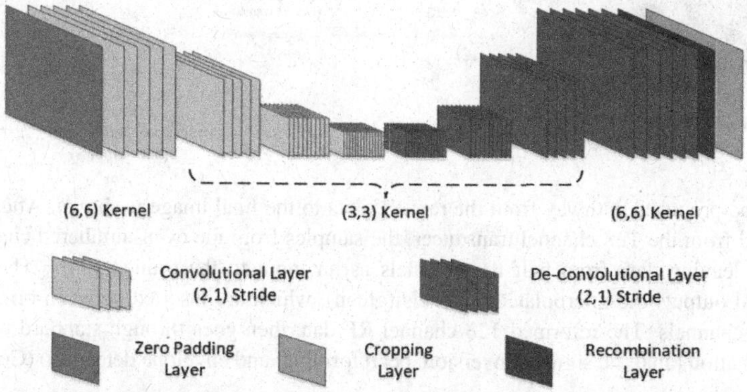

Fig. 2. The encoder-decoder sequential convolutional neural network used for RF data interpolation, with 4 encoding layers and 4 deconvolutional layers. The number of kernels for each encoding layer in order is 18, 24, 36, 48, with the reverse holding for the de-convolutional layers. The input is an image of 64 channels by 500 samples of RF data, as is the output.

3.2 Training and Testing

A total of 2093 instances of *in vivo* human carotid 0° plane wave ultrasound was acquired using an L14-5 linear probe on a SonixTouch (Analogic Ultrasound, Peabody, MA, USA) scanner, with an attached data acquisition board configured for plane wave imaging, from fifteen volunteers over several sessions. Each acquisition contained 128 channels of 3000 samples of RF data from the transducer elements – the center frequency for the RF data was at 5 MHz and the data was acquired at a 40 MHz sampling rate. The odd numbered channels are kept as set of training inputs, and the even numbered channels are left as the training. After examining the frequency spectrum, the fast-time data of each channel was then maximally down-sampled 2x to 1500 samples per channel without aliasing and then the middle 500 samples (imaging depths of 19 mm to 38 mm) were selected for the neural network input and output. The first 500 samples (0 to 19 mm depth) and last 500 samples (38 to 58 mm depth) were unused as they tended to have values in the large and small extremes respectively. Additionally, the geometry of the problem stretches with the distance from the probe, leading to slightly different feature sets at different depths, further motivating limiting the selection from the RF data. The data was then split into 1893 examples for training, with an initial 80-20 validation split for model selection, and 200 examples set aside for testing.

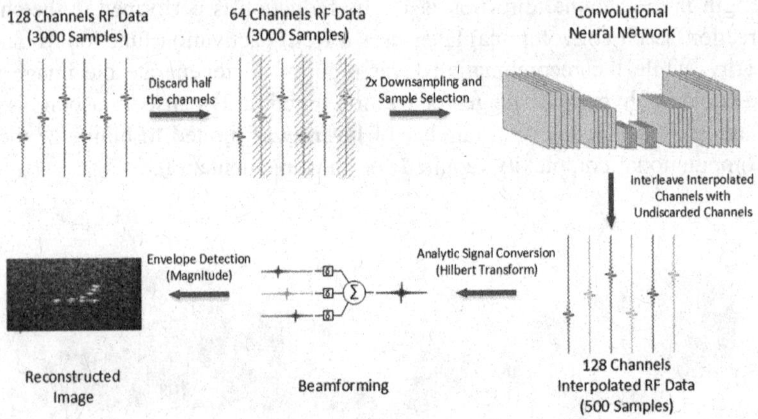

Fig. 3. The proposed pathway from the raw RF data to the final image is shown. After the data is collected from the 128 channel transducer, the samples from the even-numbered channels are discarded, leaving data from half the channels as an input to the trained CNN. The CNN is applied and outputs the interpolated channels (green), which are inserted between original odd-numbered channels. The reformed 128 channel RF data then goes through standard ultrasound image formation (analytic signal conversion, beamforming, and envelope detection) (Color figure online)

The neural network, training, and testing were programmed in Python 3.6.8 using keras with TensorFlow 1.12.0 [13] as the backend and GPU acceleration on an Nvidia GTX 1080 (Nvidia Corporation, Santa Clara, CA, USA). Because the raw data from the probe has inherent signed 12-bit resolution, the data was normalized by a factor of 2048 to bring the values to the range of –1 to 1 before training. The convolutional neural network was trained for 1500 epochs with a batch size of 128 using the Adam optimization algorithm (lr = 0.001, beta_1 = 0.9, beta_2 = 0.999, epsilon = 1e–7) and mean-squared error as the loss function. After training, the algorithm converged to an MSE loss of around 0.01 on the training data and evaluated to a loss of 0.02 on the unseen testing data. The experiments followed the system as shown in Fig. 3 to evaluate the actual performance of the CNN interpolator. To characterize the behavior of the neural network on a known ultrasound phantom, the network was also applied to RF channel data collected from a Multi-Purpose Multi-Tissue Ultrasound Phantom (Computerized Imaging Reference Systems, Inc., Norfolk, VA, USA) to compare the faithfulness of reconstruction from both interpolated and non-interpolated channels. The interpolated RF channels were also compared to the original channels to see if the structure was captured as expected.

4 Results

4.1 Improvement of Reconstructed Images

Figure 4 shows a few 128 × 256 reconstructed images based on RF data from a Multi-Purpose Multi-Tissue Ultrasound Phantom that was set apart from the training and testing data sets. The image reconstructed using all 128 original channels is shown in Fig. 4a, while b, c, and d show the reconstructions based on the 64 odd-numbered channels without interpolation, 128 channels with linearly interpolated interleaved channels, and 128 channels interpolated with the novel method with no retraining or fine tuning, respectively. The reconstruction was performed using a rudimentary

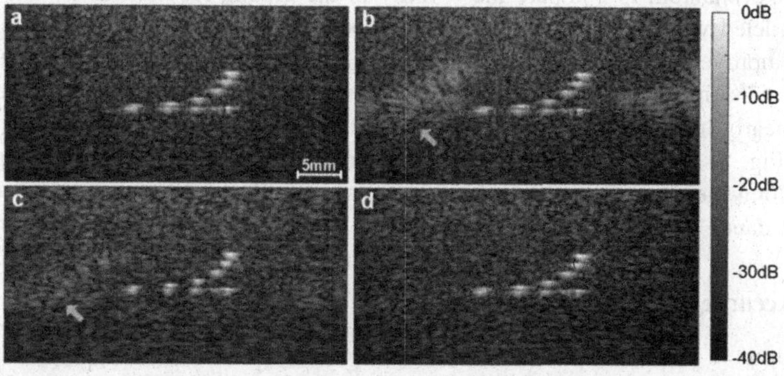

Fig. 4. 128 × 256 reconstructed images of 19.25 mm by 39 mm window using, (a) full 128 channels, (b) 64 channels without interpolation, MSE = 0.0026, (c) 128 channel reconstruction with half interleaved linear interpolated, MSE = 0.0016, (d) 128 channel reconstruction with half interleaved neural network interpolated, MSE = 0.0009. Images displayed on the same logarithm scale for a 40 dB range. Yellow arrows highlight areas with grating lobe artifacts. (Color figure online)

beamformer based on [2] and [4] without advanced apodization or image compounding techniques, and the image is approximately 19.25 mm (axial, top to bottom) by 39 mm (lateral, side to side) in its physical representation. After beamforming, each image was then scaled to the pixel of maximum magnitude and displayed on a log dB scale. The proposed method shows over 50% reduced mean-squared error (calculated before log scaling) on the phantom compared to linear interpolation. It can also be clearly seen that the proposed reconstruction visibly reduces the grating lobes (yellow arrows on Fig. 4), artifacts that arise from the beamforming process in ultrasound due to additive interference when the element pitch is larger than the acoustic wavelength, compared to the other methods.

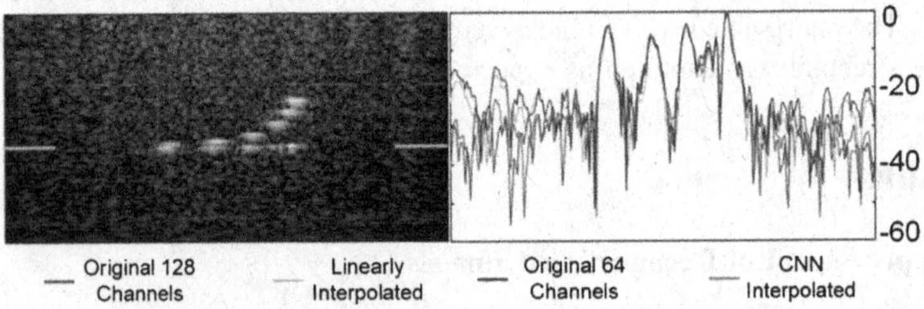

Fig. 5. A slice (axial position shown on left in yellow) taken from the same phantom as in Fig. 4 with dB values on the right. The neural network output and original 128-channel data show 10–15 dB lower grating lobe behavior on the left and right sides of the phantom. (Color figure online)

4.2 Grating Lobe Suppression

Figure 5 takes a slice of the image along the shown line of point sources in the ultrasound phantom to compare the severity of the grating lobe artifacts – the image reconstructed with the channels from the encoder-decoder interpolation shows a 10–15 dB improvement in grating lobe magnitude, comparable to the reconstructions from the full 128 channels (–30 to –35 dB on far left of Fig. 5), over the reconstructions from linearly interpolated and 64-channel non-interpolated data (–15 to –20 dB on far left of Fig. 5). For the neural network-based reconstruction, the level of the grating lobes along the slice is comparable to the image beamformed from the original 128-channel data.

4.3 Accuracy of RF Channel Data

In addition to post-beamformed image-based comparisons, the interpolated RF data was also compared to their corresponding original channels as well as the results from linear interpolation. Figure 6 shows a single channel of RF data taken from the set aside *in vivo* test data, with a window displaying the first 100 samples in additional

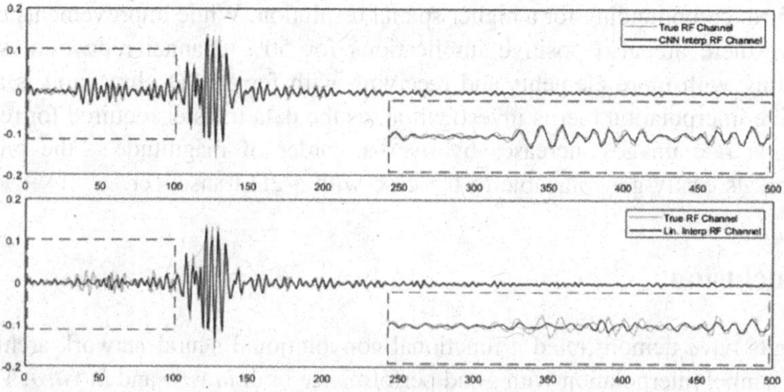

Fig. 6. Comparison of neural network output (top blue) to linear interpolation (bottom blue) for data from a single transducer for an *in vivo* example overlaid with the true RF data (red). Scaled sample values are plotted on the y-axis against sample number on the x-axis. The first hundred samples are expanded in the bottom right (Euclidean distance of 0.074 and 0.137 respectively) (Color figure online)

detail. Visually, the figure shows for this channel that the neural network interpolation follows the pattern of the original RF data more closely than linear interpolation, particularly in the first 100 samples examined (imaging depths of 19.25 mm to 23.1 mm).

5 Discussion

From our results, images reconstructed from encoder-decoder interpolated RF channels show visual improvement in clarity and grating lobe reduction while only using information from half the transducer channels. Based on the RF channel comparison, the neural network appears successful in capturing features with smaller magnitude in the RF data, which may play a role in the reduction of the grating lobes. Despite the convolutional neural network being trained only on human carotid data for a small set of depths, the performance of the network evaluated on the phantom lends credence to the idea that the network is indeed capturing the geometric details. Current directions involve applying the network on RF data at all depths using a single, related, network architecture; however, training different networks for different depths, with possible time gain compensation applied, is another approach with physical justifications.

Although the convolutional encoder-decoder network demonstrates viability, there remain many improvements that can be made. There may be benefit in training with simulated RF data through randomly generated examples in order to capture the most geometric variation. Transfer learning can also be applied to the network to potentially better characterize the network for imaging different areas of the body; however, in general the neural network relies more on the acquisition setup (transducer pitch, imaging frequency) than on the type of input data. A further avenue for improvement would be to increase the number of plane wave transmission angles used for the image and perform compounding for a higher spatial resolution. While improvements can still be made, there are also positive implications for 50% channel reduction, such as transmitting with more elements and receiving with fewer. 3D ultrasound is another area where interpolation merits investigation, as the data transfer required for real-time high frame rate images increases by over an order of magnitude – the presented framework is easily generalizable to the case with a 2D transducer.

6 Conclusion

Our results have demonstrated a functional convolutional neural network architecture for RF channel interpolation with good performance both *in vivo* and *in vitro*. The data carried between RF channels has enough redundancy for a deep learning approach to learn the appropriate features across the channels. The viability of using interpolated channels for plane wave ultrasound image reconstruction has important implications for future work, whether in reducing the physical hardware by removing channels or simply cutting the data transferring in half. As ultrasonics moves more towards real-time 3D imaging, the ability to faithfully reconstruct images based on interpolated data has even more relevance.

References

1. Garcia, D., Tarnec, L., Muth, S., Montagnon, E., Poree, J., Cloutier, G.: Stolt's f-k migration for plane wave ultrasound imaging. IEEE Trans. Ultrason. Ferroelectr. Freq. Control **60**, 1853–1867 (2013)
2. Montaldo, G., Tanter, M., Bercoff, J., Benech, N., Fink, M.: Coherent plane-wave compounding for very high frame rate ultrasonography and transient elastography. IEEE Trans. Ultrason. Ferroelectr. Freq. Control **56**, 489–506 (2009)
3. Boni, E., Yu, A., Freear, S., Jensen, J., Tortoli, P.: Ultrasound open platforms for next-generation imaging technique development. IEEE Trans. Ultrason. Ferroelectr. Freq. Control **65**, 1078–1092 (2018)
4. Yiu, B., Tsang, I., Yu, A.: GPU-based beamformer: fast realization of plane wave compounding and synthetic aperture imaging. IEEE Trans. Ultrason. Ferroelectr. Freq. Control **58**, 1698–1705 (2011)
5. Liebgott, H., Prost, R., Friboulet, D.: Pre-beamformed RF signal reconstruction in medical ultrasound using compressive sensing. Ultrasonics **53**, 525–533 (2013)
6. Yoon, Y., Khan, S., Huh, J., Ye, J.: Efficient B-mode ultrasound image reconstruction from sub-sampled RF data using deep learning. IEEE Trans. Med. Imaging **38**, 325–336 (2019)
7. Carotenuto, R., Sabbi, G., Pappalardo, M.: Spatial resolution enhancement of ultrasound images using neural networks. IEEE Trans. Ultrason. Ferroelectr. Freq. Control **49**, 1039–1049 (2002)
8. Zhou, B., Lapedriza, A., Xiao, J., Torralba, A., Oliva, A.: Learning deep features for scene recognition using places database. In: Advances in Neural Information Processing Systems, pp. 487–495 (2014)
9. Krizhevsky, A., Sutskever, I., Hinton, G.E.: Imagenet classification with deep convolutional neural networks. In: Advances in Neural Information Processing Systems, pp. 1097–1105 (2012)

10. Badrinarayanan, V., Kendall, A., Cipolla, R.: SegNet: a deep convolutional encoder-decoder architecture for image segmentation. IEEE Trans. Pattern Anal. Mach. Intell. **39**, 2481–2495 (2017)
11. Xie, J., Xu, L., Chen, E.: Image denoising and inpainting with deep neural networks. In: Advances in Neural Information Processing Systems, pp. 341–349 (2012)
12. Springenberg, J.T., Dosovitskiy, A., Brox, T., Riedmiller, M.: Striving for Simplicity: The All Convolutional Net. arXiv preprint arXiv:1412.6806 (2014)
13. Abadi, M., et al.: Tensorflow: a system for large-scale machine learning. In: 12th {USENIX} Symposium on Operating Systems Design and Implementation ({OSDI} 2016), pp. 265–283 (2016)

Segmentation of Aliasing Artefacts in Ultrasound Color Flow Imaging Using Convolutional Neural Networks

Hassan Nahas(✉), Takuro Ishii, Adrian Chee, Billy Yiu, and Alfred Yu

Research Institute for Aging and Department of Electrical and Computer Engineering, University of Waterloo, Waterloo, ON N2L3G1, Canada
hassan.nahas@uwaterloo.ca

Abstract. Color flow imaging is a biomedical ultrasound modality used to visualize blood flow dynamics in the blood vessels, which are correlated with cardiovascular function and pathology. This is however done through a pulsed echo sensing mechanism and thus flow measurements can be corrupted by aliasing artefacts, hindering its application. While various methods have attempted to address these artefacts, there is still demand for a robust and flexible solution, particularly at the stage of identifying the aliased regions in the imaging view. In this paper, we investigate the application of convolutional neural networks to segment aliased regions in color flow images due to their strength in translation-invariant learning of complex features. Relevant ultrasound features including phase shifts, speckle images and optical flow were generated from ultrasound data obtained from anthropomorphic flow models. The investigated neural networks all showed strong performance in terms of precision, recall and intersection over union while revealing the important ultrasound features that improved detection. This study paves the way for sophisticated dealiasing algorithms in color flow imaging.

Keywords: Ultrasound imaging · Color flow imaging · Convolutional neural networks · Deep learning · Cardiovascular · Doppler · Aliasing

1 Introduction

Color flow imaging (CFI) [1], a modality of biomedical ultrasound, is a color coded method for visualization of flow *in vivo* using Doppler principles. It has long been used as a diagnostic tool for conditions such as stenosis and monitoring plaque formation by detecting abnormal flow such as jets, turbulence and flow reversal [1, 2]. Moreover, CFI can be integrated with recent innovations such as high frame rate ultrasound and vector doppler [3] to analyze highly transient phenomena [4] and allow quantitative analysis [5].

One of the limitations in CFI is the presence of aliasing artefacts [6] due to the underlying pulsed echo sensing mechanism. Aliasing corrupts measurements of fast flow and this in turn hinders the analysis of complex hemodynamics. Aliasing is

F. Karray et al. (Eds.): ICIAR 2019, LNCS 11663, pp. 452–461, 2019.
https://doi.org/10.1007/978-3-030-27272-2_40

especially problematic when imaging vortices in the heart [7] and jetting in conditions of stenosis [8], where it makes the visualization of flow very challenging, thereby impacting diagnosis. Consequentially, it is imperative that aliasing artefacts are eliminated in order to study complex flow using CFI.

To address aliasing artefacts in CFI, a common approach is to segment the aliased region, then correct it by phase unwrapping to achieve smooth flow [9]. To this end, Shahin et al. [10] employed a fuzzy logic approach to identify aliased regions based on velocity and spatial information while Muth et al. [11] developed an unsupervised method with region growing segmentation followed by the optimization of a flow continuity criteria. These methods have succeeded in stationary scenarios, but segmentation failed in conditions of complex flow and low signal-to-noise ratio: particularly the scenarios where aliasing is most impactful. Alternatively, a staggered transmission sequence can be used but this can complicate ultrasound processing downstream such as clutter filtering [12]. Consequentially, a robust method to segment aliasing is needed as a basis for reliable dealiasing algorithms.

On the other hand, robust segmentation may be achieved using Convolutional Neural Networks (CNN). Indeed, Long et al. [13] demonstrated that fully convolutional neural networks can be used for semantic segmentation on a variety of datasets. More specifically, one class of CNN architectures known as encoder-decoders [14] have particularly excelled in this area. This comes from the architecture's ability to extract and combine translation-invariant patterns at multiple scales then refining them to achieve high resolution segmentation. This is appropriate for aliasing artefacts, which can form complex patterns with varying sizes and orientations. Consequentially, we hypothesize that an encoder-decoder can learn to segment aliasing artefacts in Color Flow images.

In this paper, we investigate the applicability of the encoder-decoder architecture for aliasing segmentation in CFI. To our knowledge, this is the first application of CNNs towards a robust segmentation of aliasing in CFI. Therefore, this investigation involved two stages: First, different relevant ultrasound processing steps were implemented. These were then compared on a custom encoder-decoder architecture tuned for a blood flow-related application. We shall report the most effective processing pipeline and experimental evidence that the encoder-decoder can segment aliasing in a carotid bifurcation model. The findings of this study will pave the way for more comprehensive deep-learning methods to eliminate aliasing in CFI.

2 Methodology

2.1 Strategic Overview

To meet the objectives of this study effectively, our approach to deep learning must be guided by the mechanisms underlying Aliasing. Namely, aliasing occurs when flow is too fast such that it exceeds the Nyquist limit, resulting in a wrap around, and showing up as inconsistent flow regions in the CFI. For example, obstruction at the carotid bifurcation (see Fig. 1a) leads to a flow jet where velocities are so high that the body of the jet phase wraps, suggesting incorrectly that flow is going the opposite direction (see Fig. 1b). The desired segmentation (see Fig. 1c) should therefore determine the pixels affected by this corruption.

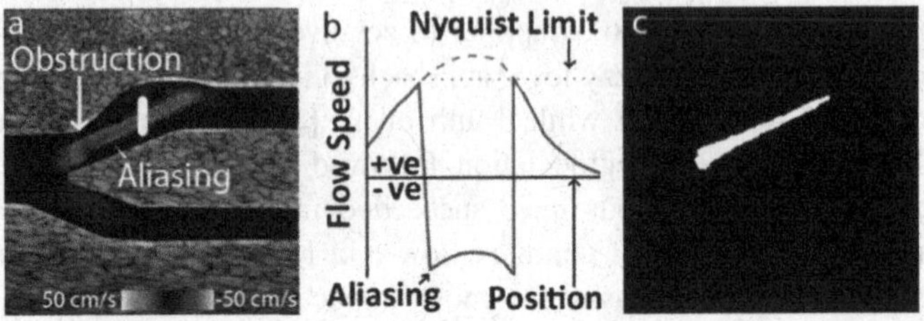

Fig. 1. Illustration of aliasing in CFI: (a) CFI with aliasing in the jet. (b) flow profile across the white line in (a) corrupted by aliasing. (c) desired segmentation of aliasing artefacts.

But while aliasing is predominantly a CFI issue, other imaging modes may compliment the CFI and allow more effective deep learning. Accordingly, we devised three approaches involving different combinations of three ultrasound image modes. The following subsections will detail the relevant imaging modes, how our CNN model was designed and how the model was trained and tested.

2.2 Imaging Modes and Configurations

Three Imaging Modes Were Investigated.

Color Flow Images. One of the most obvious markers for aliasing is the presence of sharp boundaries indicating flow inconsistency, therefore CFIs are crucial inputs for aliasing segmentation. CFI can be produced from beamformed ultrasound data using lag-one autocorrelation, after filtering to remove clutter (tissue).

Speckle Images. Recent dealiasing algorithms [15] have made use of speckle patterns (see Fig. 2b): interference of reflections from multiple scatterers in the flow region that

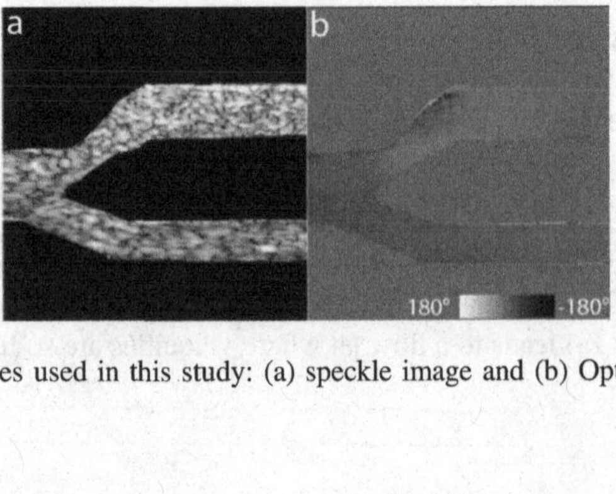

Fig. 2. Imaging modes used in this study: (a) speckle image and (b) Optical flow angle using Flownet2.0.

can be tracked to indicate flow motion. Speckle images can be produced from beamformed data through clutter filtering, envelope detection and log compression.

Optical Flow Angle. Motivated by the relevance of interframe motion of speckle patterns to aliasing segmentation, we investigated a direct approach by incorporating speckle-based optical flow as an imaging mode. While many methods exist for optical flow, we chose Flownet2.0 [16] for its performance and ability to connect with the rest of the deep learning module, allowing global optimization. Training Flownet2.0 in ultrasound images was beyond our scope and, thus, the weights were obtained from the original contribution [16]. Initial results showed the magnitude of flow predicted by Flownet2.0 was of low quality so only the optical flow angle (see Fig. 2b) was used.

Dataset Configuration. As per the overview, the three imaging modes relevant to aliasing were then combined to form three combinations (see Table 1) for testing. Since aliasing is primarily a CFI problem, all tested combinations included the CFI. To investigate the role of speckle motion in the aliasing problem, two further combinations were considered. One combination included two time-consecutive speckle images with the encoder-decoder expected to extract the relevant features. The final combination instead included the optical flow angle derived by Flownet2.0.

Table 1. Imaging mode combinations investigated in this study

Imaging mode combination	Channel count	Description
CFI	1	Normalized CFI only
CFI + speckle imaging	3	Normalized CFI; speckle image at the current frame; speckle image at a previous frame
CFI + optical flow angle	2	Normalized CFI; optical flow angle derived from flownet2.0

2.3 Network Architecture

Motivation. Having determined the relevant inputs, a custom encoder-decoder architecture was designed specifically for this study. Traditional encoder-decoder architectures such as SegNet [14] typically come with many layers. On the other hand, multiple dataset configurations had to be compared in this study, therefore the training time had to be fast. Consequentially, we devised a relatively more compact encoder-decoder for rapid training and testing.

Network Design. Figure 2 illustrates the general architecture of the neural network. First, a set of three convolutional layers + max pooling (depicted as blue + orange) were employed to extract translation-invariant features at three scales. This was then followed by another convolutional layer to process the features at that scale. Finally, three deconvolutional layers (depicted as green) were used to increase the resolution of segmentation. The number of layers and kernel sizes were chosen to produce an effective receptive field of 34 × 34, which was appropriate as the vessels used in this study were around 40 pixels wide. The filter number was increased throughout the encoder to match the increasingly complex patterns being encoded.

To match the three dataset configurations with different channel inputs, three encoder-decoder models were constructed where the filter number in the whole network was proportional to the number of input features in the combination to match the increased complexity that comes with processing more channels, denotes as i in Fig. 3.

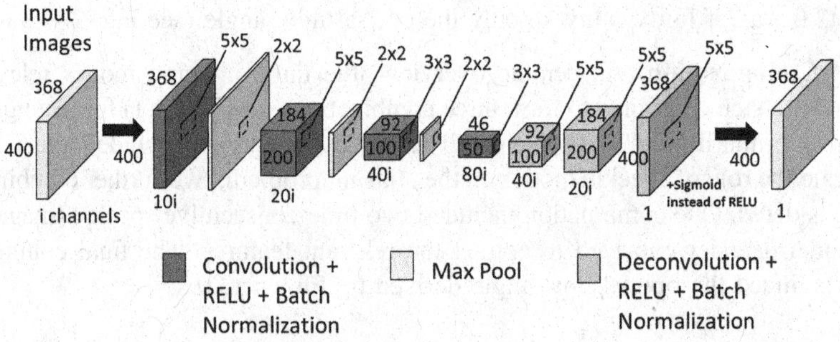

Fig. 3. An illustration of the simple encoder-decoder neural network architecture used. All layers were activated by a REctified Linear Unit (RELU) except the last layer which was activated by sigmoid activation layer. The number of filters in each layer was proportional to the number of channels, i = 1, 2, 3 depending on the dataset used

2.4 Experimental Data Generation and Training Parameters

Imaging Setup. To acquire the datasets, we utilized our research imaging platform [17]. The scanner (SonixTouch; Analogic Ultrasound, Peabody, MA, USA), combined with a custom acquisition board [17] and a L14-5 linear array transducer (Analogic Ultrasound), was configured for high frame rate ultrasound imaging and used in this study with the same imaging parameters (Imaging frequency = 5 MHz, emission type = plane wave, pulse duration = 3 cycles, transmission angle = −10° and pulse repetition frequency = 3333 Hz).

Training Set. We utilized our novel *in vitro* flow model fabrication process [18, 19] to generate data. For training, we required a dataset that contains flow with aliasing but in a variety of orientations and formations. To that end, the training datasets was acquired using the spiral model [18] (see Fig. 4a), which contains flow in all directions within the imaging view and was therefore expected to improve the generalizability of learning. Flow was chosen to be constant at 3 ml/s, to produce aliasing with at most one cycle (see Fig. 4b).

To increase the variety of aliasing artefacts, the original series for training was also down sampled by a factor of 2 along the imaging time axis, effectively reducing the PRF and producing more prominent aliasing. Data augmentation (horizontal and vertical flipping, rotation <180̊, scales: 25%–300%) was also applied to produce different patterns of aliasing. The training set ultimately contained 7000 samples where each sample was a 400 × 368 image at 0.1 mm/pixel.

Test Set. To produce the test set, the same imaging setup was used to image a second model, an anthropomorphic wall-less carotid bifurcation model based on the work by Chee *et al.* [19] (see Fig. 4c). This model possesses flow in a clinically relevant setting, with jets that are often aliased during imaging (see Fig. 4d) and is sufficiently distinct from the training set. Flow was configured to an anthropomorphic pulsatile waveform at 72 beats/min with peak flow at 5 ml/s to ensure the occurrence of aliasing artefacts but with no more than one cycle.

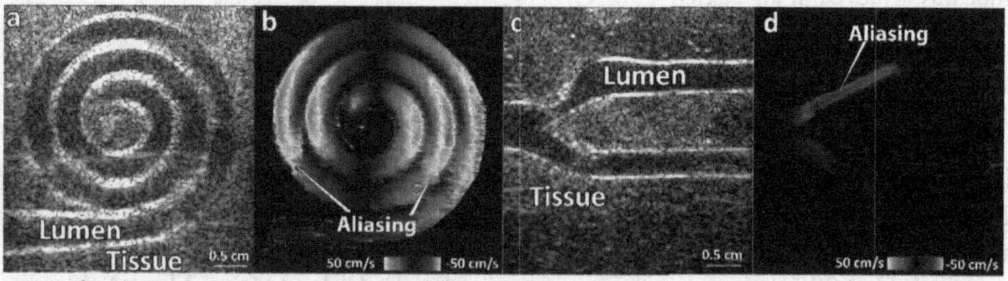

Fig. 4. Ultrasound scans of the flow models used in this study. (a) spiral model US brightness mode image, (b) spiral model normalized CFI map, (c) carotid bifurcation model US brightness mode image and (d) carotid bifurcation model normalized CFI map.

Training Parameters. To account for the effects of randomization in model training, 30 instance models were trained for each feature combination using an Adam Optimizer with default parameters using random initializations, for 5 epochs with a batch size of 8. Binary cross-entropy was the chosen loss as pixels could be segmented into one of two classes. For training and evaluation, the ground truths for the training and testing sets were generated manually.

3 Results

3.1 Aliasing Segmentation Successfully Achieved on the Test Set

The first observation in this study was that all methods provided segmentation results matching the ground truth. To illustrate the achieved segmentation, a sample at systole near the jet region in the carotid bifurcation model where aliasing is most prominent is shown in Fig. 5 for a random model from each method with errors color coded. Errors were most prevalent at the boundaries of the aliasing artefacts, but the network largely matched the aliasing boundaries.

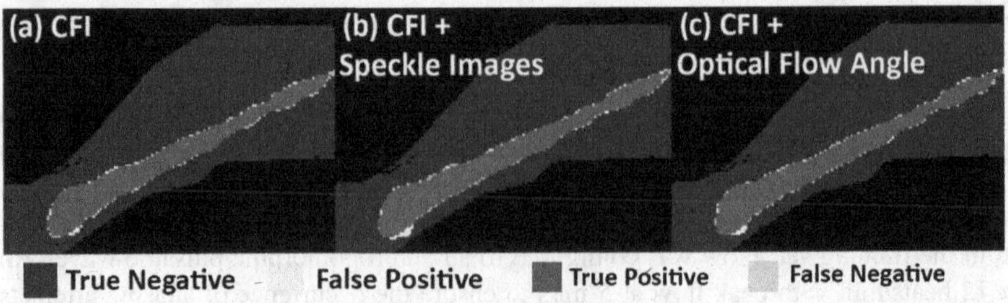

Fig. 5. Results of the three methods applied on the testing sets at systole. (a) CFI only. (b) CFI + speckle imaging. (c) CFI + optical flow angle. Segmentation matching the ground truth was achieved in all cases.

3.2 CFI + Optical Flow Angle Method Scored Highest in All Evaluation Metrics

The average performance of the three methods across thirty models was evaluated on the carotid bifurcation using precision, recall and Intersection-over-Union (IoU). The mean and standard deviations are shown in Table 2. While all three models had an average IoU at 90% or greater, the performance for the CFI + Optical Flow Angle was the highest across all metrics, with IoUs reaching 96%. Interestingly, the CFI + Blood speckle images method's performance was rather comparable to the CFI only method in all metrics, albeit with reduced variance in the precision.

Table 2. Evaluation of 30 models for each of the three experiments on the carotid bifurcation model in terms of mean metrics ± standard deviation. The CFI + optical flow angle method scored the highest.

Imaging mode combination	Precision (%)	Recall (%)	IoU (%)
CFI	88 ± 9	91 ± 6	90 ± 4
CFI + speckle imaging	91 ± 4	90 ± 6	91 ± 3
CFI + optical flow angle	94 ± 6	94 ± 3	94 ± 3

4 Discussion

4.1 Summary of Contributions

In this study, we have presented a consistent Doppler aliasing detection framework by employing a convolutional neural network with encoder-decoder structure. This is the first time that has been done using CNNs. The achieved segmentation can be further combined with existing aliasing correction methods to achieve robust performance dealiasing for CFI. Furthermore, we were able to identify the features relevant to this problem by applying the same architecture to different feature sets.

4.2 The Encoder-Decoder Can Learn Aliasing Segmentation from CFI and Optical Flow Angles

The encoder-decoder model was able to achieve strong segmentation in this study by only utilizing the information in the CFI. This suggests that the encoder-decoder was able to identify spatial features in CFI that correspond to aliasing and that the CFI itself can be sed to predict aliasing with good reliability. This is plausible for single cycle aliasing in the absence of turbulence as was the case in the carotid bifurcation model. These findings are also consistent with the success of the region growing-based segmentation of aliasing artifacts in CFI maps [11].

More interestingly, the encoder-decoder was able to extract the interaction between the CFI and optical flow angle for aliasing segmentation, achieving the highest evaluation metrics using the two imaging modes. This confirms the relevance of speckle motion to the problem of aliasing as previous studies have shown [15] and that convolutional layers are able to utilize this information when presented as optical flow.

Interestingly, this increased performance was not achieved by incorporating the speckle images as additional channels to our encoder-decoder. This may be attributed to the increased complexity of the problem when expecting the network to derive inter-frame variations from the speckle images. In particular, the encoder-decoder structure used here might have been too simple for the problem of optical flow extraction. Flownet2.0 [16] includes difference layers between the consecutive frames along with skip connections for refinement, making it more suitable for optical flow extraction than the simple encoder-decoder model. This probably explains the superior performance of the CFI + optical flow angle method.

4.3 Future Work: Beyond Single Cycle Aliasing

The limitations of this study emerge from the relative simplicity of the aliasing artefacts included in this study, whereas aliasing may include multiple cycles and sharp pressure gradients may naturally exist without aliasing. One potential solution is to incorporate higher order aliasing artefacts in the training and testing sets, with the expectation that the neural network model would be able to learn the more complex problem. Alternatively, an iterative method may be explored where aliasing artefacts are segmented, and phase unwrapped one cycle at a time until no more aliasing artefacts are found.

5 Conclusions

Aliasing is a pressing issue in flow estimation using Doppler techniques, particularly in conditions such as stenosis when flow reaches high speeds or in cardiac imaging where a reduced PRF may be necessary. With the novel aliasing segmentation techniques developed here, single cycle aliasing artefacts may be corrected to extend the range of measurable flow speeds; this approach readily extends to more advanced Doppler techniques such as vector flow imaging. Finally, as the first application of CNN's to aliasing in biomedical ultrasound, this study paves the way for more sophisticated methods capable of addressing more complex aliasing situations using deep learning, by highlighting the relevant ultrasound features and neural network design principles.

References

1. Merritt, C.R.B.: Doppler color flow imaging. J. Clin. Ultrasound **15**, 591–597 (1987). https://doi.org/10.1002/jcu.1870150904
2. Foley, W.D., Erickson, S.J.: Color doppler flow imaging. Am. J. Roentgenol. **156**, 3–13 (1991). https://doi.org/10.2214/ajr.156.1.1898567
3. Jensen, J.A., Nikolov, S.I., Yu, A.C., Garcia, D.: Ultrasound vector flow imaging-part II: parallel systems IEEE transactions on ultrasonics. Ferroelectr. Freq. Control **63**, 1722–1732 (2016)
4. Cikes, M., Tong, L., Sutherland, G.R., D'hooge, J.: Ultrafast cardiac ultrasound imaging: technical principles, applications, and clinical benefits. JACC Cardiovasc. Imag. **7**, 812–823 (2014). https://doi.org/10.1016/j.jcmg.2014.06.004
5. Hansen, K.L., et al.: Intra-operative vector flow imaging using ultrasound of the ascending aorta among 40 patients with normal, stenotic and replaced aortic valves. Ultrasound Med. Biol. **42**, 2414–2422 (2016)
6. Terslev, L., Diamantopoulos, A.P., Dohn, U.M., Schmidt, W.A., Torp-Pedersen, S.: Settings and artefacts relevant for doppler ultrasound in large vessel vasculitis. Arthritis Research and Therapy. 19 (2017). 167-017-1374-1
7. Mehregan, F., et al.: Doppler vortography: a color doppler approach to quantification of intraventricular blood flow vortices. Ultrasound Med. Biol. **40**, 210–221 (2014)
8. Hansen, K.L., Moller-Sorensen, H., Kjaergaard, J., Jensen, M.B., Jensen, J.A., Nielsen, M. B.: Aortic valve stenosis increases helical flow and flow complexity: a study of intra-operative cardiac vector flow imaging. Ultrasound Med. Biol. **43**, 1607–1617 (2017)
9. Yiu, B.Y.S., Lai, S.S.M., Yu, A.C.H.: Vector projectile imaging: time-resolved dynamic visualization of complex flow patterns. Ultrasound Med. Biol. **40**, 2295–2309 (2014). https://doi.org/10.1016/j.ultrasmedbio.2014.03.014
10. Shahin, A., Ménard, M., Eboueya, M.: Cooperation of fuzzy segmentation operators for correction aliasing phenomenon in 3D color doppler imaging. Artif. Intell. Med. **19**, 121–154 (2000). https://doi.org/10.1016/S0933-3657(00)00042-7
11. Muth, S., Dort, S., Sebag, I.A., Blais, M.J., Garcia, D.: Unsupervised dealiasing and denoising of color-doppler data. Med. Image Anal. **15**, 577–588 (2011)
12. Udesen, J., Nikolov, S., Jensen, J. A.: A simple method to reduce aliasing artifacts in color flow mode imaging. In: 2005 IEEE Ultrasonics Symposium, vol. 2, pp. 1352–1355 (2005). https://doi.org/10.1109/ultsym.2005.1603104
13. Long, J., Shelhamer, E., Darrell, T.: Fully convolutional networks for semantic segmentation. In: 2015 IEEE Conference on Computer Vision and Pattern Recognition (CVPR), pp. 3431–3440 (2015). https://doi.org/10.1109/cvpr.2015.7298965
14. Badrinarayanan, V., Kendall, A., Cipolla, R.: SegNet: a deep convolutional encoder-decoder architecture for image segmentation. IEEE Trans. Pattern Anal. Mach. Intell. **39**, 2481–2495 (2017). https://doi.org/10.1109/TPAMI.2016.2644615
15. Ekroll, I.K., Avdal, J., Swillens, A., Torp, H., Lovstakken, L.: An extended least squares method for aliasing-resistant vector velocity estimation. IEEE Trans. Ultrason. Ferroelectr. Freq. Control **63**, 1745–1757 (2016)

16. Ilg, E., Mayer, N., Saikia, T., Keuper, M., Dosovitskiy, A., Brox, T.: FlowNet 2.0: evolution of optical flow estimation with deep networks (2016). arXiv:1612.01925
17. Cheung, C.C.P., et al.: Multi-channel pre-beamformed data acquisition system for research on advanced ultrasound imaging methods. IEEE Trans. Ultrason. Ferroelectr. Freq. Control **59**, 243–253 (2012). https://doi.org/10.1109/TUFFC.2012.2184
18. You, B.Y.S., Yu, A.C.H.: Spiral flow phantom for ultrasound flow imaging experimentation. IEEE Trans. Ultrason. Ferroelectr. Freq. Control **64**, 1840–1848 (2017). https://doi.org/10.1109/TUFFC.2017.2762860
19. Chee, A.J.Y., Ho, C.K., You, B.Y.S., Yu, A.C.H.: Walled carotid bifurcation phantoms for imaging investigations of vessel wall motion and blood flow dynamics. IEEE Trans. Ultrason. Ferroelectr. Freq. Control **63**, 1852–1864 (2016). https://doi.org/10.1109/TUFFC.2016.2591946

Automatic Frame Selection Using MLP Neural Network in Ultrasound Elastography

Abdelrahman Zayed(✉) and Hassan Rivaz

Department of Electrical and Computer Engineering, PERFORM Centre, Concordia University, Montreal, QC H3G 1M8, Canada
a_zayed@encs.concordia.ca, hrivaz@ece.concordia.ca

Abstract. Ultrasound elastography estimates the mechanical properties of the tissue from two Radio-Frequency (RF) frames collected before and after tissue deformation due to an external or internal force. This work focuses on strain imaging in quasi-static elastography, where the tissue undergoes slow deformations and strain images are estimated as a surrogate for elasticity modulus. The quality of the strain image depends heavily on the underlying deformation, and even the best strain estimation algorithms cannot estimate a good strain image if the underlying deformation is not suitable. Herein, we introduce a new method for tracking the RF frames and selecting automatically the best possible pair. We achieve this by decomposing the axial displacement image into a linear combination of principal components (which are calculated offline) multiplied by their corresponding weights. We then use the calculated weights as the input feature vector to a multi-layer perceptron (MLP) classifier. The output is a binary decision, either 1 which refers to good frames, or 0 which refers to bad frames. Our MLP model is trained on *in-vivo* dataset and tested on different datasets of both *in-vivo* and phantom data. Results show that by using our technique, we would be able to achieve higher quality strain images compared to the traditional methods of picking up pairs that are 1, 2 or 3 frames apart. The training phase of our algorithm is computationally expensive and takes few hours, but it is only done once. The testing phase chooses the optimal pair of frames in only 1.9 ms.

Keywords: Ultrasound elastography · Frame selection · Multi-Layer Perceptron (MLP) classifier · Neural networks · Principal component analysis (PCA)

1 Introduction

Ultrasound elastography is a branch of tissue characterization that aims to determine the stiffness of the tissue. Elastography has a significant potential

This research was funded by Richard and Edith Strauss Foundation.

F. Karray et al. (Eds.): ICIAR 2019, LNCS 11663, pp. 462–472, 2019.
https://doi.org/10.1007/978-3-030-27272-2_41

in improving both detection and guiding surgical treatment of cancer tumors since tumors have higher stiffness values compared to the surrounding tissue [1]. Elastography can be broadly divided into dynamic and quasi-static elastography [2], where the former deals with faster deformations in the tissue such that dynamics of motion should be considered. In this paper, we focus on quasi-static elastography, and in particular, quasi-static strain imaging where the final goal is to estimate strain images. In quasi-static elastography, tissue deformations are slow and therefore motion dynamics can be ignored.

In spite of the wide range of applications that quasi-static elastography has, it is highly user-dependent, which has hindered its widespread use. A pure axial compression yields higher quality strain images compared to a compression that has both in-plane and out-of-plane displacements. Therefore, the user needs to be highly skilled in axially deforming the tissue. Even for highly skilled users, some organs are hard to reach and the probe needs to be held in angles and directions that make imaging yet more challenging. Therefore, it has become crucial to develop a method for selecting the frames that result in strain images of high quality.

In order to make the strain image quality independent of the experience the user has in applying purely axial compression, Hiltawsky et al. [3] developed a freehand applicator that can apply purely axial force regardless of the user's experience. The transducer could be put on a fixed surface moving vertically in the range of 1 to 2 mm.

Jiang et al. [4] worked on frame selection by defining a quality metric for performance assessment and maximizing it. This metric depends on the normalized cross correlation (NCC) between Radio-Frequency (RF) frames and the NCC between their corresponding strain images.

Another approach by Foroughi et al. [5] used an external tracker that gives complete information about the location of the RF frame at the time of being produced, where frames collected from the same plane are selected. Among the selected frames, they only chose some of them according to a defined cost function that maximized axial compression.

Although the previously mentioned approaches showed an improvement over the traditional way of picking up RF frames while maintaining a fixed gap between them, they also have some drawbacks, such as the need for an external mechanical applicator [3] or an external tracking device [5]. Other approaches such as [4] need to calculate the strain before determining whether the pair of frames is good or not, so we can't use it in real-time applications, especially when we have a search range for finding good frames.

Herein, we introduce a novel real-time method for determining good RF frames used to obtain high-quality strain images, without the need of any external hardware. In the training phase, we calculate a set of principal components for quasi-static elastography. In the test phase, we develop a fast technique to find any compression as a weighted sum of those principal components. We then develop a Multi-Layer Perceptron (MLP) Neural Network to classify each pair of RF data as suitable or unsuitable for elastography.

2 Methodology

Let two RF frames I_1 and I_2 be collected before and after some deformation in the tissue. Our goal is to determine whether or not they are suitable for strain estimation. However, developing a classifier that takes the RF frames as an input and outputs a binary decision is not practical, as the number of samples in each RF frame is approximately one million, and therefore, a large network with a powerful GPU is required [6,7]. To solve the problem, we calculate N principal components that describe the axial displacement as the tissue deforms. These principal components are represented by $\mathbf{b}_1$ to $\mathbf{b}_N$. Figure 1 shows some of these principal components learned from real experiments. We then calculate a coarse estimation of the axial displacement that occurred to the pixels between the two frames using Dynamic Programming (DP) [8], where we only get an integer value of the axial displacement. Due to the computational complexity of DP, we don't run it on the whole RF image, it is only run on a very small number of RF lines to get their displacement. After that we decompose the displacement into a linear weighted combination of the principal components that we computed offline. The resulting weight vector corresponds in a one-to-one relationship with the displacement image, but it has a lower dimensionality, which means that we can use it as the input to a multi-layer perceptron (MLP) classifier.

2.1 Feature Extraction

Let the dimensions of each of the RF frames I_1 and I_2 be $m \times l$, where m refers to the number of samples in an RF line and l is the number of RF lines. We start by choosing p equidistant RF lines (where $p \ll l$), then we run DP to get their integer displacement values, resulting in K estimates (where $K = m \times p$). We then form a K-dimensional vector $\mathbf{c}$ that has the displacement estimates of only a few sparse points out of the total $m \times l$ that we have in the RF image. In the next step, we form the matrix $\mathbf{A}$ such that

$$\mathbf{A} = \begin{bmatrix} \mathbf{b}_1(q_1) & \mathbf{b}_2(q_1) & \mathbf{b}_3(q_1) & \dots & \mathbf{b}_N(q_1) \\ \mathbf{b}_1(q_2) & \mathbf{b}_2(q_2) & \mathbf{b}_3(q_2) & \dots & \mathbf{b}_N(q_2) \\ \dots & \dots & \dots & \dots & \dots \\ \mathbf{b}_1(q_K) & \mathbf{b}_2(q_K) & \mathbf{b}_3(q_K) & \dots & \mathbf{b}_N(q_K) \end{bmatrix} \tag{1}$$

where q_1 to q_K refer to the 2D coordinates of our K sparse points chosen along the p RF lines. We then solve the optimization equation below:

$$\hat{\mathbf{w}} = \arg\min_{\mathbf{w}} ||\mathbf{A}\mathbf{w} - \mathbf{c}|| \tag{2}$$

This means that the linear combination of the N principal components multiplied by the weight vector $\mathbf{w} = (w_1, \dots, w_N)^T$ would result in the displacement image with the minimum sum-of-squared error. Algorithm 1 summarizes the procedure for feature extraction.

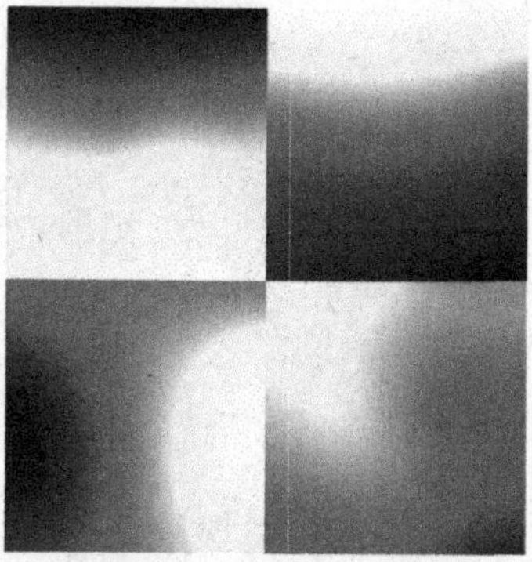

Fig. 1. Principal components of in-plane axial displacement learned from both *in-vivo* and phantom experiments. Top row represent desirable axial deformation principal components.

Algorithm 1

1: **procedure**
2: Choose p equidistant RF lines
3: Run DP to get the integer axial displacement of the p RF lines
4: Solve Eq. 2 to get the vector $\mathbf{w}$
5: Pass the vector $\mathbf{w}$ as input to the MLP classifier
6: **end procedure**

2.2 Training the MLP Classifier

We train an MPL classifier that takes the weight vector as the input feature vector, and outputs a binary decision whether the displacement is purely axial or not. Figure 2 shows the architecture of the used MLP model, which consists of an input layer, two hidden layers and an output layer. Our model is relatively simple due to having a low-dimensional input vector. The training is done by minimizing the mis-classification error using the cross-entropy loss function, and backpropagation is used to calculate the gradients. The applied optimization technique is the Adam optimizer [9] with a learning rate of 1e−3. The MLP code is written in Python using Keras [10].

2.3 Data Collection

PCA Model. For our training data, we collected 3,163 RF frames from 3 different CIRS phantoms (Norfolk, VA), namely Models 040GSE, 039 and 059 at different locations at Concordia University's PERFORM Centre using a 12R Alpinion (Bothell, WA) ultrasound machine with an L3-12H high density linear array probe. The center frequency is 8.5 MHz and the sampling frequency is 40 MHz. We allowed both in-plane and out-of-plane motion during collecting the data, where the probe could move in the 6 degrees of freedom (DOF).

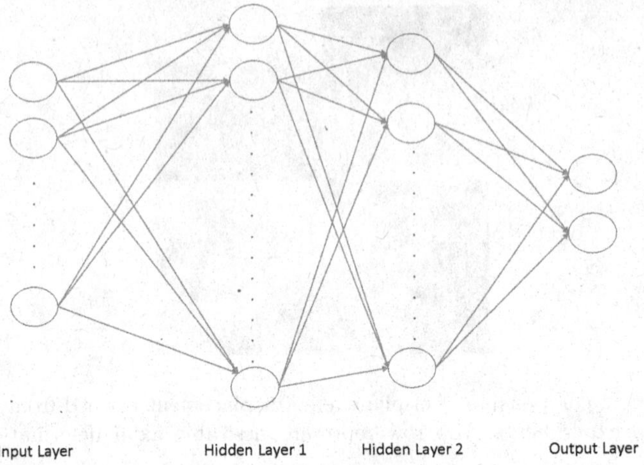

Fig. 2. The architecture of the MLP binary classifier. The network has two hidden layers and is fully connected.

In addition, we have access to 420 RF frames collected from 4 patients undergoing liver ablation, where testing is done on only one of them. The choice of the number of principal components was made so as to represent the displacement image in a simpler form while keeping most of the variance of the data. We chose N=12 which captures 95% of the variance present in the original data using only a 12-dimensional feature vector.

MLP Classifier. We trained our model using 1,012 pairs of frames from the *in-vivo* liver data through different combinations where each frame is paired with the nearest 16 frames forming 16 different pairs. We used 80% of the data for training and 20% for validation. Testing was done on a completely different dataset to ensure generalization. It is important to note that the ground truth (i.e. high or low quality strain image) was obtained by Abdelrahman Zayed through manual inspection of the strain image obtained using the Global Ultrasound Elastography technique [11]. The criteria for labelling the output as a good strain image were visual clarity and the ability to distinguish the inclusion from the surrounding tissue.

3 Results

We set $p=5$ RF lines as trials showed us that choosing a value for p more than 5 would not improve the quality of the strain image [12]. The number of hidden units in the MLP classifier is a hyperparameter that is chosen in a way so as to have the highest accuracy on the validation data. The first and second hidden layers contain 64 and 32 hidden units respectively with a Rectified Linear Unit (ReLU) as the activation function. The output layer has two neurons with a softmax activation function.

For the PCA model, the unoptimized MATLAB code takes 5 hours to train the model, but it is only done once. During test time, extracting the features for two very large RF images of size 2304 × 384 using the procedure in Algorithm 1 takes 262 ms on a 7th generation 3.4 GHz Intel core i7. As for the MLP classifier, training takes 5.57 s after extracting the features from all the training dataset. For testing, our model takes only 1.9 ms to choose the best frame by searching in a window composed of the nearest 16 frames (8 frames before and 8 frames after the desired frame), assuming that feature extraction is already done for the test dataset.

Our model is tested on both tissue-mimicking phantom data and *in-vivo* liver data. In order to be able to accurately measure the improvement in the quality of the strain image, we use two quality metrics which are the signal to noise ratio (SNR) and contrast to noise ratio (CNR) [13], calculated as follows:

$$CNR = \frac{C}{N} = \sqrt{\frac{2(\bar{s_b} - \bar{s_t})^2}{\sigma_b^2 + \sigma_t^2}}, SNR = \frac{\bar{s}}{\sigma} \tag{3}$$

where $\bar{s_t}$ and σ_t^2 are the strain average and variance of the target window (as shown in Figs. 3 and 5), $\bar{s_b}$ and σ_b^2 are the strain average and variance of the background window respectively. We use the background window for SNR calculation (i.e. $\bar{s} = \bar{s_b}$ and $\sigma = \sigma_b$). The background window is chosen in uniform areas. For the target window, we selected a window that lies completely inside the inclusion to show the contrast.

3.1 Phantom Results

We used data acquired from the CIRS elastography phantom Model 059 at a center frequency of 10 MHz and sampling frequency of 40 MHz using the 12R Alpinion E-Cube ultrasound machine. Figure 3 shows the B-mode image as well as the axial strain images calculated using both our method and the fixed skip frame pairing. Figure 4 shows the SNR and CNR of the axial strain images calculated from the same experiment. It is clear that our automatic frame selection substantially outperforms simply skipping one, two or three frames. Table 1 summarizes the data in Fig. 4 by computing the average and standard deviation of the SNR and CNR.

3.2 *In-vivo* data

Our *in-vivo* results were obtained from one patient undergoing open surgical radio frequency thermal ablation for primary or secondary liver cancers. The data was acquired at Johns Hopkins Hospital, with full details of the data collection protocol outlined in [14]. Figure 5 shows the B-mode image as well as the axial strain images using both our method and the fixed skip frame pairing. Table 2 shows the average and standard deviation of the SNR and CNR of the axial strain images computed from the same experiment. As observed in the phantom experiment, automatic frames selection substantially improves the quality of the strain images.

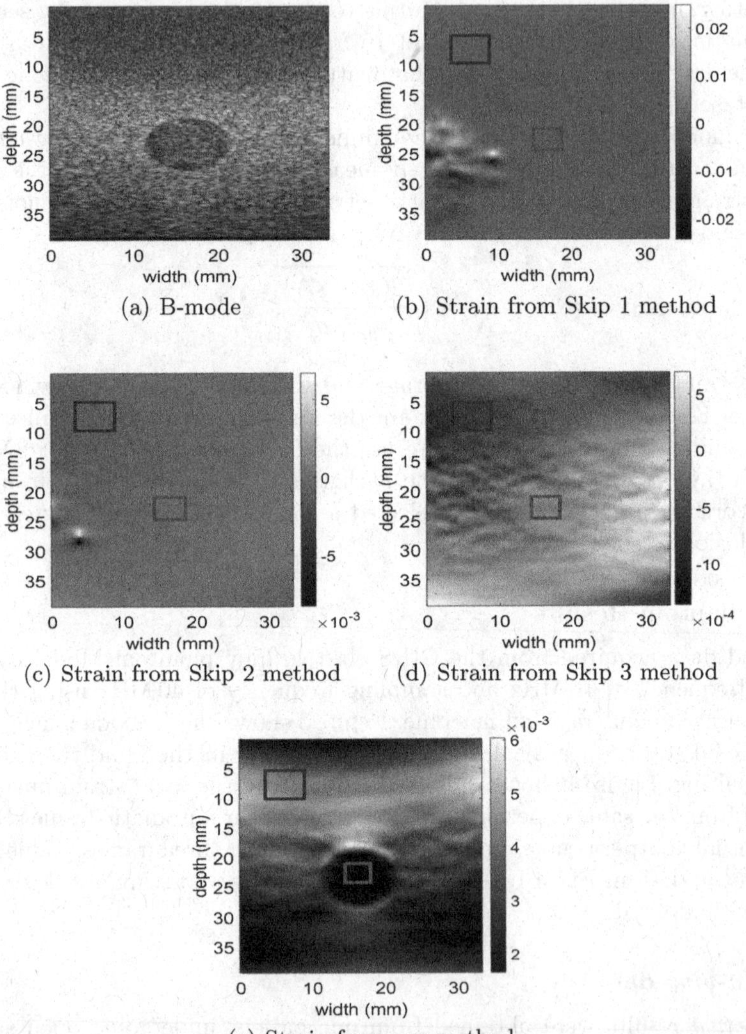

Fig. 3. The B-mode ultrasound and axial strain image for the phantom experiment.

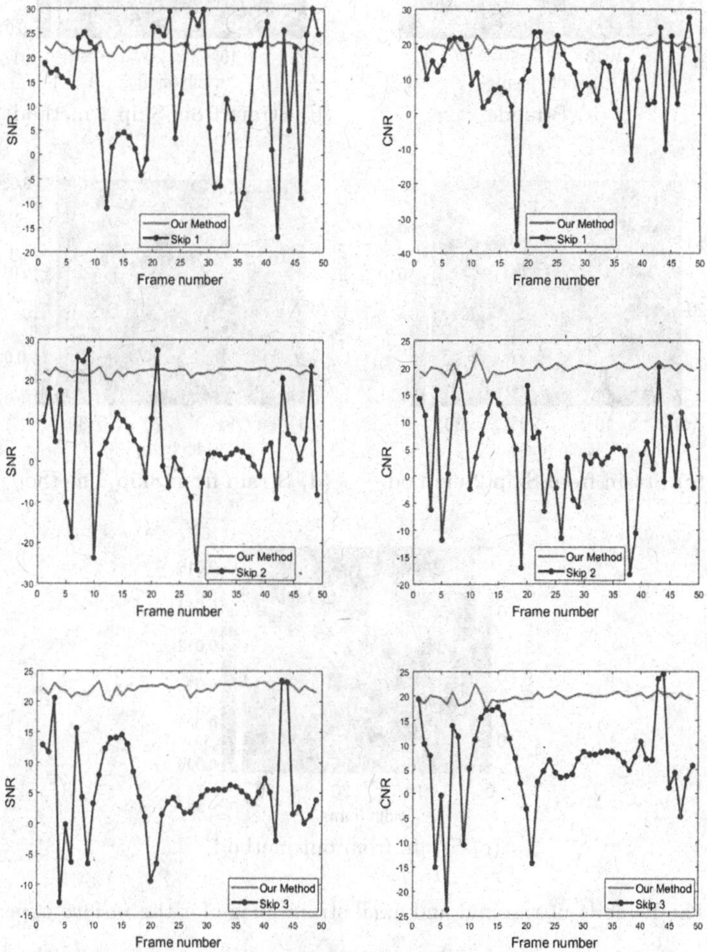

Fig. 4. A comparison between the SNR and CNR of the automatic frame selection and the fixed skip frame pairing for the phantom experiment. Rows 1 to 3 show the results for skipping 1 to 3 frames respectively.

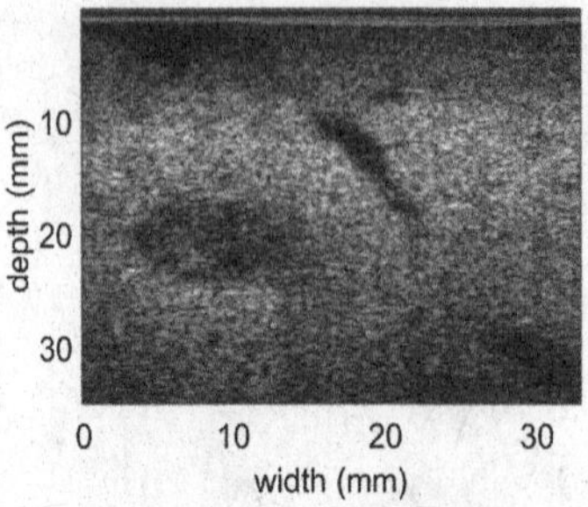

(a) B-mode

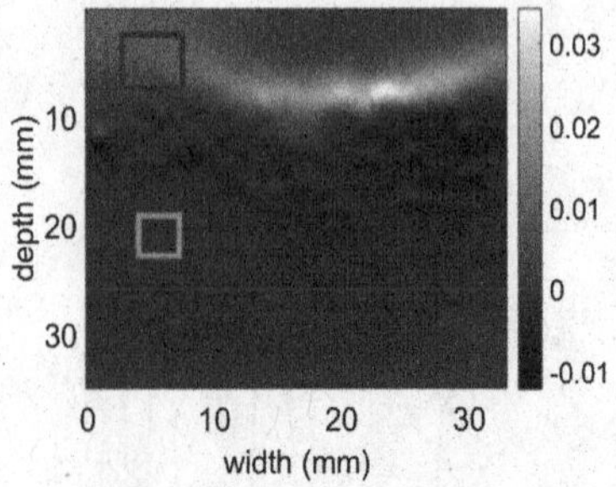

(b) Strain from Skip 1 method

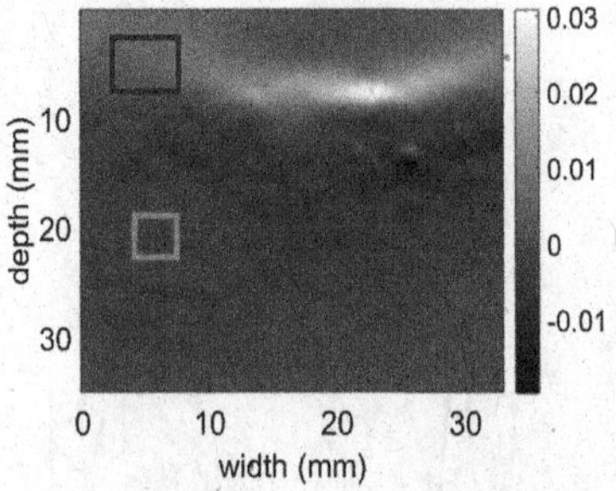

(c) Strain from Skip 2 method

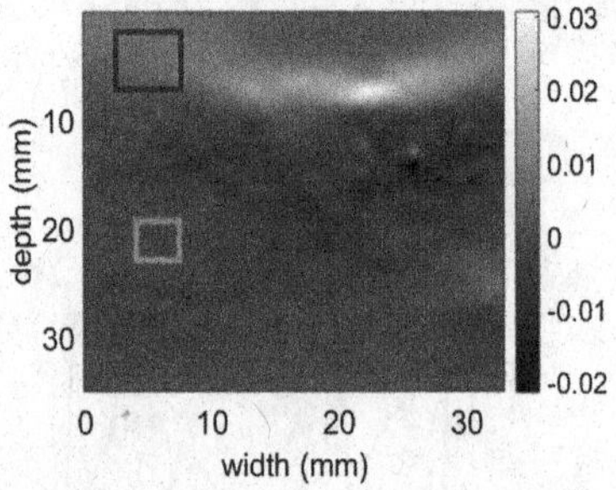

(d) Strain from Skip 3 method

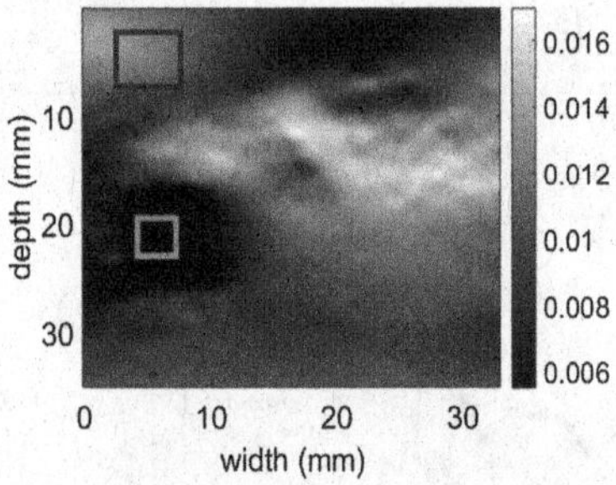

(e) Strain from our method

Fig. 5. The B-mode ultrasound and axial strain image for the *in-vivo* experiment.

Table 1. A comparison between SNR and CNR of the automatic frame selection and the fixed skip frame pairing for the phantom experiment. The numbers for each method show average ± standard deviation.

Method used	SNR	CNR
Skip 1	12.27 ± 13.31	10.11 ± 11.36
Skip 2	3.54 ± 11.78	3.80 ± 8.92
Skip 3	5.24 ± 7.45	6.34 ± 9.09
Our method	$\mathbf{22.15 \pm 0.79}$	$\mathbf{19.77 \pm 0.9}$

Table 2. A comparison between the SNR and CNR of the automatic frame selection and the fixed skip frame pairing for the *in-vivo* experiment. The numbers for each method show average $\pm$ standard deviation.

Method used	SNR	CNR
Skip 1	13.87 ± 6.23	12.92 ± 5.21
Skip 2	13.60 ± 7.11	5.30 ± 20.68
Skip 3	13.54 ± 8.74	11.05 ± 8.52
Our method	$\mathbf{21.25 \pm 2.23}$	$\mathbf{17.12 \pm 3.22}$

4 Conclusion

In this work, we presented a novel approach for real-time automatic selection of pairs of RF frames used to calculate the axial strain image. Our method is easy to use as it does not require any additional hardware. In addition, it is very computationally efficient and runs in less than 2 ms, and as such, can be used to test many pairs of RF frames in a short amount of time. Given that ultrasound frame rate is very high, and that there exist many combinations of two frames, this low computational complexity is of paramount practical importance. Our method can be used commercially where for each input RF frame, we choose the best possible frame to be paired with it among the collected frames.

Acknowledgements. The authors would like to thank the principal investigators at Johns Hopkins Hospital Drs. E. Boctor, M. Choti and G. Hager for providing us with the *in-vivo* liver data.

References

1. Gennisson, J.L., Deffieux, T., Fink, M., Tanter, M.: Ultrasound elastography: principles and techniques. Diagn. Interv. Imaging **94**(5), 487–495 (2013)
2. Hall, T.J., et al.: Recent results in nonlinear strain and modulus imaging. Curr. Med. Imaging Rev. **7**(4), 313–327 (2011)
3. Hiltawsky, K.M., Krüger, M., Starke, C., Heuser, L., Ermert, H., Jensen, A.: Freehand ultrasound elastography of breast lesions: clinical results. Ultrasound Med. Biol. **27**(11), 1461–1469 (2001)
4. Jiang, J., Hall, T.J., Sommer, A.M.: A novel performance descriptor for ultrasonic strain imaging: a preliminary study. IEEE Trans. Ultrason. Ferroelectr. Freq. Control **53**(6), 1088–1102 (2006)
5. Foroughi, P., et al.: A freehand ultrasound elastography system with tracking for in vivo applications. Ultrasound Med. Biol. **39**(2), 211–225 (2013)
6. Kibria, M.G., Rivaz, H.: GLUENet: ultrasound elastography using convolutional neural network. In: Stoyanov, D., et al. (eds.) POCUS/BIVPCS/CuRIOUS/CPM -2018. LNCS, vol. 11042, pp. 21–28. Springer, Cham (2018). https://doi.org/10.1007/978-3-030-01045-4_3

7. Peng, B., Xian, Y., Jiang, J.: A convolution neural network-based speckle tracking method for ultrasound elastography. In: IEEE International Ultrasonics Symposium (IUS), pp. 206–212 (2018)
8. Rivaz, H., Boctor, E.M., Foroughi, P., Zellars, R., Fichtinger, G., Hager, G.: Ultrasound elastography: a dynamic programming approach. IEEE Trans. Med. Imaging **27**(10), 1373–1377 (2008)
9. Kingma, D., Ba, J.: Adam: a method for stochastic optimization. In: International Conference on Learning Representations, pp. 1–13 (2014)
10. Chollet, F.: Keras (2015). https://github.com/fchollet/keras
11. Hashemi, H.S., Rivaz, H.: Global time-delay estimation in ultrasound elastography. IEEE Trans. Ultrason. Ferroelectr. Freq. Control **64**(10), 1625–1636 (2017)
12. Zayed, A., Rivaz, H.: Fast approximate time-delay estimation in ultrasound elastography using principal component analysis. In: IEEE Engineering in Medicine and Biology 41st Annual Conference (in press)
13. Ophir, J., et al.: Elastography: ultrasonic estimation and imaging of the elastic properties of tissues. Proc. Inst. Mech. Eng. H **213**(3), 203–233 (1999)
14. Rivaz, H., Boctor, E.M., Choti, M.A., Hager, G.D.: Real-time regularized ultrasound elastography. IEEE Trans. Med. Imaging **30**(4), 928–945 (2011)

Auto SVD Clutter Filtering for US Doppler Imaging Using 3D Clustering Algorithm

Saad Ahmed Waraich(✉), Adrian Chee, Di Xiao, Billy Y. S. Yiu, and Alfred Yu

Research Institute for Aging and Department of Electrical and Computer Engineering, University of Waterloo, Waterloo, ON N2L3G1, Canada
saad.waraich@uwaterloo.ca

Abstract. Blood flow visualization is a challenging task in the presence of tissue motion. Conventional clutter filtering techniques perform poorly since blood and tissue clutter echoes share similar spectral characteristics. Thus, unsuppressed tissue clutter produces flashing artefacts in ultrasound color flow images. Eigen-based filtering was recently introduced and has shown good clutter rejection performance; however, there is yet no standard approach to robustly determine the eigen components corresponding to tissue clutter. To address this issue, we propose a novel 3D clustering based singular value decomposition (SVD) clutter filtering method. The proposed technique makes use of three key spatiotemporal statistics: singular value magnitude, spatial correlation and the mean Doppler frequency of singular vectors to adaptively determine the clutter and noise clusters and their corresponding eigen rank to achieve maximal clutter and noise suppression. To test the clutter rejection performance of the proposed filter, high frame rate plane wave data was acquired in-vivo from a subject's common carotid artery and jugular vein region induced with extrinsic tissue motion (voluntary probe motion). The flow detection efficacy of the clustering based SVD filter was statistically evaluated and compared with current eigen rank estimation methods using the receiver operating characteristic (ROC) analysis. Results show that the clustering based SVD filter yielded the highest area under the ROC curve (0.9082) in comparison with other eigen rank estimation methods, signifying its improved flow detection capability.

Keywords: Clustering · Unsupervised learning · Ultrasound imaging · Doppler imaging · Singular Value Decomposition

1 Introduction

Blood flow detection in ultrasound (US) imaging is a challenging task in certain clinical scenarios e.g., slow-flow detection and assessing blood flow with fast tissue motion. Tissue clutter is a significant source of artefacts in ultrasound imaging which hampers blood flow detection since the backscattering strength of tissue can be 40 to 100 dB stronger than blood due to its relatively high acoustic impedance mismatch [1]. Tissue motion being slower than blood exhibits slow temporal variation compared to the fast fluctuations of the blood flow signal [2]. Therefore, high-pass temporal filtering is

F. Karray et al. (Eds.): ICIAR 2019, LNCS 11663, pp. 473–483, 2019.
https://doi.org/10.1007/978-3-030-27272-2_42

necessary to remove the low frequency tissue clutter and in turn preserve the blood flow signal. Clutter filtering remains a key challenge for accurate flow visualization especially when tissue and blood echoes similar spectral characteristics in some scenarios which correspond to important US imaging applications. Such as, slow flow detection becomes very difficult in microvascular networks of tumors which is necessary for cancer diagnosis [3], while imaging flow in presence of fast vessel wall pulsations is a major issue in cardiac imaging [4]. Due to fast myocardial tissue motion and small vessel diameters, acquisition of Doppler flow measurements from the coronary arteries becomes very difficult and this combination also results in flashing artefacts due to inadequate clutter suppression [5].

Conventional high-pass clutter filtering methods like the Finite Impulse Response (FIR) and Infinite Impulse Response (IIR) filters which work on the temporal dimension only, fail to sufficiently differentiate between blood flow and tissue motion when their Doppler frequency spectrums overlap significantly. Whereas, an eigen-based clutter filter builds a spatiotemporal vector basis adapted to both blood and tissue signals which offers a much better discrimination capability between them [6]. Eigen filtering benefits from the high temporal sampling rates offered by high frame rate (HFR) plane wave imaging [7]. Singular value decomposition (SVD) of ultrasonic RF data generates singular values whose magnitude distribution aids in detection and removal of the higher energy containing tissue signal. SVD also results in singular vectors which provide both spatial and temporal information that can be used to distinguish and eliminate tissue clutter from the blood signal [8].

A drawback however in the SVD filter implementation is that there is yet no standard approach to determine the eigen components corresponding to tissue clutter. Various methods have been reported in the literature to achieve clutter rank selection in eigen-based filtering. Each of these methods have limitations of its own. Arnal *et al.* developed a singular value threshold (SVT) estimator based on the spatial similarity matrix (SSM) of singular vectors [9]. Yu and Cobbold proposed a Hankel-SVD formulation which selects clutter rank based on mean frequency of singular values [10]. Kruse and Ferrara reported a fixed eigen rank cut-off for clutter based on the strength of the eigenvalues [11]. The performance of all these estimators highly depend on the quality of the local data statistics. Whereas, identifying the boundaries of tissue and blood spatial correlation squares in the SSM technique is not always possible since blood correlation can represent an elliptic shape instead of a definite square. The Hankel-SVD approach requires a hand-tuned cut-off frequency to be defined which faces issue where blood and tissue spectra overlap. It can also become difficult to compute the correct eigen rank cut-off based on the singular value strength especially for larger ensemble size [12]. Hence, there is a clear motivation to develop a robust and fully automated clutter rank estimator which makes use of all the spatial and temporal metrics to remove tissue signal efficiently. Clustering is a powerful machine learning tool for grouping data points. There are various established clustering algorithms that have been used for biomedical image segmentation [13, 14]. Moubark *et al.* used K-means clustering for classifying and eliminating tissue clutter based on its energy from ultrasound image [15].

In this paper, a novel 3D clustering based SVD clutter filtering framework is proposed to cluster the eigen-components by leveraging on three key spatiotemporal statistics: singular value magnitude distribution, spatial correlation and the mean Doppler frequency of singular vectors. The information from these parameters is combined in 3D to visualize the spatiotemporal distribution of the data points. Our guiding hypothesis is that since tissue and blood signals have different spatiotemporal characteristics, a clustering algorithm can leverage on these distinctive properties to adaptively identify and suppress eigen components corresponding to clutter, and in turn improve blood flow detection performance. Since the data involved is unlabeled, an unsupervised learning algorithm K-means is applied which adaptively determines the tissue cluster and its corresponding rank to achieve maximal clutter suppression. Moreover, this paper statistically compared the flow detection performance of the proposed 3D clustering based SVD filter with the current clutter rank estimation methods using receiver operating characteristic (ROC) analyses [16].

2 Methodology

The theoretical principles behind Auto SVD Clutter Filtering Using 3D Clustering are explained in steps in this section of the paper.

2.1 Ultrasound Doppler Signal Components

The ultrasound Doppler flow signal is composed of the sum of three components: tissue clutter, blood and thermal/electronic noise. A typical post-beamformed ultrasound raw data matrix is represented as a time series of 2D images. Mathematically, the raw data matrix is a three-dimensional complex variable $s(x, z, t)$ of size (N_z, N_x, N_t), where one dimension is time t and the other two are spatial dimensions x (lateral) and z (depth).

2.2 Singular Value Decomposition

The raw data cineloop $s(x, z, t)$ is reshaped to a spatiotemporal Casorati matrix [17] which reorders the data into a 2D space-time matrix $\boldsymbol{S}$ of size $(N_z \times N_x, N_t)$. SVD is performed on the Casorati matrix $\boldsymbol{S}$ which yields the product of the following three matrices:

$$\boldsymbol{S} = \boldsymbol{UDV}^* \tag{1}$$

Where matrices **U** and **V** are unitary matrices with dimensions $(N_z \times N_x, N_z \times N_x)$ and (N_t, N_t) respectively. * stands for the conjugate transpose and **D** is a diagonal matrix of size $(N_z \times N_x, N_t)$ with diagonal values λ_k sorted in a descending order of magnitude. S is decomposed into eigen-components λ_k and each component consists of U and V vectors scaled by D. The rows of matrix S contain the raw spatial information, while its columns represent the time dimension. Thus, the SVD of S results in the singular vectors of U that provide spatial information while singular vectors of V represent the temporal information in *S*.

2.3 Extraction of Image Statistics

Singular Value Magnitude. Tissue structures generally appear much brighter than blood scatterers in ultrasound images. The difference in energy of the tissue and blood signals can be seen in the singular value distribution curve as shown in Fig. 1(a).

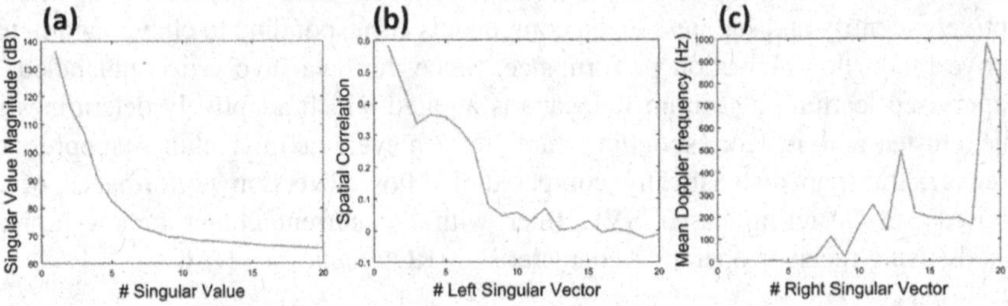

Fig. 1. (a) Singular values λ_k of matrix D expressed in dB, (b) Spatial correlation curve (correlation of the first singular vector U_1 with left singular vectors $|U_k|$ $k \in [1, N_t]$), (c) Mean Doppler frequency estimation curve of the right singular vectors, for a plane wave HFR Doppler acquisition on an in-vivo carotid region.

Spatial Correlation. In ultrasound imaging, it has been widely observed experimentally that tissue has a much higher spatial coherence relative to blood since it is far less deformable then the blood scatterers which have low viscosity and elasticity compared to the tissue [4]. This underlying difference in spatial distribution is leveraged by computing the spatial correlation of the first spatial singular vector $\mathbf{U_1}$ (typically representative of tissue clutter) with the spatial singular vectors $|\mathbf{U_k}| \boldsymbol{k} \in [1, N_t]$.

$$C = \sum_{k=1}^{N_t} \frac{\left(|U_1| - \overline{|U_1|}\right) \cdot \left(|U_k| - \overline{|U_k|}\right)}{\sigma_1 \cdot \sigma_k} \tag{2}$$

Where $\overline{\mathbf{U_k}}$ stands for the mean and $\boldsymbol{\sigma_k}$ is the standard deviation of $\mathbf{U_k}$ indexes. **C** is the spatial correlation vector of size $(1, N_t)$ which reveals the high spatial coherence of low-order singular vectors corresponding to tissue and low spatial correlation of high-order singular vectors typically corresponding to blood as shown in Fig. 1(b).

Mean Doppler Frequency. Tissue clutter being relatively slower than blood, exhibits low frequency motion compared to the high frequency flow of blood scatterers. To make use of the temporal difference between the blood and tissue signal, the mean Doppler frequency is calculated for each individual temporal (right) singular vector $\mathbf{V_k}$ using the following lag-one autocorrelation based estimator:

$$\hat{R}_k = \sum_{i=1}^{N_t - 1} V_k^*(i) \cdot V_k(i+1) \tag{3}$$

$$\hat{f}_k = \frac{PRF}{2\pi} \times \arctan\left(\frac{imag(\hat{R}_k)}{real(\hat{R}_k)}\right) \tag{4}$$

Where $\hat{f}_k$ is the mean Doppler frequency estimate for the kth temporal singular vector $\mathbf{V_k}$. PRF stands for the pulse repetition frequency which is the number of pulses fired by the ultrasound transducer per second. Mean Doppler frequency estimation curve of the right singular vectors is shown in Fig. 1(c).

2.4 3D Clustering Based Clutter Filtering

K-means clustering (Lloyd's algorithm) [18] is applied on the three-dimensional data formed from the image statistics. Each of the three statistics were computed from the SVD of five consecutive frame blocks, where each frame block contains a sequence of 100 frames. Cluster centroids were initialized using the K-means++ algorithm [19]. K-means iteratively calculates the squared Euclidean distance between the data points and cluster centroids to allocate each point to the closest cluster. The centroids are recomputed in each iteration by evaluating the mean of all points in that centroid's cluster until the centroid positions do not change and the algorithm converges to an optimal result. Number of clusters were pre-defined as three, where each cluster represents one of tissue, blood and noise component. The cluster with the highest mean singular value magnitude and spatial correlation and the lowest mean Doppler frequency is classified as tissue clutter. The eigen components corresponding to the tissue cluster points are then set to zero for clutter removal.

2.5 In-Vivo Experimental Setup

For in-vivo data acquisition, our lab's research purpose ultrasound scanning platform was used [20]. A 192-element linear array transducer (SL1543; Esaote, Genova, Italy) probe configured for plane wave imaging was placed on a subject's neck to image the common carotid artery (CCA) and jugular vein (JV) in short-axis view. Extrinsic tissue motion was induced in the dataset by voluntary probe motion to test the efficacy of the clutter filtering methods. High frame rate (HFR) raw data acquisition was performed at 5 MHz imaging frequency at a PRF of 6 kHz. HFR Doppler acquisition was done using a steering angle of $-10°$ and interleaved B-mode firings were done using 30 angles (ranging from -15 to $15°$ (excluding $0°$) with $1°$ incremental steps), resulting in an effective PRF of 3 kHz. In total 7800 frames were acquired in 2.6 s. Details of imaging parameters for the experiment can be seen in [20].

2.6 Tissue and Flow Region Identification

The acquired HFR data is beamformed to generate B-mode images (2D spatial map which represents ultrasound echoes as bright dots) [21]. The boundaries between the flow and tissue region were demarcated on the cross-sectional B-mode image of the carotid and vein for ROC analysis. MATLAB's built-in contour tool was used for selecting the regions of interest. As shown in Fig. 2, the carotid flow region (red dashed circle) and jugular vein flow region (blue dashed circle) is selected as the hypoechoic B-mode pixels inside the vessel walls, while the tissue region are all the B-mode pixels outside the flow region.

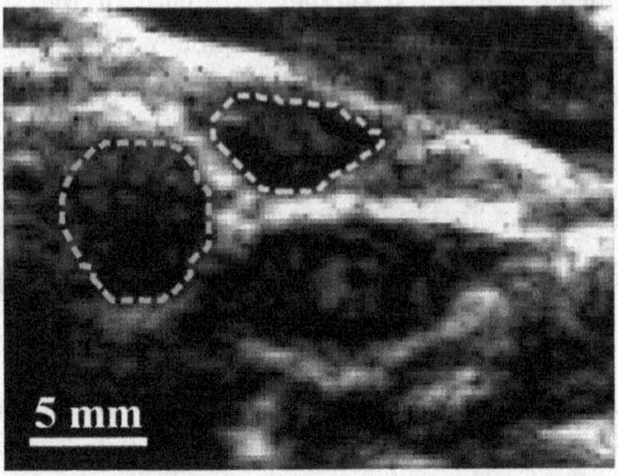

Fig. 2. Cross-sectional view of the Common Carotid Artery (CCA) flow region (red dashed circle) and Jugular Vein (JV) flow region (blue dashed circle), in the ultrasound B-mode image (Color figure online)

2.7 Computation of ROC Curves

Pixel values corresponding to the identified tissue and flow regions were extracted from the post-filtered power Doppler maps of each clutter rank estimation method. Two statistical parameters were then computed for different power Doppler thresholds (swept in 0.2 dB increments from 0 to 100 dB): true positive rate (TPR) and the false alarm rate (FAR). The TPR or sensitivity was defined as the percentage of flow pixels with post-filtered Doppler power higher than the threshold value, while the FAR (1-Specificity) was defined as the percentage of tissue pixels with post-filtered Doppler power higher than the threshold value. The ROC curves for each filter were plotted with their respective TPR against the corresponding FAR.

3 Results

3.1 K-means Clustering Yields Distinct Clusters

K-means clustered the data (convergence time: 17 ms) into discrete groups as shown in Fig. 3(a). Cluster 3 (blue) has the highest mean singular value magnitude and spatial correlation, and at the same time, the lowest mean Doppler frequency among all. These are typical properties of signals originating from tissues and hence cluster 3 can be identified as clutter. Cluster 1 (gray) has the least spatial correlation with high frequency content; both distinct features of noise. Upon identifying these two clusters, Cluster 2 (red) can therefore be confidently attributed to signals from blood flow.

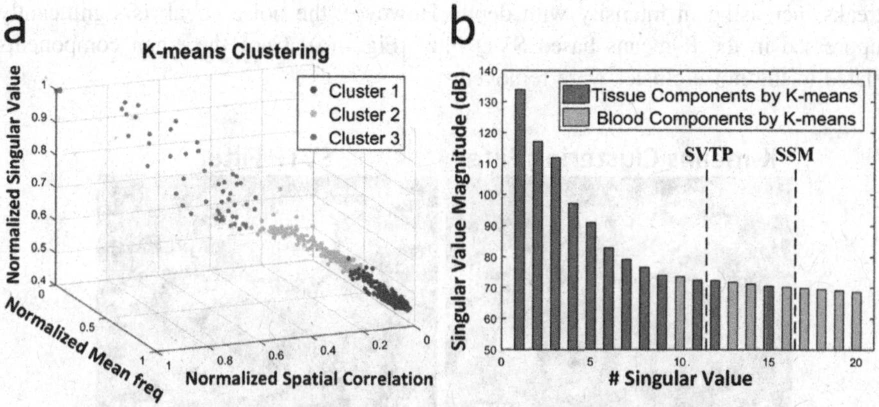

Fig. 3. (a) K-means clustering performed on the 3D distribution of image statistics acquired from in-vivo common carotid artery and jugular vein data at systolic phase of the cardiac cycle. (b) Singular value thresholds (shown in dashed lines) corresponding to tissue clutter computed by the following eigen rank estimators: Spatial Similarity Matrix (SSM) and Singular Value Turning Point (SVTP). Red bars represent the singular values identified as part of the blood flow signal by the K-means based SVD filter, while the blue bars represent the singular values identified adaptively as tissue clutter. (Color figure online)

3.2 Adaptive Eigen Rank Estimates for Clutter and Blood Achieved Using Clustering

Different eigen-based clutter filtering methods were implemented on the same in vivo dataset for comparison. Spatial Similarity Matrix (SSM) [12] and the singular value curve turning point (SVTP) [22] generated fixed singular value thresholds for removing clutter as shown by their respective dashed lines in Fig. 3(b). On the other hand, K-means clustering based SVD generates clutter rank adaptively and identifies blood eigen components that are interspersed between thresholds determined by the SSM and SVTP estimation approaches.

3.3 K-means Clustering Based SVD Achieves Strong Flow Detection and Noise Suppression

K-means based clutter filtering strongly distinguished between flow and tissue regions at the systolic phase of the cardiac cycle in presence of strong tissue motion caused by both vessel wall pulsations and extrinsic probe motion. Figure 4 shows the post-filtered power Doppler maps corresponding to different clutter filtering methods which include the K-means based SVD filter [Fig. 4(a)], SVTP filter [Fig. 4(b)] and the SSM filter [Fig. 4(c)] (with noise suppression). All power maps are rendered with a fixed dynamic range (30 dB). Figure 4(a) shows strong flow detection in the carotid and vein region for the K-means based SVD filter with limited false coloring seen in the vessel wall pixels. Figure 4(b) and (c) demonstrates that the SVTP and SSM filter achieved similar performance to the K-means filter in terms of flow identification. Another evident finding is that the SVTP and the SSM filter power maps both show parallel noise streaks increasing in intensity with depth. However, the noise streak is significantly suppressed in the K-means based SVD filter [Fig. 4(a)] since the eigen components related to the noise cluster were removed.

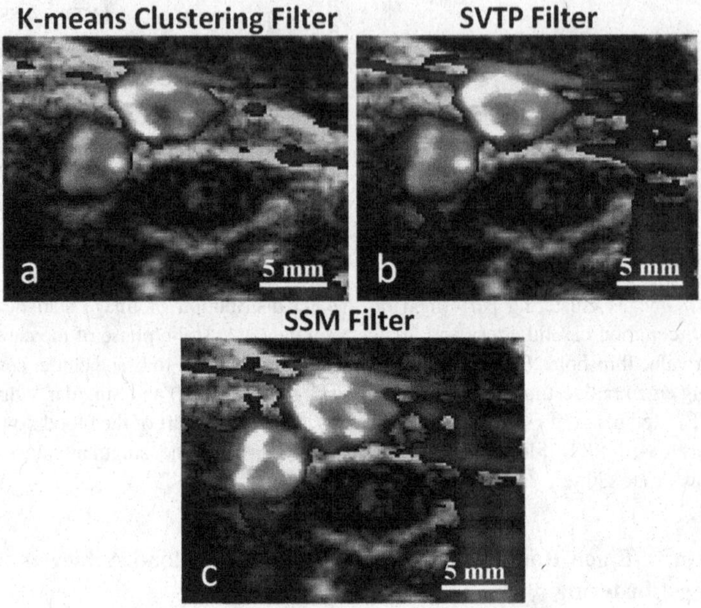

Fig. 4. Post-filtered power Doppler maps of (a) K-means clustering based SVD filter (b) SVTP filter (c) SSM filter, overlaid on the CCA and JV cross-sectional B-mode image. Enhanced flow detection and noise suppression achieved by the K-means clustering based SVD filter in comparison to all other filters at systolic phase of the cardiac cycle. Dynamic range was kept the same for all the images at 30 dB. (Color figure online)

3.4 Improved ROC Performance Gained by K-means Clustering Based SVD Filter

The improved flow detection efficacy of the K-means based SVD filter is substantiated by its high ROC performance as shown in Fig. 5. The area under the ROC curve (AUC) quantifies the diagnostic performance in ROC analysis. The higher the AUC value is the better the detection performance [16]. At systole, where tissue motion is the strongest due to strong vessel wall pulsations, the ROC curve of K-means based SVD filter yielded the largest AUC value (0.9082) in comparison to the other filters.

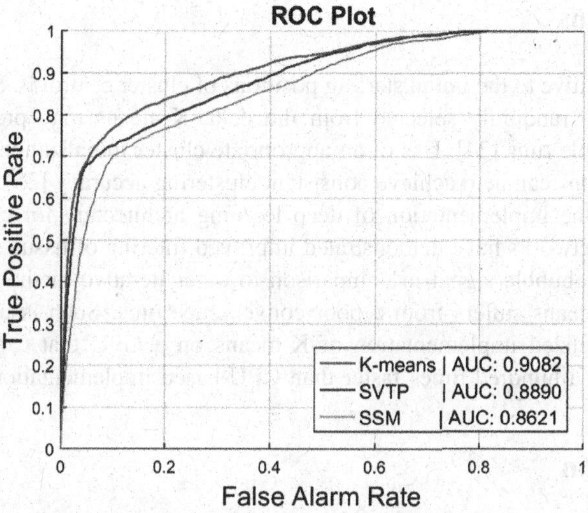

Fig. 5. K-means clustering based SVD filter achieved the highest flow detection ROC performance compared to SSM and SVTP filters.

4 Discussion

This paper presents a novel framework for 3D clustering based automatic SVD clutter filtering to address the challenge of adaptively determining the eigen rank corresponding to tissue clutter in the presence of vessel wall pulsations and extrinsic tissue motion. The proposed method combines the spatiotemporal information from the three image statistics: singular value magnitude, spatial correlation and the mean Doppler frequency which allows enhanced clutter, blood and noise detection through K-means clustering as demonstrated in Fig. 3(a). Our findings in Fig. 3(b) showed that K-means clustering based SVD adaptively determines the eigen components corresponding to clutter and blood unlike other eigen rank estimation techniques which selects a fixed singular value threshold for tissue clutter. Such adaptive clutter removal enables the K-means clustering based SVD filter to achieve improved flow detection as demonstrated in Fig. 4(a). Removal of the noise cluster enabled significant suppression of noise streaks as evident from the power Doppler map of K-means based SVD in Fig. 4(a) compared to Fig. 4(b) and (c). The vessel wall artefact in the power Doppler maps of Fig. 4(b) and (c) resulted from angled (−10°) plane wave insonification at right angle to the vessel walls were well-suppressed in the K-means based SVD power map in Fig. 4 (a). Our experimental results are statistically substantiated by the better ROC performance of the K-means based SVD technique as shown by its ROC curve with the highest AUC value (0.9082) in Fig. 5. A direct continuation of this work can be to apply this framework in a block-wise fashion [23] in which SVD is performed on local spatially overlapped segments of the image, rather than applying it globally on the entire image data. This approach can allow more localized extraction of image statistics for clustering which can lead to robust clutter reduction and potent flow visualization in many challenging clinical imaging scenarios.

5 Limitations

K-means is sensitive to the initial starting positions of cluster centroids. Since the initial cluster center is randomly selected from the data, K-means may produce different results on multiple runs [24]. Use of an appropriate cluster initialization technique and repeating K-means can help achieve consistent clustering accuracy [25]. An alternative to K-means is the implementation of deep learning architecture for clustering; deep convolutional networks have demonstrated improved filtering of tissue signal from the ultrasound microbubble signal in comparison to other iterative methods [26]. Lastly, CPU-based K-means suffers from a poor convergence time. Such issue can be overcome by parallelized implementation of K-means on a GPU that can speed up the algorithm up to a hundred times faster than CPU-based implementation [27].

6 Conclusion

This paper has shown the potential merit of K-means clustering based automatic SVD clutter filtering in achieving adaptive clutter and noise suppression and in turn improved flow detection performance in comparison with existing eigen rank estimation methods. The impact of this work is on the automated as well as adaptive (in contrast to a fixed cutoff) selection of eigen-components corresponding to tissue clutter, blood and noise.

References

1. Bjaerum, S., Torp, H., Kristoffersen, K.: Clutter filter design for ultrasound color flow imaging. IEEE Trans. Ultrason. Ferroelectr. Freq. Control **49**(2), 204–216 (2002)
2. Hoskins, P.R., McDicken, W.: Colour ultrasound imaging of blood flow and tissue motion. Br. J. Radiol. **70**(837), 878–890 (1997)
3. Jin, Z.-Q., He, W., Wu, D.-F., Lin, M.-Y., Jiang, H.-T.: Color Doppler ultrasound in diagnosis and assessment of carotid body tumors: comparison with computed tomography angiography. Ultrasound Med. Biol. **42**(9), 2106–2113 (2016)
4. Demené, C., Deffieux, T., Pernot, M., Osmanski, B.-F., Biran, V., Gennisson, J.-L.: Spatiotemporal clutter filtering of ultrafast ultrasound data highly increases Doppler and fUltrasound sensitivity. IEEE Trans. Med. Imaging **34**(11), 2271–2285 (2015)
5. Heimdal, A., Torp, H.: Ultrasound Doppler measurements of low velocity blood flow: limitations due to clutter signals from vibrating muscles. IEEE Trans. Ultrason. Ferroelectr. Freq. Control **44**(4), 873–881 (1997)
6. Yu, A.C., Lovstakken, L.: Eigen-based clutter filter design for ultrasound color flow imaging: a review. IEEE Trans. Ultrason. Ferroelectr. Freq. Control **57**(5), 1096–1111 (2010)
7. Bayat, M., Fatemi, M.: Concurrent clutter and noise suppression via low rank plus sparse optimization for non-contrast ultrasound flow Doppler processing in microvasculature. In: IEEE International Conference on Acoustics, Speech and Signal Processing (ICASSP), Calgary, AB, Canada (2018)

8. Ikeda, H., et al.: Singular value decomposition of received ultrasound signal to separate tissue, blood flow, and cavitation signals. Jpn. J. Appl. Phys. **57**(7S1), 07LF04 (2018)
9. Arnal, B., Baranger, J., Demene, C., Tanter, M., Pernot, M.: In vivo real-time cavitation imaging in moving organs. Phys. Med. Biol. **62**(3), 843–857 (2017)
10. Yu, A.C., Cobbold, R.S.: Single-ensemble-based eigen-processing methods for color flow imaging - Part I. The Hankel-SVD filter. IEEE Trans. Ultrason. Ferroelectr. Freq. Control **55** (3), 559–572 (2008)
11. Kruse, D., Ferrara, K.: A new high resolution color flow system using an eigendecomposition-based adaptive filter for clutter rejection. IEEE Trans. Ultrason. Ferroelectr. Freq. Control **49**(12), 1739–1754 (2002)
12. Baranger, J., Arnal, B., Perren, F., Baud, O., Tanter, M., Demené, C.: Adaptive spatiotemporal SVD clutter filtering for ultrafast Doppler imaging using similarity of spatial singular vectors. IEEE Trans. Med. Imaging **37**(7), 1574–1586 (2018)
13. Wu, M.-N., Lin, C.-C., Chang, C.-C.: Brain tumor detection using color-based k-means clustering segmentation. In: Third International Conference on Intelligent Information Hiding and Multimedia Signal Processing, Kaohsiung, Taiwan (2007)
14. Dolon, L.I.: Segmentation analysis on magnetic resonance imaging (MRI) with different clustering techniques: wavelet and BEMD. In: 2016 International Conference on Innovations in Science, Engineering and Technology (ICISET), Dhaka, Bangladesh (2016)
15. Moubark, A.M., Harput, S., Cowell, D.M.J., Freear, S.: Clutter noise reduction in b-mode image through mapping and clustering signal energy for better cyst classification. In: IEEE International Ultrasonics Symposium (IUS), Tours, France (2016)
16. Zweig, M.H., Campbell, G.: Receiver-operating characteristic (ROC) plots: a fundamental evaluation tool in clinical medicine. Clin. Chem. **39**(4), 561–577 (1993)
17. Candès, E.J., Sing-Long, C.A., Trzasko, J.D.: Unbiased risk estimates for singular value thresholding and spectral estimators. IEEE Trans. Signal Process. **61**(19), 4643–4657 (2013)
18. Lloyd, S.: Least squares quantization in PCM. IEEE Trans. Inf. Theory **28**(2), 129–137 (1982)
19. Arthur, D., Vassilvitskii, S.: K-means++: the advantages of careful seeding. In: ACM-SIAM Symposium on Discrete Algorithms (SODA 2007), New Orleans, Louisiana (2007)
20. Yiu, B.Y.S., Walczak, M., Lewandowski, M., Yu, A.C.: Live ultrasound color encoded speckle imaging platform for real-time complex flow visualization in vivo. IEEE Trans. Ultrason. Ferroelectr. Freq. Control **66**, 656–668 (2019)
21. Yiu, B.Y.S., Tsang, I.K.H., Yu, A.C.: GPU-based beamformer: fast realization of plane wave compounding and synthetic aperture imaging. IEEE Trans. Ultrason. Ferroelectr. Freq. Control **58**(8), 1698–1705 (2011)
22. Lovstakken, L., Bjaerum, S., Kristoffersen, K., Haaverstad, R., Torp, H.: Real-time adaptive clutter rejection filtering in color flow imaging using power method iterations. IEEE Trans. Ultrason. Ferroelectr. Freq. Control **53**(9), 1597–1608 (2006)
23. Song, P., Manduca, A., Trzasko, J.D., Chen, S.: Ultrasound small vessel imaging with block-wise adaptive local clutter filtering. IEEE Trans. Med. Imaging **36**(1), 251–262 (2016)
24. Celebi, M.E., Kingravi, H.A., Vela, P.A.: A comparative study of efficient initialization methods for the k-means clustering algorithm. Expert Syst. Appl. **40**(1), 200–210 (2013)
25. Fränti, P., Sieranoja, S.: How much can k-means be improved by using better initialization and repeats? Pattern Recogn. **93**, 95–112 (2019)
26. Cohen, R.: Deep convolutional robust PCA with application to ultrasound imaging. In: ICASSP 2019–2019 IEEE International Conference on Acoustics, Speech and Signal Processing (ICASSP), Brighton, United Kingdom (2019)
27. Li, Y., Zhao, K., Chu, X., Liu, J.: Speeding up k-means algorithm by GPUs. J. Comput. Syst. Sci. **79**(2), 216–229 (2013)

Author Index

Printed in the United States
By Bookmasters

Printed in the United States
By Bookmasters